Exercise Testing and Exercise Prescription for Special Cases

Theoretical Basis and Clinical Application

Exercise Testing and Exercise Prescription for Special Cases

Theoretical Basis and Clinical Application

James S. Skinner

Professor, Department of Exercise Science and Physical Education
Director, Exercise and Sport Research Institute
Arizona State University
Tempe, Arizona

Second Edition

LEA & FEBIGER

PHILADELPHIA/LONDON

Williams & Wilkins
Rose Tree Corporate Center, Building II
1400 North Providence Road, Suite 5025
Media, PA 19063-2043 USA

Executive Editor-George H. Mundorff
Project Editor-Frances M. Klass
Production Manager-Michael DeNardo

Library of Congress Cataloging-in-Publication Data

Exercise testing and exercise prescription for special cases :
  theoretical basis and clinical application / [edited by] James S.
Skinner. -- 2nd ed.
      p.   cm.
  Includes bibliographical references and index.
  ISBN 0-8121-1440-X
  1. Exercise therapy.   2. Exercise tests.   I. Skinner, James S.,
1936-   .
  [DNLM: 1. Exercise Test.   2. Exercise Therapy.   WB 541 E955]
RM725.R94   1993.
615.8′2--dc20
DNLM/DLC
for Library of Congress   92-10383
                                                                              CIP

Reprints of chapters may be purchased from Lea & Febiger in quantities of 100 or more. Contact Sally Grande in the Sales Department.

PRINTED IN THE UNITED STATES OF AMERICA

Print number: 5   4   3   2

A mon amie, ma chérie, et mon épouse,
MARIETTE.

PREFACE TO SECOND EDITION

The second edition reflects the continued growth of exercise science and sports medicine and their application to special populations. Although the basic principles and programs have changed little since the first edition, new developments and refinements have been reported and are incorporated in the revised chapters. The chapters on pregnancy and cystic fibrosis have been completely rewritten by different researchers and clinicians. Four new chapters on asthma, low-back pain, osteoporosis, and renal disease have been added. These revisions and additions should give the reader an even broader and deeper understanding of how exercise testing and exercise prescription can be applied to the general population and to special cases.

Tempe, AZ   James S. Skinner

PREFACE

The sedentary lifestyle so prevalent today in most developed countries is associated directly or indirectly with a number of health problems (e.g., obesity and coronary heart disease). There is a need for a reference source book that discusses the theoretical and applied aspects of exercise testing and exercise prescription for many of these special problems. As of now, one must search for and read numerous articles on each topic of interest (e.g., diabetes, pregnancy, and hypertension). One then attempts to 1) understand why certain exercise tests were used; 2) understand why certain types of exercise were emphasized or avoided; and 3) determine the efficacy of exercise programs relative to the special health state. Scientists and clinicians in the rapidly growing fields of exercise science and sports medicine have provided the research and experience needed for such a compendium. The authors of the chapters within this book were selected because they have been responsible for much of this information.

First presented are the general principles of exercise testing and exercise prescription, followed by a discussion of the importance of such general factors as age, gender, and environment. Finally, there are chapters on the specific health states. Where applicable, the authors were asked to discuss the health state and its general treatment; risk factors and associated health states; how it may affect and be affected by exercise; how to modify exercise testing procedures; how to prescribe exercise (especially the types of exercise to emphasize or avoid and why); and the effects to be expected from exercise programs.

Most physicians have studied various diseases and health states but are not as well versed in exercise testing and exercise prescription. Conversely, most physical educators and exercise specialists learn about exercise but know far less about medical problems or their signs and symptoms. Because many people seek the advice of physicians and physical educators as to what to do and what to avoid, both groups need information on what role exercise testing and exercise programs might play in modifying a person's health status. The goal of this book is to provide information for all professional groups interested in the interaction between exercise and health.

Two important findings from research in exercise science are 1) optimal exercise tests and exercise programs are those that are individualized and personalized; and 2) the effects of training are specific to the systems that are stimulated to adapt. Thus, even though the basic principles of exercise testing and exercise prescription are the same for everyone, these principles can be and may have to be modified because of the restrictions or limitations imposed by the particular health state involved. The understanding of these restrictions and the modifications that should be made form the basis for adequate functional evaluations and exercise programs that are safe and effective. It should be mentioned that although exercise testing and exercise prescriptions are based on scientific facts, the leading of *enjoyable* exercise programs is still an art.

The proper selection of activities requires communication and cooperation among the physician, the exercise specialist, and the patient. The physician should have basic information concerning exercise and should recommend exercise programs led by competent and qualified professionals. Exercise specialists should have basic information about the medical aspects of various health states so that they can receive and understand results from the medical screening (e.g., special problems and medications) and the exercise test. It is hoped that this book will help to bridge the gap, assisting each professional to understand their roles better, as well as the place that exercise testing and exercise prescription has in preventive and rehabilitative exercise programs.

Tempe, AZ   James S. Skinner

CONTRIBUTORS

Oded Bar-Or, M.D.
Professor of Pediatrics, McMaster University;
Director, Children's Exercise and Nutrition
  Centre
McMaster University
Hamilton, Ontario, Canada

Peter D. Bartkiewicz, M.C.P.A., P.T.
H.W. Lung Association program co-ordinator;
Hamilton, Ontario, Canada

Leslie B. Berman, M.D.
Clinical Associate Professor of Medicine
McMaster University;
Director, Respiratory Rehabilitation Program
Chedoke-McMaster Hospitals
Hamilton, Ontario, Canada

Elsworth R. Buskirk, Ph.D.
Professor of Applied Physiology
Director, Laboratory for Human
  Performance Research
The Pennsylvania State University
University Park, Pennsylvania

Frank Cerny, Ph.D.
Associate Professor
Department of Physical Therapy and
  Exercise Science
State University of New York at Buffalo
Buffalo, New York

Mary M. Checovich, B.S.
Department of Preventive Medicine
University of Wisconsin
Madison, Wisconsin

Gordon R. Cumming, M.D.
Vice President and Medical Director
The Great-West Life Assurance Company
Winnipeg, Manitoba, Canada

J. Larry Durstine, Ph.D.
Associate Professor, Department of Exercise
  Science
The University of South Carolina
Columbia, South Carolina

Björn Ekblom, M.D., Ph.D.
Karolinska Institutet
Department of Physiology III
Stockholm, Sweden

Kenneth D. Fitch, M.D.
Medical Consultant
Department of Human Movement and
  Recreation Studies
The University of Western Australia
Nedlands, Western Australia, Australia

Victor F. Froelicher, M.D., F.A.C.C.
Palo Alto Veterans Administration
Medical Center
Stanford University School of Medicine
Palo Alto, California

Catherine Gilligan, B.A.
Department of Preventive Medicine
University of Wisconsin
Madison, Wisconsin

William L. Haskell, Ph.D.
Associate Professor of Medicine
Stanford University School of Medicine
Stanford, California

Norman L. Jones, M.D., F.R.C.P.
Professor of Medicine
Director, Ambrose Cardiorespiratory Unit,
  McMaster University
Hamilton, Ontario, Canada

Arthur S. Leon, M.D.
H. L. Taylor Professor of Exercise and Health
  Enhancement
Division of Kinesiology
School of Kinesiology and Leisure Studies
University of Minnesota
Minneapolis, Minnesota
Chief Cardiologist, Lipid Research Clinic
Department of Medicine, University of
  Minnesota
Minneapolis, Minnesota

M. Dan McKirnan, Ph.D.
Research Physiologist
Department of Pathology, School of
  Medicine, University of California, San
  Diego
La Jolla, California

Henry S. Miller, Jr., M.D.
Professor of Medicine, Bowman Gray School
  of Medicine
Director, Section on Cardiology, and
Medical Director, Wake Forest Cardiac
  Rehabilitation Program
Wake Forest University
Winston-Salem, North Carolina

Deborah L. Morley, Ph.D.
Research Director, Heart Failure/Transplant
  Center
Assistant Professor of Medicine
Hahnemann University
Philadelphia, Pennsylvania

Alan R. Morton, Ed.D.
Professor, Department of Human Movement
  and Recreation Studies
The University of Western Australia,
  Australia
Nedlands, Western Australia, Australia

Rolf Nordemar, M.D.
Associate Professor and Assistant Head
Department of Physical Medicine and
  Rehabilitation
Karolinska Institutet
Stockholm, Sweden

Neil B. Oldridge, Ph.D.
Professor, Department of Health Sciences
University of Wisconsin, Milwaukee;
Clinical Professor, Division of BioStatistics
  and Clinical Epidemiology
Milwaukee, Wisconsin

David Orenstein, M.D.
Associate Professor of Pediatrics
Associate Professor of Instruction and
  Learning (Exercise Physiology)
Director, Pediatric Pulmonary/Cystic
  Fibrosis
Children's Hospital of Pittsburgh
Pittsburgh, Pennsylvania

Patricia Painter, Ph.D.
Transplant Rehabilitation Director
University of California at San Francisco
San Francisco, California

Kent B. Pandolf, Ph.D.
Director, Environmental Physiology and
  Medicine Directorate
United States Army Research Institute of
  Environmental Medicine
Natick, Massachusetts

Rune Sannerstedt, M.D., Ph.D.
Assistant Professor of Medicine,
University of Göteborg;
Chief Physician, Carlanderska Hospital
Göteborg, Sweden

James S. Skinner, Ph.D.
Professor, Department of Exercise Science
  and Physical Education
Director, Exercise and Sport Research
  Institute
Arizona State University
Tempe, Arizona

Everett L. Smith, Ph.D.
Department of Preventive Medicine
University of Wisconsin
Madison, Wisconsin

James E. Stoll, M.D.
Milwaukee Spinal Associates
Columbia Hospital
Milwaukee, Wisconsin

Jack H. Wilmore, Ph.D.
Department of Kinesiology and Health
  Education
The University of Texas at Austin
Bellmont Hall
Austin, Texas

Larry A. Wolfe, Ph.D.
Associate Professor, School of Physical and
  Health Education
Queen's University
Kingston, Ontario, Canada

CONTENTS

Section I.   General Considerations

Section II.   Special Cases

GENERAL CONSIDERATIONS

1
CHAPTER

General Principles of Exercise Testing

by

M. Dan McKirnan and Victor F. Froelicher

Exercise is one of the most common physiologic stressors. Exercise testing provides a unique and practical means of assessing the body's capacity for physical effort. It can define the limits of athletic performance as well as the functional capabilities of a symptomatic patient. General applications of exercise testing include 1) disease prediction, prognosis, and severity; 2) evaluation of surgical and medical treatments; 3) assessment of functional capacity or maximal oxygen consumption ($\dot{V}_{O_2max}$); and 4) exercise prescription. In this chapter, the physiology, methodology, applications, interpretations, and special considerations for exercise testing are discussed.

PHYSIOLOGIC PRINCIPLES OF TESTING THE OXYGEN TRANSPORT SYSTEMS

Oxygen Transport and Muscular Effort

The transport of oxygen from the external environment to the mitochondria of the contracting muscle cell requires the coupling of blood flow and ventilation to cellular metabolism (Fig. 1–1).[129] This transport chain is normally capable of supporting a level of metabolism 10- to 12-fold greater than that at rest. Because this coupling is not tight enough to support rapid increases in muscular activity, however, anaerobic metabolism temporarily compensates for these transitions in energy demands. Similarly, anaerobic processes make an increasing contribution to metabolism as the limit of oxygen transport is approached and is briefly exceeded at maximal exercise. These types of metabolic adjustments are observed in graded exercise testing.

Respiratory contributions to oxygen transport involve an increased minute ventilation ($\dot{V}_E$) resulting from increases in both rate (f) and tidal volume (TV), as presented in Figure 1–1. Diffusion and the ratio of alveolar ventilation ($\dot{V}_A$) to lung perfusion ($\dot{Q}_L$) also determine gas exchange. Cardiovascular adjustments include an increase in the volume of blood pumped, or cardiac output ($\dot{Q}$), which is a function of heart rate (HR) times stroke volume (SV). $\dot{V}_{O_2}$ is dependent on $\dot{Q}$ and the extraction of oxygen from the blood, the arteriovenous oxygen difference (AVD-O_2). With exercise, blood flow is directed away from inactive organs to the active skeletal muscle. The $\dot{V}_{O_2}$ of muscle then depends upon vascularity, diffusion, muscle fiber distribution, and the total oxidative potential of these muscle fibers. In normal individuals, the limitation in oxygen transport probably lies in the delivery of oxygen to active muscle by the circulation.[103]

Cardiovascular adjustments to dynamic exercise are depicted in Figure 1-2 for a hypothetical 25-year-old, non-athletic man.[12] There is a linear rise in $\dot{Q}$ versus $\dot{V}_{O_2}$, with

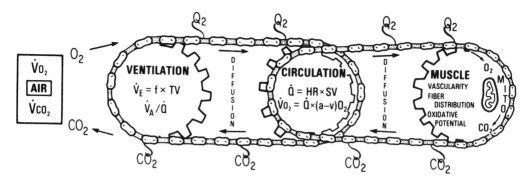

Fig. 1-1. *Transport of oxygen from the external environment to active muscle. (Modified from Wasserman and Whipp.[129])*

HR contributing most to this rise because SV increases minimally above 40 to 50% $\dot{V}_{O_2max}$. Systolic blood pressure (SBP) increases with $\dot{V}_{O_2}$, but diastolic pressure (DBP) changes are small. The mean arterial pressure (MAP) increases modestly. Predicting or directly measuring $\dot{V}_{O_2max}$ during graded exercise testing provides a noninvasive method of estimating $\dot{Q}_{max}$, because AVD-O_2 has a physiologic limit.

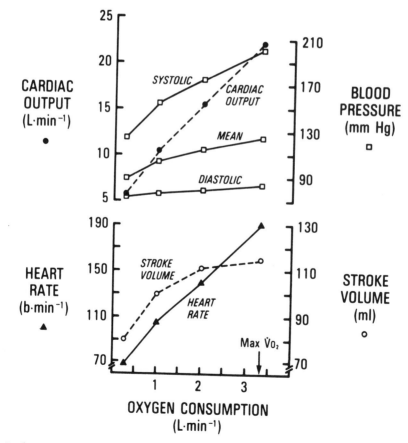

Fig. 1-2. *Cardiovascular adjustments to dynamic exercise for a 25-year-old man. (Modified from Bar-Or and Buskirk.[12])*

In contrast to dynamic exercise, static or isometric exercise results in disproportionate increases in ventilatory and cardiovascular variables relative to the external work performed. The proportional increases in $\dot{Q}$, SV, and HR and minimal change in MAP for dynamic exercise indicate a volume load for the heart. Static exercise produces a marked elevation in MAP, with relatively small increases in HR and $\dot{Q}$. This pressure load on the heart occurs in proportion to the relative muscle tension and the muscle mass involved.[83,84]

$M\dot{V}_{O_2}$ versus $\dot{V}_{O_2}$

An important physiologic principle is that total body $\dot{V}_{O_2}$ and myocardial $\dot{V}_{O_2}$ ($M\dot{V}_{O_2}$) are distinct, both in their determinants and in the way they are measured or estimated. Total body $\dot{V}_{O_2}$ is the amount of oxygen extracted from inspired air. Its accurate measurement requires gas analysis equipment, but this value can be estimated from power output, because there is relatively small variation in the $\dot{V}_{O_2}$ at a given power output. By contrast, $M\dot{V}_{O_2}$ is best estimated by the product of HR $\times$ SBP or the rate-pressure product (RPP). Accurate measurement requires the placement of catheters in an artery and in the coronary venous sinus to measure oxygen content. Its determinants include intramyocardial wall tension (left ventricular pressure $\times$ end-diastolic volume), contractility, and HR. Angina pectoris usually occurs at the same RPP, rather than at the same power output.

The relationships between estimated $M\dot{V}_{O_2}$ (i.e., RPP) and measured total body $\dot{V}_{O_2}$ for various combinations of static and dynamic exercise are illustrated in Figure 1-3.[5,64,73,74] Static exercise was handgrip exercise at various percentages of the maximal voluntary contraction. Handgrip exercise produces little change in $\dot{V}_{O_2}$, but the $M\dot{V}_{O_2}$ value increases in proportion to the relative intensity alone or in combination with dynamic exercise. Arm exercise elicits a higher $M\dot{V}_{O_2}$ than does leg exercise relative to total body $\dot{V}_{O_2}$; this may be partially attributed to a greater isometric component for arm exercise. These comparisons have important implications for exercise test selection, as well as for the prescription of physical activities.

General Principles of Challenging the Oxygen Transport Systems

Exercise tests designed to measure functional capacity, $\dot{V}_{O_2}$, or both should meet general requirements, as suggested by Åstrand and Rodahl.[4]

1. Work must involve large muscle groups.
2. Work must be measureable and reproducible.
3. Test conditions must be such that the results are comparable and repeatable.
4. Testing must be tolerated by the individuals being evaluated.
5. Mechanical efficiency (skill) required to perform the task should be as uniform as possible in the population to be tested.

These general principles should be applied in all tests designed to challenge the oxygen transport system.

CONSIDERATIONS FOR TESTING THE OXYGEN TRANSPORT SYSTEM

Type of Exercise

ISOMETRIC VERSUS ISOTONIC EXERCISE. Evaluating the cardiovascular responses to the pressure load of isometric exercise as well as to the volume load of isotonic exercise may be warranted in some clinical and occupational exercise testing. Results of several investigations have revealed that isometric exercise alone fails to elicit the myocardial ischemia produced by dynamic exercise.[30,56,63] When isometric was added to dynamic exercise, the threshold for ischemia occurred at a higher $M\dot{V}_{O_2}$.[30,63] This result was attributed to a higher coronary perfusion pressure produced by the isometric elevation of DBP.

Although induction of arrhythmias by isometric and dynamic exercise was not

5

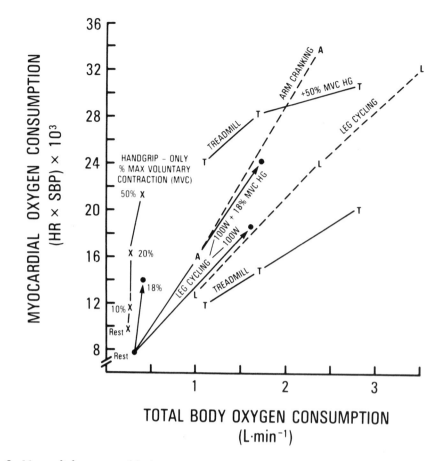

Fig. 1–3. *Myocardial versus total body oxygen consumption.*[5,64,73,74]

different in some coronary heart disease (CHD) patients, a significantly greater incidence has been reported during isometric effort.[6,29,30] In normal men, isometric exercise was effective in inducing ventricular premature beats; the induction by treadmill exercise was highly variable.[28] These differences may have been due to patient selection, e.g., CHD patients with more severe disease probably develop more dysrhythmias with isometric effort.

ARMS VERSUS LEGS. Dynamic exercise responses of individuals with lower extremity impairments or who normally engage in arm work may be evaluated by arm ergometry.[9,41,52,70,94,104,106,107] Arm ergometry effectively elicits myocardial ischemia in CHD patients.[9,70,106,107] In one group of patients, ischemic responses on ECG occurred more frequently for leg than arm ergometry, but ventricular pre-

mature beats occurred more frequently with arm exercise.[29] Arm and wheelchair ergometry have effective applications in testing and rehabilitating the disabled person.[104]

DIAGNOSTIC VALUE. In clinical testing, the type of exercise can influence the diagnostic value of the exercise test. For example, in exercise-induced bronchospasm, treadmill running has proven to be more asthmogenic than is treadmill walking or cycle ergometry.[25] Physiologic monitoring, however, is easier to perform during cycling.

For coronary patients, Niederberger and colleagues found that bicycle exercise constituted a greater stress on the cardiovascular system at any given $\dot{V}_{O_2}$ than did treadmill exercise; HR, RPP, MAP, and peripheral vascular resistance values were higher.[92] Forty post-myocardial infarction

6

patients achieved a 17% higher $\dot{V}_{O_2max}$ on the treadmill when compared to values on a cycle ergometer, but the RPP was similar (HR was higher and SBP was lower).[136] Electrocardiographic changes consistent with myocardial ischemia were similar. Leg ergometry was somewhat more effective in eliciting ischemia but was less arrhythmogenic than arm ergometry.[29] Posture can also influence the diagnostic value of an exercise test because body position alters central hemodynamics and the ventilatory and metabolic responses to dynamic exercise.[14,71,134]

MAXIMAL OXYGEN CONSUMPTION ($\dot{V}_{O_2max}$). During a progressive exercise test, $\dot{V}_{O_2max}$ is defined as a plateau in $\dot{V}_{O_2}$, in spite of an increase in the external power output. This value represents an objectively defined limit of aerobic performance, but requires expensive equipment and technical support. Reasonable estimates of $\dot{V}_{O_2max}$ can be obtained from the external power output, providing standard testing methods are employed. The highest values for $\dot{V}_{O_2max}$ have been obtained during grade walking and running. Lower values were recorded for stepping (-3%), bicycling upright (-4 to -7%), bicycling supine (-15 to -18%), and arm cranking (-30 to -35%).[3,113] Oxygen consumption is commonly expressed in METS, which represent multiples of the metabolic requirement for resting in the seated posture (Table 1–1).[1,120]

HYPERVENTILATION. The voluntary increase of $\dot{V}_E$ above normal levels at rest will cause a reduction in arterial CO_2 and may distinguish between effects of muscular and respiratory effort. This procedure

has been used prior to exercise testing to screen for potential false-positive responders in an asymptomatic population, but it has not been systematically studied to warrant routine use. Although this procedure may be used to determine labile ST-T wave changes after a test that is thought to have yielded false-positive results, the procedure can produce angina and coronary spasm. As well, the effects of hyperventilation on the ECG findings may be neurogenic rather than metabolic.

ORTHOSTATIC STRESS. Changing from the supine to upright posture produces a large shift in blood volume from the central to the peripheral circulation. This gravity-dependent shift causes blood to pool in the distensible veins of the lower extremities and acutely challenges the baroreceptor regulation of blood pressure; lightheadedness or syncope may result. Monitoring of an individual in a simple static stand may explain recent symptomatology or may reveal underlying cardiovascular disease.[103] Borderline hypertensive patients have exhibited diastolic hypertension upon standing.[60]

VALSALVA MANEUVER. The Valsalva maneuver consists of a sustained, forced expiration against an airway obstructed by a closed glottis or an external column of mercury (Flack test). Blood pressure rises at the onset of straining due to the increased intrathoracic pressure being added to the blood pressure in the aorta. The pressure then falls sharply as straining is maintained because the high intrathoracic pressure compresses the great veins, decreasing venous return and $\dot{Q}$. The reductions in arterial pressure and pulse pressure are sensed by the baroreceptors,

TABLE 1–1. **Key MET Values**

1 MET = resting $\dot{V}_{O_2}$ = 3.5 ml $\times$ kg^{-1} $\times$ min^{-1}
Equivalent METs at speeds from 2 to 5 mph:

<5 METs:	Poor prognosis
5 METs:	Minimal activities of daily living, post-MI limit for 1 month
10 METs:	Fit, no benefit for survival from CABG compared to medical management
13 METs:	Good prognosis regardless of treadmill test results
20 METs:	Aerobic master athlete
24 METs:	Aerobic athlete

resulting in reflex increases in HR and total peripheral resistance. Cessation of straining reduces intrathoracic pressure and restores $\dot{Q}$, but peripheral resistance remains high. Blood pressure levels then exhibit a distinct overshoot, followed by a baroreceptor-mediated slowing of the HR and restoration of normal pressure.

Clinically, this procedure has been used to evaluate autonomic nervous system insufficiency and syncope in patients with chronic lung disease, congestive heart failure, and left ventricular dysfunction.[36,62,72,141] This maneuver is often performed during such daily tasks as weight lifting, pushing, and the use of levers when the muscles of the chest and shoulder girdle are isometrically fixed. The use of this procedure in patient evaluation may prove beneficial prior to their resumption of similar occupational and leisure activities.

Exercise Testing Protocols

A number of testing protocols have been employed to evaluate functional capacity. Exercise protocols are illustrated in Figure 1–4. Protocol considerations should be consistent with testing objectives and include maximal versus submaximal testing, single versus multiple-stage testing, continuous versus intermittent effort, and

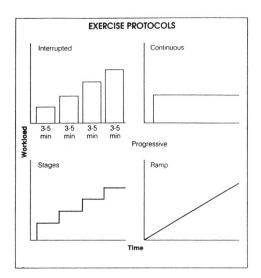

Fig. 1–4. *Types of protocols.*

stage duration. Submaximal testing has been used to predict $\dot{V}_{O_2max}$, to group individuals for studies of functional status, and to screen for latent CHD. Tests targeted to reach a specific percentage of age-predicted HR_{max} can easily be in error by ±10 b·min^{-1}. In a group of 510 normal men, 27% exhibited ECG changes consistent with ischemia during or after a maximal exercise test. Termination of the test at 85% of predicted HR_{max} would have reduced the ischemic responders by 50%.[26] A symptom-limited or sign-limited maximal test offers the advantages of direct assessment of functional capacity, accurate determination of HR_{max}, and a more complete evaluation of cardiac performance.[1,3,25] Exercise prescriptions can also be more accurately given after completion of a maximal test. The risk of complications for all types of tests is small (0.8 per 10,000 tests), and thus safety is not seriously threatened with maximal testing.[50] Although the submaximal test is more specific for CHD with fewer false-positive results, a maximal test is more sensitive, revealing a higher percentage of true-positive tests.[44] *Specificity* refers to the percentage of persons without CHD who have normal results of exercise tests; *sensitivity* is the percentage of patients with CHD who have abnormal test results.

Single-stage tests produce a wide range of HR and are more likely to result in false-negative responses and overstressing in a small proportion of the population.[124,125] A comparison of five commonly used tests revealed that the graded double Masters two-step had the highest energy cost, whereas the lowest value was measured for treadmill walking at 3 mph, 5% grade.[15] The HR for the bicycle test was disproportionately high relative to $\dot{V}_{O_2}$. The graded double Master two-step also had the highest inter-individual variability in determinations of $\dot{V}_{O_2}$ and HR. The least amount of variability in weight-adjusted $\dot{V}_{O_2}$ was noted during treadmill walking. However, fixed external power output values, expressed independent of body weight, exhibited the smallest degree of variability in $\dot{V}_{O_2}$. When screening large groups, the single-stage test has a distinct economic advantage.[118] Although single-stage tests may yield important information, the multistage test can ascertain responses to exercise that increases progressively from rest to maximal effort. The test protocol can be adapted for the elite athlete and the severely limited patient.

Tests with progressive increases in external work may be done in a continuous or intermittent fashion. The latter offers periods of rest between work bouts, a more demonstrable plateau for $\dot{V}_{O_2max}$, and performance that does not appear to be as vulnerable to local muscle fatigue.[124,125] Because rest periods can vary from minutes to a day or more between bouts, the time requirement is a major limitation. Similar values for $\dot{V}_{O_2max}$ found during continuous and intermittent testing strongly support the use of a continuous protocol for routine use.[40,123]

Generally, the duration of each stage varies from 1 to 3 minutes for most progressive, continuous testing protocols. For normal individuals, adjustments in $\dot{V}_{O_2}$ to match external power output are almost complete by 2 minutes into each stage, but this timing can be altered if the increment in exercise is large.[3,123] Whether stage duration has a significant effect on test outcome has not been determined. Post-coronary patients exhibited somewhat more ST segment depression during a rapid progressive test (1 minute per stage) than during a steady-state test (3 minutes per stage).[112] Blood pressure and HR responses for 1 to 2-minute stages lag behind those found during a more steady-state, 3-minute protocol and can result in a prescription for a higher exercise level than is desired for sustained training.

Protocols suitable for clinical testing should include a low-intensity warm-up phase, 8 to 10 minutes of continuous progressive exercise during which the myocardial oxygen demand is elevated to the patient's maximal level, and a suitable recovery or cool-down period. Today, the most widely used treadmill test employed in clinical settings is the Bruce protocol. Unfortunately, it has significant disadvantages for functional testing, especially among patients with low exercise capacities or orthopedic problems. To test low-functional-capacity patients, two preliminary, lower-intensity stages can be added to the Bruce protocol. Nevertheless, because the MET increments in the Bruce protocol are large and uneven, and because it severely limits the number of submaximal responses that may be observed in relation to exercise states, we do not recommend its use. The United States Air Force School of Aerospace Medicine modification of the Balke-Ware protocol is a particularly attractive alternative because of its constant treadmill speed of either 2.0 or 3.3 mph and grade increments of 5% applied every 2 to 3 minutes. This protocol provides good flexibility so that an optimal exercise time to maximal exertion can be achieved, thereby allowing the examination of patient responses across four or five stages. An illustration of two versions of the Balke-Ware protocol in comparison to the Bruce is presented in Figure 1–5.[19]

One recent advance in test methodology that can overcome many of the limitations of multistage exercise tests is the ramp protocol. The ramp involves a nearly continuous and uniform increase in metabolic demand that replaces the "staging" used in conventional exercise tests (Fig. 1–4). With ramping, the uniform increase in demand allows a steady rise in cardiopulmonary responses. Protocols have been developed that provide for ramping rates appropriate to patients with different functional capacities, for use both with the cycle ergometer and the treadmill.[24,81,89,96]

Deciding on an exercise protocol that will optimize test duration for each patient is important, whether the approach used involves ramping or staging. Errors in this step can advance the patient toward maximal exertion too rapidly or too slowly. The consequence of early test termination is an inadequate opportunity to observe clinically important responses, whereas the consequence of a prolonged procedure is muscular fatigue, which may limit performance before a myocardial

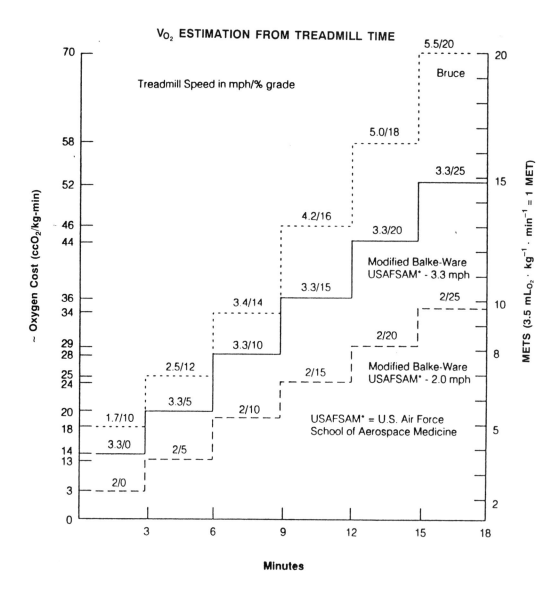

Fig. 1–5. *Two versions of the Balke-Ware treadmill protocol compared with the Bruce protocol.*

challenge adequate for diagnosis can be obtained. Thus, the protocol should be individualized to accommodate the patient's limitations. When the patient has not previously taken an exercise test, as is most often the case, it can be helpful to consult tables showing normal MET values for functional capacity graded by age, sex, and habitual physical activity level. The approach of Hlatky et al.[58] may be particularly helpful in guiding the selection of the exercise test protocol (Table 1–2). It is easily completed as a self-administered questionnaire and can be considered reasonably valid based on its correlation with measured $\dot{V}_{O_2 max}$.

Field tests provide a suitable means to assess functional capacity in large groups of people. Considerations for use of these predictive tests include equipment costs, staffing convenience, predictive accuracy, and the relative risk for the population to

TABLE 1-2. **Duke Activity Status Index**

Activity	Weight
Can You...	
1. Take care of yourself, that is, eating, dressing, bathing or using the toilet?	2.75
2. Walk indoors, such as around your house?	1.75
3. Walk a block or two on level ground?	2.75
4. Climb a flight of stairs or walk up a hill?	5.50
5. Run a short distance?	8.00
6. Do light work around the house like dusting or washing dishes?	2.70
7. Do moderate work around the house like vacuuming, sweeping floors, or carrying in groceries?	3.50
8. Do heavy work around the house like scrubbing floors, or lifting or moving heavy furniture?	8.00
9. Do yard work like raking leaves, weeding or pushing a power mower?	4.50
10. Have sexual relations?	5.25
11. Participate in moderate recreational activities like golf, bowling, dancing, doubles tennis, or throwing a basketball or football?	6.00
12. Participate in strenuous sports like swimming, singles tennis, football, basketball or skiing?	7.50

be evaluated. Running and stepping tests are the field tests used most frequently.

Running tests have been utilized to evaluate military personnel; only a stopwatch, a measured course, and a recording form are required. Accurate prediction requires motivated participants who can pace themselves at a peak level for the fixed distance or specified time period. The linear relationship between running velocity and $\dot{V}_{O_2}$ provides the empiric physiologic basis for these tests. For this reason, the 15-minute run of Balke may be favored over the 12-minute run of Cooper, because it involves a larger proportion of aerobic than anaerobic metabolism.[10,11,23] Because these tests require a maximal effort, they pose some threat to individuals at risk.

Step tests involve submaximal to maximal efforts and require single or multiple step heights, a metronome to establish stepping rate, a stopwatch for timing and counting HR, and a recording form.[43] Functional capacity can be evaluated from recovery HR by using norms and predictive equations or by extrapolation to HR_{max} from those measured at the standard submaximal levels. Fitness Canada has promoted a Canadian Home Fitness Kit containing a record that leads the indi-

vidual through a simple step test with HR counting in recovery.[110,111] This test has been criticized for inaccuracies in the counting of HR, which can be a significant limitation of any test.[27]

The Åstrand-Ryhming Step Test involves 5 minutes of stepping at 90 steps$\cdot$min^{-1} on a 40-cm bench for men and a 33-cm bench for women. Exactly 15 to 30 seconds after the test is completed, HR is taken. This test has proven useful for screening and classifying large numbers of college students.[79] In the most reliable HR counting method, two counters are employed. The Kasch Pulse Recovery Test involves the use of a 12-inch (30.5-cm) step and a rate of 24 steps$\cdot$min^{-1} for 3 minutes. A 60-second HR count begins 5 seconds after exercise, with the participant sitting. This test appears suitable for middle-aged individuals and norms are available for men.[87]

A progressive step test has been used for both submaximal and maximal testing.[69,91] The bench heights of 10, 20, 30, and 40 cm are stepped at 120 steps$\cdot$min^{-1} for 3 minutes each. Heart rate is obtained after each bout (the end point may be a "critical" HR based on age or fatigue) and is plotted against $\dot{V}_{O_2}$ estimated from a standard formula based on step height and

11

rate. Submaximal HR is then extrapolated to age-predicted maximal levels for prediction of functional capacity.[76]

Running and step tests offer alternatives to expensive laboratory testing procedures when large groups require evaluations. With careful attention to the limitations of motivation, pacing, and counting HR, reasonable data on functional capacity can be obtained.[57,90]

Selection of Exercise Testing Devices

The most commonly used devices for testing are the bicycle ergometer, treadmill, step, and arm ergometer (see Table 1–3 for an evaluation).[2] Bicycle ergometry is favored in Europe and Scandinavia, whereas the treadmill is most often used in clinical settings in North America.[7,119] Although step testing offers an inexpensive alternative, there are technical limitations. Arm ergometry offers a suitable means for testing individuals with lower extremity impairment.[52,106]

Clinical Applications of Treadmill Testing

Some applications of exercise testing are 1) to help predict whether chest pain or sensations or cardiac abnormalities are due to CHD; 2) to determine prognosis and severity of disease; 3) to assess functional capacity; 4) to evaluate surgical and medical therapy; 5) to evaluate dysrhythmias; 6) to screen for latent CHD; 7) to evaluate patients with peripheral vascular disease and those with lung disease; and 8) to evaluate patients after myocardial infarction, including testing before discharge from the hospital. The appropriate applications of exercise testing have been addressed by the ACC/AHA Task Force, as summarized in Table 1–4.[120]

The exercise test can be used to evaluate patients that currently have chest sensations, patients with a history of worrisome chest pain, or patients with other findings suggestive (but not diagnostic) of CHD. The results of exercise testing can help to establish the probability that such patients have CHD.[66]

TABLE 1–3. **Modes of Testing***

Criterion	Testing Devices			
	Treadmill	Bicycle	Step	Arm Crank
Ability to achieve highest $\dot{V}_{O_2max}$	4	2 (−10%)	3 (−2%)	1 (−20%)
Obtaining physiological data				
ECG	3	4	2	1
Blood pressure	3	4	2	1
Blood samples	3	4	2	1
$\dot{V}_E$ and $\dot{V}_{O_2}$	3	4	1	2
Performance not limited by local muscle fatigue	4	2	3	1
Familiarity and skills not required	4	3	2	1
Instrument calibration	2	3[†] 1[‡]	4	3[†] 1[‡]
Adjustment of work load	4	2[†] 3[‡]	1	2[†] 3[‡]
Cost of equipment	1	3	4	2
Maintenance	1	2	4	3
Subject compliance	4	2	3	1

* Each device was rated from 1 (lowest) to 4 (highest) in its ability to satisfy the indicated testing criterion. (Adapted from Andersen et al.[2]).
† Friction brake.
‡ Electric brake.

TABLE 1–4. **ACC/AHA Task Force on Assessment of Cardiovascular Procedures: Guidelines for Use of Exercise Testing**

CLASS I	General consensus agreement that it is justified
CLASS II	Frequently used but divergence of opinion regarding justification
CLASS III	General agreement regarding little or no value, inappropriate contraindications

Use in Patients with Signs/Symptoms of Coronary Artery Disease (CAD) or with Known CAD

CLASS I
1-To diagnose male patients with atypical signs/symptoms of CAD
2-To assess functional capacity
3-For prognosis
4-To evaluate patients with symptoms consistent with recurrent exercise induced arrhythmias

CLASS II
1-To diagnose women with chest pain
2-To diagnose patients on digoxin, with right bundle branch block
3-To evaluate functional capacity and response to therapy with drugs in CAD or congestive heart failure
4-To evaluate variant angina
5-To serially follow (1 year or longer) patients with CAD

CLASS III
1-To evaluate patients with single PVCs
2-To serially evaluate patients in rehabilitation
3-To diagnose CAD in patients with Wolf-Parkinson-White Syndrome or left bundle branch block

Use in Screening of Apparently Healty Individuals

CLASS I
None

CLASS II
To evaluate asymptomatic males over 40:
1-in special occupations
2-with 2 or more risk factors (chol > 240, high blood pressure (HBP), cigarettes, diabetes mellitus, family history of CAD, < 55 years)
3-who are sedentary and plan to enter a vigorous exercise program

CLASS III
To evaluate asymptomatic men and women:
1-with no risk factors
2-with chest discomfort not thought to be cardiac

Use Soon After Myocardial Infarction (MI)

CLASS I
To evaluate prognosis and functional capacity in uncomplicated Mis

CLASS II
1-To evaluate those with baseline ECGs or medical problems that affect responses
2-To evaluate those with complicated Mis

CLASS III
1-To evaluate acute ischemia
2-To evaluate patients who are unstable or have complicating illnesses

Use After Specific Procedures

CLASS I
To evaluate coronary artery bypass graft (CABG) surgery and PTCA patients

CLASS II
To follow asymptomatic patients with CABG or PTCA yearly

Use in Patients with Valvular Heart Disease

CLASS I
Not used

CLASS II
To evaluate functional capacity

CLASS III
To evaluate symptomatic critical aortic stenosis or asymmetrical septal hypertrophy

Use in the Management of Patients with High Blood Pressure or Cardiac Pacemakers

CLASS I
Not used

CLASS II
To evaluate BP response in patients treated for HBP who wish to exercise vigorously

CLASS III
To evaluate patients with severe HBP, to evaluate HBP patients who do not plan to exercise, to evaluate pacemaker function

Results of an exercise test help to establish the risk of morbidity and mortality and to evaluate the severity of CHD. Individuals with exercise-induced hypotension, very limited exercise capacity, inadequate HR response, ST segment elevation, and marked ST segment abnormalities (including those beginning at a low HR) have a bad prognosis.[80] Patients who are able to achieve a normal power output, HR_{max}, and a normal SBP response are more likely to have better ventricular function, less coronary obstruction, and a better prognosis than those unable to do so.

Although more than 10 follow-up studies have been completed to address this issue, none has demonstrated that the exercise test is effective in screening asymptomatic individuals to prevent cardiac events. In fact, the American College of Cardiology/American Heart Association Guidelines[120] state that the exercise test should not be used in this group unless they have two or more of the standard risk factors (i.e., cigarette smoking, hypercholesterolemia, hypertension, family history of heart disease). Sox et al.[117] suggested that exercise tests might be justifiable for screening asymptomatic individuals who have at least one clinical risk factor or a total cholesterol/HDL ratio greater than 6.0. However, Ekelund et al.[35] recently reported the results of exercise testing in a population with elevated blood cholesterol levels, and still found that an abnormal test had a very low predictive value. The first eight screening studies used angina pectoris as an endpoint, whereas later studies used only such hard endpoints as MI or death (Table 1–5). These later studies were more valid and have demonstrated that an abnormal response has a much lower predictive value. Only 1 in 20 people with an abnormal ST response will have a hard cardiac event within 5 to 8 years of the test. This means that 19 out of 20 must deal with the psychological, social, and financial problems created by a false-positive test.

An exercise test can be used to determine the appropriateness or effects of rehabilitation programs, medications, and coronary artery bypass surgery. It can be used to evaluate patients with arrhythmias or to induce such arrhythmias as premature ventricular contractions, sick sinus syndrome, paroxysmal tachycardia, and heart block.[54] The exercise test can be used to evaluate the safety of participation in an exercise program or the performance of other activities; it is essential for formulating an individualized exercise prescription based on a person's actual HR max rather than on an estimated value. In addition, the successful performance of a test after an acute myocardial infarction can be reassuring, and is the first step in rehabilitation.[116]

ABSOLUTE AND RELATIVE CONTRAINDICATIONS. Contraindications to the performance of an exercise test are listed in Table 1–6. Good clinical judgment should be foremost in any decision. For example, although the absolute contraindications are clear, testing can provide valuable information (even if performed submaximally) in selected patients with relative contraindications.

TABLE 1–5. **Screening Asymptomatic, Apparently Healthy Individuals for Silent Ischemia (St Depression) with Exercise Testing**

	Sensitivity	Specificity	Positive Predictive Value	Risk Ratio
Including angina pectoris as endpoint (N = 8)	48%	90%	26%	9X
Including only hard endpoints (N = 4)	27%	91%	6%	4X

Absolute Contraindications	Relative Contraindications
Acute myocardial infarction or any recent change in the resting ECG	Any less serious non-cardiac disorder
Unstable angina	Ventricular conduction defects
Serious cardiac dysrhythmias	Significant arterial or pulmonary hypertension
Acute pericarditis or myocarditis	Tachy- or bradydysrhythmias less than serious
Endocarditis	Moderate valvular or myocardial heart diseases
Severe aortic stenosis	Drug effect or electrolyte abnormalities
Severe left ventricular dysfunction	Fixed-rate artificial pacemaker
Acute pulmonary embolus or pulmonary infarction	Left main artery obstruction or its equivalent
Any acute or serious non-cardiac disorder	Psychiatric disease or inability to cooperate
Severe physical handicap	

METHODOLOGY. The patient should be instructed to not eat 2 to 3 hours before the test and to come dressed for exercise. A brief history and physical examination should be obtained to rule out any contraindications, and specific questioning should determine if any drugs are currently being taken or if there are possible electrolyte abnormalities. If the indications for testing are unclear, the patient should be questioned and the referring physician should be contacted. Before the exercise test is performed, it is important to obtain a 12-lead ECG (particularly in patients with known CHD), because an abnormality uncovered in the resting ECG may prohibit testing. There should be a careful explanation of the testing procedure with its risks and possible complications. The patient should be instructed on how to perform the exercise test, and it should be demonstrated.

Skin resistance must be reduced to improve the signal-to-noise ratio of the ECG because noise increases with the square of resistance. The skin must be properly prepared, even though it may cause discomfort or minor skin irritation, so that the ECG can be continuously monitored and accurately interpreted. Computer-averaging techniques should not be used to handle noise, because they can cause distortion.[130] Muscle artifact can often be decreased when patients relax their arms.

Bipolar leads have been used because of the ease of application, the relative freedom from motion and muscle artifact, and the ease with which the source of noise can be located. When using the torso-mounted lead system, the conventional ankle and wrist electrodes are replaced by electrodes mounted on the torso at the base of the limbs. The advantage of this system is that a reasonable facsimile of the standard 12-lead ECG can be obtained if the limb electrodes are kept as far as possible from the heart.[99]

Lead V5 is the most sensitive, with 75 to 90% of abnormal responses occurring in it alone or in addition to other leads. The sensitivity of exercise testing can be increased by monitoring other leads, but the specificity is decreased. It appears that inferior leads produce more false-positive results, partially due to atrial repolarization. Global subendocardial ischemia reduces the ability of ST segment depression to predict the location of coronary artery lesions, but ST segment elevation does help to localize lesions when diagnostic Q waves are not present.

Although the question of the number of leads needed during an exercise test has not been resolved, it seems advisable to

15

record as many as is practical.[21] In patients with a normal resting ECG, a precordial V5 or bipolar lead along the long axis of the heart is probably all that is necessary. In patients with dyskinetic areas, a myocardial infarction, or a history suggestive of spasm, additional leads are especially helpful over the affected area. In this situation, at least three leads should be recorded: a lateral V5-type lead; an anterior V2-type lead; and an inferior lead, such as AVF or Frank X, Y, and Z.

Maximal exercise testing is preferred to submaximal testing, except when the latter is safer. Maximal effort yields increased sensitivity and is required for estimating or measuring $\dot{V}_{O_2max}$.[26] Most problems can be avoided by having a physician standing next to the patient to take blood pressure readings, assess skin temperature, and talk to the patient during the test. The technician should operate the equipment, take the appropriate tracings, enter data on a form, and alert the physician to any abnormalities that might be missed on the monitor scope.

Patients should be discouraged from grasping the rails because the work decreases, exercise time increases, and muscle artifact results.[98] It is helpful to have the patient close the fists and extend one finger, which by touching the rail can help to maintain balance while walking.

Blood pressure readings should be taken at least at the midportion of each exercise stage and with the appearance of chest pain. Standard blood pressure measuring equipment is preferable to and is more accurate than automated blood pressure devices. The patient's arm should be held free of the treadmill siderail when blood pressure is measured.

If maximal sensitivity is to be achieved for diagnostic testing, the patient should be supine after exercise, as increased heart volume in the supine position increases $M\dot{V}_{O_2}$ and enhances ST segment abnormalities. Monitoring should be continued for 6 to 8 minutes or until changes have stabilized. In the fifth minute of supine recovery, approximately 85% of abnormal exercise tests are already abnormal (alone or in addition to other times).[47] An abnormal response occurring only in a recovery period is not unusual. A cool-down walk can delay the time at which ST segment depression occurs or can eliminate it.[55] For diagnostic purposes, therefore, the patient should stop walking immediately after completing exercise, stand still for about 10 seconds while ECG data are gathered at near maximal HR, and then lie down.

Most clinical treadmill protocols are continuous and progressive. When compared to other protocols, a modified Balke-Ware protocol (illustrated in Figure 1–5) has many advantages.[138] The test consists of a constant walking speed (2.0 to 3.3 mph) with 2 to 5% increases in grade every 2 or 3 minutes. A constant treadmill speed requires only an initial adaptation in stride and produces less ECG and blood pressure artifacts than do protocols involving higher speeds. The protocol provides a number of suitable power outputs by calling for increases in even increments. It is advisable to individualize any exercise protocol for the type of patient tested. Performance should be estimated on the basis of $\dot{V}_{O_2}$ ($ml\cdot kg^{-1}\cdot min^{-1}$) or METs associated with the maximal workload achieved, rather than on total treadmill time.[46,127] Estimates of $\dot{V}_{O_2}$ should be based on values derived for the patient population tested.

END POINTS. The following absolute and relative indications for terminating an exercise test have been derived from clinical experience. As stated previously, absolute indications are clear-cut, whereas relative indications can sometimes be disregarded if good clinical judgment is used. Absolute indications include a drop in SBP, despite an increase in power output; anginal chest pain that is more severe than usual; central nervous system symptoms; such signs of poor perfusion as pallor, cyanosis, and cold skin; serious dysrhythmias; technical problems with monitoring the patient; the patient's request to stop; and such marked ECG changes as more than 0.3 mV of horizontal or downsloping ST segment depression or 0.2 mV of ST segment elevation. Relative indications for termination include such worrisome ST or QRS changes as excessive junctional depression; increasing chest pain; fatigue; shortness of breath; wheezing; leg cramps or intermittent claudication; worrisome appearance; hypertensive response (SBP > 280 mm Hg or DBP > 115 mm Hg); and less serious dysrhythmias, including supraventricular tachycardias. In some high risk patients, as estimated by their clinical history, it may be appropriate to stop at a submaximal level because the most severe ST segment depression and/ or dysrhythmias occur only after exercise. If more information is required, the test can be repeated.

OBJECTIVE RESULTS.

Functional Capacity. Recent technical advances have made it easier to perform an expired gas analysis during exercise. Such measurement advances allow physicians to accurately assess $\dot{V}_{O_2max}$ instead of estimating it from treadmill speed and grade. $\dot{V}_{O_2max}$ is directly related to maximal $\dot{Q}$ and gives the best measurement of cardiac performance during exercise.[22,128] In addition, gas exchange parameters allow an assessment of the anaerobic threshold.[22,96,128] This submaximal measurement may be of more importance clinically than $\dot{V}_{O_2max}$ because it defines a person's limitations at submaximal levels common to daily activities. Currently, the clinical application of gas exchange variables is limited to the evaluation of treatments, athletic performance, and disability. In regard to disability evaluation, many physicians have the impression that gas exchange variables identify patients who are malingering during the test and not giving a maximal performance. Such judgments should be made cautiously because many of the parameters used to quantify maximal performance, such as plateauing, exceeding the anaerobic threshold, or exhibiting a respiratory exchange ratio of unity, are subject to considerable measurement error and intersubject variability.[88]

Heart Rate and Blood Pressure Responses. "Chronotropic incompetence" is defined as an HR response to treadmill testing below the 95% confidence limits for age and gender. With the exception of patients treated with beta blockers or aerobic athletes, patients with this response had the same incidence of CHD as patients with ST segment depression.[37] "Heart rate impairment" is defined as the percent deviation in measured HR max from the predicted value.[18] The mechanism of the failure of HR to rise normally is poorly understood, but many of these patients have poor ventricular function and multivessel disease.

An inadequate rise in SBP can be due to aortic outflow obstruction or to left ventricular dysfunction. Serious CHD is usually found in all patients who develop hypotension along with angina during exercise testing.[126] "Left ventricular impairment" is defined as the percent deviation in the RPP at maximal exercise from the predicted value.[18] Exercise-induced hypotension, defined as a drop in SBP of 10 mm Hg or more, was found to be a reliable sign of severe CHD in men, but not in women.[86] When this finding is noted, complications during testing are more likely to occur.[61] Figure 1–6 illustrates the normal HR and blood pressure responses to treadmill testing.[139]

Exertional Hypotension. Although exertional hypotension (EH) has been related to a poor prognosis in patients with CHD, various criteria have been used to define it, and little consideration has been given to the difficulties of measuring it or to its reproducibility. To determine the cutpoint or discriminant value for EH,[34] we apply the following criteria: 1) a drop of 20 mm Hg or more after an initial rise, but not a fall below rest levels, and 2) a drop in SBP below the standing rest value. A drop of 20 mm Hg was chosen to avoid the technical and reproducibility limitations of blood pressure measurement during exercise. Our population consisted of 2036 patients who underwent routine treadmill testing, 131 (6.4%) of whom exhibited EH when either cutpoint was used. We found that EH is best defined as a drop in SBP during exercise below the standing pre-exercise value, and indicates

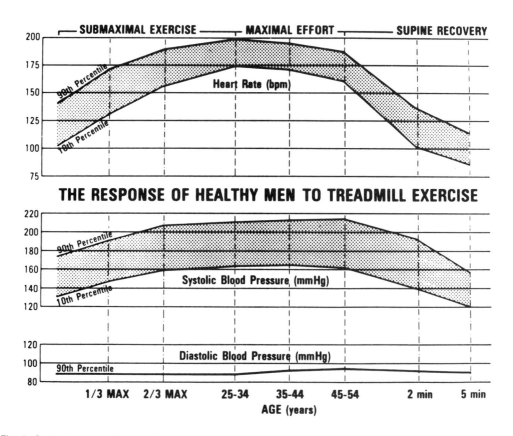

THE RESPONSE OF HEALTHY MEN TO TREADMILL EXERCISE

Fig. 1–6. *Reference or "normal" values for the physiologic response to submaximal and maximal treadmill exercise based on testing of apparently healthy men. Blocks represent the 10th and 90th percentile limits; 10% of the normals could lie above or below the blocks so that outliers are not necessarily abnormal, but are at increased risk of being abnormal. A wall chart is available on request.*

a significantly increased risk of cardiac events (three times normal) when associated with myocardial ischemia or damage. As in other studies, more than half of the patients tested who exhibited EH had left-main or triple-vessel disease.

When using a surface ECG, exercise-induced myocardial ischemia may produce one of three ST segment manifestations: ST segment elevation; ST segment normalization or no change; and ST segment depression. ST shifts are considered relative to the PR segment, rather than to the TP segment, which disappears at high HRs. Investigators correlating exercise testing and coronary angiography in hospital patients found a 3 to 11% prevalence of ST segment elevation; this elevation appears to be an insensitive but highly specific indicator of severe coronary artery occlusion.[20] The ST segment vector points

through areas of asynergy and usually occurs in an area supplied by vessels with angiographically visible lesions; [115] it does not always represent ischemia when it occurs over Q waves, but somehow the severity of the underlying aneurysm is reflected.

The frequency with which cancellation forces result in normalization or no ST segment changes in the surface ECG during exercise-induced ischemia is unknown. In one report, a patient normalized minor ST segment depression during treadmill testing, only to have an acute myocardial infarction 10 minutes after completion of the test.[121]

The classic criterion for an abnormal ST segment depression has been 0.1 mV or more of horizontal or downward sloping ST segment. The probability and severity of CHD are directly related to the amount of J junctional depression and are inversely related to the slope of the ST segment. It is preferable to call tests with a slowly upsloping ST segment (but with depression) borderline, and to place added emphasis on other responses. When one lead shows upsloping ST segment depression and another shows horizontal or downward sloping depression, the more severe changes should be reported. This disparity can even occur in adjacent precordial leads. It is uncertain whether the classic criteria have the same significance in all leads. The optimal criteria of abnormality in the inferior leads, various bipolar leads, and in the Frank X lead most likely are different than those with V5.

Heart Rate Adjustment of the ST Segment. Several investigators have improved the diagnostic accuracy of ST segment depression by using a variety of heart rate adjustment schemes. Kligfield et al.[65] demonstrated that a simple approach to heart rate adjustment (dividing the total ST segment shift by the change in HR during exercise) works better than more time-consuming methods. Hoping to validate its diagnostic accuracy, we studied 328 patients at our institution who had undergone cardiac catheterization.[68] Unfortunately, the analysis using this technique was no more diagnostically accurate than the standard analysis was, nor was it a better way to identify triple-vessel or left main coronary artery disease. Its performance characteristics were no different in patients receiving beta blockers, those with Q waves on their resting ECGs, or those who had prior MI. Until population characteristics associated with an improvement in exercise test characteristics when using this score are identified, it cannot be recommended for general application.

ST Depression Occurring in Recovery. Because of technical limitations, the first diagnostic use of the exercise ECG involved observations made only after exercise. However, the development of modern electrocardiographic techniques that could accurately record the ECG during activity shifted the testing emphasis toward changes occurring during the exercise period itself. The diagnostic accuracy of ST changes limited to the post-exercise period has been controversial. It has been proposed that such changes are more likely to represent false positives or are due to coronary artery spasm. Studies comparing nuclear procedures to the exercise ECG often do not include post-exercise ECG evaluation, so they can image as soon as possible during recovery.[32] In addition, most of the exercise test scores consider only ST segment changes that occur during exercise, thereby excluding changes occurring during recovery alone.[45] A "cool down" walk, which is known to delay or obscure recovery changes,[55] is frequently used for greater safety[50] and patient comfort.

We performed a study to determine if ST segment depression limited to the recovery period increased the diagnostic yield of the exercise test, or if these changes should be disregarded.[67] The study population was composed of 328 male patients who had undergone a sign/symptom-limited treadmill test and coronary angiography. Abnormal ST segment depression during recovery only occurred in 26 patients out of a total abnormal group of 168. Recovery-period-only ST segment depression had an 84% predictive value for angiographic disease, which was not statistically different from the 87% predictive value of ST segment depression occurring during exercise. Considering ST segment depression during recovery significantly increased the sensitivity (from 50% to 59%) without a change in predictive value. We concluded that ST segment depression that occurs only during recovery is not a false-positive indicator for angiographic disease, and that considering ST segment depression during recovery increases the diagnostic yield of the exercise test. Most exercise test scores and exercise ECG analyses performed with scintigraphy or a cool-down walk have a falsely lowered sensitivity that could be increased by considering ST segment changes that appear during recovery.

Computer Analysis of the Exercise ECG and Treadmill Scores. Computer signal averaging is now available in the standard clinical exercise laboratory thanks to microprocessor technology. Manufacturers have utilized software research to filter and average ECG signals to make exercise ECG analysis more reproducible and accurate. However, researchers utilized large mainframe computers and were not concerned with on-line analysis. Manufacturers have had to alter these programs for the real-time exercise laboratory environment. This has led to problems with the fidelity of the computer-processed ECG wave forms. Although these computer averages are very attractive, they can be distorted and represent the raw data poorly. It is extremely important that the responsible physician carefully observe the raw ECG data that are used to generate the averaged waveforms. Distortion can be caused by noise, baseline wander, aberrant beats, and changes in conduction. The measurements depend on the average wave forms and therefore can be erroneous also. The measurements are particularly problematic because, even with good averages, the algorithms can have trouble indicating ST segment onset.

We recommend using the averages by first looking at the raw data to see that this input is not grossly distorted (by inadequate skin preparation, for example), making measurements over at least three consecutive beats, and then seeing if the averages agree. The averages can be used as a summary of the results if they agree with the raw data. All too frequently, we have seen inaccuracies in the ECG algorithms produce clearly abnormal averaged complexes in healthy people with normal raw data. In short, do not rely exclusively on filtering or averaging, but look at the raw data and use adequate skin preparation.

Numerous computer scores have been recommended, most of which are very laborious. Unfortunately, none have been validated and are recommended only by the investigators who first evaluated them.

At this point, none of these scores are appropriate for clinical use.

Several computer scores have been derived using appropriate multivariate statistical techniques. Two of the best are those from Duke[77] and the University of Louvain in Belgium.[33] Of note is the angina index. When no angina occurred, the index is zero, when angina occurred during the test, the index is one, and a two is reserved for angina that caused cessation of the test. The multivariate approach of Detry et al.[33] has been demonstrated by Deckers et al.[31] to be more accurate than the ST heart rate index,[65] the Hollenberg Score,[59] and Simoon's method.[114] Although experts disagree, most studies have demonstrated that multivariate approaches to prediction are more robust than Bayesian methods.[85]

Exercise-Induced Ventricular Dysrhythmias. Premature ventricular contractions occur in approximately one third of asymptomatic men who perform a maximal treadmill test; prevalence is directly related to age. These premature beats most frequently occur at maximal exercise and often are not found when testing is repeated. A small percentage of healthy men (about 2%) have serious appearing, exercise-induced dysrhythmias. This subgroup has two to three times the risk of developing CHD, but the sensitivity and specificity of this finding are small.[47] Coronary patients usually have a higher prevalence of severe dysrhythmias, which usually occur at a lower HR than in healthy subjects. Dysrhythmias suppressed by exercise do not rule out the presence of CHD.

Inverted U waves are an insensitive, but specific, indicator of CHD.[49] Changes in the R wave do not appear to have independent diagnostic power, although the normal response is a decline in amplitude with maximal exercise.[13,140]

Subjective Results (Including Physical Examination, Appearance, and Chest Pain). Careful observation of the patient's appearance is necessary for the safe performance of an exercise test, and is helpful in clinical assessment. It is usually easy to identify patients who exaggerate their limitations or symptoms, who are unwilling to cooperate, and who have inadequate Q. Findings on physical examination can be helpful, but their sensitivity and specificity have not been demonstrated. Gallop sounds, a mitral regurgitant murmur, or a precordial bulge could be due to left ventricular dysfunction, but these findings might not always be secondary to CHD.

Ischemic chest pain induced by the exercise test predicts the presence of CHD, as do ST segment shifts; when both occur, predictive power increases.[133] Atypical chest pain is not as indicative, but classic ischemic chest pain can have a marked diagnostic impact.

Silent Ischemia During Exercise Testing. The prognostic implications of ST depression unaccompanied by angina are controversial. However, ST segment depression often signals silent ischemia, and it has been suggested that those with silent ischemia are at greater risk for cardiac death because they do not have an intact warning system. Because of the superior reliability of ST segment recording during exercise testing versus ambulatory monitoring, we performed a study to determine the prognosis of silent ischemia in an unselected population referred for exercise testing.[19] A second objective was to determine whether old or recent MI, diabetes mellitus, or age influenced the prevalence of silent myocardial ischemia. The study population was predominantly male veterans (1747 male and 26 female patients; mean age: 58 years) and excluded those with resting ST depression or left ventricular hypertrophy or those who were receiving digoxin. In approximately 60% of our patients with exercise-induced ST segment depression, the ischemia was silent. Mean maximal ST segment depression was significantly greater among patients with angina plus ST depression than it was among patients with silent ischemia. Exercise-induced ST segment depression conferred an adverse 2-year prognosis, and those with silent ischemia tended to have a better survival rate than did those with angina and ST segment depression. The prevalence of silent ischemia was not altered by recent or remote MI, an absence of previous MI, nor diabetes mellitus, but it was directly related to age.

A more rigorous follow-up study performed at Duke[78] and a Canadian study[16] have definitively demonstrated that silent ischemia tends to have a better prognosis than does ST depression accompanied by angina. An angiographic study of 586 patients[82] at our institution concurred, demonstrating milder disease in patients with silent myocardial ischemia. This was also the case in those with "true" silent ischemia; that is, in those without prior history of angina. Thus, therapy should not be more aggressive for patients with silent ischemia than for patients who have angina and ST segment depression. Since antianginal medication has not been demonstrated to improve survival in silent ischemia, there is no indication that these patients should be treated pharmacologically. However, if such patients have exercise test markers or severe disease (i.e., poor exercise capacity or marked or prolonged ST depression), then catheterization and revascularization should be considered, as for symptomatic disease.

There are many ancillary measurements that can be made in conjunction with exercise testing (e.g., radionuclide imaging, echocardiography, systolic time intervals, and apical movement), but their actual value requires further study.[51,71,102] Many computer criteria for an abnormal ST segment response have also been recommended.[130] Multivariate approaches in which hemodynamic, functional, and ST segment responses (as well as symptoms) are all considered offer the optimal approach to exercise test interpretation.

COMPLICATIONS. The major complications of exercise testing are acute myocardial infarction and sudden death. Most of these occurrences can be avoided by having an experienced physician present who is cognizant of the contraindications and termination end points to evaluate the patient and to monitor the test. Prompt and effective cardiopulmonary resuscitation must be available. Exercising testing is remarkably safe if the described guidelines are followed.[50]

SPECIAL CONSIDERATIONS. Individuals should be given proper instructions for the period prior to testing to ensure accurate and objective test results. Patients should fast for a period of 3 hours prior to testing and the previous meal should be light. This measure permits adequate time for gastric emptying and prevents the nausea and distress present when exercising muscle competes with the gastrointestinal tract for the available $\dot{Q}$. Gastric distention can impede movement of the diaphragm, and the stomach contents pose a threat of aspiration should an emergency arise. A meal can also produce such electrocardiographic changes as ST-T wave changes.

Caffeinated and alcoholic beverages and smoking should also be avoided prior to testing. Caffeine ingestion elevates plasma catecholamines, increases SBP and DBP, and alters HR at rest.[101] The effects of caffeine during exercise are not clearly known, but those measurements in a group of CHD patients were not significantly altered.[17] Alcohol has a negative effect on myocardial contractility and may produce temporary vasoconstriction.[131] Arrhythmias have also been associated with holiday drinking episodes.[32]

Cigarette smoking significantly increases cardiac index, MAP, and HR at rest.[53] During exercise, stroke index is lower and the HR is higher after smoking. Supine measurements at rest reveal an augmented $M\dot{V}_{O_2}$ (HR, contractility, preload, and afterload) after a high nicotine cigarette.[97] Exposure to cigarette smoke (passive smoking) should also be avoided prior to testing.

The exercise laboratory should be maintained at a thermoneutral temperature of 72 to 75° F (22 to 24° C), with the relative humidity less than 60%. Temperatures greater than 24° C can result in an elevated HR in unacclimated men by 1 beat $\cdot$ min$^{-1} \cdot$ °C^{-1}.[95] A high relative humidity or water vapor pressure increases the heat load of exercise by impeding heat loss through evaporation of sweat. Demands for thermoregulation via increases in skin blood flow elevate $\dot{Q}$ during exercise and may result in competition between skin and active muscle for a limited $\dot{Q}$.

The individual should be requested to report to the exercise laboratory with comfortable, loose-fitting clothing and a pair of soft-soled athletic shoes. A pleasant waiting room and exercise laboratory as well as a thorough explanation of testing procedures can reduce emotional stress. Elevations in plasma catecholamines have been observed in response to emotional stress.[122] A good history taken prior to testing should detect any factor known to alter the test results.

Legal Implications of Exercise Testing

The legal aspects of exercise testing include several considerations. Establishing good communication between tester and patient before and after the exercise test should be the first consideration. A test should not be performed without first obtaining the patient's informed consent, preferably in writing. The patient should be made aware of the potential risks and benefits of any procedure. Even if the test is carefully performed, a tester may be held responsible for a major untoward effect if consent was not first obtained. The position can be taken that a patient would not have undergone the procedure had he or she been aware of the associated risks. After the test is completed, the physician is responsible for prompt interpretation and consideration of the implications of the test. Communication of these results to the patient is essential and advice concerning adjustments in lifestyle should be made without delay. It would be of major concern if an untoward event occurred during such a delay.

The second consideration should be adherence to proper standards of care during the test. Every test should be preceded by a physical examination and an ECG performed by the supervising or referring physician. Testing should be carried out only by persons thoroughly trained in the administration of exercise tests, in recognizing signs and symptoms that may arise, and in cardiopulmonary resuscitation. The patient must be instructed to report symptoms (e.g., angina or lightheadedness) that may require test termination. A physician trained in exercise testing and resuscitation should be immediately accessible during the test to make the judgment to stop. Resuscitative equipment and medications should always be available.

Testing the body's capacity for physical effort has many applications, ranging from clinical medicine to competitive athletics. Progressive dynamic exercise is the most appropriate means to challenge the oxygen transport system. There exist many testing protocols, but a symptom or sign-limited maximal test administered in a continuous, progressive fashion efficiently provides the most objective information. Clinical treadmill testing has been extensively discussed, but many of the principles and procedures have widespread application.

Essential to the understanding of testing principles is the knowledge of the metabolic, respiratory, and cardiovascular adjustments made during dynamic and static exercise. The body and myocardial $\dot{V}_{O_2}$ are distinct variables. When compared with dynamic exercise, static exercise produces a disproportionately greater myocardial than total body oxygen demand. For normal individuals, oxygen transport during dynamic exercise is probably limited by the circulation in delivering oxygen to the active muscle.

In spite of newer technologies, the use of exercise testing continues to increase. Based on a recent survey by the American College of Physicians,[137] 50% of internists now perform the test in their office. This means that it serves as a gatekeeper in the process of deciding who should be referred to the cardiologist. Up-to-date application of testing methods and interpretation is critical to appropriate and timely referral for therapeutic intervention.

The purpose of this chapter is to provide an overview of many factors of exercise testing. The reader is referred to several other references for a more extensive review.[8,42,45,48,75,93,102,104,120,132]

ACKNOWLEDGMENT. The authors acknowledge the excellent editorial assistance of Julie A. Scharf.

REFERENCES

1. American College of Sports Medicine: Guidelines for Graded Exercise Testing and Exercise Prescription. 4th ed. Philadelphia, Lea & Febiger, 1990.
2. Andersen, K.L., et al.: Fundamentals of Exercise Testing. Geneva, World Health Organization, 1971.
3. Åstrand, P.-O.: Quantification of exercise capability and evaluation of physical capacity in man. Prog. Cardiovasc. Dis., 19:51, 1976.
4. Åstrand, P.-O., and Rodahl, K.: Textbook of Work Physiology. New York, McGraw-Hill, 1970.
5. Åstrand, P.-O., et al.: Intra-arterial blood pressure during exercise with different muscle groups. J. Appl. Physiol., 20:253, 1965.
6. Atkins, J.M., et al.: Incidence of arrhythmias induced by isometric and dynamic exercise. Br. Heart J., 38:465, 1976.
7. Atterhog, J., Jonsson, B., and Samuelsson, R.: Exercise testing in Sweden: a survey of procedures. Scand. J. Clin. Invest., 39:87, 1979.
8. Atwood, J.E., et al.: Exercise testing in patients with aortic stenosis. Chest, 93:1083, 1988.
9. Balady, G.J., et al.: Arm exercise-thallium imaging testing for the detection of coronary artery disease. J. Am. Coll. Cardiol., 9:84, 1987.
10. Balke, B.: A Simple Field Test for the Assessment of Physical Fitness. Civil Aeromedical Research Institute Report 63–6, pp. 1–8, 1963.
11. Balke, B., and Ware, R.W.: An experimental study of "physical fitness" of Air Force personnel. U.S. Armed Forces Med. J., 10:657, 1959.
12. Bar-Or, O., and Buskirk, E.R.: The cardiovascular system and exercise. In Science and Medicine of Exercise and Sport. 2nd Ed. Edited by W.R. Johnson, and E.R. Buskirk. New York, Harper and Row, 1974.
13. Battler, A., et al.: Relationship of QRS amplitude changes during exercise to left ventricular function and volumes and the diagnosis of coronary artery disease. Circulation, 60:1004, 1979.
14. Bevegård, S., et al.: The effect of body position on the circulation at rest and during exercise, with special reference to the influence on the stroke volume. Acta Physiol. Scand., 49:279, 1960.
15. Blackburn, H., et al.: Exercise tests. In Medicine and Sport: Physical Activity and Aging. Vol. IV. Edited by D. Brunner, and E. Jokl. Baltimore, University Park Press, 1970.
16. Bogaty, P., et al.: Prognosis in patients with a strongly positive exercise electrocardiogram. Am. J. Cardiol., 64:1284, 1989.
17. Brink, L.S. et al.: Caffeine ingestion by cardiac patients prior to ECG monitored exercise training. Med. Sci. Sports Exerc., 12:111, 1980.
18. Bruce, R.A.: Exercise testing for evaluation of ventricular function. N. Engl. J. Med., 296:671, 1977.
19. Callaham, P.R., et al.: Exercise-induced silent ischemia: age, diabetes mellitus, previous myo-

cardial infarction and prognosis. J. Am. Coll. Cardiol., *14*:1175, 1989.

20. Chahine, R.A., Raziner, A.E., and Ishimori, T.: The clinical significance of exercise-induced ST segment elevation. Circulation, *54*:209, 1977.

21. Chaitman, B.R., et al.: Improved efficiency of treadmill exercise testing using a multiple lead ECG system and basic hemodynamic exercise responses. Circulation, *57*:71, 1978.

22. Cohn, J.N.: Quantitative exercise testing for the cardiac patient: the value of monitoring gas exchange. Circulation, *76*(Suppl. 6):vi–1, 1987.

23. Cooper, K.H.: A means of assessing maximal oxygen intake. Correlation between field and treadmill testing. JAMA, *203*:201, 1968.

24. Cox, N.J.M., et al.: Reproducibility of incremental maximal cycle ergometer tests in patients with mild to moderate obstructive lung diseases. Lung, *167*:129, 1989.

25. Cropp, G.J.: The exercise bronchoprovocation test: standardization of procedures and evaluation of response. J. Allergy Clin. Immunol., *64*:627, 1979.

26. Cumming, G.R.: Yield of ischaemic exercise electrocardiograms in relation to exercise intensity in a normal population. Br. Heart J., *34*:919, 1972.

27. Cumming, G.R., and Glenn, J.: Evaluation of the Canadian Home Fitness Test in middle-aged men. Can. Med. Assoc. J., *117*:346, 1977.

28. DeBacker, G., et al.: Ventricular premature beats: screening and induction tests in normal men. Cardiology, *65*:23, 1980.

29. DeBusk, R., et al.: Cardiovascular responses to dynamic and static effort soon after myocardial infarction. Circulation, *58*:368, 1978.

30. DeBusk, R., et al.: Comparison of cardiovascular responses to static-dynamic effort and dynamic effort alone in patients with chronic ischemic heart disease. Circulation, *59*:977, 1979.

31. Deckers, J.W., et al.: A comparison of methods of analyzing exercise test for diagnosis of CAD. Br. Heart J., *62*:428, 1989.

32. Detrano, R., et al.: Factors affecting sensitivity and specificity of a diagnostic test: The exercise thallium scintigram. Am. J. Med., *84*:699, 1988.

33. Detry, J.M.R., et al.: Diagnostic value of computerized exercise testing in men without previous myocardial infarction. A multivariate, compartmental and probabilistic approach. Eur. Heart J., *6*:227, 1985.

34. Dubach, P., et al.: Exercise-induced hypotension in a male population. Criteria, causes, and prognosis. Circulation, *78*:1380, 1988.

35. Ekelund, L.G., et al.: Coronary heart disease morbidity and mortality in hypercholesterolemic men predicted from an exercise test: The Lipid Research Clinics Coronary Primary Prevention Trial. J. Am. Coll. Cardiol., *14*:556, 1989.

36. Elisberg, E.I.: Heart rate response to Valsalva maneuver as a test of circulatory integrity. JAMA, *186*:120, 1973.

37. Ellestad, M.H., and Wan, M.K.: Predictive implications of stress testing. Follow-up of 2700 subjects after maximum treadmill stress testing. Circulation, *51*:363, 1975.

38. Eschenbacher, W.L., and Mannina, A.: An algorithm for the interpretation of cardiopulmonary exercise tests. Chest, *97*:263, 1990.

39. Ettinger, P.O., et al.: Arrhythmias and the "holiday heart": alcohol-associated cardiac rhythm disorders. Am. Heart J., *95*:555, 1978.

40. Fardy, P.S., and Hellerstein, H.K.: A comparison of continuous and intermittent progressive multistage exercise testing. Med. Sci. Sports, *10*:7, 1978.

41. Fletcher, G.F., et al.: Exercise testing in patients with musculoskeletal handicaps. Arch. Phys. Med. Rehabil., *69*:123, 1988.

42. Fletcher, G.F., et al.: Exercise Standards. A statement for health professionals from the American Heart Association. Circulation, *82*:2286, 1990.

43. Francis, K.T.: Fitness assessment using step tests. Compr. Ther., *13*:36, 1987.

44. Froelicher, V.F.: The application of electrocardiographic screening and exercise testing to preventive cardiology. Prev. Med., *2*:592, 1973.

45. Froelicher, V.F.: Exercise and the Heart. Clinical Concepts. Chicago, Year Book, 1987.

46. Froelicher, V.F., et al.: A comparison of three maximal treadmill exercise protocols. J. Appl. Physiol., *36*:720, 1974.

47. Froelicher, V.F., et al.: Value of exercise testing for screening asymptomatic men for latent coronary artery disease. Prog. Cardiovasc. Dis., *43*:265, 1976.

48. Froelicher, V.F., and Marcondes, G.: A Manual of Exercise Testing. Chicago, Year Book, 1989.

49. Gerson, M.C., et al.: Exercise-induced U wave inversion as a marker of stenosis of the left anterior descending coronary artery. Circulation, *60*:1014, 1979.

50. Gibbons, L., et al.: The safety of maximal exercise testing. Circulation, *80*:846, 1989.

51. Gibbons, R.J., et al.: Supine exercise electrocardiography compared with exercise radionuclide angiography in noninvasive identification of severe coronary artery disease. Ann. Intern. Med., *112*:743, 1990.

52. Glaser, R.M., et al.: Physiological responses to maximal effort wheelchair and arm crank ergometry. J. Appl. Physiol., *48*:1060, 1980.

53. Goldbarg, A.N., Krone, R.J., and Resneko, L.: Effects of cigarette smoking on hemodynamics at rest and during exercise. I. Normal subjects. Chest, *60*:531, 1971.

54. Goldschlager, N., Cohn, K., and Goldschlager, A.: Exercise-related ventricular arrhythmias. Mod. Concepts Cardiovasc. Dis., *48*:67, 1979.

55. Gutman, R.A., et al.: Delay of ST depression after maximal exercise by walking for two minutes. Circulation, *42*:229, 1970.

56. Haissly, J., et al.: Comparative response to isometric (static) and dynamic exercise tests in coronary disease. Am. J. Cardiol., *33*:791, 1974.

57. Harrison, M.H., et al.: A comparison of some indirect methods for predicting maximal oxygen uptake. Aviat. Space Environ. Med., *51*:1128, 1980.

58. Hlatky, M.A., et al.: A brief self-administered questionnaire to determine functional capacity (The Duke Activity Status Index). Am. J. Cardiol., *64*:651, 1989.

24

59. Hollenberg, M., et al.: Comparison of a quantitative treadmill exercise score with standard electrocardiographic criteria in screening asymptomatic young men for coronary artery disease. N. Engl. J. Med., 313:600, 1985.

60. Hull, D.H., et al.: Borderline hypertension versus normotension: differential response to orthostatic stress. Am. Heart J., 94:414, 1977.

61. Irving, J.B., and Bruce, R.A.: Exertional hypotension and postexertional ventricular fibrillation in stress testing. Am. J. Cardiol., 39:849, 1977.

62. Judson, W.E., Harcher, J.D., and Wilkins, R.W.: Blood pressure responses to the Valsalva maneuver in cardiac patients with and without congestive failure. Circulation, 11:889, 1955.

63. Kerber, R.E., Miller, R.A., and Najjar, S.M.: Myocardial ischemic effects of isometric, dynamic and combined exercise in coronary artery disease. Chest, 67:388, 1975.

64. Kilbom, A., and Brundin, T.: Circulatory effects of isometric muscle contractions, performed separately and in combination with dynamic exercise. Eur. J. Appl. Physiol. 36:7, 1976.

65. Kligfield, P., et al.: Heart rate adjustment of ST segment depression for improved detection of coronary artery disease. Circulation, 79:245, 1989.

66. Koppes, G., et al.: Treadmill exercise testing. Curr. Prob. Cardiol., 7:1, 1977.

67. Lachterman, B., et al.: "Recovery only" ST segment depression and the predictive accuracy of the exercise test. Ann. Intern. Med., 112:11, 1990.

68. Lachterman, B., et al.: Comparison of the ST segment/heart rate index to standard ST criteria for analysis of exercise electrocardiogram. Circulation, 82:44, 1990.

69. Larson, L.A. (ed.): International Committee for the Standardization of Physical Fitness Tests: Fitness, Health, and Work Capacity. New York, Macmillan, 1974.

70. Lazarus, B., Cullinane, E., and Thompson, P.D.: Comparison of the results and reproducibility of arm and leg exercise tests in men with angina pectoris. Am. J. Cardiol., 47:1075, 1981.

71. Lear, J.L.: Effect of exercise position during stress testing on cardiac and pulmonary thallium kinetics and accuracy in evaluation of coronary artery disease. J. Nucl. Med., 27:788, 1986.

72. Levin, A.B.: A simple test of cardiac function based upon the heart rate changes induced by the Valsalva maneuver. Am. J. Cardiol., 18:90, 1966.

73. Lind, A.R., and McNicol, G.W.: Circulatory responses to sustained hand-grip contractions performed during other exercise, both rhythmic and static. J. Physiol., 192:595, 1967.

74. Lind, A.R., et al.: The circulatory effects of sustained voluntary muscle contraction. Clin. Sci., 27:229, 1964.

75. Lollgen, H., et al.: Recommendations and Standard Guidelines for Exercise Testing: a report of the Task Force Conference on Ergometry. Eur. Heart J., 9(Suppl.):3, 1988.

76. Louhevaara, V., Ilmarinen, J., and Oja, P.: Comparison of the Åstrand nomogram and the WHO extrapolation methods for estimating maximal oxygen uptake. Scand. J. Sports Sci., 2:21, 1980.

77. Mark, D.B., et al.: Exercise treadmill score for predicting prognosis in coronary artery disease. Ann. Intern. Med., 106:793, 1987.

78. Mark, D.B., et al.: Painless exercise ST deviation on the treadmill: long-term prognosis. J. Am. Coll. Cardiol., 14:885, 1989.

79. Marley, W.P., and Linnerud, A.C.: A three-year study of the Åstrand-Ryhming step test. Res. Q., 47:211, 1976.

80. McNeer, J.F., et al.: The role of the exercise test in the evaluation of patients for ischemic heart disease. Circulation, 57:64, 1977.

81. Michelsen, S.: Reproducibility of cumulative work, heart rate and blood pressure response during stepwise versus continuous load increment during a maximal bicycle ergometer test. Scand. J. Clin. Lab. Invest., 50:409, 1990.

82. Miranda, C., et al.: Comparison of angina without ST-depression versus ST-depression without angina during exercise testing. J. Am. Coll. Cardiol., 15:81A, 1990.

83. Mitchell, J.H., and Wildenthal, K.: Static (isometric) exercise and the heart: physiological and clinical considerations. Annu. Rev. Med., 25:369, 1974.

84. Mitchell, J.H., et al.: The role of muscle mass in the cardiovascular response to static contractions. J. Physiol. (Lond.), 309:45, 1980.

85. Morise, A.P., and Duval, R.D.: Comparison of three Bayesian methods to estimate post-test probability in patients undergoing exercise stress testing. Am. J. Cardiol., 64:1117, 1989.

86. Morris, S.N., and McHenry, P.L.: The incidence and significance of decreases in systolic blood pressure during graded treadmill exercise testing. Am. J. Cardiol., 41:221, 1978.

87. Myers, C.R., Golding, L.A., and Sinning, W. (eds): Y's Way to Physical Fitness. Chicago, IL, National Council of YMCA, 1973.

88. Myers, J., et al.: Can maximal cardiopulmonary capacity be recognized by a plateau of oxygen uptake? Chest, 96:1312, 1989.

89. Myers, J., and Froelicher, V.F.: Optimizing the exercise test for pharmacological investigations. Circulation, 82:1839, 1990.

90. Myles, W.S., Brown, T.E., and Pope, J.I.: A reassessment of a running test as a measure of cardiorespiratory fitness. Ergonomics, 23:543, 1980.

91. Nagle, F.J., Balke, B., and Naughton, J.P.: Gradational step tests for assessing work capacity. J. Appl. Physiol., 20:745, 1965.

92. Niederberger, M., et al.: Disparities in ventilatory and circulatory responses to bicycle and treadmill exercise. Br. Heart J., 36:377, 1974.

93. Noakes, T.D.: Implications of exercise testing for prediction of athletic performance: a contemporary perspective. Med. Sci. Sports Exer., 20:319, 1988.

94. Owens, G.R., et al.: Comparison of arm and leg ergometry in patients with moderate chronic obstructive lung disease. Thorax, 43:911, 1988.

95. Pandolf, K.B., et al.: Hyperthermia: effect on exercise prescription. Arch. Phys. Med. Rehabil., 56:524, 1975.

96. Pina, I.L., and Karalis, D.G.: Comparison of four exercise protocols using anaerobic threshold

25

measurement of functional capacity in congestive heart failure. Am. J. Cardiol., 65:1269, 1990.

97. Rabinowitz, B.D., et al.: Acute hemodynamic effects of cigarette smoking in man assessed by systolic time intervals and echocardiography. Circulation, 60:752, 1979.

98. Ragg, K.E., et al.: Errors in predicting functional capacity from a treadmill exercise stress test. Am. Heart J., 100:581, 1980.

99. Rautaharju, P.M., et al.: The effect of modified limb electrode positions on electrocardiographic waveform amplitudes. J. Electrocardiol., 13:109, 1980.

100. Riff, D., and Carleton, R.: Effect of exercise on the atrial recovery wave. Am. Heart J., 82:759, 1971.

101. Robertson, D., et al.: Effects of caffeine on plasma renin activity, catecholamines and blood pressure. N. Engl. J. Med., 298:181, 1978.

102. Rozanski, A., and Berman, D.S.: The efficacy of cardiovascular nuclear medicine exercise studies. Semin. Nuclear Med., 14:104, 1987.

103. Saltin, B., and Rowell, L.B.: Functional adaptations to physical activity and inactivity. Fed. Proc., 39:1506, 1980.

104. Sawka, M.N.: Upper body exercise: physiology and practical considerations. Med. Sci. Sports Exer., 21:S119, 1989.

105. Schaaning, J.: Value of simple parameters during exercise in chronic obstructive lung disease. Bull. Eur. Physiopathol. Respir., 13:441, 1977.

106. Schwade, J., Blomqvist, C.G., and Shapiro, W.: A comparison of the response to arm and leg work in patients with ischemic heart disease. Am. Heart J., 94:203, 1977.

107. Shaw, D.J., et al.: Arm-crank ergometry: a new method for the evaluation of coronary artery disease. Am. J. Cardiol., 33:801, 1974.

108. Sheffield, L.T.: Key references: clinical exercise stress testing. Circulation, 61:1053, 1980.

109. Sheikh, K.H., et al.: Relation of quantitative coronary lesion measurements to the development of exercise-induced ischemia assessed by exercise echocardiography. J. Am. Coll. Cardiol., 15:1043, 1990.

110. Shephard, R.J.: Current status of the Canadian Home Fitness Test. S. Afr. J. Sports Sci., 2:19, 1979.

111. Shephard, R.J.: A critique: coronary disease and exercise stress tests. Can. Fam. Physician, 26:555, 1980.

112. Shephard, R.J., and Kavanagh, T.: On the stage duration for a progressive exercise test protocol. In Physical Fitness Assessment. Principles, Practice and Application. Edited by R.J. Shephard, and H. Lavallée. Springfield, Charles C Thomas, 1978.

113. Shephard, R.J., et al.: The maximum oxygen intake. Bull. WHO, 38:757, 1968.

114. Simoons, M.L.: Optimal measurements for detection of coronary artery disease by exercise ECG. Comput. Biomed. Res., 10:483, 1977.

115. Simoons, M.L., Brand, M., and Hugenholtz, P.G.: Quantitative analysis of exercise ECGs and left ventricular angiograms in patients with abnormal QRS complexes at rest. Circulation, 55:55, 1977.

116. Sivarajan, E.S., et al.: Progressive ambulation and treadmill testing of patients with acute myocardial infarction during hospitalization: a feasibility study. Arch. Phys. Med. Rehabil., 58:241, 1977.

117. Sox, H.C., et al.: The role of exercise testing in screening for coronary artery disease. Ann. Intern. Med., 110:456, 1989.

118. Stamford, B.A.: Step increment versus constant load tests for determination of maximal oxygen uptake. Eur. J. Appl. Physiol., 35:89, 1976.

119. Stuart, R.J., and Ellestad, M.H.: National survey of exercise stress testing facilities. Chest, 77:94, 1980.

120. Subcommittee on Exercise Testing. Guidelines for Exercise Testing. A report of the American College of Cardiology/American Heart Association Task Force on Assessment of Cardiovascular Procedures. J. Am. Coll. Cardiol., 8:725, 1986.

121. Sweet, R.L., and Sheffield, L.T.: Myocardial infarction after exercise-induced ECG changes in patients with variant angina pectoris. Am. J. Cardiol., 33:813, 1974.

122. Taggart, P., Parkinson, P., and Carruthers, M.: Cardiac responses to thermal, physical, and emotional stress. Br. Med. J., 3:71, 1972.

123. Taylor, H.L., Buskirk, E., and Henschel, A.: Maximal oxygen intake as an objective measure of cardio-respiratory performance. J. Appl. Physiol., 8:73, 1955.

124. Taylor, H.L., et al.: The standardization and interpretation of submaximal and maximal tests of working capacity. Pediatrics II (Suppl.): 703, 1963.

125. Taylor, H.L., et al.: Exercise tests: a summary of procedures and concepts of stress testing for cardiovascular diagnosis and function testing. In Measurement in Exercise Electrocardiography. Edited by H. Blackburn. Springfield, Charles C Thomas, 1969.

126. Thompson, P.D., and Keleman, M.H.: Hypotension accompanying the onset of exertional angina. Circulation, 52:28, 1975.

127. Tonino, R.P., and Driscoll, P.A.: Reliability of maximal and submaximal parameters of treadmill testing for the measurement of physical training in older persons. J. Gerontol., 43:M101, 1988.

128. Wasserman, K.: Measures of functional capacity in patients with heart failure. Circulation, 81(Suppl. II):ii–1, 1990.

129. Wasserman, K., and Whipp, B.J.: Exercise physiology in health and disease. Am. Rev. Respir. Dis., 112:219, 1975.

130. Watanabe, K., Bhargave, M., and Froelicher, V.: Computer analysis of the exercise ECG: a review. Prog. Cardiovasc. Dis., 22:423, 1980.

131. Webb, W.R., and Degerli, I.U.: Ethyl alcohol and the cardiovascular system. JAMA, 191:1055, 1965.

132. Weber, K.T., and Janicki, J.S.: Cardiopulmonary Exercise Testing: Physiologic Principles and Clinical Application. Philadelphia, Saunders, 1986.

133. Weiner, D.A., et al.: Correlations among history of angina, ST-segment response and prevalence of coronary-artery disease in the coronary ar-

tery surgery study (CASS). N. Engl. J. Med., *301*:230, 1979.

134. Wetherbee, J.N., et al.: Comparison of ST segment depression in upright treadmill and supine bicycle exercise testing. J. Am. Coll. Cardiol., *11*:330, 1988.

135. White, N.J.: Heart-rate changes on standing in elderly patients with orthostatic hypotension. Clin. Sci., *58*:411, 1980.

136. Wicks, J.R., et al.: Comparison of the electrocardiographic changes induced by maximum exercise testing with treadmill and cycle ergometer. Circulation, *57*:1066, 1978.

137. Wigton, R.S., et al.: Procedural skills of the general internist: a survey of 2500 physicians. Ann. Intern. Med., *111*:1023, 1990.

138. Wolthuis, R., Froelicher, V., and Fischer, J.: A new practical clinical treadmill protocol. Am. J. Cardiol., *39*:697, 1977.

139. Wolthuis, R.A., et al.: The response of healthy men to treadmill exercise. Circulation, *54*:209, 1976.

140. Wolthuis, R.A., et al.: Normal electrocardiographic waveform characteristics during treadmill exercise testing. Circulation, *60*:1028, 1979.

141. Zema, M.J., et al.: Left ventricular dysfunction—bedside Valsalva manoeuvre. Br. Heart J., *44*:560, 1980.

2
CHAPTER

General Principles of Exercise Prescription

by
James S. Skinner

According to the American College of Sports Medicine, "exercise prescription is the process whereby a person's recommended regimen of physical activity is designed in a systematic and individualized manner."[1] This chapter will attempt to outline some of the knowledge required and the basic components of good programs, as well as general principles and factors to consider when prescribing exercise.

GENERAL KNOWLEDGE

Physicians and exercise leaders find variations in motivation, attitude, and responses to exercise in any group of people they encounter and advise; these variations may be due to such factors as age, health status, social class, and previous experience. Therefore, physicians and allied health professionals need to be knowledgeable about many factors and the potential of each for modifying an exercise prescription. Some of the more important factors are subsequently discussed.

Exercise Physiology

A good understanding of exercise physiology is necessary for prescribing individualized exercise programs. This knowledge includes such factors as steady-state, efficiency, sources of energy, and mechanisms of energy production; differences and similarities between kilocalories and METs; and the relationship between work performed and oxygen intake ($\dot{V}_{O_2}$) or heart rate (HR). The person prescribing

exercise should also know how prescriptions can be affected by specific characteristics of an activity, i.e., whether it is static or dynamic, brief or prolonged, intermittent or continuous, and whether it is done with the arms or legs or while supine, sitting, or standing. It is assumed that the reader has this knowledge, as it is the basis for another important aspect in exercise prescription—the measurement and quantification of exercise.

Effects of Age, Gender, and Environment

Each of these factors, discussed in more detail in subsequent chapters, can modify the selection and performance of activities. Physiologic (functional) age is more important than chronologic age in the type of activity chosen, but age is a risk factor in itself and must be considered. Physiologically, there is little difference in the mechanisms used by men and women to respond to exercise or to adapt to training. Any differences are more likely to be quantitative (partly related to body size). There will also be differences in the types of activities selected. Because environment (heat, cold, and altitude) can affect the capacity to perform exercise, it can also modify an exercise prescription.

Knowledge About Health and Fitness

HEALTH STATUS. Exercise may be contraindicated for some people who have certain diseases or medical conditions. For more detailed information related to persons to be tested and the tests to be performed, the reader is referred to other chapters in this book and to publications by the American College of Sports Medicine and the American Heart Association.[1-4] If there is any doubt about a person's health status, a comprehensive medical examination should be performed, especially for those individuals who plan to increase their activity level significantly. Musculoskeletal status is as important as cardiovascular-respiratory health; orthopedic problems are common in adults and are a major reason for patients dropping out in the initial stages of an exercise program. A person's health status also influences the frequency, intensity, duration, type, and progression of exercise.

FITNESS PROFILE. After a medical examination has been performed for those persons at possible risk, a comprehensive fitness profile can be given. This profile could include such variables as body composition, physical working capacity, responses to a series of submaximal work loads, flexibility, strength and muscle endurance, as well as information on each person's needs, interests, and objectives. As will be detailed later, persons who are more active and fitter tend to be able to exercise more often, at higher intensities, and for longer durations (i.e., they do more total exercise), and will probably progress more rapidly.

The evaluations of health and fitness and subsequent consultations can be useful for teaching people about the benefits and risks of exercise and for motivating them to begin or to continue exercising. Specific and reasonable goals can then be given to each individual. Information regarding a person's health status and his/her responses to exercise forms the basis for prescribing an exercise program that will be safe and effective. Another important factor, enjoyment, can be promoted by understanding the needs, interests, and goals of the individual. Thus, a comprehensive approach is needed to promote regular and continued participation in safe, effective, and enjoyable programs.

NEED FOR EXERCISE PRESCRIPTION

Once a person's functional capacity, medical status, and interests are known, individualized exercise prescriptions can be given. The physician or exercise leader should define the major purposes of the exercise program and plan accordingly. Because the reasons for exercising can vary greatly, however, the need for precision in exercise testing and prescribing exercise will also vary.

As suggested by Balke, only two categories of people need careful and precise prescriptions: athletes and those who have a disease that adversely affects their ability to exercise (e.g., coronary heart disease or emphysema).[5] Figure 2–1 is a schematic representation of the need for precision in prescribing exercise for different types of people according to their reasons for exercising.

Although health, fun, and fitness may come about as a result of intense training, the primary goal of most athletes is to improve performance. The exercise leader is more involved than the physician with this type of person. The exercise leader should determine the specific characteristics of the activity in which the athlete competes, decide on the relative importance of pertinent physiologic factors, and design a detailed program geared specifically to develop those factors in particular athletes so that they can perform as closely as possible to their genetic potential.

At the other end of the fitness continuum, disease-limited persons are probably most interested in improving their health. Fun and fitness are generally secondary; performance, per se, is unimportant. The physician is more involved with these persons because of the medical nature of their problems and because they need guidance on how to improve their functional reserves and possibly to counteract further degeneration. As well, medication can affect responses to exercise and training. Not only do patients need precise prescriptions to know the types of exercises to be emphasized and avoided, they may

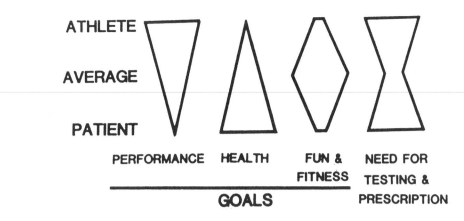

ATHLETE

AVERAGE

PATIENT

PERFORMANCE   HEALTH   FUN &   NEED FOR
                              FITNESS   TESTING &
GOALS   PRESCRIPTION

Fig. 2-1. *The goals and need for precise exercise testing and exercise prescription in different types of people.*

have to exercise under varying degrees of supervision.

It appears that persons of below-average health and fitness are often the ones who 1) need exercise most, 2) do less, 3) are less motivated to exercise, 4) have more problems and limitations when they do exercise, 5) need more guidance, and 6) have been studied less.[18]

Between these two extremes are the "average" persons. Fun and fitness are generally the main reasons why they exercise, although performance, health, and appearance may be important considerations. Often, the health status of this group is not known, i.e., they may not have signs or symptoms and may not know or recognize any limitations. Only when average persons migrate to either end of the continuum do they need more assistance. In other words, the more risk factors these apparently healthy adults have, the longer and the more sedentary they have been, or the more they wish to compete, the more important is their need for exercise testing and precise prescriptions. If it is assumed that these individuals are healthy, however, precision is rarely needed and general principles of exercise and training are adequate. Most such people select activities that they enjoy or that allow them to have social, recreational, or competitive interaction.

The important point to remember is that the same principles of training apply to everyone. Modifications are usually as-

sociated with the absence or presence of medical restrictions or contraindications, types of activities to be emphasized or avoided, the initial level of fitness, the intensity of participation, and the rate of improvement expected.

PRINCIPLES OF TRAINING

It should be emphasized that there is no one program or set of programs that is best for everyone or even for the same person over time as interests, needs, goals, and capabilities change. People also respond differently to exercise and adapt differently to training. Nevertheless, programs can be individualized if the prescriptions are modified using the general principles outlined in this chapter.

It is axiomatic that the body tries to adapt to the habitual demands placed on it. Training is a form of adaptation to the repeated stimulation of exercise. When one has no difficulty adjusting to these demands, adaptation is said to be complete. When the demands placed on the body are too great or are applied too rapidly, too often, or too long, the adaptation will then be incomplete; this partial adjustment usually manifests itself in the form of fatigue, soreness, pain, or injury.

The two major principles of training that apply to all individuals are overload and specificity. Related to overload are the principles of reversibility and maintenance.[17]

31

Overload

If the body is not required to adapt, it will not. For adaptation to occur, the body and its various parts and systems must be stimulated at levels greater than those they habitually encounter. A safe and effective training program is one that progressively overloads the body and allows adequate time for adaptation to each level of stimulation. There is a minimal amount (threshold) of activity that is effective. There is also an upper limit that may require more adaptation than is possible and may be unsafe. The key is to find the upper and lower limits for each individual. As a person adapts to a higher level of activity, these limits also rise.

Specificity

The effects of training are specific to those parts and systems of the body that are overloaded. As an example, weight lifting produces muscle hypertrophy and strength, whereas distance running produces cardiorespiratory endurance but no hypertrophy. Adaptation is specific to the muscle groups that are stimulated (e.g., arms versus legs), as well as to the energy-producing systems that are stimulated (e.g., running sprints, middle distance, or marathons). In other words, the effects of training depend greatly on the activities that are selected. The principle of specificity is probably most important for those persons with specific goals (e.g., to lose weight or to run 10 km), but becomes less important for those who exercise for fun and general fitness.

Reversibility

Because the body adapts to its habitual level of stimulation, the changes brought about by training reverse if the individual becomes more sedentary. In other words, the effects of training are transient and reversible. The opposite of overload, this principle states that the body can also adapt to inactivity.

Maintenance

It takes less time and effort to maintain an improved level of fitness than it does to attain it. Once people adapt to a level of stimulation and there is no overload, further adaptation is not required. If they are satisfied with their current level of fitness, they may be able to maintain it by continuing to do the same amount of training per week and even by slightly reducing their training for brief periods.

BASIC COMPONENTS OF EXERCISE PROGRAMS

The five components of exercise programs are frequency, duration, intensity, type of exercise, and progression. Training is the product of frequency, duration, and intensity of exercise, i.e., the total amount of stimulation or overload. Type of activity is associated with the principle of specificity, as are duration and intensity, because high intensity activities tend to be brief and anaerobic and low intensity activities tend to be prolonged and aerobic.

With all the possible combinations of the first four components, training can be as general or as specific as is desired. The key to a good exercise program is the selection of activities that the individual enjoys and will do often enough, long enough, and at an intensity sufficient to produce a training effect. For the general population, cardiorespiratory endurance is the most important objective of an exercise program, followed by strength, muscular endurance, and flexibility.[16] With the proper selection of activities, all of these objectives can be attained.

Frequency

The inactive person should exercise one to three times per week during the first few weeks to allow adequate time for adaptation. Exercise should not be done on consecutive days because the chances of soreness, fatigue, and possible injury are greatest during the first few weeks of overload. If there are no problems, frequency can be gradually increased to three to four times per week over the next few months. The eventual goal should be three to five times per week, as this frequency is associated with significant gains in fitness and losses in body fat.[2]

32

Frequency may be reduced after reaching the desired fitness level. How much of a reduction depends primarily on the fitness level one wishes to maintain. An athlete who has been training daily may be able to maintain a very high level on four to five times per week, whereas a below average level of fitness may be maintained by exercising one to two times per week. For the general population, it appears that three times per week is optimal. Twice per week is the minimum for maintaining a good level of fitness but only for brief periods (e.g., 2 to 4 weeks) or the fitness level may drop.[1,2]

Duration

Sedentary, asymptomatic and symptomatic persons can tolerate low-intensity exercise for a long duration better than they can high-intensity exercise for brief periods. They are also less likely to have musculoskeletal problems. Therefore, exercise sessions should last 20 to 30 minutes, gradually increasing to 40 to 60 minutes. An optimal program has three phases: warm-up (5 to 10 minutes), overload (15 to 40 minutes), and cool-down (5 to 10 minutes), for a total of 25 to 60 minutes.

The warm-up phase includes walking, slow jogging, stretching exercises, and moderate exercises for muscular strength and endurance. This phase allows the body to increase its metabolism gradually, and to prepare for the more strenuous exercise to follow. The older and the less fit is the individual, the more important is this phase, and the longer it should be.[14,17]

Activities during the overload phase should be at intensities that are safe and effective, i.e., high enough to provide an overload but not so high that they are unsafe or cannot be done for 15 to 20 minutes. Once a person has worked up to it, the minimal duration of the overload phase should be 20 minutes; this amount is especially important in programs designed to increase maximal aerobic power and to control weight.

The cool-down phase should include slow movements, similar to those in the warm-up. Less fit and older persons require more time to recover from exercise. The cool-down time will also be longer if the overload exercises were difficult, were done for a long time, or were done in a hot environment.

Intensity

Exercise intensity is a critical factor in exercise prescriptions and is the most difficult to adjust. Duration and frequency are absolute values that can be the same for persons differing greatly in fitness, whereas intensity is a relative term. The intensity of an activity is the energy required to do that activity relative to the maximal amount of energy that can be provided aerobically; this amount is expressed as a percent of $\dot{V}_{O_2max}$. Therefore, a precise prescription presumes a determination or estimation of a person's $\dot{V}_{O_2max}$, i.e., that an exercise tolerance test has been given. Even without a test, it is possible to give general guidelines.

During the 5 to 15 minutes of the warm-up and cool-down phases, intensity should be 30 to 50% $\dot{V}_{O_2max}$. Because this level of exercise can be done for as many as 8 hours daily, it can be easily done for these brief periods. To overload the cardiorespiratory systems, however, the minimal intensity must be higher.

For sedentary people with low fitness levels, improvements have been obtained with intensities of 50 to 60%.[2] Although there is a suggestion that the threshold intensity for the elderly is about 40% $\dot{V}_{O_2max}$,[7] it seems that 50% is the threshold for most adults and is a good level of intensity during the first weeks of increased activity. If there are no problems, the average intensity during the overload phase can be gradually increased to 60 to 70% and then to 70 to 85%. At intensities greater than 90%, the anaerobic system provides significant amounts of the required energy. The resulting fatigue and lactic acid accumulation reduce exercise duration to less than 15 to 20 minutes. For the general population, the optimal intensity is about 60 to 80%.[2,16,17]

Results from large-scale epidemiologic studies suggest that regular participation in light or moderate exercise reduces the risk of developing coronary heart disease.[15] Similarly, training programs requiring no more than 55% of initial functional capacity have produced significant increases in the $\dot{V}_{O_2max}$ of men whose initial fitness levels were low.[8] Thus, more research is needed to determine threshold levels for stimulating adaptations and for improving health.

Total Amount of Exercise

Training is the product of frequency, duration, and intensity, or the total amount of exercise done. Table 2–1 is an example of how these components might be increased to overload the aerobic system. By gradually increasing one or two components for a 2-week period, a sedentary person can adapt over 3 to 4 months. Depending on how each person reacts and feels, the rate at which the total is increased can be modified. Interestingly, once the frequency, duration, and intensity are above certain levels and the total amount of exercise done per week is similar, the effects of aerobic training are also similar.[2,16] Training programs and sessions within these programs can thus vary widely and apparently still produce similar results.

Type of Exercise

Work is defined as force times distance. For example, if 154 lbs (70 kg) are lifted 33 ft (10 m), $154 \times 33 = 5082$ ft-lbs or 70 $\times$ 10 = 700 kgM of work is done. Power is work done per unit of time, e.g., 700 kgM done in 30 seconds or in 1 minute is 1400 and 700 kgM·min^{-1}, respectively. Given amounts of power require given amounts of energy, although the source of that energy may differ. As an example, 700 kgM·min^{-1} requires 45 to 50% $\dot{V}_{O_2max}$ in an average young man and is primarily aerobic. On the other hand, 1400 kgM·min^{-1} requires 90 to 100% $\dot{V}_{O_2max}$ in the same person, a part of which comes from anaerobic sources.

These facts are important for exercise prescription. The same number of kilocalories are needed to run 10 miles, whether a person runs the 10 miles in 1 day or runs 1 mile per day for 10 days. Speed of running has little effect on total energy expenditure per mile, i.e., the same amount of energy is required to run each mile, even though the intensity or power output will vary with the speed. Thus, the total amount of work done is more important for weight loss, whereas power output is more important for training because it affects the intensity and duration of exercise and the relative stimulation of the aerobic and anaerobic systems.

To overload the aerobic system specifically, it is best to use prolonged, continuous, and moderate intensity activities involving rhythmic contractions of large muscle groups. Strength and speed tend to be anaerobic and are best developed

TABLE 2–1. **Example of Gradually Increasing Overload with Aerobic Training**

	Week Since Onset of Training								
	0	2	4	6	8	10	12	14	16
Frequency (sessions / week)	2	3	3	3	3	4	4	4	4
Duration (min)									
Warm-up	5	5	6	6	7	7	7	8	8
Overload	10	10	15	15	20	20	25	25	30
Cool-down	5	5	5	6	6	7	7	7	7
Total	20	20	26	27	33	34	39	40	45
Intensity (% $\dot{V}_{O_2max}$)	50	55	60	60	65	65	70	70	75

by brief, intermittent, and high intensity activities.

Exercise Progression

The older participants are, the longer they have been sedentary, and the more limitations they have, the slower should be the rate of progression in the total amount of exercise done per week (frequency × duration × intensity). The main goals when beginning an exercise program are to avoid injuries, to allow the participants to tolerate and adapt to each increase in activity, and to make exercise part of their lifestyle. Once participants have adjusted to a regular program (e.g., week 8 in Table 2–1), a good rule of thumb is to increase the total amount of exercise done per week by no more than 10%.

At the onset of an exercise program, it is important for each individual to set a number of realistic goals that can be evaluated periodically. Participants should also be instructed to pay attention to how they are feeling so that they can look for signs and symptoms that suggest that they stop exercising or that another evaluation is needed before they should continue.

REFINEMENTS AND INDIVIDUALIZATION OF EXERCISE PROGRAMS

Level of Fitness

People who are older, less fit, less healthy, and less active generally have more problems when beginning an exercise program. As noted earlier, exercise intensity is usually expressed as a percentage of each person's functional capacity (e.g., % $\dot{V}_{O_2max}$). However, the percentage of $\dot{V}_{O_2max}$ that a given person is able to sustain for a given duration is quite variable and is associated with the level of fitness. For example, well-trained endurance athletes can often exercise at 80 to 90% $\dot{V}_{O_2max}$ for 2 hours, whereas less fit, inactive persons may become fatigued after only 5 to 10 minutes at these same relative intensities. For this reason, Balke suggests a sliding scale for prescribing average training intensities: Average inten-

sity (% $\dot{V}_{O_2max}$) = (60 + $\dot{V}_{O_2max}$ in METs)/100.[5] According to this scale, sedentary persons with a maximum of 10 METs should exercise at (60 + 10)/100 = 70% of their lower capacity or 7 METs, and endurance athletes with a maximum of 20 METs should work at (60 + 20)/100 = 80% or 16 METs. Similar to Balke's sliding scale, another method for estimating exercise intensity and for possibly equating the exercise stimulus among people with different levels of fitness is available. This method uses the concept of the lactate threshold, which is identified by the power output at which ventilation and blood lactate levels rise markedly. This threshold generally occurs from 60 to 90% $\dot{V}_{O_2max}$, with the higher percentages being more prevalent in well-trained endurance athletes. If one assumes that the power output associated with this threshold represents a similar stimulus for change in cellular homeostasis, then exercise requiring the same $\dot{V}_{O_2}$ may produce a different stimulation in people with similar $\dot{V}_{O_2max}$ values but different thresholds.[11] It is obvious that the whole area of what constitutes adequate and equal stimulation needs more research, especially in persons with different levels of fitness.

Although well-trained athletes can and should train regularly at higher percentages of their maximum, high intensity activities are associated with a greater incidence of orthopedic and cardiovascular complications and tend to cause a greater number of dropouts.[2] Therefore, sedentary and less-fit individuals are better off working at low to moderate intensities for longer durations, especially during the initial part of their program.

Controlling Intensity

The intensity of an exercise program should be above the threshold for effectiveness but below some upper value to ensure safety and adequate duration. One way to control intensity is to prescribe exercise on the basis of energy required for an activity. Reasonable estimates of energy cost are available for a whole range of such standardized activities as walking, running, rowing, and cycling, for which the exercise can be done for a long enough period, and at a constant speed to reach a metabolic steady-state.[1,17] When there are changes in wind or water resistance, in the slope or firmness of the terrain, or in mechanical efficiency, these estimates are less accurate. Similarly, accurate estimates are not available for activities that are anaerobic, intermittent, done at variable speeds, or have wide variations in skill and efficiency (e.g., games). In these cases, averages and ranges are usually presented.[1,16,17]

Intensity can also be controlled by the linear relationship between HR and $\dot{V}_{O_2}$ for each individual.[21] If HR and $\dot{V}_{O_2}$ have been measured during a progressively increasing exercise test, participants can estimate their $\dot{V}_{O_2}$ by measuring their steady-state HR. With this method, they can stay within the prescribed range of intensity (e.g., 60 to 80%) by knowing the HRs associated with this range. When HR and $\dot{V}_{O_2}$ have not been measured, participants can measure their HR after 4 to 5 minutes of walking or running at constant speeds or doing any standardized activity in which $\dot{V}_{O_2}$ can be estimated with reasonable accuracy.

Even if exercise testing has not been performed, a fair estimate of intensity can be made by using a percentage of the maximal HR reserve:[10,17]

$$\text{Intensity (\% } \dot{V}_{O_2\text{max}})$$
$$= \frac{(\text{Exercise HR} - \text{resting HR})}{(\text{Maximal HR} - \text{resting HR})}$$

As an example, for a person with a maximal HR of 200 and a resting HR of 80, exercise requiring a HR of 164 represents an intensity of $(164 - 80)/(200 - 80) = 84/120 = 0.70$ or 70%. Whereas resting HR is easy to obtain, most people have little idea of their maximal HR unless they have been tested to maximum or have pushed themselves to exhaustion and measured their HR. As a rule of thumb, maximal HR decreases 1 beat·min^{-1} each year after age 20 to 25 years, and can be esti-

mated by subtracting present age from 220. Thus, the average 40-year-old individual has a maximal HR of $220 - 40 = 180$. This estimate may not be accurate, however, because maximal HR varies by about 10%, i.e., although the average for a 40-year-old person is 180, values may vary from 160 to 200 beats·min^{-1}. As with any estimate, one should obtain accurate measurements taken under standardized conditions and realize their limitations.

Another method to determine the training HR range is to take a fixed percentage of the estimated or determined maximal HR. For comparative purposes, it has been shown that 60 to 80% $\dot{V}_{O_2\text{max}}$ corresponds to approximately 60 to 80% of the HR reserve and 70 to 85% of the maximal HR.[1]

If a given HR is associated with a given intensity for each person, exercise HR is a useful and convenient way to control intensity. For example, HR at a given power output usually drops with aerobic conditioning. Because relatively minor changes occur in maximal and resting HRs with training, it appears that $\dot{V}_{O_2\text{max}}$ has risen and that the power output represents a lower relative intensity. The power output should then be raised to reach the desired HR and intensity. With increasing altitude or temperature, HR will increase at a given level of exercise. Using the same training HR range as a guide, a person will be able to do less exercise but will still be at the same relative stress. Similarly, if people stop training due to such factors as lack of interest, injury, or job pressures, they will use a lower power output to exercise at the same HR and relative intensity when they resume exercise.

Ratings of Perceived Exertion

Even though such objective physiologic indices as HR and $\dot{V}_{O_2}$ change minimally from day to day during standard exercise, subjective feelings of psychologic strain may vary and should also be considered. Borg developed a scale for rating perceived exertion (RPE) associated with a given amount of exercise.[6] This RPE scale can be helpful in exercise prescription when ratings are obtained with HR and

$\dot{V}_{O_2}$ during exercise testing or with HR during standardized exercise tasks for which the energy costs are known. Once people perceive the effort associated with various exercise intensities, they may have a better understanding of how hard they should exercise. After training regularly at a prescribed intensity, the subjective feelings can then be transferred to other activities, e.g., it can be used to estimate fatigue and the varying intensities associated with games or other non-steady state activities.[6,12,16]

Exercise intensity can be controlled reasonably well throughout an exercise session without having to stop, just on the basis of subjective RPEs.[6,16] Using Borg's 15-point scale, RPEs of 12 to 13 (somewhat hard) and 16 (hard) correspond to 60% and 85% of the HR reserve, respectively.[1] The respective ratings on the Borg 10-point scale are 4 and 6.

Periodic Evaluation

Periodic testing is useful to assess the effectiveness of an exercise program, to modify an exercise prescription, and to motivate those persons who have improved. There is a small percentage of the population that may not respond appropriately to exercise, however. A trained exercise leader may observe small signs and symptoms (changes in fatigue, gait, or comments) that suggest the need for re-evaluation, resulting in a modified prescription and, in a few cases, termination of the exercise program. All exercise staff should be aware of these signs and symptoms.

How often people should be re-evaluated depends on their need for a precise prescription. As shown in Figure 2–1, athletes and patients may need to be evaluated more often than the average person. As the needs, interests, and goals of these three groups change, however, so might the need for evaluation. For example, the average person who becomes interested in running a marathon or who develops chest pain should be evaluated more than the average person who continues to exercise for fun and general fitness. Likewise,

patients who improve their health status or athletes who stop or reduce training may need less evaluation than was required previously.

OTHER CONSIDERATIONS

Problems Associated With Overuse

Many problems associated with exercise programs arise from overuse or overtraining, i.e., overstimulation from exercise that is more intense, more frequent, or longer than the demands to which the body has adapted. The signs and symptoms of this inadequate adaptation are fatigue, soreness, pain, and injury.

FATIGUE. Fatigue is a general feeling of weariness that can produce performance decrements due to slower reaction and movement times and reduced levels of speed, agility, strength, and neuromuscular coordination. Thus, people who are tired are more prone to injury. Because the amount of fatigue and its onset are related to the relative intensity of exercise, proper training can reduce the chance of injury by increasing a person's maximum. Some fatigue is normal after exercise, especially during the first few weeks of increased activity. If fatigue persists, the individual should stop exercising for several days or exercise at a lower intensity or duration until the body has recovered.

SORENESS. Soreness is a dull ache that comes on gradually due to overuse. General soreness lasts 4 to 8 hours, followed by localized, specific soreness that may last for several days. The degree of overuse and the resulting soreness is associated with a person's present level of adaptation. Thus, people who are older, less fit, less healthy, and who have been sedentary longer tend to have more soreness after exercise.

The type and amount of exercise is also a contributing factor, i.e., too much of the same or different type of exercise can cause overstrain and soreness. As a general rule, one should continue to exercise with lighter work loads, change the type of exercise for a few days, or both to reduce the soreness. It should be remembered, however, to start at a lower intensity and duration to avoid soreness in the new muscle groups.

PAIN. Pain is a localized, sharp feeling of discomfort that usually comes on rapidly. If pain develops, one should stop immediately and attempt to determine whether it is due to muscle, joint, or cardiovascular problems. It is neither necessary nor advisable to continue with pain. Although "no pain, no gain" may be an acceptable motto for an elite athlete committed to excellence who is willing to put forth the time and effort needed to attain it, the same principle is not valid for the average person or patient.

INJURY. The severity of an injury is associated with the past history of injury, the type and speed of the movement causing the injury, and the present level of fitness and habitual activity. The risk of injury is usually greatest during the first few months of exercise or any time there are abrupt increases in the total amount of exercise done.[2] First, beginning exercisers are often overweight and unfit, such that the low maximum and excess weight increase the relative intensity of exercise. Second, beginners often have inadequate levels of strength, endurance, and flexibility, making them more prone to injury. Third, many beginners do not know what exercises to do or how to do them; this fact emphasizes the need for and importance of individualized exercise prescriptions as well as qualified people to lead exercise programs.

Exercising Alone or With Others

Exercise is a social activity for many people. Belonging to a group may fill a strong social need and is an excellent way to receive the positive reinforcement that is so critical in the initial stages of increased exercise. Qualified instructors can lead, educate, and motivate individuals to ensure that the appropriate exercises are done properly to avoid problems of overuse and to improve the chances of progress. Another advantage of group programs is that there is usually a fixed

routine that may help some people make exercise a regular part of their lifestyle.

There are, however, some disadvantages to group exercise. Some people prefer to exercise alone, may have difficulty with regular schedules, or may not know what to do when they are away from the group. If a group program attempts to have one program for persons with varying degrees of fitness and ability, the intensity is not optimal for all participants. As a result, the rate of progress also varies. Individualized exercise prescriptions, flexibility within the programs, and qualified leadership can avoid some of these problems.

One compromise that has been found useful, easier to schedule, and more individualized is to exercise with one or two other persons. This approach works best when the members of the group have similar interests and fitness levels.

Degree of Supervision

Whether supervision is required or suggested depends mainly on the degree of risk associated with exercise. The important thing is to provide effective and enjoyable programs that are also safe but not too restrictive in terms of the participants' work schedules or economic situations.[1] Those individuals who have a functional capacity of less than 8 METs, who are known to be at high risk for coronary heart disease, or who have cardiovascular disease (regardless of their functional capacity) should exercise in a group under the supervision of a qualified leader (see Chapter 17).[1]

Qualified and creative instructors can make the program more diversified, more individualized, more interesting, and safer by demonstrating appropriate exercises and their proper sequences. Instructors can provide a degree of health surveillance, can monitor changes in intensity and duration of exercise, and can educate the group so that its members know what to do, how to do it, and why.[13,19,20] As an example, the group can be taught how to measure HR and then can be informed that their highest training HR during non-supervised exercise should not be greater than the mean HR attained during supervised exercise.[1] Another advantage of supervised exercise programs is that people with similar medical problems or risks can help each other understand and cope with the restrictions imposed by their medical condition.

Starting versus Continuing an Exercise Program

Most people drop out of exercise programs in the first few months. Although the highest incidence of injuries also occurs at this time, it is not the only or major factor. Factors that influence an individual to begin exercising are usually quite different from those associated with continuing an exercise plan.[9] In oversimplified terms, many people begin because of other persons, e.g., their appearance, it is the "in" thing to do, or to improve their health when others (physician, family, or friends) think it is the best thing to do. These people continue to exercise, however, because of themselves and how they perceive that the program helps them, e.g., the program has an effective leader who makes the activities enjoyable, they feel better, and they can see improvements.

There are so many reasons why people decide to start or to continue to exercise that health professionals should not try to impose their own reasons; people should be allowed to decide what is important in their particular case. As well, participants should set short-term, realistic goals to increase the chances of having many small successes that will motivate them to continue. Periodic evaluations also can be used to monitor progress and to motivate continued participation.

At the onset of training, games and sports are not the ideal choice for those individuals who are older and less fit, because these activities tend to be more intermittent and less well controlled. People should train to play a sport and not use sports as the main way to train. Sports and games are better used during the maintenance phase when the fitness level is adequate and when enjoyment is more important to continued participation.

Successful exercise programs are based on sound exercise prescription and qualified leadership. This statement implies that there is communication and cooperation among exercisers, physicians, and exercise leaders so that the exercisers are taught what to do and why and are then motivated to follow through on their own initiative. The best activities during any phase of a program are those that are safe, effective, and enjoyable. If the frequency, duration, and intensity of exercise are adequate to stimulate adaptation but are not so high as to cause incomplete adaptation or be unsafe, then it makes little difference which activities are selected. Once these conditions are met, a more important factor is whether the activity is fun so that it will be continued. In other words, programs can and should vary, because there is no one program that is correct for all or even for the same person over time as interests, needs, goals, health, or fitness change.

REFERENCES

1. American College of Sports Medicine: Guidelines for Graded Exercise Testing and Exercise Prescription. 4th Ed. Philadelphia, Lea & Febiger, 1991.
2. American College of Sports Medicine: Position statement on the recommended quantity and quality of exercise for developing and maintaining cardiorespiratory and muscular fitness in healthy adults. Med. Sci. Sports Exerc., 22:265–274, 1990.
3. American College of Sports Medicine: Position statement on proper and improper weight loss programs. Med. Sci. Sports Exerc., 15:ix, 1983.
4. American Heart Association: Exercise Testing and Training of Individuals with Heart Disease or at High Risk for its Development: A Handbook for Physicians. New York, American Heart Association, 1975.
5. Balke, B.: Prescribing physical activity. In Sports Medicine. Edited by A. Ryan, and F. Allman. New York, Academic Press, 1974.
6. Borg, G.: Psychophysical bases of perceived exertion. Med. Sci. Sports Exerc., 14:377, 1982.
7. DeVries, H.: Physiology of physical conditioning for the elderly. In Guide to Fitness After Fifty. Edited by R. Harris, and L. Frankel. New York, Plenum Press, 1977.
8. Gossard, D., Haskell, W., Taylor, C., et al.: Effects of low- and high-intensity home-based exercise training on functional capacity in healthy middle-aged men. Am. J. Cardiol., 57:446, 1986.

9. Heinzelmann, F.: Social and psychological factors that influence the effectiveness of exercise programs. *In* Exercise Testing and Exercise Training in Coronary Heart Disease. Edited by J. Naughton, and H. Hellerstein. New York, Academic Press, 1973.

10. Karvonen, M., Kentala, K., and Musta, O.: The effects of training on heart rate: a longitudinal study. Ann. Med. Exp. Biol. Fenn., *35*:307, 1957.

11. McLellan, T., and Skinner, J.: Submaximal endurance performance related to the ventilatory thresholds. Can. J. Appl. Sport Sci., *10*:81, 1985.

12. Noble, B.: Clinical applications of perceived exertion. Med. Sci. Sports Exerc., *14*:406, 1982.

13. Oldridge, N.: What to look for in an exercise class leader. Physician Sportsmed., *5*:85, 1977.

14. Oldridge, N., Wicks, J., and McIntosh, J.: Exercise in coronary rehabilitation: prescription and program design (part II). Physiother. Can., *30*:69, 1978.

15. Paffenbarger, R., Hyde, R., Wing, A., and Hsieh, C.: Physical activity, all-cause mortality, and longevity of college alumni. N. Engl. J. Med., *314*:605, 1986.

16. Pollock, M., Wilmore, J., and Fox, S.: Exercise in Health and Disease. Philadelphia, W.B. Saunders, 1984.

17. Skinner, J.: Body Energy. Mountain View, CA, Anderson World, 1981.

18. Skinner, J.: Exercise research on persons of below-average health and fitness: a commentary. *In* Future Directions in Exercise and Sport Science Research. Edited by J. Skinner, C. Corbin, D. Landers, P. Martin, and C. Wells. Champaign, Human Kinetics, 1986.

19. Stoedefalke, K.: The principles of conducting exercise programs. *In* Exercise Testing and Exercise Training in Coronary Heart Disease. Edited by J. Naughton, and H. Hellerstein. New York, Academic Press, 1973.

20. Wilmore, J.: Individual exercise prescription. Am. J. Cardiol., *33*:757, 1974.

21. Wilmore, J., and Haskell, W.: Use of the heart rate-energy expenditure relationship in the individual prescription of exercise. Am. J. Clin. Nutr., *24*:1186, 1971.

3
CHAPTER

Importance of Differences Between Men and Women for Exercise Testing and Exercise Prescription

by

Jack H. Wilmore

The decade of the 1970s and the first half of the 1980s produced considerable interest in the physical abilities and limitations of women, both in the work place and in the athletic arena. In the United States, passage of the Civil Rights Act of 1964 prohibited job discrimination on the basis of sex. The Women's Equal Rights Amendment of 1972, although never ratified, increased the awareness of women's rights under the law. Finally, the passage in 1972 of the U.S. Education Amendment (Title IX) forbade sex discrimination in any institution receiving federal funds. The first two legislative acts opened many employment opportunities for women that were previously unavailable. Women are now found in such occupations as commercial airline pilots, law enforcement officers, telephone linemen, construction workers, and heavy equipment operators, and hold combat assignments in the military. The U.S. Education Amendment (Title IX) has also had a major impact on athletic programs in public and private schools at all grade levels. In the past, when compared to programs for boys and men, girls and women were denied the opportunity for quality athletic experiences. Title IX accomplished much in a relatively short period of time, equalizing athletic opportunities for the sexes.

The sudden changes brought about by this federal legislation have created considerable confusion and many questions. Are girls and women physically capable of assuming these new roles as they take advantage of these new opportunities? Can girls and women physically cope with the rigors of high level athletic competition? Can girls and women obtain the traditional benefits of exercise and sport that boys and men have enjoyed for centuries? Finally, can girls and women be trained for sport or conditioned for fitness by using a format identical to that for boys and men, or are there special considerations that dictate a unique training or conditioning format? The intent of this chapter is to probe the similarities and differences between the genders relative to their physique and body composition, as well as their physiologic responses to acute exercise and physiologic adaptations to chronic exercise, so to determine how these differences and similarities influence exercise testing and exercise prescription.

PHYSIQUE AND BODY COMPOSITION

From the data of McCammon, which summarizes the Child Research Council's

This chapter was adapted from Wilmore, J.H., and Costill, D.L.: Training for Sport and Activity. Dubuque, IA, Wm. C. Brown, 3rd Ed., 1988, with permission of the publisher.

longitudinal growth study in Denver, it appears that differences in height, weight, circumferences, diameters, and skinfold thicknesses between the genders do not appear until the age of 12 to 14 years, i.e., approximately at the time of puberty.[20] Before puberty, there is a striking similarity between boys and girls of the same socioeconomic background for all indices of size and maturity. Forbes estimated lean body mass (LBM) from [40]K assessment in 609 normal boys and girls 7.5 to 20.5 years of age and found no sex differences prior to adolescence in LBM expressed per unit of height.[14] At 12 to 13 years of age, the LBM to height ratio began to plateau in girls, but continued to increase in boys until the age of 20 years. The LBM tended to peak in males at 18 to 20 years of age and was approximately 1.4 times greater than the peak value attained by females at 15 to 16 years of age. Body density data from hydrostatic weighings are somewhat inconsistent with the preceding data, as girls typically demonstrate lower body density values at all ages, including the preadolescent period. Lohman has shown that lower body density values in girls do not indicate a higher relative body fat.[19] Somatotype data are generally lacking for the preadolescent ages. The limited data that have been published indicate a similarity in somatotype between the genders at age 12 years, with girls exhibiting a slightly higher degree of endomorphy and a lesser degree of ectomorphy.

At puberty, rather major differences in body composition begin to develop between the genders, due largely to the associated endocrine changes. Testosterone secretion by the testes, which stops at birth, is reinstituted in the male at puberty, producing an increased deposition of protein in muscle, bone, skin, and other parts of the body. The ultimate result is the male adolescent being larger and more muscular than the female adolescent, characteristics that carry over into adulthood. Before puberty, the anterior pituitary gland is unable to secrete any gonadotrophic hormones. Thus, in girls, at the time when a sufficient quantity of follicle-stimulating hormone

begins to be secreted, the ovaries develop and estrogen secretion begins. Estrogen has a significant influence on body growth, broadening the pelvis, increasing the size of the breasts, and proliferating the deposition of fat, particularly in the thighs and hips. Additionally, estrogen increases the growth rate of bone, allowing the ultimate bone length to be reached within 2 or 4 years after the onset of puberty. As a result, the female adolescent grows rapidly for the first few years after puberty and then ceases to grow. Boys have a much longer growth phase, allowing a greater height to be attained. As a result of these endocrine changes at puberty, the male at full maturity is nearly 13 cm (5 in.) taller, 14 to 18 kg (30 to 40 lbs) heavier in total weight, 18 to 22 kg (40 to 50 lbs) heavier in LBM, 3 to 6 kg (7 to 13 lbs) lighter in fat weight, and 8 to 10 percentage units less in relative body fat, i.e., 15 versus 23 to 25% fat. With respect to somatotype at the age of 17 years, the female adolescent exhibits a substantially greater degree of endomorphy, whereas the male adolescent has a greater degree of mesomorphy and ectomorphy.

There are rather substantial gender differences in anthropometric measurements at maturity, as illustrated in Table 3–1. These data were synthesized from the studies of Wilmore and Behnke and Pollock et al. for young men and women.[24,25,39,40] Men have broader shoulders, narrower hips, and a greater chest girth relative to total body size. Men also tend to carry body fat in the abdominal and upper regions of the body, whereas women pattern their fat in the hips, buttocks, and thighs.

With aging, both men and women tend to accumulate fat and decrease LBM. In one of the few longitudinal studies conducted, Forbes found an average decrease in LBM of approximately 3 kg per decade or more than 0.6 lb per year.[15] These data confirm previous cross-sectional data indicating a loss in LBM of 0.3 to 0.5 lb per year. This decline is associated with lower levels of physical activity and testosterone. Apparently, the concomitant increase in total body fat with aging is also associated

TABLE 3–1. **Anthropometric Measurements for Young and Middle-aged Men and Women**

	Men			Women		
	Young		Middle-aged	Young		Middle-aged
	Wilmore (n = 133)	Pollock (n = 95)	Pollock (n = 84)	Wilmore (n = 128)	Pollock (n = 83)	Pollock (n = 60)
Skinfolds (mm)						
Scapula	14.1	13.9	20.2	13.2	15.3	17.3
Triceps	7.9	13.6	18.5	12.8	18.8	22.2
Mid-axillary	11.7	15.5	24.8	10.7	13.3	16.9
Chest	–	11.4	20.6	–	14.0	14.0
Suprailiac	19.3	15.2	22.0	17.2	15.3	17.3
Abdominal	16.0	20.6	30.0	15.1	22.8	29.6
Thigh	14.9	17.4	22.2	31.8	28.8	33.1
Knee	5.3	–	–	7.0	17.4	17.3
Circumferences (cm)						
Head	57.5	–	–	55.0	–	–
Neck	38.5	–	–	31.8	–	–
Shoulders	117.0	112.5	114.8	101.9	99.7	100.9
Chest	97.4	91.4	96.3	85.2	84.6	87.1
Bust	–	–	–	87.8	87.7	90.8
Abdomen	84.0	81.0	91.1	75.3	75.0	82.7
Hips	96.9	94.4	98.4	95.9	93.1	97.5
Thigh	58.0	57.1	59.0	57.0	56.5	57.6
Knee	37.7	–	–	36.1	–	–
Calf	37.6	36.5	36.9	35.1	33.9	34.4
Ankle	22.7	22.1	22.1	21.1	20.8	20.8
Deltoid	36.3	–	–	30.7	–	–
Biceps, flexed	33.2	32.6	34.0	27.2	27.0	28.6
Biceps, extended	29.1	–	–	25.0	–	–
Forearm	27.6	28.3	29.2	23.5	23.8	24.4
Wrist	17.0	16.7	17.4	14.9	14.8	15.1
Diameters (cm)						
Head length	19.9	–	–	19.0	–	–
Head width	15.5	–	–	14.9	–	–
Biacromial	40.4	41.1	41.5	36.5	36.8	36.7
Bideltoid	47.6	46.9	47.4	42.1	41.4	41.8
Chest	29.3	31.8	33.0	25.8	27.8	28.6
Bi-iliac	28.4	29.6	31.4	28.4	29.9	31.2
Bitrochanteric	32.9	33.6	35.1	32.1	34.0	35.3
Knee	9.5	9.8	10.1	8.9	9.3	9.6
Ankle	7.1	–	–	6.3	–	–
Elbow	7.0	–	–	6.0	–	–
Wrist	5.6	5.9	6.0	4.9	5.1	5.2
Arm span	181.7	–	–	165.8	–	–
Foot length	26.7	–	–	24.1	–	–
Hand length	19.1	–	–	17.3	–	–

with the general decline in physical activity, without an equivalent decrease in caloric intake. Table 3–2 outlines the changes in relative body fat with aging for both genders.

The aforementioned normative data can be misleading. As an example, the average difference in relative body fat between young men and women of 18 to 24 years of age is 6 to 10 percentage units,

TABLE 3–2. **Relative Body Fat Values for Men and Women of Various Ages and in Various Sports***

Group	% Relative Fat	
	Men	Women
General population by age (yrs)		
15–19	13–16	20–24
20–29	15–20	22–25
30–39	18–26	24–30
40–49	23–29	27–33
50–59	26–33	30–36
60–69	29–33	30–36
Athletic population		
Baseball/softball	8–15	12–18
Basketball	6–13	16–22
Canoeing	10–14	–
Football	8–18	–
Gymnastics	5–9	8–12
Ice hockey	10–15	–
Jockeys	8–12	12–16
Skiing	8–14	10–16
Ski jumping	12–16	–
Soccer	7–12	–
Speed skating	8–12	14–18
Swimming	5–12	10–16
Tennis	8–12	14–18
Track and field		
Track	5–12	8–14
Field	14–20	16–24
Volleyball	8–12	14–20
Weight lifting	8–18	–
Wrestling	5–10	–

* Adapted from Wilmore, J.H., and Costill, D.L.: Training for Sport and Activity. 3rd Ed. Dubuque, IA, Wm. C. Brown, 1988.

i.e., 13 to 16% for men versus 20 to 25% for women. At first, this difference was thought to be the result of gender-specific differences in fat depots, e.g., breast tissue and hips. Subsequent research with female athletes, however, particularly women distance runners, indicated that these women were exceptionally lean, well below the average woman, and even below the average for young men. Many of the better runners were below 10% body fat. These low values can be the result of either a genetic predisposition toward leanness or the high training mileage run by these women each week, which in some cases exceeded 100 miles per week. In any event, it is obvious that women can reduce their fat stores to levels well below those considered normal for women of this age.

Differences between the genders have also been noted for body fluids. In the newborn, total body water (TBW), expressed as a percentage of total body weight, is approximately 77%, with the extracellular water (ECW) and intracellular water (ICW) contributing 44 and 33%, respectively. By 1 year of age, the infant has achieved the adult fraction of TBW (58 to 64%), composed of approximately 25% ECW and 36% ICW. Gender differences are evident by the age of 18 years, with the TBW of girls dropping to approximately 47 to 54% of total body weight. This difference comes almost totally from the ICW, which is only 23 to 29%. It is quite possible that the decreases in TBW and ICW are due to the increased levels of body fat, because adipose tissue contains only a small fraction of water and because both TBW and ICW are expressed relative to total body weight. Fluid levels are also altered considerably consequent to menstruation. Weight gains of 4 to 8 lb caused by fluid retention are common.

PHYSIOLOGIC RESPONSES TO ACUTE EXERCISE

When male and female subjects are exposed to an acute bout of exercise, whether it be an all-out run to exhaustion on the treadmill or a one time attempt to lift the heaviest weight possible, there are characteristic responses that differentiate the sexes.

Neuromuscular Responses

Females have typically been regarded as the weaker sex. In previous studies, female subjects have been found to be 43 to 63% weaker than their male counterparts in upper body strength, but only 25 to 30% weaker in lower body strength. Because there is a considerable size difference between the sexes, as noted in the previous section, several studies have expressed strength relative to body weight (absolute strength / body weight) or relative to LBM as a reflection of the muscle mass (absolute strength / LBM). When lower body strength is expressed relative to body weight, there is still a 5 to 15% difference between the sexes. When expressed relative to LBM, however, the difference between the sexes disappears, which indicates that the histologic and biochemical qualities of muscle and its motor control properties are similar for the two sexes. Although the differences in upper body strength are reduced somewhat when expressed relative to TBW and LBM, substantial differences remain. There are at least two possible explanations for the different findings in upper and lower body strength. First, a woman has a higher percentage of her LBM in the lower body. Second, and probably related, she uses the muscle mass in her lower body to a greater extent than she uses her upper body muscle mass, particularly when compared to patterns of use in men. Some women of normal body size have phenom-enal strength, exceeding even that of the average man. This fact points to the importance of neuromuscular recruitment and synchronization of motor unit firing in determining ultimate levels of strength.

Recently, there has been a great deal of interest in muscle fiber typing. In the 1960s, researchers started using the muscle biopsy technique to investigate several aspects of muscle physiology. Through various staining techniques, it was possible to identify the different muscle fiber types, which led to an interest in how athletes might differ in various sports. Over the years, biopsies have become more common among female athletes. This has led to a natural interest in the differences and similarities between male and female athletes participating in the same sport or event. The classification system most commonly used identifies three basic fiber types: slow-twitch oxidative (Type I), fast-twitch oxidative (Type II_a), and fast-twitch glycolytic (Type II_b). A Type II_c fiber has also been identified but is not considered in this discussion. Athletes who participate in events or activities requiring a high degree of aerobic activity (e.g., distance runners and cross-country skiers) have a high proportion of Type I fibers (typically 70% or higher). Those athletes who participate in speed or anaerobic-type activities (e.g., sprinters) have a predominance of Type II fibers (again, usually 70% or higher). Interestingly, weight event athletes have nearly an equal distribution of Type I and Type II fibers, even though these sports are generally considered to be short-burst, power activities. Male and female athletes in the same sport or event have similar distributions of fiber types, although the men appear to reach greater extremes (i.e., > 90% type I or > 90% Type II), as well as to have larger fiber areas.[37]

Cardiovascular Responses

When placed on a cycle ergometer, for which the power output can be precisely controlled independent of body weight, men generally have a lower heart rate (HR) response at each absolute level of submaximal exercise. Maximal heart rate

(HR max), however, does not appear to be different for men and women. Because cardiac output ($\dot{Q}$) is nearly identical for the same absolute submaximal power output for the two genders, the lower HR response in men is associated with a higher stroke volume (SV). The enhanced SV is primarily the result of at least three factors. First, a man has a larger heart and therefore a larger left ventricle, both advantages of a larger body size. Second, and also related to body size, he has a greater blood volume. Finally, the average man is typically less sedentary and will therefore exhibit the classic alterations (to be discussed in the next section) that are associated with physical training. When the power output is controlled to provide the same relative level of exercise, usually expressed as a fixed percentage of the maximal oxygen uptake ($\dot{V}_{O_2max}$), the HR of the female exerciser is still elevated when compared to that of the male. At 50% $\dot{V}_{O_2max}$, $\dot{Q}$, SV, and $\dot{V}_{O_2}$ are generally less and the HR is slightly higher in women.

In one of the first studies designed to investigate the response of $\dot{Q}$ to exercise in boys and girls, Bar-Or et al. exercised 29 girls and 27 boys, ranging in age from 10 to 13 years, at levels that varied from 40 to 70% of their respective $\dot{V}_{O_2max}$ values.[3] For a given submaximal $\dot{V}_{O_2}$, the girls had a higher $\dot{Q}$, a higher HR, and a lower arteriovenous oxygen difference (AVD-O_2). Stroke volume (SV) was higher in the boys at the low work loads, but was the same as that of the girls at the higher work loads. Becklake et al. measured $\dot{Q}$ in men and women, ranging in age from 20 to 85 years at three different power outputs on the cycle ergometer.[4] From the age of 20 to 39 years, $\dot{Q}$, HR, and SV were higher, and the AVD-O_2 was lower in the women at identical power outputs. For those 40 years of age or older, the women had higher HR, similar $\dot{Q}$, and lower SV. Miyamura and Honda conducted a study of maximal $\dot{Q}$ responses to exercise in 233 male subjects (9 to 53 years of age) and in 102 female subjects (9 to 20 years of age).[21] Whereas $\dot{Q}_{max}$ was similar for boys and girls up to the age of 15 years, by 18 years,

the boys achieved values that were approximately 30% higher than those of the girls.

As stated previously, the differences in SV response to exercise between the sexes are primarily the result of differences in heart size, blood volume, and level of physical conditioning. In addition, the differences noted in AVD-O_2 are considered to be the result of a lower hemoglobin content in girls and women, resulting in a lower arterial oxygen content. This fact is an important consideration when discussing differences in values of $\dot{V}_{O_2max}$ in male and female subjects.

Respiratory Responses

The differences between the genders in the respiratory responses to exercise are largely the result of differences in body size. There appears to be little difference in breathing frequency when working at the same relative power output, although the female tends to breathe at a higher frequency at the same absolute power output. This latter response is probably due to the fact that she is working at a higher percentage of her $\dot{V}_{O_2max}$. Tidal volume and ventilation volume are generally smaller in the female at both the same relative and absolute power outputs, up to and including maximal levels. Highly trained male athletes have maximal ventilation volumes of 150 L·min^{-1} and higher (some exceeding 250 L·min^{-1}); most female athletes have maximal values below 125 L·min.$^{-1}$. Again, these differences in volume are closely associated with differences in body size.

Metabolic Responses

The $\dot{V}_{O_2max}$ is regarded by most exercise scientists as the single best index of an individual's cardiorespiratory endurance capacity. For this reason, numerous studies have been conducted to compare $\dot{V}_{O_2max}$ values of male and female subjects, both untrained and trained. Åstrand conducted the first study and compared a large population of males and females, from 4 years of age up to adulthood.[1] Subsequently, additional data have been published confirming the original work of Åstrand and adding considerably to the data pool.

Before puberty, there are no significant differences in $\dot{V}_{O_2max}$ for boys and girls when expressed relative to body weight, i.e., $ml \cdot kg^{-1} \cdot min^{-1}$. Girls tend to reach their peak $\dot{V}_{O_2max}$ between the ages of 13 and 15 years, whereas boys do not reach their peak until 18 to 22 years of age. Beyond puberty, the $\dot{V}_{O_2max}$ of women is only 70 to 85% of that found in normal untrained men.[32]

Differences in $\dot{V}_{O_2max}$ between the genders must be interpreted carefully. In 1965, Hermansen and Andersen published data indicating that there is considerable variability within each gender and that there is considerable overlapping of values between sexes.[17] Taking a group of men and women, 20 to 30 years of age, they compared the physiologic responses to submaximal and maximal exercise of four subgroups: male athletes, male non-athletes, female athletes, and female non-athletes. First, for the same absolute level of work, they found that there was a tendency for athletes to have slightly higher $\dot{V}_{O_2}$ values at submaximal levels and for men to have slightly higher values than women. With respect to $\dot{V}_{O_2max}$ expressed relative to body weight, average values for the male athletes were 61% higher than those of male non-athletes, whereas those of the female athletes were 45% higher than those of female non-athletes. Values of male athletes were 29% higher than those of the female athletes, but the mean $\dot{V}_{O_2max}$ of female athletes was 25% higher than the mean value for the male non-athletes. From this study, Drinkwater calculated that 76% of the female non-athletes overlapped 47% of the male non-athletes, and that 22% of the female athletes overlapped 7% of the male athletes.[9] These data demonstrate the importance of considering both the level of physical conditioning in the sample and of looking beyond mean values to the extent of overlapping between samples that are being compared.

Because $\dot{V}_{O_2}$ is the product of $\dot{Q}$ and AVD-O_2, $\dot{V}_{O_2max}$ represents that point during exhaustive exercise at which the subject has maximized oxygen delivery and utilization capabilities. Typical values range from less than 20 $ml \cdot kg^{-1} \cdot min^{-1}$ in deconditioned, aging individuals to values in excess of 85 $ml \cdot kg^{-1} \cdot min^{-1}$ in superbly conditioned, endurance athletes. The highest recorded value (94 $ml \cdot kg^{-1} \cdot min^{-1}$) for a man was found in a champion Norwegian cross-country skier; the highest recorded value for a woman was 77 $ml \cdot kg^{-1} \cdot min^{-1}$ for a Russian cross-country skier.

In 1984, Drinkwater conducted an extensive review of the existing research literature relative to $\dot{V}_{O_2max}$ values for female subjects of varying age and athletic ability.[10] Although $\dot{V}_{O_2max}$ values of boys and girls are similar until puberty, there is a question as to the validity of the values when comparing male and female subjects beyond the age of 12 years. The data might reflect an unfair comparison of relatively sedentary females with relatively more active male subjects. Thus, the differences would reflect the level of conditioning, as well as possible gender differences. To overcome this potential problem, investigators began to look at highly trained male and female athletes, with the assumption that the level of training would be similar for the sexes. Saltin and Åstrand compared $\dot{V}_{O_2max}$ values of male and female athletes who participated on Swedish national teams.[29] In comparable events, the men had 15 to 30% higher values. Wilmore and Brown, in their study of 11 women long-distance runners of national and international caliber, found $\dot{V}_{O_2max}$ values (mean = 59.1 $ml \cdot kg^{-1} \cdot min^{-1}$) that were considerably higher than those of the average woman or man of similar age.[41] Still, when compared to equally trained male distance runners, the women had values 15.9% lower when expressed relative to body weight and 8.6% lower when expressed relative to LBM. The three best runners from this study had an average value of 67.4 $ml \cdot kg^{-1} \cdot min^{-1}$, which is similar to the average value of 70.3 $ml \cdot kg^{-1} \cdot min^{-1}$ reported for nationally ranked marathon runners of similar age. Table 3–3 details $\dot{V}_{O_2max}$ values for

TABLE 3-3. $\dot{V}_{O_2max}$ Values for Male and Female Populations of Different Ages and in Various Sports*

Group	$\dot{V}_{O_2max}$ (ml·kg⁻¹·min⁻¹)	
	Males	Females
General population by age (yrs)†		
10–14	47–51	47–51
15–19	49–56	44–52
20–29	43–52	37–46
30–39	39–48	33–42
40–49	36–44	30–38
50–59	34–41	28–35
60 and above	31–38	25–32
Athletic population		
Baseball/softball	48–54	40–46
Basketball	44–50	40–46
Bicycling, competitive	65–72	48–56
Canoeing	60–68	54–60
Football	48–54	–
Gymnastics	50–58	46–52
Ice hockey	52–60	–
Jockey	52–60	46–52
Orienteering	48–58	–
Skiing, cross-country	66–80	58–70
Ski jumping	66–72	–
Soccer	54–62	–
Speed skating	58–74	48–56
Swimming	56–70	48–64
Track and field		
Track	60–80	50–70
Field	46–54	40–50
Volleyball	50–60	46–56
Weight lifting	40–50	–
Wrestling	54–65	–

* Adapted from Wilmore, J.H., and Costill, D.L.: Training for Sport and Activity. 3rd Ed. Dubuque, IA, Wm. C. Brown, 1988.
† Data are desirable values rather than population norms.

male and female athletes of different ages and in different sports.

A number of investigators have attempted to scale $\dot{V}_{O_2max}$ values relative to height, weight, LBM, or limb volume in an attempt to compare these values in men and women more objectively. Several studies have yielded results that show differences between the genders disappear when $\dot{V}_{O_2max}$ is expressed relative to fat-free body weight (LBM) or active muscle mass, but there are also studies that continue to demonstrate differences, even when one accounts for differences in body fat. A study by Cureton and Sparling involved the use of a novel approach to in-

vestigate this problem.[7] They studied the submaximal and maximal responses to treadmill runs under various conditions in 10 male and 10 female adults who regularly engaged in distance running. The men were studied at normal weight and under an artificial condition in which they had to run with external weight added to the trunk so that the total percent of excess weight was equal to the percent fat of matched females. The women exercised only under normal weight conditions. Equating the genders for excess weight resulted in a reduction of 32% in the original mean sex differences in treadmill run time, of 38% in the oxygen required per unit fat-free weight to run at various submaximal speeds, and of 65% in $\dot{V}_{O_2max}$. Cureton and Sparling concluded that the greater amount of sex-specific, essential body fat stores of women is a major determinant of the sex differences in the metabolic responses to running.[7] Finally, Davies found that when the $\dot{V}_{O_2max}$ of 116 boys and girls was expressed relative to body weight or to LBM, definite gender differences were observed.[8] When expressed relative to the volume of the leg, however, these differences disappeared. Davies concluded that $\dot{V}_{O_2max}$ is directly related to the volume or mass of active tissue involved in the exercise.

With respect to submaximal $\dot{V}_{O_2}$ values, there appears to be little, if any, difference between the genders for the same absolute power output. Bunc and Heller found no significant differences in the net energy cost of treadmill running of similarly trained men and women athletes representing various sports.[5] It should be remembered, however, that at the same absolute submaximal load, women usually work at a higher percentage of their $\dot{V}_{O_2max}$. As a result, blood lactate levels are higher and the anaerobic or lactate threshold occurs at a lower absolute power output. Peak blood lactate values are generally higher in men, but there is a paucity of data for female athletes who would be more inclined to exert themselves to higher values. There is no obvious reason to expect differences between the sexes in peak blood lactate values. With respect to anaerobic or lactate threshold, there are only limited data available on female athletes. It would appear, however, that anaerobic or lactate threshold values would be similar between equally trained male and female subjects, providing the values were expressed in relative and not absolute terms. Anaerobic or lactate threshold appears to be more related to the mode of testing and to the state of training of the individual. Thus, gender differences would not be expected. There are also limited data available for equally trained men and women with respect to anaerobic power tests, such as the Wingate test, mak-

ing gender comparisons at this time meaningless. With untrained subjects, gender differences in anaerobic power appear to reflect differences in muscular strength and power,[22] which were previously discussed.

With the increase in popularity of distance running in the United States during the 1970s and 1980s, an interesting theory was proposed that implied women were natural distance runners due to their inherently better ability to utilize fat as the energy substrate for endurance activity. Further, it was stated that with proper training, women might be even better distance runners than men because of their unique ability to mobilize and utilize free fatty acids, thus sparing glycogen. Costill et al. put this theory to the test in 1979.[6] These investigators took muscle biopsies from the gastrocnemius muscle of 13 male and 12 female distance runners matched for $\dot{V}_{O_2max}$ and training mileage. Although male and female runners had similar fiber types, male runners exhibited significantly greater activity of the muscle enzyme succinate dehydrogenase and carnitine palmitoyl transferase. They also found that male and female runners derive similar fractions of their energy from lipids during treadmill running at 70% $\dot{V}_{O_2max}$.

PHYSIOLOGIC ADAPTATIONS TO CHRONIC EXERCISE

With physical training, there are substantial alterations in basic physiologic function, both at rest and during exercise. This section is a discussion of how girls and women adapt to chronic exercise, emphasizing those areas in which their responses might be different from those of boys and men.

Body Composition, Bone, and Connective Tissue

With exercise training, emphasizing either cardiorespiratory endurance activities or strength training, all individuals experience losses in total body weight, fat weight, and relative fat, in addition to small to moderate gains in LBM.[38] The gains in LBM are generally less for female participants. The magnitude of change in body composition, with the exception of LBM, appears to be more related to the total energy expenditure associated with training activities, rather than to gender. Increases in LBM are of much greater magnitude in response to strength training when compared to endurance training, but again, the changes in females are generally small when compared to those seen in males.

Alterations in bone and connective tissue with training are not well understood. In general, results of studies with animals and limited studies with humans support an increase in the density of the weight-bearing long bones; this adaptation appears to be independent of gender, at least in young and middle-aged populations. There are exceptions to this conclusion, which are discussed in detail in the last section of this chapter. Connective tissue appears to be strengthened with endurance training; gender-specific differences in response have not been identified. There has been some concern that female subjects are more susceptible to injury while participating in physical activity and sport. This susceptibility has been largely attributed to gender-specific differences in joint integrity, as well as to the strength of ligaments, tendons, and bones. Unfortunately, few published reports serve to confirm or deny the validity of such concerns. When differences in the rate of injury have been observed, it is highly possible that the injury was related more to the level of conditioning than to the gender of the participant. Objective data are difficult to obtain, but this area is nevertheless an important one that needs to be better defined.

Neuromuscular Adaptations

For a number of years, it was not considered appropriate to prescribe strength training programs for female athletes. During the 1960s and 1970s, it became evident that many of the better female athletes in the United States were not doing well in international competition and that this was mainly due to the fact that they were weaker than their competitors. Slowly, research demonstrated that considerable benefit could be gained from strength training programs, and that strength gains were usually not accompanied by large increases in muscle bulk. One study compared the training response of 47 women and 26 men who volunteered to participate in identical progressive-resistance, weight-training programs.[35] The program was conducted two times per week, 40 minutes per day, for a total of 10 weeks. Bench press and leg press strength increased by 28.6 and 29.5%, respectively, in the women and increased 16.5 and 26.0%, respectively, in the men. There were only small increases in muscle girth in the female subjects, whereas the men exhibited classic muscle hypertrophy. Thus, it is apparent that hypertrophy is neither a necessary consequence nor a prerequisite of gains in muscular strength. Several studies have confirmed these results.

From the aforementioned results, it appears that women have the potential to develop substantially higher levels of strength than those normally identified in the average, typically sedentary female. Will women ever be able to attain the same levels of strength as men for all major regions of the body? From the similarity of leg strength to weight ratios between the two sexes, it appears that the quality of muscle is the same, irrespective of gender. Because of the higher levels of testosterone in men, however, they will continue to have a larger total muscle mass. If muscle mass is the major determinant of strength, then men have a distinct advantage. If neural factors are as important, or even more important, than size, then the potential for absolute strength gains in girls and women is considerable. Because the basic mechanisms that allow the expression of greater levels of strength have not yet been clearly resolved, it is premature to draw conclusions.

Cardiovascular and Respiratory Adaptations

Rather major cardiovascular and respiratory adaptations accompany cardiorespiratory endurance training; these adaptations do not appear to be gender-specific. In a review article, Saltin and Rowell describe the classic cardiovascular, respiratory, and metabolic adaptations to physical activity and inactivity.[30] With training, there are major increases in maximal $\dot{Q}$. Because HR_{max} does not change with training, this increase in $\dot{Q}_{max}$ is the result of a large increase in SV, which is the result of both a greater end-diastolic volume and a reduced end-systolic volume. The former is related to an increased blood volume and a more efficient venous return, and the latter is the result of a stronger myocardium, i.e., a stronger contraction and a reduction in peripheral resistance. At submaximal levels of work, there is minimal or no change in $\dot{Q}$, although SV is considerably higher for the same absolute level of work. Consequently, HR for any given level of work is reduced. Resting HR can be reduced to 50 beats·min^{-1} or less. Several female distance runners have had a resting HR below 36 beats·min^{-1}.[41] This rate reduction is considered a classic training response and corresponds to an exceptionally high SV.

The increases in $\dot{V}_{O_2max}$ that accompany cardiorespiratory endurance training are discussed subsequently, but they are primarily the result of the large increases in $\dot{Q}_{max}$, with only small increases in AVD-O_2. Saltin and Rowell, however, state that the major limitation to $\dot{V}_{O_2max}$ resides in the transport of oxygen to the working muscles.[30] Whereas $\dot{Q}$ is important in this respect, it is the position of these researchers that the increases in maximal aerobic power that accompany training are attributed primarily to increased maximal muscle blood flow and muscle capillary density. There is no reason to suspect that girls and women would differ in this response to training. In fact, Ingjer and Brodal recently demonstrated that endurance-trained women have considerably higher capillary-to-fiber ratios than do untrained women, i.e., 1.69 and 1.11, respectively.[18]

With respect to respiration, women experience considerable increases in maximal ventilation, which reflect increases in both tidal volume and breathing frequency. These changes are generally assumed to be unrelated to the increase in $\dot{V}_{O_2max}$.

Metabolic Adaptations

With cardiorespiratory endurance training, women experience the same relative increase in $\dot{V}_{O_2max}$ that has been observed in men. The magnitude of increase is highly related to the initial level of fitness, i.e., those with low fitness levels prior to the start of training will generally experience a greater percentage increase. Each person, theoretically, has a genetically established upper limit of $\dot{V}_{O_2max}$ that they cannot exceed, irrespective of the duration or intensity of training. Consequently, the closer one is to this upper limit, the more difficult it is to obtain large improvements with subsequent training. Thus, it would be expected that most women would experience rather substantial improvements in $\dot{V}_{O_2max}$ with endurance training, because they have relatively low initial values. On the basis of findings in the research literature, women can improve their $\dot{V}_{O_2max}$ by 10 to 30% with cardiorespiratory endurance training, the magnitude of change being dependent on the initial level of fitness, the intensity and duration of the individual exercise sessions, the frequency of sessions per week, and the length of the study.[10]

Oxygen uptake at the same absolute submaximal work load does not appear to change, although several studies have reported decreases. Blood lactate levels are reduced for the same absolute submaximal work levels and peak lactate levels are generally increased. The anaerobic or lactate threshold in men does increase with training but this increase has not been verified in women. Finally, endurance training also improves the ability to utilize free fatty acids, an adaptation that is important for glycogen sparing.

Therefore, it appears that women respond to physical training in exactly the same manner as their male counterparts. Whereas the adaptations to training may

51

differ somewhat in magnitude (e.g., lean body weight), the trends do appear to be identical. This consideration is extremely important when exercise is to be prescribed to a female population.

SPECIAL CONSIDERATIONS

Although men and women respond to acute exercise and adapt to chronic exercise in much the same manner, there are several areas that must be considered when prescribing exercise to a female population. Although there is a possibility of some overlap with other chapters in this book, replication will be minimized.

Aging

Once full maturity is reached, there is generally a gradual decline in $\dot{V}_{O_2max}$. This fact was first noted in men by Robinson in 1938.[28] I. Åstrand conducted a similar study on women in 1960 and noted the same decline.[2] The decrease with age is linear, and although the slopes detailing this decline are nearly identical for men and women, the intercept for the women's curve is approximately 9 ml·kg^{-1}·min^{-1} lower than that for men.[36] In addition, men and women tend to both increase the amount of total body fat and decrease LBM as they age. Thus, the woman is fatter and has less LBM at any given age. These differences in endurance capacity and body composition definitely influence both exercise testing and exercise prescription.

Are the changes in endurance capacity and body composition a necessary consequence of aging or are other factors involved? With respect to body composition, there is accumulating evidence that the increases in body fat and decreases in LBM are primarily the result of physical inactivity, and overeating to a lesser extent. Likewise, the $\dot{V}_{O_2max}$ of trained individuals is considerably higher than those values for untrained individuals of similar age at all ages. Maintaining an active lifestyle will not, however, prevent the decrease in $\dot{V}_{O_2max}$ with age, for the slope of the regression line is similar for trained and untrained individuals alike. Vaccaro

et al. compared trained and untrained female swimmers from ages 20 to 69 years, and found that although the trained swimmers had a significantly higher $\dot{V}_{O_2max}$, they demonstrated a 7% decrease per decade in $\dot{V}_{O_2max}$.[34] The untrained group demonstrated a similiar 8% decrease per decade. Therefore, maintaining an active lifestyle will promote a healthier and more attractive physique and body composition, and may also allow the individual to have the endurance capacity equal to that of a sedentary person of the same gender who is 30 to 40 years younger.

Osteoporosis

There is evidence that maintaining a healthy lifestyle may also retard one of the detrimental aging processes that is a major health concern of women—osteoporosis. Osteoporosis is characterized as an increase in bone porosity, a decrease in bone mineral content, and an increase in the risk of fractures that typically begins in their late thirties and is accelerated two to five times that rate at the onset of menopause. Although there is still a good deal to discover concerning the etiology of osteoporosis, three major contributing factors in post-menopausal women appear to be an overall reduction in calcium intake, an estrogen deficiency, and a reduction in physical activity.

In addition to post-menopausal women, women with amenorrhea and those with anorexia also suffer from osteoporosis, the results of either decreased calcium intake or a reduction in serum estrogen levels, or possibly both. Rigotti et al. assessed the skeletal mass of 18 women who were known anorexics and 28 normal controls by direct photon absorptiometry, and found that the patients with anorexia had significantly reduced bone densities when compared to the control subjects.[27] Drinkwater et al. compared radial and vertebral bone densities of 14 athletic amenorrheic women to 14 athletic eumenorrheic women and discovered that physical activity did not protect the amenorrheic group from significant bone density losses.[13] When bone density values of the amenorrheic women were compared with the age-related regression equation of Riggs et al.,[26] their values (mean age 24.9 years) were equivalent to those of women of 51.2 years of age. It should also be noted that normally menstruating runners tend to exhibit higher bone mineral content values than those of menstruating control subjects. Drinkwater et al. while finding that reversal of this bone mineral loss in amenorrheic athletes accompanies resumption of normal menses, have now reported that these losses may not be fully recovered, that is, the ability to regain bone mineral may be limited.[11]

As of yet, there do not appear to be enough data to draw any firm conclusions in regard to the effects exercise and amenorrhea may have on osteoporosis. It does seem logical, however, that increased physical activity (and adequate calcium intake combined with an adequate caloric intake) is a sensible approach to maintaining the integrity of the skeletal system at any age.

Menstruation

Two questions foremost in the minds of many women, particularly women athletes, relate to the influence of their menstrual cycle on athletic performance and the influence of their physical activity and competition on menstruation and childbirth. The question of childbirth will be addressed in a later discussion. With respect to alterations in athletic performance during different phases of the menstrual cycle, there appears to be considerable individual variability. Some women have absolutely no noticeable change in their ability to perform at any one time in their monthly cycle, whereas other women have considerable difficulty in the pre-flow and initial flow phases. The limited research that has been conducted tends to suggest that performance ability is best in the immediate post-flow period up to the fifteenth day of the cycle, with the first day of the cycle corresponding to the initiation of the flow or menstrual phase, and ovulation occurring on about day 14. The number of women who report impaired performance during the flow phase is approximately the same as those who experienced no difficulty. In fact, some women athletes have reportedly set world records during the flow phase.

With respect to the question concerning the influence of various training programs and intense competition on the menstrual cycle, existing data are limited. Several long-term studies have been reported that involved former competitive swimmers, with findings to suggest that intense training at an early age has no serious consequences relative to future gynecologic problems. One possible problem has surfaced recently, although it is possibly not a problem but rather is a very natural response of the body. Athletes who have trained and competed intensely in such sports as figure skating, ballet dancing, gymnastics, cycling, and distance running have reported the absence of menses for months or even years. Secondary amenorrhea, as well as oligomenorrhea (abnormally infrequent or scanty menses) among female athletes is not well documented, but its occurrence is estimated to be approximately 20% or higher in certain sports or events, which is considerably higher than the estimated 5% in the general population. The actual percentage of women involved varies according to the sport and to the intensity of training. The occurrence appears to be greater in those women who train for many hours each day and in those women who work at high intensities.

Neither the cause nor the long-term consequences of secondary amenorrhea or oligomenorrhea are known. Some of these women have become pregnant during this phase of amenorrhea, which is indicative of the fact that fertility is possibly not influenced in the absence of menstruation. This latter point is an important one, for many women assume that they have a simple but effective form of birth control while amenorrheic. It is tempting to assume that exercise in itself is responsible for changes in menstrual dysfunction in female athletes, but the cause may be related to low levels of body weight or body fat, to the acute effects of stress, or to changes in the levels of circulating hormones.

It has been known for some time that excessive fatness, undernutrition, or both are associated with amenorrhea. It has been estimated that a loss of one third of an individual's body fat or a 10 to 15% decrease in body weight will induce amenorrhea.[16] The reason for this occurrence is that aromatization of androgens and estrogen takes place in adipose tissue and abdominal fat, and any decrease in adipose tissue influences the storage and metabolism of estrogen. More recently, investigators have challenged the theory that there is a critical body fat level that must be achieved or maintained to assure normal menses.[31]

Although many investigators have reported menstrual irregularities in athletes, it is apparently difficult to separate the effects of exercise per se from the effects of the physical and emotional stresses of training, the stress of excessive weight loss, hormonal alterations associated with exercise training, and a low body fat or low body weight, which have all been associated with menstrual irregularities.[31] Fortunately, athletically induced amenorrhea is reversible, usually occurring during periods of reduced training, injury, or vacation.[33]

Environmental Factors

Exercise in the heat or cold or at altitude provides an additional stress or challenge to the body's adaptive abilities. Results of many early studies indicated that women are less tolerant to heat than men, particularly when physical work is involved. Much of this difference, however, is the result of lower levels of fitness in those women who were tested, because the men and women were tested at the same absolute level of work. When work load is adjusted relative to the individual's capacity ($\dot{V}_{O_2max}$), women respond in an almost identical manner. Women generally have lower sweat rates for the same exercise and heat stress, although they do possess a larger number of active sweat glands.

When exposed to repeated bouts of heat stress, the body undergoes considerable adaptation (acclimatization), which enables it to survive future heat stress more efficiently. Recent evidence suggests that men and women undergo similar reductions in the internal temperature thresholds for sweating and vasodilation and an increase in the sensitivity of the sweating response per unit of internal temperature increase after both physical training and heat acclimation.[23] Any differences noted between the sexes were attributed to the initial differences in physical conditioning and not to gender. With respect to cold exposure, women do have a slight advantage as a result of their higher levels of subcutaneous body fat. Their smaller muscle mass, however, is a disadvantage in exposure to extreme cold, because shivering is the major adaptation for generating body heat. The greater the active muscle mass, the greater will be the subsequent generation of heat. An excellent review on this subject was published in 1984 by Drinkwater.[10]

Several investigators have reported differences between the genders in response to hypoxia, both at rest and during submaximal exercise. Although there is a reported 26.7% decrease in $\dot{V}_{O_2max}$ during hypoxic work, the differences between men and women are small and do not seem to have an adverse effect on the ability of women to work at high altitude.[12] Studies of maximal exercise at high altitude demonstrate no difference in response between the genders.

Exercise Testing and the Prescription of Exercise

In reviewing the acute responses and chronic adaptations to exercise, it is apparent that few differences exist between male and female subjects. Consequently, few adjustments need to be made when testing or prescribing exercise for the female population. The most important point to consider was reviewed in the section on aging. When compared with men of the same age, the average woman is fatter, has less LBM, and has a lower endurance capacity. This difference is probably more related to physical inactivity than to gender, although sex differences must still be recognized. When selecting a protocol for exercise testing, women may require a protocol that has a lower ramp, i.e., the step increments should progress more slowly. Also, when using the same test protocol, different regression equations should be applied when test duration is used to estimate $\dot{V}_{O_2max}$. With respect to the interpretation of the exercise electrocardiogram, it is important to recognize that women exhibit a higher percentage of false-positive tests. In several studies, as many as one half (50%) of a sample of asymptomatic women were found to have S-T segment changes indicative of myocardial ischemia.

In the prescription of exercise, it is important to match the intensity of the exercise to the capacity of the individual. When prescreening exercise testing precedes the exercise prescription, it is relatively easy to prescribe intensity on the basis of a training HR that has been determined from the results of the exercise test. When exercise testing is not conducted prior to prescribing exercise, it is best to be conservative in the prescription of exercise intensity. Because women are fatter and have less LBM to support their total body weight, in addition to their lower endurance capacity, they must have their exercise intensity adjusted accordingly. It might also be appropriate to reduce exercise duration and frequency during the first few months, because the exercise program will probably constitute a considerable physical stress, with a potentially greater risk of injury. Consideration should be given to walking or swimming programs, in which the potential for injury is minimized and success is a more likely outcome. Another excellent activity that is popular with women of all ages is aerobic dance. Aerobic dance classes, however, must be graded according to endurance capacity, as well as dancing ability.

It is important not to misconstrue the aforementioned statements to imply that women should be pampered or coddled.

Women who have the same body composition and endurance capacity as men of similar age should be given a similar exercise prescription. The preceding advice simply recognizes that most women are not similar to their male counterparts when they initiate their program, and that these precautions are taken to provide the participant with the best conditions in which to be successful.

REFERENCES

1. Åstrand, P.-O.: Experimental Studies of Physical Working Capacity in Relation to Age and Sex. Copenhagen, Munksgaard, 1952.
2. Åstrand, I.: Aerobic work capacity in men and women with special reference to age. Acta Physiol. Scand. [Suppl.], 49:169, 1960.
3. Bar-Or, O., Shephard, R.J., and Allen, C.L.: Cardiac output of 10- to 13-year-old boys and girls during submaximal exercise. J. Appl. Physiol. 30:219, 1971.
4. Becklake, M.R., et al.: Influence of age and sex on exercise cardiac output. J. Appl. Physiol., 20:938, 1965.
5. Bunc, V., and Heller, J.: Energy cost of running in similarly trained men and women. Eur. J. Appl. Physiol., 59:178, 1989.
6. Costill, D.L., et al.: Lipid metabolism in skeletal muscle of endurance trained males and females. J. Appl. Physiol., 47:787, 1979.
7. Cureton, K.J., and Sparling, P.B.: Distance running performance and metabolic responses to running in men and women with excess weight experimentally equated. Med. Sci. Sports Exerc., 12:288, 1980.
8. Davies, C.T.M.: Body composition in children: a reference standard for maximum aerobic power output on a stationary ergometer. Acta Paediatr. Scand. [Suppl.], 217:136, 1971.
9. Drinkwater, B.L.: Physiological responses of women to exercise. Exerc. Sport Sci. Rev., 1:125, 1973.
10. Drinkwater, B.L.: Women and Exercise: Physiological Aspects. Exerc. Sport Sci. Rev., 12:21, 1984.
11. Drinkwater, B.L., Bruemner, B., and Chesnut, C.H. Menstrual history as a determinant of current bone density in young athletes. JAMA, 263:545, 1990.
12. Drinkwater, B.L., et al.: Response of women mountaineers to maximal exercise during hypoxia. Aviat. Space Environ. Med., 50:657, 1979.
13. Drinkwater, B.L., et al.: Bone mineral content of amenorrheic and eumenorrheic athletes. N. Engl. J. Med., 311:277, 1984.
14. Forbes, G.B.: Relation of lean body mass to height in children and adolescents. Pediatr. Res., 6:32, 1972.
15. Forbes, G.B.: The adult decline in lean body mass. Hum. Biol., 48:161, 1976.
16. Frisch, R.E.: Body fat, puberty, and fertility. Biol. Rev., 59:161, 1984.

17. Hermansen, L., and Andersen, K.L.: Aerobic work capacity in young Norwegian men and women. J. Appl. Physiol., *20*:425, 1965.
18. Ingjer, F., and Brodal, P.: Capillary supply of skeletal muscle fibers in untrained and endurance-trained women. Eur. J. Applied Physiol., *38*:291, 1978.
19. Lohman, T.G.: Applicability of body composition techniques and constants for children and youths. Exerc. Sport Sci. Rev., *14*:325, 1986.
20. McCammon, R.W.: Human Growth and Development. Springfield, IL, Charles C Thomas, 1970.
21. Miyamura, M., and Honda, Y.: Maximum cardiac output related to sex and age. Jpn. J. Physiol., *23*:645, 1975.
22. Murphy, M.M., Patton, J.F., and Frederick, F.A.: Comparative anaerobic power of men and women. Aviat. Space Environ. Med., *57*:636, 1986.
23. Nadel, E.R., Roberts, M.F., and Wemger, C.B.: Thermoregulatory adaptation to heat and exercise: comparative responses of men and women. *In* Environmental Stress. Edited by L.J. Folinsbee, et al. New York, Academic Press, 1978.
24. Pollock, M.L., et al.: Prediction of body density in young and middle-aged men. J. Appl. Physiol., *40*:300, 1976.
25. Pollock, M.L., et al.: Prediction of body density in young and middle-aged women. J. Appl. Physiol., *38*:745, 1975.
26. Riggs, B.L., Wahner, H.W., and Seeman, E.: Changes in bone mineral density of the proximal femur and spine with aging: differences between the postmenopausal and senile osteoporosis syndromes. J. Clin. Invest., *70*:716, 1982.
27. Rigotti, N.A., Nussbaum, S.R., Herzog, D.B., and Neer, R.M.: Osteoporosis in women with anorexia nervosa. N. Engl. J. Med., *311*:1601, 1984.
28. Robinson, S.: Experimental studies of physical fitness in relation to age. Arbeitsphysiol., *10*:251, 1938.
29. Saltin, B., and Åstrand, P.-O.: Maximal oxygen uptake in athletes. J. Appl. Physiol., *23*:353, 1967.
30. Saltin, B., and Rowell, L.B.: Functional adaptations to physical activity and inactivity. Fed. Proc., *39*:1506, 1980.
31. Shangold, M.M.: Exercise and the adult female: hormonal and endocrine effects. Exerc. Sport Sci. Rev., *12*:53, 1984.
32. Shvartz, E., and Reibold, R.C.: Aerobic fitness norms for males and females aged 6 to 75 years: a review. Aviat. Space Environ. Med., *61*:3, 1990.
33. Stager, J.M.: Reversibility of amenorrhea in athletes. Sports Med., *1*:337, 1984.
34. Vaccaro, P., et al.: Body composition and physiological responses of masters female swimmers 20 to 70 years of age. Res. Q., *55*:278, 1984.
35. Wilmore, J.H.: Alterations in strength, body composition, and anthropometric measurements consequent to a 10-week weight training program. Med. Sci. Sports, *6*:133, 1974.
36. Wilmore, J.H.: Inferiority of female athletes: myth and reality. J. Sports Med., *3*:1, 1975.
37. Wilmore, J.H.: The application of science to sport: physiological profiles of male and female athletes. Can. J. Appl. Sport Sci., *4*:103, 1979.
38. Wilmore, J.H.: Body composition in sport and exercise: directions for future research. Med. Sci. Sports Exerc., *15*:21, 1983.
39. Wilmore, J.H., and Behnke, A.R.: An anthropometric estimation of body density and lean body weight in young men. J. Appl. Physiol., *27*:25, 1969.
40. Wilmore, J.H., and Behnke, A.R.: An anthropometric estimation of body density and lean body weight in young women. Am. J. Clin. Nutr., *23*:267, 1970.
41. Wilmore, J.H., and Brown, C.H.: Physiological profiles of women distance runners. Med. Sci. Sports, *6*:178, 1974.

4
CHAPTER

Importance of Differences Between Children and Adults for Exercise Testing and Exercise Prescription

by
Oded Bar-Or

Most knowledge of the physiologic responses of humans to exercise is based on studies with adults. Less data are available on the effects of acute or chronic exercise on children and adolescents. To a certain point, our considerations regarding exercise testing and prescription for children can be borrowed from those available for adults. Yet, there are some specific characteristics of the young individual that require a special approach. In the first place, a child's metabolic, cardiopulmonary, thermoregulatory, and perceptual responses to acute or chronic exercise are somewhat different from those of mature individuals. Secondly, methods and protocols used for testing of adults are not always applicable to children, whether due to differences in size, mental ability, attention span, and emotional maturity, or to ethical constraints. Additional differences are in the clinical context, i.e., the major pediatric diseases are different from those prevalent in young or middle-aged adults. The questions, guidelines, and precautions relevant for exercise testing or rehabilitation of, for example, an adult patient with coronary heart disease are not applicable for most pediatric patients. Inversely, the rationale for exercise provocation in such conditions as congenital heart defects, growth hormone deficiency, bronchial asthma, cystic fibrosis, or progressive muscular dystrophy is of little relevance to adults.

The purpose of this chapter is to highlight the main differences in exercise testing and prescription between children and adults. In spite of a growing number of original publications in the field, little information has been synthesized in review form. Readers interested in testing of children for clinical purposes could consult the book, *Exercise Testing of Children*.[47] *Pediatric Sports Medicine for the Practitioner: From Physiologic Principles to Clinical Application* includes information concerning physiologic characteristics of the exercising child, the uses of exercise in diagnosis and in prescription, the detrimental effects of exercise, and protocols for exercise testing.[11] The chapter "Diagnostic Use of Exercise Testing in Pediatric Cardiology: the Noninvasive Approach" summarizes the rationale and the specific categories of exercise tests in pediatric cardiology.[37] The book *Exercise and Children's Health* provides insight into exercise prescription in various pediatric chronic diseases and strategies for motivating the young sedentary child to become more active.[84]

TYPICAL RESPONSES TO EXERCISE

The basic physiologic responses to a single bout of exercise or to repeated exercise stimuli are similar in people of all ages. There are, however, age- or development-related *quantitative differences* in the reaction to exercise stress of certain body tissues and systems.

Methodologic and ethical constraints, coupled with the short period that pediatric exercise physiology has been systematically studied, delineate our current knowledge on the child's response to exercise. Information is available on some cardiovascular, pulmonary, metabolic, and thermoregulatory phenomena, but hormonal, renal, and cellular (especially subcellular) processes in muscle have barely been studied. There also are no data on changes within the nervous system. A brief discussion of some physiologic characteristics peculiar to the exercising child follows, in which the metabolic, cardiopulmonary, and thermoregulatory differences between children and adults are emphasized.

Aerobic and Anaerobic Characteristics

In physical activities that require sustained or intense energy turnover, children can seldom compete at par with adolescents or young adults. Such is the case in tasks that comprise long or short distance running, jumping, cycling, rowing, or skiing. A basic question is whether this handicap of children is primarily due to a deficiency in their maximal aerobic power or their anaerobic capacity.

MAXIMAL AEROBIC POWER. Taking maximal oxygen uptake ($\dot{V}_{O_2max}$) as a criterion, one might conclude that maximal aerobic power is distinctly lower in children. An 8-year-old boy, for example, may have a $\dot{V}_{O_2max}$ of 1.3 to 1.5 $L \cdot min^{-1}$ when that of an 18-year-old boy is 3.0 to 3.5 $L \cdot min.^{-1}$ However, because many tasks require the translocation of the whole body from one place to another, a child whose body weight is low may not *need* as high a $\dot{V}_{O_2max}$ as that needed by a heavier adolescent. It has been customary, therefore, to describe $\dot{V}_{O_2}$ per kilogram of body weight, rather than in absolute values, whenever individuals who differ in body weight are to be compared. Studies done on thousands of subjects have shown that when expressed per kilogram of body weight, the $\dot{V}_{O_2max}$ of young children is the same as that of adolescents and young adults. $\dot{V}_{O_2max}$ per kilogram is even higher in prepubescent girls than in older girls and women.[11]

Thus, maximal aerobic power (as reflected by $\dot{V}_{O_2max}$ per kilogram of body weight) is not deficient in children. The metabolic cost of walking and running (and possibly other activities) at a given speed, however, is distinctly higher in children than in older individuals.[2,31,66] At a running speed of 10 $km \cdot hr^{-1}$, for example, 7-year-old boys consume about 47 $ml \cdot kg^{-1} \cdot min^{-1}$; the respective $\dot{V}_{O_2}$ for 17-year-old boys is 40 $ml \cdot kg^{-1} \cdot min^{-1}$. Such a marked difference cannot be explained by the higher resting metabolic rate in children that is 1 to 1.5 $ml \cdot kg^{-1} \cdot min^{-1}$ higher than in adults, but probably reflects a mechanically "wasteful" running or walking style in smaller children. Whatever its cause, the end result of greater O_2 cost of locomotion leaves the child with a lower energy "reserve" between a submaximal task and maximal aerobic power.[11] Thus, children are definitely inferior in aerobic activities.

Another question to consider is whether scaling data to body weight is the method of choice for expressing maximal aerobic power in individuals who vary in size, i.e., is $\dot{V}_{O_2max}$ ($ml \cdot kg^{-1} \cdot min^{-1}$) the correct variable to use? The number of opponents to this customary approach is growing.[3,4,20,41,81,99] An alternative approach, based on geometric and dimensionality principles, has been suggested. If one assumes that body proportions remain fairly constant during childhood, adolescence, and adulthood, changes in body dimensions and functions can be predicted by knowing the respective changes in body length (L).[4] Thus, length of body segments will be proportional to L, area (cross-sectional and other) to L^2, and volume or mass to L^3. For example, stroke volume (SV) or vital capacity should be related to L^3, whereas muscle strength (which is proportional to the cross-sectional area of the muscle) should be related to L^2. Time is proportional to L according to dimensionality principles.[99] Thus, work will be re-

58

lated to L^3, but power will be related to L^2. Along the same lines, $\dot{V}_{O_2}$ (which is volume per time unit) can be expressed as L^3/L^1 or L^2.

How would scaling of $\dot{V}_{O_2max}$ to L^2 affect the interpretation of growth-related changes in maximal aerobic power? If, for example, a 6-year-old boy is 117 cm tall and has a $\dot{V}_{O_2max}$ of 1.0 L·min^{-1}, his *expected* $\dot{V}_{O_2max}$ at age 17 years, when he is 175 cm tall, is 2.25 L·min^{-1}. This determination, however, is only some 75% of those values commonly found in sedentary young men. Based on such geometric and dimensionality principles, therefore, it seems that a child's maximal aerobic power is lower than that of adults. The actual exponent of L found in longitudinal studies is not identical with the theoretical L^2. In a 7-year follow-up study of 51 boys who were first examined at 8 years of age, Bailey et al. concluded that their $\dot{V}_{O_2max}$ increase during the 7 years was proportional to $L^{2.46}$, i.e., a greater rise than the theoretical L^2.[6] In contrast, in a 4-year follow-up survey of 26 girl and boy athletes (initial testing at age 11 years), an exponent of only 1.5 to 1.6 was found.[90] For further elaborations on scaling and dimensionality, see the review by Cooper.[24]

ANAEROBIC CAPACITY. Unlike maximal aerobic power, anaerobic capacity of children, even when expressed per kilogram of body weight, is distinctly lower than that of older age groups. When such short-term, all-out power output tasks as the Margaria running step test or the Wingate 30-second cycling test are undertaken, performance rises continuously with age.[10,11,32,63] As found in the author's laboratory, an 8-year-old boy produces only 45 to 50% of the mechanical power produced by a 14-year-old boy. When normalized for body weight, the figure is still 65 to 70% (it will be lower if performance is scaled to L^2). With girls, the same trend exists, although the performance per kilogram of body weight does not increase beyond 11 to 12 years.

Biochemical data based on muscle biopsies suggest that the concentrations of CP, ATP, and glycogen in the resting muscle of children are the same as, or only slightly lower than, those of young adults.[40,44] Although there is no age-related difference in the utilization rate of ATP or CP, the utilization rate of glycogen is greatly diminished in the child. This difference is reflected in the rate of lactate production, e.g., 13- to 15-year-old boys may reach only 65 to 70% of that concentration in muscle reached by adults during maximal exercise.[43] Younger children reach even lower muscle lactate levels. Muscle lactate production was suggested to be related to the sexual maturity level of pubescent boys and to the testosterone level in the blood of rats.[43,62] Activity of phosphofructokinase in muscle is lower in children than in adults; this enzyme is considered rate-limiting in glycolysis.

Work under anaerobic conditions induces an increased H^+ concentration in body fluids and a reduction in base excess. Trained individuals who can push themselves hard to work anaerobically may reach blood pH levels as low as 6.9 to 7.0, whereas those individuals who are less capable of exerting anaerobically will seldom reach a pH value of 7.2. Characteristically, the ability to reach low pH values is age-dependent.[58,68,98] Similarly, children cannot lower their base excess to the extent found in adults.[46,68,98] This fact is just one additional indication that children are less suitable for anaerobic tasks, especially those dependent on their rate of glycolysis.

Typical for children is their ability to reach steady-state faster than adults. The O_2 deficit incurred with the transition from rest to exercise, or when power load increases, is thus lower in the child.[67,91] During the first 30 seconds of submaximal exercise at an intensity above the anaerobic threshold, for example, a 10-year-old boy can reach 50 to 60% of his steady-state $\dot{V}_{O_2}$, as compared with only 30 to 35% in a young adult. Such findings are in line with the low lactate levels reached by exercising children. An intriguing question is whether, thanks to their shorter $\dot{V}_{O_2}$ transients, children do not *need* to resort much to anaerobic energy pathways, or whether their short $\dot{V}_{O_2}$ transients are a compensatory phenomenon for their low glycolytic capacity. No clue is so far available to answer this question.

Cardiopulmonary Response to Exercise

Qualitatively, hemodynamic and respiratory adjustments to exercise are similar in children and adults. There are *quantitative differences,* however, as summarized in Table 4–1.

HEMODYNAMIC ASPECTS. A distinct hemodynamic characteristic of the child is a low SV at rest and during submaximal and maximal exercise.[39] Although heart rate (HR) is higher, cardiac output ($\dot{Q}$ or HR × SV) is about 1 to 3 L·min^{-1} lower than in adults at any given $\dot{V}_{O_2}$. This "hypokinetic" response seems to be more pronounced in younger children.[72] Based on the Fick principle, the calculated arteriovenous difference in O_2 content (AVD-O_2) is higher in children at submaximal, but apparently not at maximal, exercise.[11,16,39] Blood flow (BF) to the exercising muscle is greater in children than in adults. Children also have a greater reserve for BF increase beyond the metabolic needs of maximal exercise, i.e., when ischemic changes are superimposed.[60,61] Such better peripheral BF adjustment in children

can be considered compensatory for their lower $\dot{Q}$ and explains their higher AVD-O_2. Yet it is premature to infer that such a peripheral advantage is an end result of a "hypokinetic" central mechanism or vice versa. During exercise, arterial blood pressure (BP), especially the systolic (SBP), is relatively low in children.[57,79,93] A mean difference of 20 mm Hg, for example, was found between the SBP of 14-year-old adolescents and that of 9- and 12-year-old children who walked on a treadmill under identical conditions.[79] Such low BP values seem neither beneficial nor detrimental to the working capacity of the child.

RESPIRATORY ASPECTS. The ventilatory apparatus of exercising children seems less efficient than that in adults. The major difference is a greater minute ventilation ($\dot{V}_E$) at any given level of $\dot{V}_{O_2}$[2,80] and of $\dot{V}_{CO_2}$.[26] This phenomenon is more pronounced in younger children and represents a lower utilization of O_2 from the inspired air. A possible reason for such inefficient respiration in children could be the shorter time period of each respiratory cycle, caused by a higher respiratory frequency. Indeed, a child's breathing pattern is relatively shallow, as reflected by a low ratio of tidal volume to vital capacity during maximal exercise.[80] In spite of this

TABLE 4–1. **Hemodynamic and Respiratory Characteristics of Children's Responses to Exercise**

Function	Typical for Children (Compared with Adults)
Hemodynamic	
HR at submaximal power load	Higher, especially at first decade
HR$_{max}$	Higher
SV$_{submax\ and\ max}$	Lower
$\dot{Q}$ at given $\dot{V}_{O_2}$	Somewhat lower
AVD-O_2 at given $\dot{V}_{O_2}$	Somewhat higher
Blood flow to active muscle	Higher
SBP,DBP$_{submax\ and\ max}$	Lower
Respiratory	
$\dot{V}_E$ at given $\dot{V}_{C_2}$ and $\dot{V}_{CO_2}$	Higher
$\dot{V}_E$ "breaking point"	Similar
Respiration rate	Higher
Vt/VC	Lower

60

breathing pattern, the dead space to tidal volume ratio is similar in exercising children and adults, and the alveolar ventilation of the former is adequate.[87] The major disadvantage of excessive $\dot{V}_E$ in children is the greater O_2 cost of respiration, which could contribute in part to their overall higher $\dot{V}_{O_2}$ during exercise. When defined per percent $\dot{V}_{O_2max}$, the ventilatory threshold is somewhat higher in children than in adolescents and adults.[77]

Thermoregulatory Response to Exercise

For a recent review of this topic, see reference number 12. The major task of the thermoregulatory system during exercise is to dissipate the metabolic heat (M) that is produced in proportion to exercise intensity and duration. The amount of M per kilogram of body mass is greater in children during such activities as running and walking. Thus, a greater thermal load is a priori imposed upon the thermoregulatory apparatus of the child. The major avenue for heat dissipation during exercise is the evaporation of sweat, especially on a hot day, when other heat dissipation avenues become less effective. Sweating rate (SR) of children is much lower than that in adults, even when corrected for body surface area. In one study, 8- to 10-year-old boys produced 300 ml sweat per square meter of skin per hour while exercising intermittently at 50% of their maximum in 43°C, 20% relative humidity.[54] The corresponding rate for young adults was 460 ml·m^{-2}·hr^{-1}. Such a low SR is not because children activate fewer sweat glands. Even though children have a greater population density of active sweat glands, each gland produces less sweat. Whether at rest or during exercise, the gland of an adult produces some 2.5 times as much sweat.[9] Furthermore, the threshold for perspiration (expressed as the core temperature at which sweating starts) was found to be higher in children.[1]

Additional avenues for heat exchange with the environment are conduction, convection, and radiation, all of which depend on the surface area of the skin and on the temperature gradient between the skin and the environment. On the basis of geometric principles, the surface area of a child *relative to body mass* is greater than that of an adult. Heat exchange to and from the environment is therefore greater in children. Although this is an advantage for the child in neutral or warm climates, it can become a major handicap when ambient temperature exceeds skin temperature or whenever the body is exposed to a cold environment.

The "hypokinetic" circulation of children could limit their skin blood flow, thus interfering with their ability to convect heat from the core to the skin. At high levels of exercise (especially on an extremely humid day when sweat evaporation is inefficient), this limited skin BF is one more potential handicap to the child. Inversely, low central blood volume may become the limiting factor.[36]

The aforementioned geometric and functional differences make the child an inefficient thermoregulator during exercise. Will that, in fact, interfere with his well-being and performance capacity in hot, humid, or cold climates? Research in this area has only begun, but some answers are already available.

HEAT TOLERANCE. Children cannot sustain activity for as long a time as adults whenever the ambient temperature exceeds 40°C.[36,51,100] Their tolerance to swimming in cool water is also deficient.[89]

ACCLIMATIZATION TO EXERCISE IN THE HEAT. Children acclimatize to hot climates somewhat less efficiently than do adults.[54,100] Their main handicap is the *slower rate of acclimatization*.[9] A practical implication of this fact is that upon transition to a hot climate, children require more days to acclimatize. If they pursue intense athletic activities before reaching acclimatization, they are at a potential risk of a heat-related illness, including heatstroke and death.[45]

HYPOHYDRATION. Clinical reports indicate that hypohydrated children are at a risk of heatstroke and other heat-related illnesses during climatic heat waves. Yet, scant information is available on the effect of hypohydration on the performance and

61

well-being of the exercising child. The core temperature of progressively dehydrating 10- to 12-year-old boys who exercise intermittently in a hot climate was found to rise in proportion to the level of fluid deficit.[14] The rate of rise in core temperature was greater in these children than in young adults. As with adults, it was further shown that the only way to prevent hypohydration in a child who exercises for prolonged periods is to *force fluid replenishment* every 15 to 20 minutes. Otherwise, "voluntary dehydration" takes place. Although perspiration causes electrolyte loss, the perspiring child has a lower salt content in his or her sweat.[1,33,69]

CHILDREN AT SPECIAL RISK. Some juvenile populations are at a special risk when exerting in a hot climate. These include children with such diseases as anorexia nervosa (due to low insulative protection, inadequate peripheral circulation, and vomiting); cyanotic heart disease (excessive sweating); cystic fibrosis (excessive salt loss); juvenile diabetes (hypohydration); febrile states; gastroenteritis (fast dehydration); hypocaloric malnutrition (low insulative protection); mental retardation (insufficient drinking); and obesity (for details, see Bar-Or[9,11]).

Exercise Perception and Post-Exercise Recovery

An interesting feature of a child's response to exercise is a low rating of perceived exertion (RPE). In a study of some 1300 individuals ranging in age from 7 to 68 years, the Borg scale was used to determine RPE at various power loads of cycle ergometer exercise.[8,22] For a given HR (or percent HR_{max}), children rated the exertion level to be lower than did adolescents, who rated it lower than did adults. An exception were children of the 7- to 9-year-old group, who rated the level higher than the 10- to 12-year-olds.

A lower RPE could be one manifestation of the lower lactate, acidosis, and O_2 deficit levels that are typical for the exercising child. No data are available, however, to show that a child's RPE is related to the lactate concentration in the blood. When confirmed by other investigators, this age-related trend could help to explain the greater spontaneous activity levels of children.

An additional characteristic of children is their fast recovery rate after a strenuous task. Adults completing such an all-out task as a long distance race or an aerobic power test are often exhausted and cannot exert again for many hours. In contrast, children who have completed a similar all-out task are often willing to exert again as early as 30 to 45 minutes after the initial effort. No systematic studies are available to determine whether such a fast recovery is real (in terms of ability to perform well again after a short resting period) or whether it is merely subjective. The lower O_2 deficit and lactate accumulation incurred by children suggest that their faster recovery rate may be a real physiologic characteristic. Their lower RPE at an objectively strenuous activity, however, suggests that at least some component of a child's fast recovery is subjective.

Trainability of Children

Similar to adults, adolescents and children have been found to respond to conditioning or specific training regimens.[7,38,42,48] There are results of studies, however, that suggest the aerobic trainability of children in the first decade of life is lower than would be expected from changes in their athletic performance. A case in point is a study in which 91 children, ages 9 to 10 years, underwent various conditioning regimens for 9 weeks.[19] Even strenuous interval runs of 145 m, undertaken four times per week, did not induce any improvement in their $\dot{V}_{O_2max}$, although their running performance markedly improved. Similar results were obtained by other researchers.[30,73,91,106] Yoshida et al. studied 5-year-old girls and boys who ran 750 to 1500 m, five times per week for 14 months and did not raise their $\dot{V}_{O_2max}$ (per kilogram of body weight), in spite of an impressive improvement in performance.[106] Improved performance in the reported studies can be attributed to either a more efficient running style or a better anaerobic capacity. Other studies are available in which $\dot{V}_{O_2max}$ of children did increase with aerobic training, as reviewed by Rowland,[83] Vaccaro and Mahon[97] and Bar-Or.[13] Apparently, when the training regimen complies with instructions established for adults, the aerobic system of prepubescents is trainable, although to a lesser extent than in adults.

Eleven- to 13-year-old boys underwent anaerobic conditioning (sprint running or cycling) for 6 weeks.[48] Their performance in the Wingate Anaerobic Test improved significantly, but only by 3 to 5%. Such a mild improvement, even if also found among younger children, could not fully explain a better running performance. In conclusion, although children under 10 years of age are trainable, a question remains regarding their ability to improve maximal aerobic power. It is also quite possible that $\dot{V}_{O_2max}$ is not a valid criterion of maximal aerobic power in children.

Is there a specific developmental age at which trainability is especially high (or low)? Such a question is most important to the coach who wishes to maximize results, or to the health practitioner who is interested in rehabilitation by exercise. No definitive answers can be found in the literature. The various reports, in fact, are quite contradictory, perhaps because of the complicated methodology involved. A certain direction has been pointed out by Kobayashi et al., who conducted a mixed longitudinal, cross-sectional study on Japanese boys at various levels of habitual activity.[59] No regularity could be shown regarding the chronologic age at which training was most effective. When subjects were aligned according to the age at which height velocity was at its peak (PHV), however, it became apparent that effectiveness of aerobic training was much greater around PHV than at any earlier stage. A similar experimental approach was recently taken regarding local muscle endurance.[65] The preliminary report suggests that trainability of this component of fitness is *lowest* 6 months before PHV in boys and at PHV in girls.

TESTING FOR WHAT? WHO SHOULD BE TESTED?

The rationale for the use of exercise testing in children is summarized in Table 4–2. As with adults, exercise testing in the pediatric age group can be done in both healthy and sick individuals. Healthy children and adolescents are usually tested to assess their physical working capacity. In addition, several authors have suggested the potential value of stress testing of healthy children for the detection of risk factors for coronary heart disease and hypertension.[52,103] The latter approach needs further validation by longitudinal follow-up studies.

With the sick child or adolescent, exercise testing can be used to assess physical working capacity, but also as an adjunct method of clinical evaluation (see Table 4–3). Specific pathophysiologic responses to the stress of exertion can be detected, e.g., the degree of ST segment depression in aortic stenosis (which reflects the pressure gradient across the narrowing), the occurrence of ventricular dysrhythmias in complete congenital heart block, or the degree of bronchoconstriction in exercise-induced asthma.[49,86,104] Some pediatric cardiologists use information generated

TABLE 4–2. **Exercise in Pediatric Testing— For What?**

Determine physical working capacity ("effort tolerance")
Identify or evaluate *specific* pathophysiologic characteristics (ST depression in aortic stenosis)
Provide indications for surgery (congenital heart disease)
Evaluate functional post-surgical success
Evaluate need for specific procedure (pacing in heart block and catheterization in aortic stenosis)
Assess adequacy of medication (asthma, diabetes, and Addison's disease)
Identify "risk factors" for future disease
Diagnose disease (growth hormone deficiency and asthma)
Instill confidence in child and parents

TABLE 4-3. Pediatric Diseases in Which Exercise has been Used for Diagnosis or Clinical Evaluation

Cardiovascular diseases	Metabolic and hormonal disturbances
Aortic coarctation	Addison's disease
Aortic stenosis	Anorexia nervosa
Complete congenital A-V block	Diabetes mellitus
Coronary risk	Growth hormone deficiency
Ebstein's anomaly	Obesity
Hypertension	Locomotor diseases
Neurocirculatory asthenia	Cerebral palsy
Pulmonary stenosis	Muscle dystrophies
Atrial septal defect	Poliomyelitis
Single ventricle	Spina bifida
Ventricular septal defect	
Tetralogy of Fallot	
Transposition of the great arteries	
Ventricular dysrhythmias	
Respiratory tract	Miscellaneous
Bronchial asthma	Atopy
Cystic fibrosis	Drug evaluation
	Epilepsy
	Renal failure
	Scoliosis, idiopathic
	Thalassemia major

during exercise as an indication for surgery in congenital heart disease. Such is the case in pulmonary stenosis when the right ventricular end-diastolic or the right ventricular systolic pressures are inappropriately high or the SV is low during exercise.[74] Another example is an inappropriate rise of left ventricular end-diastolic pressure or an insufficient rise of SV in aortic stenosis. The functional success of cardiac surgery can also be evaluated better during exercise than at rest. Such is the case, for example, with monitoring of pressures after pulmonary valvotomy, the correction of Fallot's tetralogy, or coarctation of the aorta.[56,70,92]

Children are habitually more active than adults. Thus, adequacy of medication in some young patients can, and should be, evaluated by exercise testing and not only at rest; the main examples are bronchial asthma and diabetes mellitus. It is probable that with future research, investigators will identify the need for exercise testing to evaluate medication in a variety of other childhood diseases, e.g., maintenance therapy by thyroid or adrenocortical hormones, beta-adrenergic blockers and other anti-hypertensive drugs, sedatives, tranquilizers, and anti-epileptic medication.

As a rule, the purpose of exercise testing is not to diagnose disease, but rather to evaluate a child whose basic diagnosis has already been made. There are, however, two exceptions: growth hormone deficiency and bronchial asthma. Exercise provocation was found sensitive and quite specific for the diagnosis of growth hormone deficiency in short-statured children.[11,23] If such provocation does not induce a rise in serum growth hormone beyond 6 to 8 $ng \cdot ml^{-1}$, a positive diagnosis can be assumed. Some health professionals start therapy as a result of such a finding, whereas others seek further confirmation by pharmacologic provocation. In Canada, for example, three positive tests are required: two with pharmacologic stimuli and one with an exercise provocation.

Asthmatic children most often come to the exercise laboratory with a confirmed diagnosis. There are, however, cases in which a presumably healthy child is tested to evaluate exercise-induced cough, shortness of breath, or even chest pain and is found to have exercise-induced asthma.

A final, and most important, reason for exercise testing of children is to demonstrate to the child, and especially to the parent, that the child is capable of physical exertion. Very often, whether due to real or assumed pathologic findings, the parents and the child are apprehensive about the consequences of high intensity exertion. Such may be the case in epilepsy, hemophilia, diabetes mellitus, bronchial asthma, cystic fibrosis, hypertension, chronic renal disease, congenital heart defects, or even an innocent murmur. A sound policy whenever such children are evaluated is to invite the parent to attend the exercise test. The mere fact that their child can reach high levels of exercise with no adverse reaction is most revealing to the parents. Much self-confidence can be instilled or regained as a result of such a session.

METHODOLOGIC CONSIDERATIONS OF TESTING

Choice of an Ergometer

In principle, ergometers and testing protocols used for adults are also suitable for children. Young children, however, have some physical and psychologic characteristics that warrant the need for special methodologic considerations. Although a treadmill, a cycle ergometer, or a step can be used with most children 8 years of age or older, the ergometer of choice for younger children is the treadmill, especially when an all-out test is attempted. Often a young child starts a progressive all-out protocol on the cycle ergometer and after a while can no longer pedal, although the HR is only 170 to 180 beats·min^{-1}. The same child, if tested on a treadmill, can reach a HR of 200 to 210 beats·min^{-1} and a measured $\dot{V}_{O_2max}$ that is 20 to 30% higher than the peak value obtained on the cycle ergometer. The apparent cause of such a marked discrepancy is the relatively undeveloped muscle mass of the thighs (especially the knee extensors) in the young child, which results in an early local fatigue during cycling.

Another reason why a cycle ergometer (or a step) test is less suitable for the young child is that some children cannot conform to a rhythm set by the metronome. In addition, the attention span is short in many young children, or in older ones with a low mental age.[17] Even if such individuals start pedalling or stepping at the right cadence, they soon become distracted, much to the dismay of the examiner.

Cycle ergometers have the obvious advantage over treadmills as far as cost, portability, space, and safety are concerned. As a result, many clinicians still prefer the use of the former, even when studying children. Special attention should then be paid to the dimensions of the ergometer (specifically, the length of the pedal shaft, the distance between the seat and the pedals, the height of the handle bar, and its distance from the seat). The standard-sized ergometer for adults seldom can be modified for optimal use by children. A brand of ergometer is now available (Monark, Sweden) that is especially constructed for children. In this model, the seat height and the length of the pedal shaft can be adjusted to fit a wide range of children's sizes. No published data are available to recommend the optimal dimensions of a cycle ergometer setting for each body height.

Choice of Protocols

Many protocols have been suggested for the testing of children by either a cycle ergometer, a treadmill, or a step. It is beyond the scope of this chapter to review all of them, especially when the rationale for selection of an exercise protocol is only slightly different from that which is valid for adults.

MAXIMAL AEROBIC POWER TESTS. Two principles should govern the selection of a protocol: the overall task should last at least 6 minutes and preferably should not

65

exceed 10 minutes, and care should be taken in selecting exercise intensities to account for the wide variations in body dimensions among children of different ages. Due to the wide range in lean body mass of children and adolescents, it is hard to predict the power load for each individual that will elicit maximal aerobic demands. A progressively increasing load is therefore preferable to a single-stage protocol. The selection of the initial load and the increments should be determined according to the body height (or surface area) of each individual.

How long should each stage last? The considerations in children are not different from those for adults, with two exceptions. Due to the short attention span of children, it is best to keep the test short. As well, children seem to reach steady-state faster than adults. Thus, 2-minute stages seem adequate (see Skinner et al. for comparison of 2, 3, and 4-minute stages[88]). If the final load only is of interest, 1-minute stages can also be used.[76]

Table 4–4 outlines a protocol for treadmill use that has been found suitable for determination of submaximal and maximal HR, $\dot{V}_{O_2}$, and related variables in 6 to 15-year-old children. A corresponding protocol for all-out cycle ergometry is shown in Table 4–5 and one for step testing (ages 6 to 12 years) is detailed in Table 4–6. For adolescents, the double-step Canadian Home Fitness Test can be used.[5] Testing of 3 to 6-year-olds is feasible by using a 25 to 30-cm step at a rate of 30 ascents·min^{-1} in a test comprised of 5-minute stages.[75] In a clinical set-up, the

Bruce treadmill test has been used with success, and norms have been established for 4 to 18-year-old girls and boys.[29] This test is a 3-minute stage protocol that allows the investigator ample time to determine whether to continue to a higher load or to terminate the test for clinical or other reasons.

PITFALLS IN PREDICTION PROTOCOLS. As with adults, the use of submaximal tests to determine maximal aerobic power has been widespread for children. Both the W_{170} and the prediction of $\dot{V}_{O_2max}$ have been advocated.[71,85] Although these methods are adequate for surveys among healthy children, they have an inherent limitation when used with sick children. Both submaximal tests are valid as indicators of maximal aerobic power, as long as the maximal HR is within normal limits; this will not be the case when a child reaches lower than expected peak HR. An extreme example is a patient with complete congenital heart block. Such a child will have a low ventricular HR at each power load, leading to an erroneous prediction of an extremely high aerobic power. In reality, this child may have a distinctly deficient maximal aerobic power due to his inability to raise ventricular HR adequately and, therefore, $\dot{Q}$.[94] Other conditions in which peak HR is low are pulmonary (cystic fibrosis) or musculoskeletal (muscular dystrophy) diseases, in which the child is exhausted by exercise even though his heart is not fully stressed. Medication that lowers the maximal HR (such as propranolol) is another example

TABLE 4–4. **Suggested Progressive, Continuous Protocol for an All-Out Treadmill Walking Test, Determined by Body Height of the Child***

Body Height (cm)	Speed (km · hr^{-1})	Initial Slope (%)	Slope Increments (%)	Stage Duration (min)
≤109.9	4	10	2.5	2
110–129.9	5	10	2.5	2
130–149.9	6	10	2.5	2
≥150	6	♀10	2.5	2
		♂12.5		

* Speed should be kept constant until slope reaches 22.5%. Slope then remains constant and speed increases by 1 km · hr^{-1} with each stage.

TABLE 4–5. **Suggested Progressive, Continuous Protocol for All-Out Cycle Ergometry, Determined by Body Height of the Child**

Body Height (cm)	Initial Load (W)	Increments (W)	Stage Duration (min)
≤119.9	12.5	12.5	2
120–139.9	12.5	25	2
140–159.9	25	25	2
≥160	25	♀25	2
		♂50	

TABLE 4–6. **Recommended Progressive Protocol for a Step Test to be Used with 6- to 12-Year-Old Girls and Boys***

Stage	Rate (Ascents/min)	Step Height (cm)	Power Load (W/kg)
1	15	30	1.0
2	22.5	30	1.5
3	30	30	2.0

* Each stage should last 5 minutes, with a 5- to 10-minute resting interval between stages (based on data by Hanne[50]).

of when prediction methods should not be used.[95]

PEAK POWER OUTPUT AS AN INDEX OF FITNESS. When $\dot{V}_{O_2max}$ cannot be measured directly, an attempt should be made to bring the child to peak load for the monitoring of maximal HR and, especially, determination of peak power output. Although such an index cannot differentiate between aerobic and anaerobic characteristics, it definitely reflects the fitness of the child. Norms have been established for the index, which can be applied in the laboratory or in the field.[11] If the overall duration of the test is kept within 10 minutes, non-standard climates should hardly affect the results, which are independent of HR.

ANAEROBIC THRESHOLD. Criteria for the attainment of the anaerobic threshold, whether based on ventilatory changes or on levels of blood lactate, are similar in children and adults. One exception is that the criterion of 4 mmol blood lactate may be too high for many children[82] because children's blood lactate is lower at all exercise intensities. When collecting expired gases breath by breath, a "ramp" protocol (in which power increases continuously at 10 to 20 watts per minute) has been found useful for the detection of ventilatory

threshold in 6- to 17-year-old girls and boys.[25] The younger the child, the slower the rate of increase in power. When breath-by-breath collection is not feasible or when the ergometer is not suitable for a ramp protocol, one can use stages of 1-min duration.[77,78] When measuring blood lactate during the test, the duration of each stage is usually longer (2 to 4 min), with rest periods in between.[82]

ANAEROBIC PERFORMANCE. Although children habitually perform "anaerobic" activities (i.e., those lasting a few seconds at a supramaximal intensity), most fitness studies have been limited to the maximal *aerobic* power of the child. In point of fact, "physical working capacity" has often been used as a synonym for maximal aerobic power. One reason for the paucity of data on anaerobic characteristics of children has been the lack of a widely accepted method. Some authors have used a test in which the maximal level of acidosis reached by the child is taken as an index of anaerobic capacity.[46] Other investigators have used the Margaria step-running test.[32] In neither case have norms been established for children.

A test was developed in the author's laboratory (The Wingate Anaerobic Test) in which the subject pedals at top speed for 30 seconds. An ergometer should be used with which resistance is kept constant; this resistance is preselected to exhaust the child (or adult) during the prescribed time period.[11, 34] Reliability at various conditions and validity against other "anaerobic" characteristics have been determined, as has the sensitivity to training regimes in children and adults as well as the specificity of the test (i.e., its ability to determine anaerobic capacity and not maximal aerobic power).[15,48] The test can be used with the arms or the legs.[55] Peak power output in 5 seconds, the mean power in 30 seconds, and a fatiguability index are assessed. The optimal load found in girls to yield the highest mean power output is 3.92 joule (J) per pedal revolution (rev) per kilogram of body weight for the legs and 2.60 $J \cdot rev^{-1} \cdot kg^{-1}$ for the arms; the respective resistance for boys is 4.13 and 2.89 $J \cdot rev^{-1} \cdot kg^{-1}$ (Dotan and Bar-Or[35]; Bar-Or et al., unpublished data). Table 4-7 details the suggested resistances to be used in two mechanical cycle ergometers for healthy girls and boys whose body weight ranges between 20 and 60 kg. No optimal resistance has been established for children with such diseases as muscular dystrophy, cerebral palsy, or marked obesity.

The feasibility and reliability of the Wingate test were determined recently in 5- to 18-year-old subjects with cerebral palsy, spina bifida, muscular dystrophy, and muscular atrophy. Many of them had severe motor disabilities.[96] The arm and the leg tests were feasible for 94% and 61% of these subjects, respectively. For most groups, test-retest reliability was r = 0.93 to 0.95. It is therefore apparent that the Wingate Anaerobic Test is feasible and highly reliable for patients with neuromuscular diseases.

EXERCISE TESTS FOR SPECIAL PURPOSES. Sometimes, mostly in clinical laboratories, the purpose of exercise testing is for other than the determination of maximal aerobic power or anaerobic capacity. To provoke *exercise-induced bronchoconstriction (EIB)*, the exercise protocol should not be progressive, but rather should consist of a single load. In using a progressive protocol, the initial load may cause a warm-up effect, which could counteract the triggering of EIB. The intensity, as judged from HR, should exceed 160 beats $\cdot min^{-1}$, and the recommended duration should be 6 to 8 minutes. Running was found preferable to walking, although it is the minute ventilation, air humidity, and temperature rather than the nature of the task that determine its asthmogenicity.[11]

Diagnosis of *growth hormone (GH) deficiency* in short-statured children can be done through exercise provocation. Concentration of GH in the plasma is determined pre-exercise and again some 30 minutes after the beginning of the exercise.

TABLE 4-7. **Optimal Resistance for the Wingate Anaerobic Test, According to Body Weight**

Body Weight (kg)	Resistance with Monark Ergometer (kp)		Resistance with Fleisch Ergometer (kp)	
	Legs	Arms	Legs	Arms
20	1.50	1.00	0.90	0.60
25	1.88	1.25	1.13	0.75
30	2.25	1.50	1.35	0.90
35	2.63	1.75	1.58	1.05
40	3.00	2.00	1.80	1.20
45	3.38	2.25	2.03	1.35
50	3.75	2.50	2.25	1.50
55	4.23	2.83	2.54	1.70
60	4.80	3.20	2.88	1.92

If the post-exercise GH concentration does not rise beyond 6 to 8 ng·ml⁻¹, GH deficiency is strongly suspected. No single exercise protocol has been universally approved, but most investigators advocate running or walking for 10 to 20 minutes at a high, but not exhausting, intensity.[64,105] The tendency of some investigators to use such non-standardized protocols as running up and down stairs should be discouraged.

Testing *in conjunction with cardiac catheterization* is usually done with the child supine.[28,53] There is no agreement among investigators as to the duration or intensity of protocols. Some researchers bring the patients to exhaustion, whereas other individuals use a single-stage test of low intensity.

EXERCISE PRESCRIPTION

As a rule, a healthy child does not require an exercise prescription. Children are generally more habitually active than adults or adolescents and their spontaneous activity seems sufficient to maintain a fair level of fitness. The two subgroups of children that do require guidance and planned regimens of activity are some sick (or disabled) children and those aspiring to athletic excellence.

A major difference to recognize while planning activity programs for adults and children is that the latter group does not require special motivation. A sedentary adult recruited to an activity program must first undergo a "campaign" to modify his awareness and attitude toward physical activity. Extrinsic motivational tactics are taken, such as threatening him with risk of coronary heart disease or letting him be active during work hours at the expense of his employer. This need for motivational tactics is not so with children. Most healthy children (and many sick ones) have a built-in urge to stay active whenever they are not inhibited or distracted by their environment. Physical activity is a way of expression and an integral part of play. The games they select often include such elements as running, jumping, and climbing.

It is seldom that a child will voluntarily pursue such prolonged, monotonous activity as long distance walking, running, or swimming. More typically, children select intermittent-type exercise, during which bouts of intense exertion are interspersed with short rest periods or less strenuous activities. Their fast rate of recovery after a strenuous task enables children to sustain such intermittent activities for many hours.

It is beyond the scope of this chapter to analyze the activities that should be prescribed for a child who undertakes an athletic career. Considerations are similar to those prevailing for the older athlete and vary among sports and coaches. Still, one must take into account the difference in trainability between young children and adults. Specific problems, not yet resolved, in athletic conditioning of children relate to the risk in the premature use of weight training; the earliest age at which endurance training should be initiated; and the stage at which "specialized" training (rather than general conditioning) can be started. No doubt, such questions merit more research. Another related question, still under research in various countries, is how to select those talented children who will mature into elite athletes and how to direct them to the "right" sports specialties.

One segment of the pediatric population that merits special attention is the one with real or presumed physical or mental handicaps. Such children are often hypoactive when compared with their healthy peers. A summary of causes of hypoactivity in the sick child is given in Table 4–8. The main message to be derived from these data is that conditions in which there is a definite, objective cause for hypoactivity are outnumbered by those in which hypoactivity is imposed by fear, shame, overprotection, or sheer ignorance. In addition, a given disease can be accompanied by hypoactivity because of more than one cause.

To prescribe an activity regimen for the sick child, one should first identify the specific reason for the hypoactivity. For ex-

TABLE 4–8. Causes of Hypoactivity in Sick Children

Cause	Related Condition
Handicap causes motor limitation	Paralysis, muscle dystrophy or atrophy, advanced arthritis, extreme obesity, amputation, and cerebral palsy
Handicap causes cardiopulmonary or metabolic limitation	Advanced cyanotic heart disease, cystic fibrosis or kyphoscoliosis, and extreme obesity or undernutrition (anorexia)
Child is ashamed and is afraid of being active	Obesity, kyphoscoliosis, cerebral palsy, blindness, hemophilia, bronchial asthma, diabetes mellitus, epilepsy, Down's syndrome, and other types of mental retardation
Overprotection by parents and educators	Any "heart disease" (also benign murmur), cystic fibrosis, bronchial asthma, diabetes mellitus, epilepsy, and hemophilia
"Take-it-easy" approach by uninitiated physicians and school nurses	Dysrhythmia, congenital heart disease, diabetes mellitus, bronchial asthma, cystic fibrosis, epilepsy, and hemophilia

ample, it is only logical that an obese child who is inhibited by shame and peer rejection will not be forced to join a team sport at school, but rather will be able to join special programs with other obese children. Such programs can be carried out at school[101] or elsewhere. An asthmatic child with a history of repeated episodes of exercise-induced bronchoconstriction should be directed to swim rather than run. On the other hand, another asthmatic youth who is simply detrained due to hypoactivity can be given a variety of activities to increase his general fitness level. One hemophiliac child may choose to be inactive due to fear of bleeding; another is habitually active but has undergone recent muscle atrophy due to knee hemarthrosis. The approach to these two hemophiliacs should obviously be individualized. A diabetic youth can perform any kind of activity, but an attempt must be made to keep the total calorie output similar from one day to another.

Unlike healthy children, the child with a disease must often be motivated to assume an active way of life. More important, however, and often more difficult to accomplish is the modification of the *parental attitude, involvement and action*. Parents must first be convinced of the need for increased physical activity, as well as of its benefits and lack of hazard to their child. Otherwise, chances are slim that the child will assume an adequate activity pattern. Parents are often reluctant to allow their children to be active because of sheer ignorance of the health consequences of exertion. Such ignorance may stem from prejudice, but also from a misinterpretation of the physician's instructions or even from wrong medical advice. It has been shown, for example, that 53% of parents who curtailed the activity of their child with a *benign* cardiac murmur did so because of a physician's instructions![21] Seventy percent of these parents expressed doubt and confusion about their child's health status. Thus, to be successful in the institution of adequate activity patterns among sick (or presumed sick) children, the physician and physical educator must first and foremost obtain parental cooperation. The parents' fear should be alleviated and their level of uncertainty about the benefits and hazards of physical exertion should be reduced.

As with adults, exercise prescription should be well defined in terms of the intensity, duration, frequency, and content of each element. A major challenge is to describe to the child the notion of "intensity." An attempt has been made in the author's laboratory to use a rating of perceived exertion scale to prescribe intensity. This seems to be feasible with obese children,[102] as well as with those who are bound to their wheelchair.[18] Because of the greater spontaneity of children and their shorter attention span, one can a priori assume that adherence to a preset program may not be as expected from them. Nevertheless, good adherence can be achieved when activities are administered by an instructor. Whenever the *calorie equivalent* of activities is the main issue in exercise prescription (such as in obesity, diabetes mellitus, or anorexia), consideration must be given to the body weight of each individual. Caloric-equivalent tables constructed for adults should not be used, unless allowance for differences in weight have been made, especially in regard to such activities as walking, running, or cross-country skiing, in which the whole body is translocated from one place to another. Detailed tables of caloric equivalents constructed for a variety of body weights are available.[11] Fitting an exercise program to the child with motor disability must be based on his residual functional capacity rather than merely on classification of pathologic findings. A detailed selection of programs can be found in textbooks of *adapted physical education,* such as that by Cratty.[27]

REFERENCES

1. Araki, T., et al.: Age differences in sweating during muscular exercise. Jpn. J. Phys. Fitness Sports Med., 28:239, 1979.
2. Åstrand, P.-O.: Experimental Studies of Physical Working Capacity in Relation to Sex and Age. Copenhagen, Munksgaard, 1952.
3. Asmussen, E.: Development patterns in physical performance capacity. *In* Fitness, Health and Work Capacity, International Standards for Assessment. Edited by L. Larson. New York, Macmillan, 1974.
4. Asmussen, E., and Heebøll-Nielsen, K.R.: A dimensional analysis of physical performance and growth in boys. J. Appl. Physiol., 7:593, 1955.
5. Bailey, D.A., and Mirwald, R.L.: A children's test of fitness. *In* Pediatric Work Physiology. Edited by J. Borms, and M. Hebbelinck. Basel, Karger, 1978.
6. Bailey, D.A., et al.: Size dissociation of maximal aerobic power during growth in boys. *In* Pediatric Work Physiology. Edited by J. Borms, and M. Hebbelinck. Basel, Karger, 1978.
7. Banister, E.W.: A comparison of fitness training methods in a school program. Res. Q. Am. Assoc. Health Phys. Ed., 36:387, 1965.
8. Bar-Or, O.: Age-related changes in exercise perception. *In* Physical Work and Effort. Edited by G. Borg. New York, Pergamon Press, 1976.
9. Bar-Or, O.: Climate and the exercising child—a review. Int. J. Sports Med., 1:53, 1980.
10. Bar-Or, O.: Le test anaérobique de Wingate. Caractéristiques et applications. Symbioses, 13:157, 1981.
11. Bar-Or, O.: Pediatric Sports Medicine for the Practitioner—From Physiologic Principles to Clinical Application. New York, Springer, 1983.
12. Bar-Or, O.: Temperature regulation during exercise in children and adolescents. *In* Perspectives in Exercise Science and Sports Medicine, Volume 2: Youth, Exercise and Sport. Edited by C.V. Gisolfi, and D.R. Lamb. Indianapolis, Benchmark Press, 1989.
13. Bar-Or, O.: Trainability of the prepubescent child. Physician Sportsmed., 17:65, 1989.
14. Bar-Or, O., et al.: Voluntary hypohydration in 10- to 12-year-old boys. J. Appl. Physiol., 48:104, 1980.
15. Bar-Or, O., and Inbar, O.: Relationships among anaerobic capacity, sprint and middle distance running of school children. *In* Physical Fitness Assessment. Edited by R.J. Shephard, and H. Lavallée. Springfield, IL, Charles C Thomas, 1978.
16. Bar-Or, O., Shephard, R.J., and Allen, C.L.: Cardiac output of 10- to 13-year-old boys and girls during submaximal exercise. J. Appl. Physiol., 30:219, 1971.
17. Bar-Or, O., et al.: Maximal aerobic capacity of 6– 15-year-old girls and boys with subnormal intelligence quotients. Acta Paediatr. Scand., 217:108, 1971.
18. Bar-Or, O., Ward, D.S., and Longmuir, P.: Use of the RPE scale for exercise prescription with wheelchair-bound children and adults. Med. Sci. Sports Exerc., 22:S2, 1990.
19. Bar-Or, O., and Zwiren, L.D.: Physiological effects of increased frequency of physical education classes and of endurance conditioning on 9- to 10-year-old girls and boys. *In* Pediatric Work Physiology. Edited by O. Bar-Or. Natanya, Wingate Institute, 1973.
20. Bar-Or, O., Zwiren, L.D., and Ruskin, H.: Anthropometric and developmental measurements of 11- to 12-year-old boys, as predictors of performance 2 years later. Acta Paediatr. Belg. [Suppl.], 28:214, 1974.
21. Bergman, A.B., and Stamm, S.J.: The morbidity of cardiac nondisease in schoolchildren. N. Engl. J. Med., 276:1008, 1967.
22. Borg, G.: Physical Performance and Perceived Exertion. Lund, Gleerup, 1962.
23. Buckler, J.M.H.: Exercise as screening test for growth hormone release. Acta Endocrinol. (Copenh.), 69:219, 1972.
24. Cooper, D.M.: Development of the oxygen transport system in normal children. *In* Advances in Pediatric Sport Sciences, Volume III. Edited by O. Bar-Or. Champaign, IL, Human Kinetics, 1989.

25. Cooper, D.M., et al.: Growth-related changes in oxygen uptake and heart rate during progressive exercise in children. Pediatr. Res., *18*:845, 1984.
26. Cooper, D.M., et al.: Coupling of ventilation and CO_2 production during exercise in children. Pediatr. Res., *21*:568, 1987.
27. Cratty, B.J.: Adapted Physical Education for Handicapped Children and Youth. Denver, Love Publishing, 1980.
28. Cumming, G.R.: Supine bicycle exercise in pediatric cardiology. *In* Pediatric Work Physiology. Edited by J. Borms, and M. Hebbelinck. Basel, Karger, 1978.
29. Cumming, G.R., Everatt, D., and Hastman, L.: Bruce treadmill test in children: normal values in a clinic population. Am. J. Cardiol., *4*:69, 1978.
30. Daniels, J., and Oldridge, N.: Changes in oxygen consumption of young boys during growth and running training. Med. Sci. Sports, *3*:161, 1971.
31. Daniels, J., et al.: Differences and changes in $\dot{V}_{O_2}$ among young runners 10 to 18 years of age. Med. Sci. Sports, *10*:200, 1978.
32. Davies, C.T.M., Barnes, C., and Godfrey, S.: Body composition and maximal exercise performance in children. Hum. Biol., *44*:195, 1972.
33. Dill, D.B., Hall, F.G., and Van Beaumont, W.: Sweat chloride concentration: sweat rate, metabolic rate, skin temperature and age. J. Appl. Physiol., *21*:99, 1966.
34. Dotan, R., and Bar-Or, O.: Climatic heat stress and performance in the Wingate Anaerobic Test. Eur. J. Appl. Physiol., *44*:237, 1980.
35. Dotan, R., and Bar-Or, O.: Load optimization for the Wingate Anaerobic Test. Eur. J. Appl. Physiol., *51*:409, 1983.
36. Drinkwater, B.L., et al.: Response of prepubertal girls and college women to work in the heat. J. Appl. Physiol., *43*:1046, 1977.
37. Driscoll, D.J.: Diagnostic use of exercise testing in pediatric cardiology: the non-invasive approach. *In* Advances in Pediatric Sport Sciences, Volume III. Edited by O. Bar-Or. Champaign, IL, Human Kinetics, 1989.
38. Ekblom, B.: Effect of physical training in adolescent boys. J. Appl. Physiol., *27*:350, 1969.
39. Eriksson, B.O.: Cardiac output during exercise in pubertal boys. Acta Paediatr. Scand., *217*:53, 1971.
40. Eriksson, B.O.: Muscle metabolism in children—a review. Acta Paediatr. Scand. [Suppl.], *283*:20, 1980.
41. Eriksson, B.O., Berg, K., and Taranger, J.: Physiological analysis of young boys starting intensive training in swimming. *In* Swimming Medicine. Edited by B. Eriksson, and B. Furberg. Baltimore, University Park Press, 1978.
42. Eriksson, B.O., Gollnick, P.D., and Saltin, B.: Muscle metabolism and enzyme activities after training in boys 11–13 years old. Acta Physiol. Scand., *87*:485, 1973.
43. Eriksson, B.O., Karlsson, J., and Saltin, B.: Muscle metabolites during exercise in pubertal boys. Acta Paediatr. Scand., *217*:154, 1971.
44. Eriksson, B.O., and Saltin, B.: Muscle metabolism during exercise in boys aged 11 to 16 years compared to adults. Acta Paediatr. Belg. [Suppl.], *28*:257, 1974.
45. Fox, D.L., et al.: Effects of football equipment on thermal balance and energy cost during exercise. Res. Q. Am. Assoc. Health Phys. Ed., *37*:332, 1966.
46. Gaisl, G., and Buchberger, J.: The significance of stress acidosis in judging the physical working capacity of boys aged 11 to 15. *In* Frontiers of Activity and Child Health. Edited by H. Lavallée, and R.J. Shephard. Quebec, Pelican, 1977.
47. Godfrey, S.: Exercise Testing in Children. Applications in Health and Disease. Philadelphia, W.B. Saunders, 1974.
48. Grodjinovsky, A., et al.: Training effect on the anaerobic performance of children as measured by the Wingate Anaerobic Test. *In* Children and Exercise. Vol. IX. Edited by K. Berg, and B. Eriksson. Baltimore, University Park Press, 1980.
49. Halloran, K.H.: The telemetered exercise electrocardiogram in congenital aortic stenosis. Pediatrics, *47*:31, 1971.
50. Hanne, N.: A step-test for 6- to 12-year-old girls and boys (in Hebrew). Research Report. Natanya, Wingate Institute, 1971.
51. Haymes, E.M., et al.: Heat tolerance of exercising lean and heavy prepubertal girls. J. Appl. Physiol., *36*:566, 1974.
52. Hohn, A.R., et al.: Blood pressure and humoral factors in children of hypertensive parents. Pediatr. Res., *12*:383, 1978 (Abstract).
53. Hugenholtz, P.G., and Nadas, A.S.: Exercise studies in patients with congenital heart disease. Pediatrics, *32*:769, 1963.
54. Inbar, O.: Acclimatization to dry and hot environment in young adults and children 8–10 years old. Ed.D. dissertation, Columbia University, 1978.
55. Inbar, O., and Bar-Or, O.: Relationships of anaerobic and aerobic arm and leg capacities to swimming performance of 8–12 year old children. *In* Frontiers of Activity and Child Health. Edited by H. Lavallée, and R.J. Shephard. Quebec, Pelican, 1977.
56. James, F.W., and Kaplan, S.: Systolic hypertension during submaximal exercise after correction of coarctation of aorta. Circulation, *49*:50 (Suppl. II):27, 1974.
57. James, F.W., et al.: Responses of normal children and young adults to controlled bicycle exercise. Circulation, *61*:902, 1980.
58. Kindermann, V.W., Huber, G., and Keul, J.: Anaerobe Kapazität bei Kindern und Jugendlichen in Beziehung zur Erwachsenen. Sportarzt. Sportmed., *6*:112, 1975.
59. Kobayashi, K., et al.: Aerobic power as related to body growth and training in Japanese boys: a longitudinal study. J. Appl. Physiol., *45*:666, 1978.
60. Koch, G.: Muscle blood flow after ischemic work and during bicycle ergometer work in boys aged 12 years. Acta Paediatr. Belg. [Suppl.], *28*:29, 1974.
61. Koch, G.: Muscle blood flow in prepubertal boys— effect of growth combined with intensive physical training. *In* Pediatric Work Physiology. Edited by J. Borms, and M. Hebbelinck. Basel, Karger, 1978.

62. Krotkiewski, M., Kral, J.G., and Karlsson, J.: Effects of castration and testosterone substitute on body composition and muscle metabolism in rats. Acta Physiol. Scand., *109*:233, 1980.
63. Kurowski, T.T.: Anaerobic power of children from ages 9 through 15 years. M.Sc. thesis, Florida State University, 1977.
64. Lacey, K.A., Hewison, A., and Parkin, J.M.: Exercise as a screening test for growth hormone deficiency in children. Arch. Dis. Child., *48*:508, 1973.
65. Lammert, K., et al.: The effect of training in relation to chronological age and developmental stages in children 9 to 17 years of age. Acta Physiol. Scand., *105*:61A, 1979 (Abstract).
66. MacDougall, J.D., et al.: Maximal aerobic capacity of Canadian school children: prediction based on age-related oxygen cost of running. Int. J. Sports Med., *4*:194, 1983.
67. Maček, M., and Vávra, J.: The adjustment of oxygen uptake at the onset of exercise: a comparison between prepubertal boys and young adults. Int. J. Sports Med., *1*:70, 1980.
68. Matějková, J., Kopřivová, Z., and Placheta, Z.: Changes in acid-base balance after maximal exercise. *In* Youth and Physical Activity. Edited by Z. Placheta. Brno, J.E. Purkyne University, 1980.
69. Meyer, F., et al.: Sweat electrolytes during exercise in the heat, among pre-pubescent, pubescent and young adult females. Med. Sci. Sports Exerc., *22*:S88, 1990.
70. Mocellin, R., et al.: Exercise performance in children and adolescents after surgical repair of tetralogy of Fallot. Eur. J. Cardiol., *4*:367, 1976.
71. Mocellin, R., et al.: Determination of W_{170} and maximal oxygen uptake in children by different methods. Acta Paediatr. Scand. [Suppl.], *217*:13, 1971.
72. Mocellin, R., Sebening, W., and Buhlmeyer, K.: Cardiac output and oxygen uptake at rest and during submaximal loads in 8–14-year-old boys (in German). Z. Kinderheilk., *114*:323, 1973.
73. Mocellin, R., and Wasmund, U.: Investigations on the influence of a running-training programme on the cardiovascular and motor performance capacity in 53 boys and girls of a second and third primary school class. *In* Pediatric Work Physiology. Edited by O. Bar Or. Natanya, Wingate Institute, 1973.
74. Moller, J.H., Rao, S., and Lucas, R.V.: Exercise hemodynamics of pulmonary valvular stenosis (study of 64 children). Circulation, *46*:1018, 1972.
75. Pařízková, J.: Longitudinal study of somatic and functional development of preschool children. Bibl. Nutr. Dieta, *27*:65, 1979.
76. Pětajoki, M.L., Arstila, M., and Välimäki, I.: Pulse-conducted exercise test in children. Acta Paediatr. Belg. [Suppl.], *28*:40, 1974.
77. Reybrouck, T.M., et al.: The use of the anaerobic threshold in pediatric exercise testing. *In* Advances in Pediatric Sport Sciences, Volume III. Edited by O. Bar-Or. Champaign, IL, Human Kinetics, 1989.
78. Reybrouck, T.M., et al.: Ventilatory anaerobic threshold in healthy children. Age and sex differences. Eur. J. Appl. Physiol., *54*:278, 1985.

79. Riopel, D.A., Taylor, A.B., and Hohn, A.R.: Blood pressure, heart rate, pressure-rate product and electrocardiographic changes in healthy children during treadmill exercise. Am. J. Cardiol., *44*:697, 1979.
80. Robinson, S.: Experimental studies of physical fitness in relation to age. Int. Z. angew. Physiol. Arbeitsphysiol., *10*:251, 1938.
81. Ross, W.D., et al.: Body composition and cadaver validation: essential information for the sport sciences. Presented at the Annual Meeting, Canadian Association of Sport Sciences, Toronto, Ontario, 1978.
82. Rotstein, A., et al.: Effect of training on anaerobic threshold, maximal aerobic power and anaerobic performance of preadolescent boys. Int. J. Sports Med., *7*:281, 1986.
83. Rowland, T.W.: Aerobic response to endurance training in prepubescent children: a critical analysis. Med. Sci. Sports Exerc., *17*:493, 1985.
84. Rowland, T.W.: Exercise and Children's Health. Champaign, IL, Human Kinetics, 1990.
85. Rutenfranz, J.: Entwicklung und Beurteilung der körperlichen Leistungsfähigkeit bei Kindern und Jungendlichen. Basel, Karger, 1964.
86. Shephard, R.J.: Exercise-induced bronchospasm—a review. Med. Sci. Sports, *9*:1, 1977.
87. Shephard, R.J., and Bar-Or, O.: Alveolar ventilation in near maximum exercise. Data on preadolescent children and young adults. Med. Sci. Sports, *2*:83, 1970.
88. Skinner, J.S., et al.: Comparison of continuous and intermittent tests for determining maximal oxygen intake in children. Acta Paediatr. Scand. [Suppl.], *217*:24, 1971.
89. Sloan, R.E.G., and Keatinge, W.R.: Cooling rates of young people swimming in cold water. J. Appl. Physiol., *35*:371, 1973.
90. Šprynarová, Š., and Reisenauer, S.: Body dimensions and physiological indicators of physical fitness during adolescence. *In* Physical Fitness Assessment. Edited by R.J. Shephard, and H. Lavallée. Springfield, IL, Charles C Thomas, 1978.
91. Stewart, K.J., and Gutin, B.: Effects of physical training on cardiorespiratory fitness in children. Res. Q. Am. Assoc. Health Phys. Ed., *47*:110, 1976.
92. Stone, F.M., et al.: Pre- and postoperative rest and exercise: hemodynamics in children with pulmonary stenosis. Circulation, *49*:1102, 1974.
93. Strong, W.B., et al.: Blood pressure response to isometric and dynamic exercise in healthy black children. Am. J. Dis. Child., *132*:587, 1978.
94. Taylor, M.R.H., and Godfrey, S.: Exercise studies in congenital heart-block. Br. Heart J., *34*:930, 1972.
95. Thorén, C.: Effects of beta-adrenergic blockade on heart rate and blood lactate in children during maximal and submaximal exercise. Acta Paediatr. Scand. [Suppl.], *177*:123, 1967.
96. Tirosh, E., Bar-Or, O., and Rosenbaum, P.: New muscle power test in neuromuscular disease. Feasibility and reliability. Am. J. Dis. Child., *144*:1083, 1990.
97. Vaccaro, P., and Mahon, A.: Cardiorespiratory responses to endurance training in children. Sports Med., *4*:352, 1987.

73

98. Von Ditter, H., et al.: Das Verhalten des Säure-Basen-Haushalts nach erschöpfender Belastung bei untrainierten und trainierten Jungen und Mädchen im Vergleich zu Leistungssportlern. Sportarzt. Sportmed., 28:45, 1977.

99. von Döbeln, W., and Eriksson, B.O.: Physical training, maximal oxygen uptake and dimensions of the oxygen transporting and metabolizing organs in boys 11–13 years of age. Acta Paediatr. Scand., 61:653, 1972.

100. Wagner, J.A., et al.: Heat tolerance and acclimatization to work in the heat in relation to age. J. Appl. Physiol., 33:616, 1972.

101. Ward, D.S., and Bar-Or, O: Role of the physician and the physical education teacher in the treatment of obesity at school. Pediatrician, 13:44, 1986.

102. Ward, D.S., and Bar-Or, O.: Use of the Borg scale in exercise prescription for overweight youth. Can. J. Sports Sci., 15:120, 1990.

103. Wilmore, J.H., and McNamara, J.J.: Prevalence of coronary heart disease risk factors in boys, 8 to 12 years of age. J. Pediatr., 84:527, 1974.

104. Winkler, R.B., Freed, M.D., and Nadas, A.S.: Exercise-induced ventricular ectopy in children and young adults with complete heartblock. Am. Heart J., 99:87, 1980.

105. Wise, P.H., et al.: Selective impairment of growth hormone response to physiological stimuli. Arch. Dis. Child., 50:210, 1975.

106. Yoshida, T., Ishiko, I., and Muraoka, I.: Effect of endurance training on cardiorespiratory functions of 5-year-old children. Int. J. Sports Med., 1:91, 1980.

5
CHAPTER

Importance of Aging for Exercise Testing and Exercise Prescription

by

James S. Skinner

GENERAL EFFECTS OF AGING

Functional and structural changes occur in most cells of the body throughout life. Although the aging process actually begins before birth, its effects are generally counterbalanced by growth. Once maturity is reached at age 20 to 25 years and growth stops, however, the effects become noticeable, usually around the age of 30 years. The rate with which the age-related changes occur varies from one person to another and from one body system to another within the same person,[27] but the changes seem to be inevitable and irreversible.

With aging, there is a loss in size, number, or both of functional units within every system of the body, as well as a loss in function of those units that remain. As a result, aging can be characterized by a decreased ability to adapt to and to recover from physiologic displacing stimuli. It seems that the greater the intensity of the stimulus and the larger the number of physiologic mechanisms involved in adjusting to that stimulus, the greater will be the loss of function with age.

Because exercise is a form of physiologic stimulation requiring complex forms of regulation and interaction among many systems, it is not surprising that the performance of certain types of exercise diminishes with age. Similarly, because training is a form of adaptation to repeated exercise stimulation, it is logical to assume that adaptation to training also will be at a lower level. Therefore, people who test and prescribe exercise for middle-aged and older persons should be aware of the effects of aging on the various systems and on the ability to exercise and train, as well as the general characteristics and specific needs of older people. For more detailed descriptions of age-related changes in each system, the reader is referred to published reviews.[13,26,27,34,40]

As a result of the loss of body cells within all systems, body weight and body cell mass decrease. With age, there is a gradual loss of bone mass in almost all humans, beginning at age 30 to 35 years and accelerating after menopause in women and at age 50 to 55 years in men. These weaker bones are more susceptible to fracture spontaneously or after mild trauma.[39] Along with a decrease in bone mass, the amount of body fat tends to increase and muscle mass (size and number of muscle cells) decreases. Although the diminished muscle mass is more profound than is the overall loss of body weight, this difference is partially masked by an increased amount of body fat.

The increase in body fat appears to be more related to lifestyle than to age per se. Skrobak-Kaczynski and Andersen found that Norwegian lumberjacks had mean values of about 13% body fat from age 20 to 70 years.[35] It is not known how much exercise was needed to maintain these "younger" levels but it is clearly more than most people do in our technological society. With age, the pattern of fat distribution changes, such that more fat is deposited internally and on the torso than under the skin and on the limbs.[6] Thus, estimates of body fat based on skinfolds should be age- and population-specific. Although some equations of this type have been developed,[10,15,22,43] there is still a debate as to whether population-specific equations are better than general ones.[23] Using quadratic regression analysis, general equations independent of age and body composition have been developed for men[14] and for women.[16] Unfortunately, the upper age in these two studies was 61 years for the men and 55 for the women, suggesting the need to develop the same type of equations specific to elderly men and women. It should also be mentioned that there are problems determining body composition by hydrostatic weighing in old age. For example, there are age-related and variable decreases in bone density among men and women, as well as a rise in the amount of connective tissue within the body and a higher residual volume with increasing age.

There appears to be a greater reduction in the number and size of fast-twitch, glycolytic muscle fibers used for strength and speed than that in slow-twitch, oxidative, endurance fibers,[11] as well as a decreased ability to recruit fast-twitch fibers.[18] Along with the loss of functional units in muscle cells, there are smaller stores of ATP, CP, and glycogen and less effective enzymes needed with all three mechanisms for energy production, i.e., use of stored energy (ATP and CP), anaerobic glycolysis, and the aerobic metabolism of fats and carbohydrates.

Within the nervous system, there is a decrease in the number and size of neurons, nerve conduction velocity, and maximal conduction frequency, as well as an increase in the amount of connective tissue in the neurons and in the excitability threshold of muscle. As a result, the control of movement is less precise, less harmonious, more hesitant, and seems to require more attention.[11,34]

Cartilage, tendons, and ligaments become stiffer and more rigid with age. Although decreased flexibility has also been reported, Adrian found a minimal amount of evidence that the primary cause was an alteration in connective tissue, and suggested that it might be more related to disuse or to degenerative changes associated with osteoarthrosis and osteoarthritis.[1]

Changes in the respiratory system have little effect on the function of healthy lungs at rest, but do make it more difficult for the lungs to supply adequate levels of oxygen to the body during intense exercise. As stated by Reddan, the older person has less reserve and has less room for error in the systems that control ventilation.[24]

With increasing amounts of connective tissue, decreased elasticity, higher total peripheral resistance (TPR), and higher blood pressures (BP), the heart has to work harder to pump the same amount of blood. The higher BP and TPR and somewhat lower cardiac output ($\dot{Q}$) at rest are of little consequence, however, unless disease is present.

With increasing amounts of exercise, the aging cardiovascular and respiratory systems are less capable of adapting. At the same moderate submaximal work load, aging is characterized by 1) little change in oxygen intake ($\dot{V}_{O_2}$) and heart rate (HR); 2) higher values for ventilation ($\dot{V}_E$), BP, arteriovenous difference for oxygen (AVD-O_2), blood lactic acid concentration (LA), and oxygen debt; 3) lower values for $\dot{Q}$ and stroke volume (SV); and 4) a lower *rate* of adaptation to and recovery from exercise. The effects of age are most evident at maximal levels of exercise. With the exception of increased BP and TPR, there are reductions in maximal values of $\dot{V}_{O_2}$, $\dot{V}_E$, $\dot{Q}$, HR, SV, AVD-O_2, and LA. With the decrease in maximal aerobic power, a given amount of submaximal exercise becomes relatively more strenuous.[33]

From this brief review, it is clear why the aged are weaker, slower, and less powerful, and why there is a reduction in those performances requiring the regulating and coordinating functions of the nervous system, e.g., balance, reaction time, agility, and coordination. It is also easy to understand why older people cannot perform as well in almost any type of activity, except for low-intensity activities in which energy demands are easily met.

AGE, DECONDITIONING, AND DISEASE

When a middle-aged or older person comes for assistance, the physician or exercise leader must determine the relative effects of age, deconditioning, and disease. For example, dyspnea with moderate exercise may be due to age, poor fitness, or pulmonary disease. The structural and functional changes that occur with age and deconditioning tend to be more "normal," whereas those associated with disease are not.

Although aging and disuse are not diseases, all three factors are often treated in the same manner.[7] Not only can the aged, the deconditioned, and the sick have similar physiologic traits, they are often similar psychologically. While disuse and aging are not synonymous, they do have common attributes. In fact, Smith states that disuse and aging each account for about one half the "normal" functional decline occurring from age 30 to 70 years.[36]

Different diseases affect people at different ages, and age can have a modifying effect on various disease processes. Therefore, the ability to distinguish deconditioning and age-related changes from disease processes is a major challenge for physicians, and such a distinction will influence the type of exercise test that is given and the exercise programs that are prescribed.

Certain diseases are found more frequently with advancing age, e.g., arthritis, cardiovascular diseases, diabetes mellitus, dyslipoproteinemia, emphysema, and hypertension. For more detailed descriptions of these disorders and their effects on exercise testing and exercise prescription, the reader is referred to the specific chapters in this book.

EXERCISE TESTING OF THE ELDERLY

Whether an exercise tolerance test is needed depends on the patient's health status, present level of habitual activity, and the level of activity desired. In other words, low-risk, nonsymptomatic patients with no evidence of cardiovascular disease may not need to be tested if walking or mild calisthenics will be their main form of exercise. On the other hand, high-risk patients with a history of clinical problems that might be aggravated by exercise or patients who want to do more vigorous exercise should be tested for their personal safety.

The main purposes of exercise testing are the same for the elderly as they are for all adults: to define the degree of risk associated with varying work loads and to establish the appropriate intensities for the exercise prescription.

Assuming that the physician 1) is familiar with the patient's prior and current status in terms of health and physical activity and 2) understands the contraindications for exercise testing,[2] the Council on Scientific Affairs of the American Medical Association recommends exercise tests for the elderly "when appropriate."[3] Thus, not all older people can or should be given exercise tests to determine their fitness. For example, Sidney and Shephard found that medical screening eliminated 21% of elderly volunteers for a training program.[29] Because older people are at greater risk (even those who are apparently healthy), a physician should be in visual contact or in close proximity at all times. Interpretation of exercise test results also can be a problem. Schlenker reported that 77% of older adults take at least one prescription medication on a regular basis, whereas 65% take one to three and 20% take four to nine.[25] Depending on the interactions of these medications with each other, as well as their possible interaction with exercise, test results may be affected.

Except for research purposes, there is little reason to do maximal exercise tests with older adults. Thomas et al. found test-retest reliability coefficients of 0.67, 0.87, and 0.90 for three treadmill protocols with 224 men aged 55 to 68 years.[42] Although higher $\dot{V}_{O_2max}$ values were found when tests were repeated, only one-third of the men reached a plateau in $\dot{V}_{O_2}$; this raises more doubts about the value of and the need for maximal tests. A better approach would be to estimate fitness from submaximal tests so that more people can be evaluated with less risk.

Two practical questions arise, however. Most submaximal tests determine heart rate (HR) at several levels of $\dot{V}_{O_2}$ or power output. By extrapolating the linear relationship between HR and either of these two variables to that individual's known or estimated maximal HR, the maximal $\dot{V}_{O_2}$ or power output can be predicted. However, because of the large variation in maximal HR[29] and the concern about approaching or going to maximum, how does one select the correct maximal HR to which one should extrapolate? Similarly, if older subjects are limited by muscular weakness and cannot push themselves to maximal levels of V_{O_2} (or are not motivated to do so), of what practical significance are these "maximal" values to their health, well-being, and independence? Submaximal tests of progressively-increasing intensity to some fixed end-point (e.g., to a known HR or to the onset of predetermined signs and symptoms) may be more useful.

Many normative values are based on data on young men and may not be directly applicable to an older population, especially one with more women. Thus, more information on typical values in the young-old (65 to 75 years), the old-old (75+ years), and the athletic old are needed.[40] Perhaps more important would be information on 1) how much and what types of physical activity are needed to increase and maintain functional ability in the older person and 2) those fitness tests that best measure these abilities.

Factors Influencing Exercise Testing

As mentioned previously, age is a risk factor in the development of various diseases. The effects of each of these diseases should therefore be considered when a suitable exercise test is selected. Nevertheless, common characteristics of the elderly can modify the type of test given (Table 5–1).

With age, there is a reduction in the average values of maximal aerobic power or $\dot{V}_{O_2max}$. Starting at about 12 to 13 METs at age 25 years (men tend to have average values about 1 MET higher), there is a drop of approximately 1 MET each 7 years or a $\dot{V}_{O_2}$ of 0.5 ml·kg^{-1}·min^{-1} each year.[31] Thus, the average 60-year-old individual has a $\dot{V}_{O_2max}$ of 7 to 8 METs; this value drops to 5 to 6 METs in the average healthy 75-year-old person. Smith reports average values of 5 to 7 METs in the young-old (65 to 75 years) living in the community, 2 to 4 METs in the old-old (75+ years) living in nursing homes, and about 10 METs in the athletic old.[36] Given the low values in all but the athletic old, the initial work load should have a fairly low energy requirement. Thus, the Bruce test is not the test of choice because the second work load (2.5 mph, 12% grade) requires 7 METs and is at or near the $\dot{V}_{O_2max}$ of most elderly people.[2,17]

Older people require more time to reach a relative steady-state in $\dot{V}_E$, $\dot{V}_{O_2}$, and HR. An ideal test therefore incorporates a long period of warm-up, i.e., the intensity of the initial work load is low (2 to 3 METs) and is continued for at least 3 minutes or longer until the steady-state is attained. Increases in exercise intensity should be small (0.5 to 1.0 MET) and the time at each work load should not be too brief (at least 2 to 3 minutes). Again, the big increase in intensity found from one stage to the next in the Bruce test argues against its use. Even the modified Balke test, which starts at 3 mph, 0% grade (3 METs) and increases by 2.5% grade (1 MET) every 2 minutes, may not always be the test of choice because of the inadequate time at each work load. Smith and

TABLE 5-1. **Exercise Testing for the Elderly**

Characteristic	Suggested Test Modification
Low $\dot{V}_{O_2max}$	Start at low intensity (2–3 METs)
More time required to reach a steady state	Long warm-up (3+ min). Small rise in power output (0.5–1 MET) and/or 2–3 min at each stage
Increased fatiguability	Reduce total test time to 12–15 min or use an intermittent protocol
Increased need to monitor ECG, BP, and HR	Bike > treadmill > step test
Poor balance	Bike > treadmill > step test. Use treadmill built into floor
Poor strength (especially upper thighs)	Treadmill > bike or step test
Less ambulatory ability	Increase treadmill grade rather than speed (maximum of 3–3.5 mph)
Poor neuromuscular coordination	Increase amount of practice. May require more than one test
Difficulty holding mouthpiece with dentures	Add support or use face mask to measure $\dot{V}_{O_2}$
Impaired vision	Bike > treadmill or step test
Impaired hearing	Treadmill > bike or step test, if person needs to follow a cadence. Difficulty understanding and responding in a noisy environment (use electronic bike)
Senile gait patterns and foot problems (e.g., bunions and calluses)	Bike > treadmill or step test

Gilligan recommend another modification of the Balke test starting at 2 mph, 2% grade (2 METs) and increasing by 2% (0.55 MET) each 2 minutes.[37] For nursing home patients with a very low maximum, they suggest a four-stage chair step test that allows patients to sit while raising their legs to various heights.[37] This test begins at 2.3 METs and increases by about 0.5 MET after 2 to 5 minutes at each stage, to a maximum of 3.9 METs.

Because fatiguability increases with age, total test time should not be too long. Of course, duration will depend on the objectives of the test, on the ability to estimate an individual's fitness before testing, and on the ability to modify a protocol depending on the test results.

With advancing age, medical problems are more likely to occur, suggesting that the need for monitoring is greater. Although it is easier to monitor BP with the use of the bicycle ergometer than with the treadmill and step test, there is no problem recording HR with the electrocardiographic systems available today.

Poor balance and poor muscular strength are characteristics of the older, sedentary person. In terms of balance, weight-supported exercise on a bicycle ergometer is easier than is exercise on the treadmill or step test. Nevertheless, the treadmill is preferred for those persons with poor muscle strength, especially those with weakness in the upper thigh. Those individuals with poor balance probably feel more comfortable walking on a treadmill that is not too high off the ground. Although many people are allowed to hold the treadmill railing, the energy cost of a particular work load can be greatly altered. Whereas this effect may not be a problem if $\dot{V}_{O_2}$ is measured, it can cause significant errors when HR is used to predict maximal working capacity or maximal $\dot{V}_{O_2}$.[12]

Associated with the lack of balance is a decrease in ambulatory ability and neuromuscular coordination with age. Increasing treadmill grade rather than speed should therefore be easier. Older persons may require more practice before they feel comfortable keeping the proper cadence during a bicycle ergometer or step test and while walking on the treadmill. As a result, more than one testing session may be required before the tester is confident that the results are indicative of the older person's responses to that amount and type of exercise.

Other characteristics of the elderly should be considered when deciding on the need for exercise testing and the type of test to be given. People with dentures may have difficulty holding a mouthpiece, so that added support or use of a face mask will be needed for the direct determination of $\dot{V}_{O_2}$. Impaired vision may reduce the ability to perform treadmill and step tests adequately and safely. Persons with hearing loss may not be able to follow the proper cadence in bicycle ergometer and step tests or to respond as well to questions during a test, especially in a noisy environment. People with senile gait patterns and such foot problems as bunions and calluses may have difficulty walking on a treadmill or performing a step test.

It would appear, therefore, that there is much heterogeneity among the elderly, and that no one exercise test protocol or apparatus is optimal. Nevertheless, with consideration of the factors previously discussed, as well as of the reasons why exercise testing is done with each person, suitable alternatives may be found.

More emphasis should be placed on evaluating factors important to health and well-being, such as flexibility, endurance, strength, and body fat. In other words, fitness testing for the older adult should relate more to health and independent living than to performance. As well, their results should not be compared to "average" values. Given that "average" is not always satisfactory and that performance per se is less important to most older people, evaluations should use such terms as "desirable," "acceptable," "minimal," and "undesirable" to inform the aged about the possible interrelationships among certain aspects of fitness, health, and independence.

EXERCISE PRESCRIPTION FOR THE ELDERLY

The general principles of exercise prescription for the aged are not much different from those used with younger people, except that the principles may have to be modified because of restrictions caused by the normal effects of aging. Smith has found that the "young-old" have few problems, while the "old-old" are hindered by a variety of age-related disorders.[36] Additional modifications should be made when clinical problems or disabilities common to the elderly are present (e.g., atherosclerosis, hypertension, emphysema, arthritis, and neuromuscular incoordination). Thus, there is a wide spectrum of ability and need among the elderly. Generally speaking, the longer individuals have been sedentary and the more restrictions or limitations they have, the higher will be the number of modifications that should be made in their exercise prescription.

Aging of the cardiovascular system is almost always associated with atherosclerosis.[13,17,33,34] In addition, aging and cardiovascular disease have similar effects on exercise capacity.[30] As a result, patients with coronary disease could be considered to have advanced aging of the arterial system. Given these similarities, most principles of exercise prescription for these heart disease patients would also apply to older persons; programs for both groups require a more systematic and cautious approach.

Objectives of Exercise Programs

Depending on the health status and level of habitual activity, which can vary greatly, the goals of the elderly can be quite different. Whereas young people are more interested in performance and appearance, health and general well-being become more important with age. The primary goal of exercise programs for the elderly (see Table 5–2) should be to improve general well-being, to increase their ability to take care of themselves, and to feel better during the later years of life.

Because a loss in cardiovascular endurance, strength, or flexibility is associated with a loss of independence and a diminished ability to adjust to the requirements of daily living, improvement of these factors should be emphasized. Unless pro-

TABLE 5-2. Objectives of Exercise Programs for the Elderly

Improve self-care capabilities and general well-being

Improve cardiovascular condition and general endurance

Increase muscular strength and endurance

Maintain or improve flexibility, coordination, and balance

Maximize social contact and enjoyment of life

Improve weight control and nutrition

Aid digestion and reduce constipation

Promote relaxation

Relieve anxiety, insomnia, and depression

Sustain sexual vigor

TABLE 5-3. Considerations in Prescribing Exercise for the Elderly

Medical-physiologic factors
  Reduced cardiorespiratory capacity
  Less ability to perform moderate and high intensity exercise
  Decreased ability to adapt to and to recover from exogenous physiologic stimuli (e.g., exercise, heat, and cold)
  Reduced adaptability to physical training (degree and/or rate of improvement)
  Muscle weakness and increased fatiguability
  Degenerative bone, joint, and tendon problems
  Increased susceptibility to soreness and injury
  Impaired balance and neuromuscular coordination
  Impaired vision and hearing
  Senile gait disorders and foot problems

Psychologic factors
  Lack of encouragement to be active
  Inaccurate perception by young and old of how active the elderly are, can be, or should be
  Increased inhibitions and depression
  Negative attitudes toward physical activity
  Distorted self-image

grams also attempt to increase socialization and enjoyment, however, it is unlikely that older people will continue to participate in what should be a regular part of their lifestyle. Although the other objectives listed in Table 5–2 may be secondary for program planning, they are still associated with self-care and general well-being.

A good exercise prescription is one that sets realistic goals for persons of all ages. As with younger people, the elderly want success. This can be accomplished by setting many small and attainable short-term goals and by selecting goals with a high probability of success (e.g., improved performance of such basic motor skills as walking, instead of better performance of complex movements that require practice and are difficult to master). Because the elderly have a desire to be wanted and to have their advice sought and valued, the prescription should involve setting goals[41]; this should improve the chances that the elderly patient will adhere to the prescribed program.

Considerations in Prescribing Exercise

There are factors to consider when prescribing exercise for the aged (Table 5–3). Because the same amount of exercise requires the same amount of energy, and because there is a marked drop in $\dot{V}_{O_2max}$

with age, a given submaximal work load becomes more intense relative to the maximum. With moderate and high intensity exercise, the older person has a slower rate of increase in $\dot{V}_{O_2}$, $\dot{V}_E$, and HR, must provide more energy via the anaerobic mechanism, and cannot exercise for as long a time.[30,34] Aging appears to have a minimal effect on the ability to work at or below 50% $\dot{V}_{O_2max}$, however. People can work at these lower intensities for as many as 8 hours with little problem.[4] Thus, the elderly have more difficulty if the intensity is moderate or high and if the pace is imposed; less difficulty can be expected when they can select their own work rate.

Given that the functional ability of many sedentary elderly people is so low, such simple activities as walking, housework, and gardening may be of sufficient intensity to stimulate improvements.

Thus, even a small increment in habitual activity may improve their functional ability, independence, and quality of life.

An exercise prescription should include the frequency, duration, intensity, and types of activity that the older person can do. It should also include instructions on what to do if the patient develops such effort-related symptoms as marked dyspnea with moderate exercise, chest pain, dizziness, claudication, or extreme fatigue.[38]

INTENSITY. The risks of cardiovascular and musculoskeletal problems are much greater with intense exercise, especially in older people with bone, joint, and neuromuscular ailments. The elderly also are more easily fatigued and are more susceptible to injury. Therefore, training programs should start with exercise at a low intensity to allow a more gradual increase in activity.

The longer that individuals have been sedentary and the more restrictions or limitations they have, the lower should be the starting intensity, e.g., 30 to 40% $\dot{V}_{O_2max}$. Because average 65-year-old persons have a maximum of 7 METs, they should begin at 2 to 3 METs (walking 2 to 3 mph). After an interval that is longer than that usually required for younger people, intensity can be gradually raised to 50 to 70% $\dot{V}_{O_2max}$. DeVries suggests that the minimal intensity for a training response in older men is about 40% $\dot{V}_{O_2max}$.[9] Smith and Gilligan recommend an intensity of 40 to 70% $\dot{V}_{O_2max}$.[37]

DURATION. Because the older person is less able to adapt to and to recover from physiologic stimuli, any major increase in activity should be preceded and followed by prolonged periods of mild, gradually increasing (or decreasing) exercise. The older and more sedentary the individual, the longer should be the warm-up and cool-down periods. By avoiding rapid or major changes (up or down) in intensity, the older person has more time to adapt to and to recover from activities of higher intensity.

With prolonged periods of lower intensity exercise, the total duration of each session will have to be longer to produce a significant total energy turnover. Balke suggests that the amount of energy expended during an exercise session be at least 10% of the person's daily caloric intake.[5] For most older people, this amount would be 10% of 1800 to 2200 kcal, or about 200 kcal per day of exercise, and would require approximately 1 hour of walking in those persons with a low maximum. Less time is needed with correspondingly greater work loads. Once an individual is exercising regularly, the minimal duration of each session should be 30 minutes. If the exercise sessions go much longer than 30 minutes, the older person should consider doing two shorter sessions rather than one long session.

FREQUENCY. As with individuals of any age who wish to improve cardiovascular endurance and to control better the composition of body weight, the elderly should exercise at least three times per week. Because the aged are also trying to improve general well-being and the ability to take care of themselves, however, they need to be mentally and physically active every day. By finding ways to be active and by incorporating these activities into a given lifestyle, significant amounts of exercise can be performed. As well, it will be possible to improve such important aspects as flexibility, strength, and balance and to avoid or reduce the loss of function usually associated with disuse.

TYPE. In programs for the elderly, rhythmic, continuous exercise involving the use of large muscle groups should be emphasized. Activities of low to moderate intensity, such as walking, jogging, cycling, and swimming, are excellent for weight control and to improve general muscular and cardiovascular endurance. Games of low organization are an excellent means to improve hand-eye coordination, balance, and flexibility while having fun.

The keys to maintaining adequate joint function are movement to the joint's range of motion and adequate levels of strength. Therefore, exercise programs should include rhythmic stretching of all joints (especially during warm-up and cool-down phases) to improve flexibility; this stretching will help to maintain the ability to stoop, bend, and reach. Rhythmic calisthenics are ideal to increase strength and muscle tone, especially in those areas (thighs, back, abdomen, and arms) in which muscle weakness is common in the older adult.[19] This type of exercise with light to moderate resistance is also potentially less dangerous. As with coronary disease patients, lifting of heavy weights, isometric exercise, and arm exercises should be avoided or carefully controlled because they cause marked increases in HR and BP.[2]

Little is known about the longitudinal or cross-sectional changes in the strength of various muscle groups with age, especially in active and inactive people. Thus, age- and gender-specific norms for strength and muscular endurance are needed. It would be useful if these norms could be related to minimal and acceptable levels for independence. It is interesting that many exercise programs for the aged emphasize aerobic activities when the higher incidence of falls and changes in the neuromuscular system suggest that strength training should also be included to reduce some of these age-related problems.

In general, the activities selected for the elderly will depend on the number and type(s) of limitations they possess. For example, if an older person has a problem with balance, exercise can be performed with some sort of support (sitting, lying on the floor, standing while holding a chair, or in warm water). The usual limitations of the aged generally preclude activities involving bodily contact, rapid or complicated movements, sharp turns, excessive competition, and environmental extremes (heat, cold, or altitude).[31] Table 5–4 describes different types of exercise suitable for the elderly and gives examples of how programs can be modified in relation to characteristics of many older people.[32]

PROGRESSION. Because the older adult is generally less adaptable, more time should be spent at each level of exercise to allow for a more complete adaptation before increasing frequency, duration, or intensity. Due to the potential problems associated with high-intensity exercise, it is usually better to exercise longer, more often, or both. Nevertheless, increases in any of these three important components of training should be made gradually and without major changes in the total amount of work done.

OTHER CONSIDERATIONS. People tend to become less active with advancing age. Cunningham et al. studied the activity patterns of 1695 men, aged 20 to 70 years, and found that their frequency of participation in active leisure time activities decreased with age.[8] More importantly, the average and peak energy expenditures also declined. Although part of these reductions in activity might be associated with the effects of aging on the ability to exercise, there are also sociopsychologic factors to consider.

The general stereotype of the older person in North America is not one of an active individual. Young people are taught that a reduction in habitual activity is an inevitable process of aging.[21] The general population also believes that older people are less active than the older people say they are.[28] Thus, inactivity among the aged is perceived to be "natural."

There is also a problem in perception among the elderly themselves. Sedentary people over the age of 50 years tend to have a distorted image of their bodies, i.e., they feel broader and heavier than they actually are.[33] Sidney and Shephard asked Canadians over age 65 years if they felt that they got enough physical activity.[28] Although most individuals said that they had more than enough and were more active than other persons in their age group, most respondents were below average in their level of fitness when tested on the treadmill. Thus, older people appear to believe that their activity levels are adequate and do not perceive the need to do more, that is, that they are just as active as their friends. Unfortunately, they are probably correct. Some of this perception problem may be due to the fact that results from

TABLE 5–4. **Medical-Physiological Considerations in Prescribing Exercise for the Elderly and Examples of Possible Modifications**

Characteristic	Example of a Possible Modification
Greater chance of diseases that put patients at high risk	Increased monitoring for safety. Changes depend on limitations (e.g., avoid intense isometrics and Valsalva maneuver in patients with hypertension)
Lower cardiovascular ability	Start at lower work loads
Less ability to perform moderate to high-intensity exercise	Decrease intensity and allow patients to select their own pace
Less able to adapt to and recover from exercise	Longer warm-up and cool-down periods
Reduced adaptability to training (degree and/or rate of improvement)	More gradual progression in frequency, duration, and intensity of exercise
Muscle weakness	Moderate strength training
Increased fatiguability	Short intervals with more rest periods
Degenerative bone, joint, and tendon problems	No activities with bodily contact
Increased susceptibility to injury and soreness	No fast turns or movements
Poorer flexibility	Emphasize stretching
Poorer coordination and balance	Hold on to chair and exercise while seated or supine; exercise in warm water
Impaired vision and hearing	Exercise on a stationary bicycle
Senile gait disorder and foot problems	Use supportive, shock-absorbing shoes with good traction

most fitness tests are compared to "average" values. Even though an average rating may not reflect an acceptable or desirable level, a person might feel that average is adequate and see no reason to take corrective action. Because people of all ages tend to overestimate what they do and to underestimate what they eat, this inaccurate self-perception is probably not limited to the elderly.

Coupled with the stereotype that one is not supposed to be active and the fact that there is lack of encouragement to become active, the attitudes and perceptions previously mentioned promote a sedentary lifestyle for the aging adult. As a result, the distorted stereotype is reinforced and a vicious cycle is created. Unfortunately, many older people feel that they have little or no control over the aging process and therefore do not try to prevent or delay many of the functional losses that occur.[34,36] Increasing the habitual activity of the elderly might reinforce the idea that they are capable of doing more. If they then attempt to do more, the downward

spiral of the vicious cycle might be reversed. Perhaps by emphasizing the possible relationships between desirable fitness levels and independence, by giving fitness tests that evaluate those factors important to health and well-being, and by showing the elderly the types and amounts of activity needed to maintain functional ability, these perceptions can be changed and the overall health of the older population improved.

Several sociocultural factors can influence how well the elderly will accept and participate in exercise programs. The experiences, lifestyle, beliefs, and attitudes of young people today are not the same as those of older people. In other words, older individuals have different values and norms and may not easily accept those of a young exercise leader or physician. As an example, an older woman may feel uncomfortable exercising in a class and wearing shorts, leotards, or even slacks. Older people also tend to be more inhibited. Therefore, these feelings and inhibitions should be considered when planning exercise programs.

Finally, it should be remembered that exercise is a form of social activity for people of all ages. Exercise sessions should emphasize fun, enjoyment, social contact, and regular participation more than fitness, performance, or health, even though these benefits might and should result.

TRAINABILITY OF THE ELDERLY

Aging is characterized by a loss in number, size, and performance of functional units within the body and by a reduced adaptability to physiologic stimuli. Thus, it is logical that the adaptability to training is also impaired with age. In fact, many training studies have shown that older humans and animals require more time to improve and that less improvement occurs in such variables as strength, $\dot{V}_{O_2max}$, mitochondrial volume in muscle, and activity of oxidative enzymes.[20,30]

There are differences of opinion among researchers whether trainability is affected by age. Some investigators state that the elderly can adapt because significant improvements occur with training.[9] On the other hand, because the extent and rate of improvement are less than in younger people, other authors believe that the elderly have less adaptability.[30] This controversy is confused further by the fact that most training programs for the elderly are less strenuous, i.e., they do not require either the same absolute (e.g., running at 6 mph) or relative (75% $\dot{V}_{O_2max}$) work loads as those for younger people. Thus, it is difficult to discuss trainability unless similar programs are given to young and old alike and then a direct comparison is made.

Nevertheless, the main goal of an exercise program is not to train the elderly to become athletes. Improved psychologic and physiologic functioning are the usual results of systematic, progressive programs of increased exercise. Although some of these changes may not be as great or come as rapidly, especially in older persons who have been sedentary for many years, self-sufficiency and the ability to move with relative ease are attainable and are probably more important for daily living and independence than the high maximal aerobic power often seen in those who train intensely to improve their fitness. Those involved with the older patient should emphasize that the *process* of being active is more important than the *product* of being fit. That is, some people can train regularly and intensely but not improve their strength or endurance very much, whereas others 1) may train irregularly and get marked improvements or 2) do not train at all and are still fitter and can perform better. The important thing to remember is that at any age it is possible to improve the ability to exercise.[34]

REFERENCES

1. Adrian, M.J.: Flexibility in the aging adult. *In* Exercise and Aging: The Scientific Basis. Edited by E.L. Smith, and R.C. Serfass. Hillside, NJ, Enslow Publishing, 1981.
2. American College of Sports Medicine: Guidelines for Graded Exercise Testing and Exercise Prescription. 4th Ed. Philadelphia, Lea & Febiger, 1991.
3. American Medical Association Council on Scientific Affairs: Indications and contraindications for exercise testing. JAMA, *246*:1015, 1981.
4. Åstrand, I.: Degree of strain during building work as related to individual work capacity. Ergonomics, *10*:293, 1967.
5. Balke, B.: Prescribing physical activity. *In* Sports Medicine. Edited by A.J. Ryan, and F.L. Allman. New York, Academic Press, 1974.
6. Borkan, G., and Norris, A.: Fat redistribution and the changing body dimensions of the adult male. Hum. Biol., *49*:495, 1977.
7. Bortz, W.M.: Disuse and aging. JAMA, *248*:1203, 1982.
8. Cunningham, D.A., et al.: Active leisure time activities as related to age among males in a total population. J. Gerontol., *23*:551, 1968.
9. deVries, H.A.: Physiology of physical conditioning for the elderly. *In* Guide to Fitness after Fifty. Edited by R. Harris, and L.J. Frankel. New York, Plenum Press, 1977.
10. Durnin, J., and Womersley, J.: Body fat assessed from total density and its estimation from skinfold thickness: measurements on 481 men and women aged from 61 to 72 years. Br. J. Nutr., *32*:77, 1974.
11. Fitts, R.H.: Aging and skeletal muscle. *In* Exercise and Aging: The Scientific Basis. Edited by E.L. Smith, and R.C. Serfass. Hillside, NJ, Enslow Publishing, 1981.
12. Haskell, W.: Factors influencing estimated oxygen uptake during exercise testing soon after myocardial infarction. Am. J. Cardiol., *50*:299, 1982.

13. Holloszy, J.O.: Exercise, health and aging. A need for more information. Med. Sci. Sport Exerc., *15*:1, 1983.
14. Jackson, A., and Pollock, M.: Generalized equations for predicting body density of men. Br. J. Nutr., *40*:497, 1978.
15. Jackson, A., and Pollock, M.: Steps toward the development of generalized equations for predicting body composition in adults. Can. J. Appl. Sports Sci., *7*:189, 1982.
16. Jackson, A., Pollock, M., and Ward, A.: Generalized equations for predicting body density of women. Med. Sci. Sport Exerc., *12*:175, 1980.
17. Kasser, I.S., and Bruce, R.A.: Comparative effects of aging and coronary heart disease on submaximal and maximal exercise. Circulation, *39*:759, 1969.
18. Larsson, L.: Morphological and functional characteristics of the aging skeletal muscle in man. Acta Physiol. Scand. Suppl., *457*, 1978.
19. Morse, C.E., and Smith, E.L.: Physical activity programming for the aged. *In* Exercise and Aging: The Scientific Basis. Edited by E.L. Smith, and R.C. Serfass. Hillside, NJ, Enslow Publishing, 1981.
20. Orlander, J., and Aniansson, A.: Effects of physical training on skeletal muscle metabolism and ultrastructure in 70 to 75-year-old men. Acta Physiol. Scand., *19*:149, 1980.
21. Ostrow, C., Jones, D.C., and Spiker, D.D.: Age role expectations and sex role expectations for selected sport activities. Res. Q. Exerc. Sport, *52*:216, 1981.
22. Pollock, M., et al.: Prediction of body density in young and middle-aged men. J. Appl. Physiol., *40*:300, 1976.
23. Pollock, M., and Jackson, A.: Research progress in validation of clinical methods of assessing body composition. Med. Sci. Sport Exerc., *6*:606, 1984.
24. Reddan, W.: Respiratory system and aging. *In* Exercise and Aging: The Scientific Basis. Edited by E.L. Smith, and R.C. Serfass. Hillside, NJ, Enslow Publishing, 1981.
25. Schlenker, E.: Nutrition in Aging. St. Louis, Mosby College Publishing, 1984.
26. Shephard, R.J.: Physical Activity and Aging. Chicago, Year Book, 1978.
27. Shock, N.W., et al.: Normal Human Aging: The Baltimore Longitudinal Study on Aging. NIH Publication No. 84-2450. Washington, D.C., U.S. Department of Health and Human Services, 1984.
28. Sidney, K., and Shephard, R.J.: Activity patterns of elderly men and women. J. Gerontol., *32*:25, 1977.
29. Sidney, K., and Shephard, R.J.: Maximum and submaximum exercise tests in men and women in the seventh, eighth, and ninth decades of life. J. Appl. Physiol., *43*:280, 1977.
30. Skinner, J.S.: Aging and performance. *In* Limiting Factors of Physical Performance. Edited by J. Keul. Stuttgart, Thieme, 1973.
31. Skinner, J.S.: Body Energy. Mountain View, CA, Anderson World, 1981.
32. Skinner, J.S.: Exercise programmes for the over 60s. Recreational Healthcare, *3*:4, 1990.
33. Skinner, J.S.: The cardiovascular system with aging and exercise. *In* Physical Activity and Aging. Edited by D. Brunner, and E. Jokl. Basel, Karger, 1970.
34. Skinner, J.S., Tipton, C.M., and Vailas, A.C.: Exercise, physical training and the aging process. *In* Lectures on Gerontology. Vol. 1B. Edited by A. Viidik. London, Academic Press, 1982.
35. Skrobak-Kaczynski, J., and Andersen, K.: The effect of a high level of habitual physical activity in the regulation of fatness during aging. Int. Arch. Occup. Environ. Health, *36*:41, 1975.
36. Smith, E.L.: Age: The interaction between nature and nurture. *In* Exercise and Aging: The Scientific Basis. Edited by E.L. Smith, and R.C. Serfass. Hillside, NJ, Enslow Publishing, 1981.
37. Smith, E.L., and Gilligan, C.: Physical activity prescription for the older adult. Physician Sportsmed., *11*:91, 1983.
38. Smith, E.L., and Gilligan, C.: Exercise, sport, and physical activity for the elderly. *In* Sport and Aging. Edited by B. McPherson. Champaign, IL, Human Kinetics, 1986.
39. Smith, E.L., Sempos, C.T., and Purvis, R.W.: Bone mass and strength decline with age. *In* Exercise and Aging: The Scientific Basis. Edited by E.L. Smith, and R.C. Serfass. Hillside, NJ, Enslow Publishing, 1981.
40. Smith, E.L., and Serfass, R.C. (eds.): Exercise and Aging: The Scientific Basis. Hillside, NJ, Enslow Publishing, 1981.
41. Stoedefalke, K.G.: Motivating and sustaining the older adult in an exercise program. Topics Geriatr. Rehabil., *1*:78, 1985.
42. Thomas, S., et al.: Protocols and reliability of maximal oxygen uptake in the elderly. Can. J. Sport Sci., *12*:144, 1987.
43. Womersley, J., et al.: Influence of muscular development, obesity and age on the fat-free mass of adults. J. Appl. Physiol., *41*:223, 1976.

6
CHAPTER

Importance of Environmental Factors for Exercise Testing and Exercise Prescription

by

Kent B. Pandolf

The clinical use of exercise testing to evaluate an individual's cardiorespiratory reserve and to enable the appropriate prescription of aerobic activity has attained wide medical acceptance. The physiologic stress that results from the metabolic intensity imposed by exercise, however, is only one consideration in the testing and prescription process. An equally important stress to consider is that imposed by the environment (heat, cold, altitude, and air quality). Both exercise and environment alter the physiologic responses of the cardiorespiratory and thermoregulatory systems. These environmental factors, either singly or in combination with exercise, can result in potentially hazardous health conditions.

TEMPERATURE REGULATION AND ENERGY BALANCE

The control mechanisms of temperature regulation within the human body for dealing with overcooling (cold stress) are not as effective as those for regulation against overheating (heat stress). Consequently, humans are thought of as tropical animals. Such behavioral modifications as increased food intake and adequate clothing are typical human reactions to overcooling. In contrast, the control mechanisms for thermoregulation are primarily structured to protect the body against overheating. This fact becomes readily apparent when one considers that variations in core temperature greater than $\pm 4°C$ are associated with reductions in physiologic and psychologic performance, whereas deviations of about $+6°C$ or $-12°C$ from $37°C$ (normal deep body temperature) are usually lethal. Combined exercise and heat stress can result in greater strain on the thermoregulatory system than either stress alone, whereas exercise stress may counteract cold stress and result in less overcooling. Fortunately, the human thermoregulatory system has a remarkable ability to maintain physiologic control through appropriate adjustments over an extremely wide range of different heat productions, heat losses, and environmental temperatures.

Physical exercise dramatically alters the rate of metabolic energy (heat) production (M), with resultant physiologic adjustments for heat loss. Heavy exercise can result in a metabolic energy production in excess of 30 times the basal rate. The three major physical avenues of heat loss and attempted energy balance depend primarily on the particular environmental conditions, and are radiation (R), convection (C), and evaporation (E). The classic energy balance equation for evaluating heat gain or heat loss from the body is $S = M - (\pm W) + Q_s \pm (R + C) - E$, in which S = rate of body heat storage; M = rate of metabolic energy

The views, opinions, and/or findings contained in this report are those of the author and should not be construed as an official Department of the Army position, policy, or decision, unless so designated by other official documentation.

(heat) production estimated from measured oxygen uptake ($\dot{V}_{O_2}$); W = mechanical work, either concentric (positive) or eccentric (negative) exercise; Q_s = rate of solar radiative energy absorbed (differentiates between heat loss in sunlight and that lost from the skin in an environment without solar flux); R + C = rate of radiant and convective energy exchanges; and E = rate of evaporative loss.

The level of exercise and the particular environmental conditions determine the rate of sweat production by the body and dictate a certain required rate of evaporative cooling (E_{req}). The maximal evaporative capacity of the environment (E_{max}), however, determines the maximal possible evaporative loss. For individuals exercising outdoors, the solar radiant load becomes an important consideration. The three separate sources of solar radiation to consider are the intensity of direct sunlight, intensity of diffuse radiation on a horizontal plane, and intensity of any terrain-reflected sunlight on a vertical plane. In addition to the three major avenues for heat gain and loss, energy exchange may occur by respiratory nonevaporative heat loss, insensible evaporative loss through the lungs and skin, and conductive energy exchange (K). Although these are generally less important physical channels for energy exchange during exercise, K becomes of major importance during swimming because of the greater heat transfer capacity of water.

The relative importance of the three major avenues of heat gain or heat loss can be altered by the particular ambient temperature (T_a) and by other environmental factors. Figure 6–1 illustrates the interaction of these avenues of heat exchange for a wide range of T_a through the computer prediction of energy exchange for an exercising runner assumed to weigh 70 kg and wearing shorts, T-shirt, and running shoes. The runner is assumed to be exercising at 66% $\dot{V}_{O_2max}$, which for an average man would be 2.0 L·min^{-1} ($\sim$700 W). The T_a range is from 5 to 35°C, all at a relative humidity (rh) of 60%. All running is done in the sun; the absorbed solar heat load was taken to be 150 W.

The mean skin temperature ($\overline{T}_{sk}$) would be expected to rise ($\sim$15°C) as T_a increases. This figure clearly shows that R+C exchanges account for approximately 70% of the heat dissipation at the lower T_a, whereas E is of major importance at higher T_a in order to maintain the same rate of heat exchange. The increased gradient between $\overline{T}_{sk}$ and T_a at the lower ambient temperatures potentiates the R+C heat exchange. In contrast, $\overline{T}_{sk}$ is closer to T_a at the higher ambient temperatures, reducing the importance of R+C heat exchange. Changes in relative humidity, wind velocity, cloud cover, and exercise intensity will alter the interactions among these major avenues of heat exchange, but to a far lesser degree than changes in T_a. In 1938, Nielsen demonstrated the increased importance of R+C heat exchange at lower T_a and the greater importance of E at higher T_a.[73]

It is beyond the scope of this chapter to present a detailed essay on temperature regulation and exercise. The reader is directed to other reviews and books.[43,44,61,67,70,92,107]

EXPOSURE TO HIGH ENVIRONMENTAL TEMPERATURES

Human Physiologic Responses to Heat

The two physiologic systems primarily concerned with dynamic regulation against overheating are the cardiovascular and sweat systems. The main function of the former is the transport of heat from the deep body to the surface. Sweat glands are responsible for producing and secreting adequate amounts of sweat for the required evaporative cooling at the skin surface. During exercise, regulation by these systems is increasingly challenged when the T_a rises from temperate ($\sim$22°C) to hotter conditions.

Metabolic (exercise-induced) and environmental heat stress can result in normal or expected physiologic responses to the particular stress, but may also produce a variety of abnormal heat disorders, as

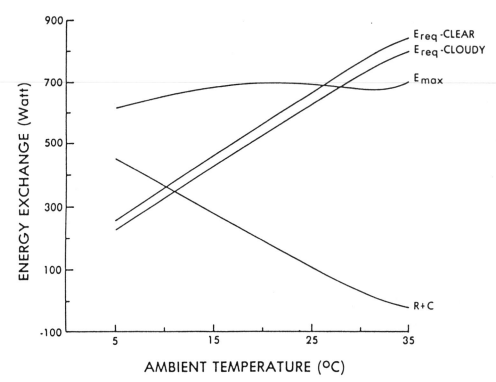

Fig. 6-1. *Avenues of heat exchange during exercise for a wide range of ambient temperatures.*

shown in Figure 6-2. Although the primary purpose of this section is not to detail the pathologic manifestations of excessive heat exposure, a few comments concerning the prevention of these heat disorders are warranted. Exercise-induced heat exhaustion can be minimized by providing proper prior heat acclimation, by grading

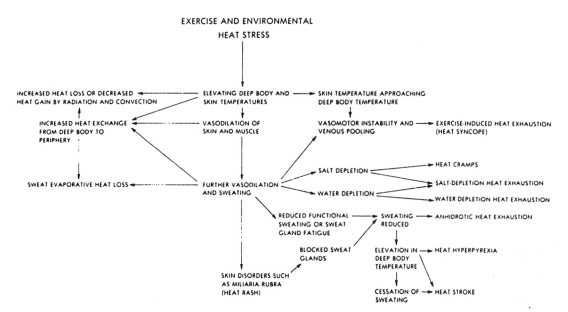

Fig. 6-2. *Mechanisms of thermoregulation during exercise and environmental heat stress, and causes for the various heat disorders. (Modified from Lind.[64])*

the exercise to consider hot climatic extremes, and by avoiding sudden postural changes or maintenance of upright static exercise situations. Obviously, heat cramps and salt-depletion heat exhaustion can be prevented by adequate salt (10 to 15 g/day) and water intake, with the latter of extreme importance in avoiding water-depletion heat exhaustion. The two former disorders, however, are more prevalent in chronically hot climates where salt and water needs are enhanced; caution should be used to avoid excessive salt intake. Anhidrotic heat exhaustion, which is related to reduced functional sweating, has been linked to certain skin disorders such as heat rash. Heat rash has been associated with exercise-heat intolerance, as depicted by elevations in core temperature and reductions in performance time.[78,79] Heat intolerance was demonstrated with as little as 20% of the body surface involved and persisted for up to 3 weeks after the clinical rash had resolved. Heat rash is prevented by drying the skin when possible and by wearing clean, dry clothing that allows unimpeded evaporation. Heat hyperpyrexia and heat stroke present dramatic elevations of core temperature, normally in the range of 41 to 42°C. The former disorder is usually characterized by the lower core temperatures in this range, with the individual still capable of sweating; the latter condition presents the higher core temperatures and generalized anhidrosis. Elevations in core temperature, however, may not be causally related to these disorders, because both marathon runners and patients with passively induced hyperthermia tolerate core temperatures of 41.8 to 42°C with minimal side-effects.[15,66] Both heat hyperpyrexia and heat stroke can be prevented by adapting exercise to the climate, by ensuring proper heat acclimation and, most importantly, by screening for individuals with a past history of heat illness.

Cardiovascular and Thermoregulatory Adjustments to Exercise in Dry and Humid Heat

EFFECTS OF SOLAR HEAT LOAD. The importance of quantifying the physiologic effects of solar radiation becomes apparent when exercise prescriptions for outdoor environments are considered. The effect of simulated solar heat load in hot-dry (40°C, 32% rh) and hot-wet (35°C, 75% rh) environments has been reported for heat-acclimated men while walking at 1.34 m·sec^{-1} (0 and 5% grade).[80] Evaluation of solar load by copper manikin predicted the delivery of an effective 300 W (semi-nude) and 120 W (clothed) of radiant heat load to the skin. Individuals were evaluated with or without this solar load while wearing either shorts, socks, and running shoes (semi-nude) or a slightly heavier clothing ensemble. After 100 minutes of exercise, final physiologic responses were greater while exercising with solar load (range of mean differences: heart rate (HR), 22 to 42 beats·min^{-1}; rectal temperature (T_{re}), 0.45 to 1.48°C; sweat rate ($\dot{m}_{sw}$), 145 to 314 g·m^{-2}·hr^{-1}). At more strenuous exercise intensities, the effects of solar heat load are even more pronounced in elevating these cardiovascular and thermoregulatory responses, and may necessitate marked alterations in outdoor exercise prescriptions.

PROBLEMS WITH FLUID BALANCE. In general, dehydration degrades endurance exercise performance, whereas there is absolutely no evidence that dehydration can benefit exercise performance.[96] In addition, man does not appear to adapt to chronic dehydration. Physical work capacity is diminished even at marginal levels of dehydration (1%), with alterations in $\dot{V}_{O_2max}$ requiring at least a 2% deficit in body water loss. Greater body water deficits are associated with progressively larger reductions in physical work capacity. Furthermore, dehydration results in larger reductions in physical work capacity in a hot as compared to a thermally neutral environment. Prolonged exercise that places large demands on aerobic metabolism is more likely to be adversely affected by dehydration than short-term exercise.

As reported by Adolph, the increment in T_{re} increases predictably as percent dehydration (water deficit) increases.[1] These data show that T_{re} rises about 0.2°C for each 1% increase in dehydration or an increment of 1°C for each 5% dehydration. The HR was found to increase about 6 beats·min^{-1} for each 1% increase in dehydration.

Strydom and Holdsworth report differences in physiologic responses to standard heat stress when individuals are kept fully hydrated rather than being allowed to drink ad libitum.[100] Drinking ad libitum was associated with higher T_{re}, slightly higher HR, and lower $\dot{m}_{sw}$. Thus, individuals exercising in the heat should be encouraged to drink in excess of their normal desired amounts. When exercise is expected to cause an increase of more than 2% in dehydration, target HR modifications are desirable.

ROLE OF CARDIORESPIRATORY TRAINING AND PHYSICAL FITNESS. The importance of training and cardiorespiratory physical fitness on physiologic responses to exercise in the heat and on the rate of heat acclimation is controversial, but there are several detailed reviews on this subject.[5,27,75] Although most authors agree that training in a cool environment improves exercise-heat tolerance, the degree of improvement remains controversial. To achieve optimal gains, researchers suggest the use of intensive interval or continuous training at an intensity greater than 50% $\dot{V}_{O_2max}$.[26,48,68,91] Improvements in performance produced by mild to moderate training at less than 50% $\dot{V}_{O_2max}$ are questionable.[98] It seems that training must exceed 1 week; Gisolfi and Henane et al. report the best improvement occurs after 8 to 12 weeks.[26,48] It seems that training should increase $\dot{V}_{O_2max}$ by 15 to 20% to improve tolerance. Improvement in exercise-heat tolerance after appropriate training appears to apply to both dry and wet heat. Individuals with high $\dot{V}_{O_2max}$ values and such athletes as marathoners (whose endurance training programs cause high levels of body hyperthermia and regulatory sweating) seem to be at an advantage.

Another debatable issue is whether $\dot{V}_{O_2max}$ is related to either improved exercise-heat tolerance or to a more rapid rate of heat acclimation. Two different authors utilizing different climates independently report that an individual's $\dot{V}_{O_2max}$ accounts for 42 to 46% of the variability that determines the T_{re} level during 3 hours of exercise in the heat or the acclimation day for a plateau in T_{re}.[76,99] In contrast, other authors report insignificant relationships between $\dot{V}_{O_2max}$ and either exercise endurance or final T_{re}.[19,35,108] In most of the studies in which a lack of relationship was shown, however, relatively few subjects or homogeneously fit subjects were evaluated. The $\dot{V}_{O_2max}$, per se, may not be important, but the physiologic adaptations associated with various fitness levels may play a vital role in determining exercise-heat tolerance. For instance, improved aerobic fitness by endurance training must be associated with significant elevations in core temperature during the training process in order to improve exercise-heat tolerance.[5]

ADVANTAGES OF HEAT ACCLIMATION. Repeated exposure to heat while exercising results in a gradual acclimation, with improved physiologic performance and tolerance.[103] The physiologic improvements seen during the first 4 days are dramatic and acclimation is virtually complete after about 10 days. During acclimation, the major physiologic changes are a heightened sweating response, lowered HR, and lowered internal body temperature during exercise in the heat.[68,107] This series of changes is probably the result of increased blood volume, increased venous tone, and increased activity of the adrenopituitary system; lowered metabolic demands from repeated exposures; and possibly increased sweating activity either through a greater number of active sweat glands at a given $\overline{T}_{sk}$ or from greater activity per gland.[64,107] No single cause explains the adaptive process; acclimation probably results from the interplay of many mechanisms.

The full development of exercise-heat acclimation need not involve daily 24-hour exposure. A continuous, daily 100-minute period of exposure appears to produce an optimal response.[107] The acclimation response is somewhat specific to the particular climatic condition and exercise intensity; it appears to be well retained for 2 weeks after the last heat exposure, but is rapidly lost during the next 2 weeks.[104] Some authors, however, report greater retention of the acclimation benefits in physically trained persons than in sedentary individuals.[76]

CLOTHING INTERACTION. Traditionally, clothing has been decorative and protective.[106] During exercise in the heat, protective considerations may be far more important, e.g., black clothing and possibly other dark colors are usually associated with a greater solar radiative absorption than white or lighter colors. Generally, clothing serves as a physical barrier that reduces heat exchange by radiation and convection, and simultaneously lowers the maximal evaporative exchange to the environment. The more impermeable the clothing ensemble (e.g., a sweat suit or rubberized suit), the greater the reduction in evaporative heat loss and the associated increase in cardiovascular and thermoregulatory strain. From a comfort standpoint, cotton clothing is generally more effective than polyester during exercise in the heat.

In hot-wet environments, when T_a is less than $\overline{T}_{sk}$, exercising individuals should wear the least amount of clothing possible. When T_a is greater than $\overline{T}_{sk}$, some additional clothing may protect individuals from the ambient heat load, but will interfere more with body heat loss. In hot-dry environments, it is particularly advisable to wear loose fitting clothing that allows greater air flow between the skin and the environment, with resultant greater evaporative cooling. In either hot-wet or hot-dry environments, a thin layer of white clothing will markedly reduce the solar heat load and should be worn when exercising under the sun. Proper clothing helps to optimize endurance exercise performance in the heat. Associated concepts have been recently reviewed in detail elsewhere.[34]

Impact of Heat on Exercise Testing and Exercise Prescription

The exercise prescription often takes the form of a target HR, intended to be within "safe" limits and to provide a beneficial training stimulus. Heat stress is known to accelerate HR independently of the exercise stress, largely as a result of cutaneous vasodilation with an increased non-nutritive blood flow. During submaximal exercise of short duration (<1 hour), elevated HR is associated with a fall in stroke volume (SV). Cardiac output ($\dot{Q}$) and arteriovenous oxygen difference (AVD-O_2) are not altered comparing hot to neutral conditions, as long as venous return is maintained and the elevated HR does not approach maximal levels. Although the suggested modifications of exercise prescription given subsequently are mostly for outdoor environments, modifications are equally applicable when exercise testing or prescription is conducted indoors in a non-thermally controlled environment.

The American College of Sports Medicine (ACSM) has published a position stand on the prevention of thermal injuries during distance running based in part on the wet bulb, globe temperature (WBGT) index, which may also be adaptable for exercise testing and prescription.[3] For instance, when WBGT is greater than 28°C (82°F), the ACSM suggests that prolonged exercise be curtailed or rescheduled until a lower WBGT is prevalent. When the WBGT is at or below 28°C, the ACSM proposes the use of color-coded flags to alert individuals of the existing risk of thermal stress. A red flag denotes high risk and is associated with a WBGT of 23 to 28°C (73 to 82°F), whereas an amber flag represents moderate risk when WBGT is 18 to 20°C (65 to 73°F), and a green flag represents low risk when WBGT is below 18°C (65°F). These WBGT values are representative for individuals dressed in running shorts, shoes, and a T-shirt; different clothing systems would necessitate further adjustments in the WBGT values associated with each level of risk. Finally, the ACSM recommends that where environmental heat stress is prevalent, all exercise should begin in the early morning (before 8 a.m.) or in the evening (after 6 p.m.) to lessen the effects of the solar load.

It has been shown in young male subjects (~21 years of age) that after 30 minutes of moderate exercise (40% $\dot{V}_{O_2max}$), HR increases predictably about 1 beat·min^{-1} for each 1°C increase in T_a (dry heat) above temperate (24° versus 44°, 54°C).[77] Because heat tolerance is generally reduced in older individuals, the cardiovascular strain can also be expected to be somewhat greater, in part because of a suspected inability to partition and regulate blood flow effectively.

Recently, more quantitative predictions of equilibrium exercise HR response were made for typical hot-dry (40°C, 20% rh) and hot-humid (35°C, 75% rh) environments in contrast to a temperate (21°C, 50% rh) environment.[28–30] It was assumed that the subject weighed 70 kg, wore shorts and a T-shirt, exercised at 700 W, and was not heat acclimated. When compared to values in a temperate climate, the HR was about 30 beats·min^{-1} higher (~1.5 beats·min^{-1} per 1°C rise in T_a) in the hot-dry and 50 beats·min^{-1} higher (~3.5 beats·min^{-1} per 1°C rise in T_a) in the hot-wet climate. Thus, whereas adjustments are necessary in dry climates, particular concern should be given to the target HR in humid climates. These prediction equations should be utilized for the *individualized* adjustments of the exercise prescription target HR when considering the particular environmental conditions, exercise intensity, and clothing interactions.[28,29] A mathematical model based on the above prediction equations has been developed to prognosticate human performance in the heat and may be useful in the establishment of the exercise prescription.[81] This prediction model allows for the calculation of sustainable exercise-rest cycles, the maximal single exercise time (if appropriate), and the associated water requirements.

Further reductions in exercise intensity and target HR are necessary when the individual becomes significantly dehydrated (>2%) or exercises on a hot-clear (solar load) day. It is suggested that target HR responses be adjusted and re-evaluated periodically to consider seasonal effects. Obviously, when the level of environmental stress necessitates precautions during exercise for healthy persons, exercise activities for cardiovascularly impaired individuals should be curtailed.

EXPOSURE TO LOW ENVIRONMENTAL TEMPERATURES

Human Physiologic Responses to Cold

Human physiologic defenses to combat cold are limited mainly to alterations in peripheral circulation to reduce heat loss and to increase heat production. The initial response to cold stress is peripheral vasoconstriction and deep splanchnic vasodilation to decrease heat exchange from the deep body to the periphery. The next major response involves increased activity of skeletal muscles, producing increased muscle tone and subsequently shivering, and increased metabolic heat production (three to four times the resting level). Moderate exercise easily results in a 10-fold increase in heat production and can be an effective counteractant to moderate cold stress, if carried out intelligently. The regulatory adaptations to cold stress and their associations with muscular exercise are illustrated in Figure 6–3. Also presented are the peripheral and central cold disorders that may result from improper physiologic regulation.

The pathophysiology of peripheral and central cold injury is not a major consideration of this chapter. However, a few comments concerning prevention of these cold disorders during muscular exercise are warranted. The pathophysiology of cold disorders can be categorized by either non-freezing (muscle cramps, chilblains, and immersion/trench hand or foot) and freezing cold injuries (frostnip and frostbite) or whole body hypothermia. A major consideration in prevention is an adequate definition of the cold stress, i.e., the particular ambient temperature and

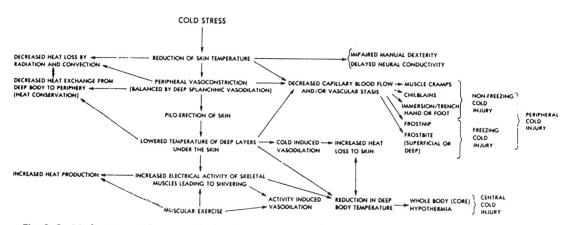

Fig. 6-3. *Mechanisms of thermoregulation during exercise and environmental cold stress, and causes for the various peripheral or central cold injuries.*

wind velocity, as well as any sweat on the skin or in the clothing. To provide maximal protection, clothing should be layered and thick and it *must* be kept dry. In the prevention of cold injuries, methods to enhance heat supply to the periphery must be considered. Auxiliary heating of the extremities through battery-charged gloves and socks (5 W per hand or foot) should help maintain safe extremity temperatures. Use of hot or alcoholic drinks produces peripheral vasodilation and added circulatory heat input. Moreover, alcohol increases the rate of deep body heat loss, thus enhancing the risk of hypothermia.[32,33] Gradual acclimation to cold over 2 to 3 weeks may induce peripheral physiologic changes that help the individual to resist local cold injury. Because exercisers seldom spend more than 2 to 10% of any given day outdoors and because exercise increases heat production, the risk of whole body hypothermia is minimal, provided the individual does not stay in the cold in a sweat-soaked state.

A variety of factors are known to alter cold tolerance.[59] Size and shape of the body alter heat loss to the environment. For a given cold stress, smaller individuals (children and women) must have a relatively greater heat production to maintain thermal equilibrium. In addition, short individuals who weigh the same as those taller lose less heat, principally because they have less exposed surface area (shorter arms, legs, and trunk). Another important factor is the thickness of subcutaneous fat deposits. Generally, subcutaneous fat acts as an effective insulator, with greater amounts being negatively related to the fall in skin or rectal temperature.[59] The advantages of increased subcutaneous fat are apparent for all types of cold exposure, but are particularly important in cold water immersion. Endurance training may be an important factor because regular exercise is known to result in hypertrophy and increased vascularization of skeletal muscle. More importantly, however, an increased level of maximal aerobic power allows an individual to sustain relatively higher exercise intensities, thus generating more heat. Respiratory heat losses can be considerable during exercise in extreme cold, with most of the loss occurring as evaporation to humidify the very dry cold air that is inhaled. The respiratory tree is sufficiently effective at heat exchange that there is almost no danger of freezing respiratory tissues, but severe drying may lead to cracking or bleeding during exercise at very low temperatures. Obviously, clothing is a crucial factor and should vary with the ambient temperature, wind velocity, solar load, and exercise level. Proper cold weather clothing should be wind resistant, but must provide adequate ventilation to reduce sweat accumulation. As mentioned previously, a multilayer system that can be opened or closed at the neck to eliminate or conserve heat is ideal for cold weather use. Proper protection of the face and extremities may be of greater concern.

Cardiovascular and Thermoregulatory Responses to Exercise in the Cold

Cooling of the body can result in marked systemic alterations.[49] The most apparent alteration is perhaps peripheral vasoconstriction, which leads to both a reduction in local circulation and reduced perfusion of various vascular beds, producing vascular stasis and local tissue anoxia. Initially, there is a paradoxical increase in HR, pulmonary ventilation, and mean arterial pressure. As deep body temperature drops, however, HR, ventilation, and blood pressure fall. Neurohumoral activation leads to release of the anterior pituitary hormones and catecholamines to conserve body heat further and perhaps to produce a slight "non-shivering" thermogenesis. Other than physical exercise, however, the major reflex response for increased heat production involves increased muscle tone and shivering. In certain circumstances, cold-induced vasodilation is seen in superficial capillaries of the limbs when $\overline{T}_{sk}$ falls below about 18°C.[63] This nervous reflex appears to act as a primary mechanism in protecting peripheral tissue from freezing injury.

Mild to moderate cold stress of a less prolonged nature (~1 hour) is more likely to be encountered by the exerciser than is prolonged severe cold stress. Even less severe cold stress alters cardiovascular performance and produces circulatory changes that tend to augment myocardial oxygen requirements, thus placing some individuals at added risk while exercising. For instance, mild cold stress (15°C) during rest and light exercise causes a consistently higher total peripheral resistance (TPR), higher systemic arterial pressure, and greater left ventricular work in individuals with and without coronary heart disease (CHD).[22] These increases in TPR occurred in the absence of reflex bradycardia; $\dot{Q}$ and SV were not altered by cold exposure.

Exposure of the face to a moderate cold stress (4°C) has been associated with bradycardia, resulting from a vagal reflex through trigeminal nerve stimulation.[59] Sympathetic nervous system stimulation produces a rise in systolic and diastolic pressures. Thus, facial exposure to cold winds and whole body exposure might be expected to precipitate angina in an individual with CHD. Exercise would only accentuate this risk by demanding further increases in left ventricular work and myocardial oxygen demands.

Cold Acclimation or Adaptive Habituation

The human physiologic adjustments to prolonged cold stress are less effective than those to heat. Cold acclimatization or acclimation must be differentiated from adaptation or habituation. Acclimatization and acclimation are functional alterations established over days or weeks in response, respectively, to either complex, natural environmental factors or artificially controlled, usually simple environmental factors.[13,21] In contrast, adaptation suggests physiologic changes that develop over generations and are genetically transmitted to help promote survival in hostile environments.[21] Habituation to cold stress seems to be associated more with nervous system regulation. Boutelier states that there are two types of habituation: specific or local habituation, which involves familiarization of a specific region of the body to a repeated cold stimulus, and general habituation, which results in a lowering of total body responses to a repeated stimulus.[13] The physiologic adjustments during human adaptation or acclimation to cold have recently been reviewed elsewhere.[109]

PROPOSED MECHANISMS FOR HUMAN COLD ACCLIMATION. It is difficult to demonstrate definitive evidence of a general (or central) physiologic acclimatization or acclimation to cold in humans. Some authors report a reduced metabolic rate (~20 to 25%) due to less shivering after repeated cold exposures[16,60] other authors describing an increased metabolic response ($\sim 20\%$).[55,97] Newman reports a reduction in shivering but a constant metabolic rate with repeated cold exposure, suggesting the development of non-shivering thermogenesis.[71,72] These divergent findings may reflect two patterns of general acclimatization or acclimation: the insulative type, with a lower peripheral tissue conductance and lower metabolic rate, and the metabolic type, with a higher metabolic response and warmer extremities, illustrative of peripheral circulatory adjustments.[13] In contrast to the question of central acclimation, local or peripheral acclimation to cold (particularly in the hands) appears to be quite possible. Upon repeated exposure of the hands to a given cold stress for a few weeks, increased local $\overline{T}_{sk}$ and blood flow have been noted, with improved mobility of the fingers and improved tactility (i.e., less numbness).[59] More recently, Young et al. demonstrated that repeated cold water immersion (5 times/week for 5 consecutive weeks) at 18°C for 90 minutes produces acclimation to cold air (5°C, 30% rh) in humans.[110] This cold acclimation is primarily of the insulative type in that $\overline{T}_{sk}$ is lower, probably because of greater sympathetic nervous system activation mediating stronger cutaneous vasoconstriction. The existence of this insulative type of cold acclimation does not necessarily refute the existence of a metabolic or a hypothermic type of cold acclimation in humans.

ADAPTIVE HABITUATION TO COLD IN MAN. Cold adaptation has been studied during continuous exposure to moderate cold and during intermittent exposure to severe cold. Evaluations of both primitive native and Caucasian populations show that continuous exposure to moderate cold reduces shivering; this functional alteration seems to be the essential feature of cold adaptation.[59] LeBlanc speculates that this type of adaptation is linked to some form of habituation.[59] Other investigators suggest a greater oxidation of free fatty acids, utilized metabolically as ketone bodies, during continuous exposure to moderate cold.[54]

The adaptive alterations of humans to intermittent exposure to severe cold appear to be somewhat different. Eskimo and Caucasian populations display enhanced peripheral circulation and reduced cold sensation upon immersion of the hand in cold water (~ 10°C) or exposure to -22°C cold air.[59] Reduced activation of the sympathetic nervous system is also evident from the markedly lower systolic blood pressure during exposure. Again, the implication of changes in nervous system regulation suggests some form of adaptive habituation.

Impact of Cold on Exercise Testing and Exercise Prescription

Upon exposure, cutaneous cold receptor stimulation through afferent nerve impulses leads to sympathetic reflex activity; this activity can result in an increased TPR, arterial pressure, myocardial inotropic state, and cardiac work during rest or exercise.[22,62,69] These altered responses were observed even during very mild cold stress (~ 15°C) in one detailed series of experiments.[22] Even localized facial exposure to moderate cold (4°C) has been associated with vagally mediated, reflex bradycardia and sympathetically increased systolic and diastolic blood pressures.[59] Thus, both localized and more total body cold receptor activity can lower the threshold and provoke an attack of angina pectoris in individuals with CHD, the result of an increase in TPR and arterial pressure, and the consequent augmentation of myocardial oxygen demands. No evidence has been found that coronary vasoconstriction, per se, contributes to the development of myocardial hypoxia during cold stress. During cold exposure, exercise would only further increase the work of the heart through added myocardial oxygen requirements. Thus, an individual with CHD would be at even greater risk because of far less functional myocardial reserve capacity.

Local or total body exposure to cold results in systemic responses that are indicative of an activated sympathetic nervous system. Therefore, an added screening test for individual cold sensitivity may become necessary if the individual is expected to be exposed to even mild cold stress ($\sim 15°C$ or less). The cold pressor test, which was designed for detecting persons who were potentially hypertensive, might be utilized effectively to classify individuals in terms of the degree of reactivity to a cold stimulus.[50,105] During immersion of the hand in cold water, individual sympathetic activity can be graded by the rise in arterial pressure (systolic and diastolic), elevation of HR, and degree of systemic vasoconstriction, as implied by the reduction in $\overline{T}_{sk}$ of the immersed hand. Extreme reactivity would contraindicate exercising in the cold for those with signs of CHD.

The use of proper clothing should be stressed in the prescription of outdoor exercise in cold air. The two basic principles are that the clothing should be thick and multilayered, while providing adequate ventilation to keep it dry. All areas of the body (particularly the face, ears, neck, hands, and feet) should be covered adequately and kept warm. Special precautions should be used for those individuals at risk who employ swimming as a form of exercise. Swimming in unheated or improperly heated pools and in the ocean (50% of which is less than 20° C) should be approached with extreme caution.

EXPOSURE TO TERRESTRIAL ALTITUDE

Exercise Performance

MAXIMAL EXERCISE. Man cannot attain as high a maximal oxygen uptake ($\dot{V}_{O_2max}$) during exercise at high altitude. Results of many studies show a progressive reduction in $\dot{V}_{O_2max}$ with increasing altitude.[14] Grover reported this relationship in graphic form, a slightly modified version of which is illustrated in Figure 6–4.[37] A major alteration in $\dot{V}_{O_2max}$ does not occur between sea level and about 1500 m. Above 1500 m, it decreases about 3% per 300 m in this pooled group of fit and unfit men.[14] The decrement in $\dot{V}_{O_2max}$ for fit men only is approximately 2% per 300 m;

other authors report a greater decrement in more physically fit men.[38,93] The decrease in $\dot{V}_{O_2max}$ persists at that altitude, provided the level of cardiorespiratory physical fitness is not altered. Upon return from higher altitude, $\dot{V}_{O_2max}$ returns to the sea level value.

The greatest reduction in $\dot{V}_{O_2max}$ usually occurs during the first few days of altitude exposure, with a small but significant increase seen with persistent residence.[58] Hartley attributes the early reduction to the low arterial oxygen content and the persistent decrease to a reduction in maximal $\dot{Q}$.[45] Reduced $\dot{Q}_{max}$ results from a decrease in SV combined with a lower maximal HR. Maintenance of plasma volume at altitude may maintain ventricular filling pressure and prevent a decrease in SV.[36,39] An increase in vagal tone has been associated with the reduction in maximal HR.[36,46] Finally, $\dot{V}_{O_2max}$ at 4300 m was reduced by 30%, whereas $\dot{Q}_{max}$ decreased only 20%.[94] This disparity suggests the involvement of other factor(s). Grover suggests an association with reduced arterial oxygen saturation.[36] The cardiovascular adaptations to exercise at high altitude have recently been reviewed in detail.[40]

SUBMAXIMAL EXERCISE. Submaximal exercise performance is also reduced at altitude, but the relative impairment is not as great as that seen in the $\dot{V}_{O_2max}$.[36] At the same absolute submaximal intensity, performance is limited at high altitude. When endurance capacity at the same relative percent ($\sim 75\%$) $\dot{V}_{O_2max}$ was compared, endurance performance was markedly greater after 12 days at 4300 m.[65] Recently, endurance time at 4300 m for the same relative exercise intensity ($\sim 85\%$ $\dot{V}_{O_2max}$) increased by 60% after a 16-day sojourn.[51] Therefore, the same relative percentages of $\dot{V}_{O_2max}$ at sea level and high altitude may be physiologically unequal, i.e., a relatively higher exercise intensity appears necessary after chronic altitude exposure. In these same experiments, however, endurance times did not differ between sea level and acute altitude exposure (2 days) at the same relative percent $\dot{V}_{O_2max}$, suggesting different physio-

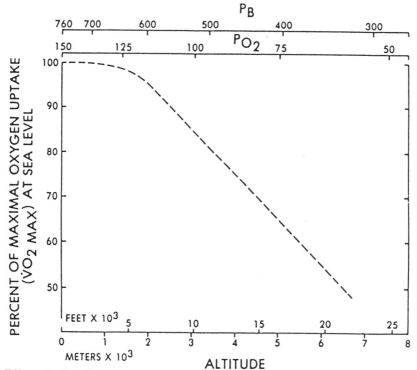

Fig. 6-4. *Effects of reduced partial pressure of oxygen at altitude on maximal oxygen uptake ($\dot{V}_{O_{2}max}$) when expressed as percent of ($\dot{V}_{O_{2}max}$) at sea level. (Modified from Grover.[37])*

logic adjustments with initial exposure to high altitude.[51,65] Some authors report a reduction in $\dot{Q}$ during rest and submaximal exercise after chronic exposure to altitude, whereas other investigators detail that the submaximal $\dot{Q}$ is similar to that found at sea level.[2,94] These findings seem to indicate that individual variability plays a major role in determining the physiologic responses to submaximal exercise at altitude. Within this framework, limitations are greater for acute than chronic altitude exposure. Whereas the limitations imposed by the cardiovascular system primarily alter maximal exercise responses at altitude, differences in the utilization rate of glycogen stores and anaerobic metabolism appear to influence submaximal exercise responses during both acute and chronic altitude exposure.

ACUTE AND SUBACUTE EXPOSURE TO HIGH ALTITUDE. The physiologic alterations at altitude that help to improve tissue oxygen delivery when oxygen availability is reduced may be classified into three separate stages: acute, subacute, and chronic adaptation. Acute adaptation occurs during the first 72 hours of exposure; subacute adaptations are seen over the next 10 to 11 days. Chronic adaptation to altitude involves changes observed after 2 weeks of exposure. Although the adaptations are presented as three distinct stages, they really represent a continuum of change with considerable individual overlap and variability.

The most prominent adaptation to acute exposure is an increased pulmonary ventilation ($\dot{V}_E$) at a given exercise $\dot{V}_{O_2}$.[9,42] This hyperpnea results in an elevated respiratory exchange ratio (R), reflective of increased CO_2 elimination from the lungs and an associated rise in blood pH.[9] In contrast to chronic altitude exposure, increased $\dot{Q}$ is noted during the first few days at altitude and is attributed mainly to an increase in HR.[37,42] These cardiopulmonary alterations are an attempt to enhance oxygen transport and delivery, and thus help to compensate for the reduction in oxygen pressure. These compensatory mechanisms are not adequate, however, and exercise performance is usually severely limited relative to the other two adaptive stages. Other factors that seem to be related to performance alterations are an uncompensated alkalosis, altered endocrine function, body fluid changes, and disturbed metabolic function.[9] During acute exposure, mountain sickness can develop with such symptoms as headache, lethargy, drowsiness, fatigue, sleep disturbances, loss of appetite, digestive disorders, and, less frequently, nausea and vomiting.[9,37] A more serious but rare disorder is high altitude pulmonary edema, associated with fluid accumulation in the lungs.[37]

The functional changes observed during subacute altitude exposure are also transient in nature.[42] The subacute stage is associated with adaptations that increase the oxygen-carrying capacity of the blood, i.e., increased hematocrit secondary to decreased plasma volume.[9,37,42] Although there may be greater blood oxygen content due to this hemoconcentration, these alterations are also associated with decreased blood flow and increased blood viscosity.[9,37] The second major change seen involves a decrease in submaximal and maximal $\dot{Q}$ attributable to a reduction in SV.[2,42] Kollias and Buskirk suggest that the reduction in plasma volume seen during this stage causes a reduction in SV via a decrease in ventricular filling.[58] A further transient increase in $\dot{V}_E$ (particularly at heavier exercise intensities) has been found during this adaptive stage and is referred to as ventilatory acclimatization.[9,18,56] At a constant $\dot{V}_{O_2}$, $\dot{V}_E$ at altitude may increase by nearly 100%. Other transient changes during the subacute stage of altitude adaptation might include a redistribution of blood flow from less to more vital areas of the body and functional alterations in the tissues possibly leading to increased capillary formation.

CHRONIC EXPOSURE TO HIGH ALTITUDE. Although the functional alterations seen during chronic exposure (~2 weeks) appear similar in many ways to those seen during subacute adaptation, Hannon and Vogel state that these functional alterations differ in four major respects.[42] "First, they develop far more slowly. Second, they are not transient; rather they approach and assume steady-state values that are maintained as long as the individual remains at altitude. Third, they are associated with most and probably all system components rather than just a few. And, fourth, they impart functional capabilities to the system that far exceed those observed during" subacute adaptation.

Although initiated during the acute adaptive stage, the effects of increased erythropoiesis become most pronounced during the chronic stage.[90] While increasing hemoglobin content, the greater number of circulating red blood cells can further decrease blood flow and increase blood viscosity; cardiac work may then be further increased at any given $\dot{Q}$.[9] Biochemical and histologic changes become more apparent after chronic exposure, which may facilitate the increase of either or both oxygen conductance and transport. For example, when compared to the other two adaptive stages, a more pronounced capillary density, an increased myoglobin content in the skeletal muscles, and other modifications of enzymatic activity that may facilitate oxygen transport have been reported after chronic exposure to hypoxia.[17,89] It should be remembered that these functional alterations require different periods of time for complete chronic adaptation. Finally, these same functional changes may necessitate significantly greater time periods when exercise responses are considered.[42,84]

Impact of Altitude on Exercise Testing and Exercise Prescription

Exercise at an altitude of 1500 to 2000 m produces no significant reduction in functional ability at submaximal intensities. Some individuals experience symptoms of respiratory distress (dyspnea and breathlessness) more readily when exercising at near maximal intensities. Exercise performance is limited at altitudes near 4000 m; survival during *acute* exposure to 7000 m or higher altitude for those individuals not accustomed to such levels is questionable.[11] Therefore, all individuals must realize that exercise performance is reduced at submaximal and particularly at maximal levels of high terrestrial elevations (2000 to 5000 m) and an exercise prescription should be adjusted accordingly. For many individuals, these adjustments can be made by utilizing the information in Figure 6–4, when the prescription is based on relative exercise intensity.

The issue of an added impairment for individuals with cardiovascular disease who exercise at altitude is debatable. Grover implies that as long as the individual with cardiovascular disease recognizes his limitations and maintains exercise intensity within these limits, cardiac performance will not be compromised.[37] Other authors report no difference in cardiac performance with the double Master's test between exercise and exercise plus hypoxia (4592 m) in subjects with stabilized CHD.[57] On the other hand, asymptomatic subjects with abnormal resting electrocardiograms (non-specific ST segment changes or T wave changes) had better results while exercising in the hypoxic environment than with exercise alone. The authors conclude that, "it is quite safe to subject persons with stabilized ischaemic heart disease to exercise in an hypoxic environment."[57] Some authors even infer an added degree of protection from cardiovascular disease by residence and proper physical activity at high altitude.[12,37]

In contrast, some authors report such electrocardiographic disturbances during exercise as atrial and ventricular ectopic beats and prolonged QT interval, as well as diphasic, inverted, or flat T wave and lowered ST segment in nonadapted individuals at altitudes of 3000 to 5000 m.[83,108] In both of these studies, the effects of altitude, per se, are confounded by the addition of cold stress. Also, it has been shown that exposure to high altitude places greater demands on the right ventricle of the heart, resulting in increased total cardiac work (i.e., greater coronary blood flow), particularly during physical exercise.[11] Whether these responses are of particular importance and are potentially dangerous for those persons with CHD is not yet known. It is known that individuals with abnormal lung function (e.g., with emphysema and chronic bronchitis) are at even greater risk at altitude.[37] Thus, it seems that individuals with respiratory and cardiovascular diseases are at particular risk during exercise at high altitude.

EXPOSURE TO ATMOSPHERIC POLLUTANTS

Relatively little is known about the effects of single agents or combinations of atmospheric air pollutants on either submaximal or maximal exercise performance. Even less is known about the particular concentration levels and critical exposure durations of these air pollutants necessary for a decrement in exercise performance. Of the various air pollutants, only carbon monoxide (CO) has been evaluated with any thoroughness regarding cardiovascular responses to exercise. In healthy individuals, CO does not alter submaximal exercise responses, but slightly reduces maximal exercise performance. Individuals with cardiovascular impairments show marked decreases in submaximal exercise time to angina onset while breathing CO.

Among the remaining atmospheric air pollutants evaluated, the photochemical oxidants ozone (O_3), nitrogen dioxide (NO_2), and peroxyacetylnitrate (PAN), and the sulfur oxides, represented by sulfur dioxide (SO_2), and PANCO have no demonstrable cardiovascular effects during submaximal exercise in healthy individuals. There are questionable effects, however, in healthy individuals during maximal exercise and in CHD patients during submaximal exercise. Table 6–1 is a summary of the effects of the various air pollutants on exercise performance for healthy and cardiovascularly impaired individuals. Although this topic is subsequently discussed in some detail, the reader is directed for further information to reviews by Hack-

TABLE 6-1. **Effects of Air Pollutants on Exercise Performance of Normal and Cardiovascularly Impaired Individuals**

Subject Group Air Pollutant Exercise Intensity	Performance Decrement	No Effect	Selected References
Normal population			
CO			
•Submaximal exercise		X	31, 101
•Maximal exercise	X		53, 87
O₃			
•Submaximal exercise		X	23, 24
•Maximal exercise	?		25, 95
NO₂			
•Submaximal exercise		X	52, 85
•Maximal exercise	?		85
PAN			
•Submaximal exercise		X	31, 88
•Maximal exercise	?		20, 85, 86
PANCO			
•Submaximal exercise		X	31, 88
•Maximal exercise	?		20, 85, 86
SO₂			
•Submaximal exercise	?		85
•Maximal exercise	?		85
Cardiovascularly impaired population*			
CO	X		7, 8
O₃	?		85
NO₂	?		85
PAN	?		20, 85
PANCO	?		20, 85
SO₂	?		85

* Denotes submaximal effects only.

ney,[41] Raven,[85] and most recently Pandolf.[74]

Exercise Performance

HEALTHY INDIVIDUALS. Carbon monoxide (CO) appears to impair cardiovascular function, particularly during exercise, by binding with hemoglobin (COHb) to impede oxygen transport. Minimal impairment of cardiorespiratory function and no major performance decrements were observed in healthy individuals at COHb levels less than 15% at submaximal exercise intensities of 35 to 60% $\dot{V}_{O_2max}$ of short and prolonged duration.

HR, however, was significantly increased with CO, and added respiratory distress was noted at slightly higher submaximal intensities ($\sim$70% $\dot{V}_{O_2max}$).[31,82,101] In contrast, $\dot{V}_{O_2max}$ was inversely related to CO concentration.[20,53,82,86,87,101] The critical level at which COHb significantly influences $\dot{V}_{O_2max}$ has been reported to be 4.3%, but even lower COHb levels (2.7%) have been associated with significant decrements in maximal exercise time.[20,53,86,87]

The photochemical oxidants primarily seem to cause lung and respiratory tract dysfunction, with questionable effects on the cardiovascular system during exercise.[85] Of these oxidants, O_3 has been studied most thoroughly. During submaximal exercise (40 to 70% $\dot{V}_{O_2max}$) after or during exposure to 0.37, 0.50, or 0.75 ppm O_3, no significant alterations in submaximal $\dot{V}_{O_2}$, HR, or $\dot{V}_E$ were reported.[23,24] Other measurements of pulmonary function, however, appeared to be somewhat disturbed.[24] The limited observations concerning a true decrement in $\dot{V}_{O_2max}$ with O_3 exposure are debatable. Whereas some authors report no change in exercise capacity or $\dot{V}_{O_2max}$ while breathing filtered air (FA) or 0.15 or 0.30 ppm O_3, other investigators show an 11% reduction in $\dot{V}_{O_2max}$ while exposed to 0.75 ppm O_3 when compared to FA.[25,95] Thus, the critical concentration level for reduced performance is questionable, particularly during maximal exercise. Raven suggests that exercise performance decrements can be predicted as a function of $\dot{V}_E$ and exposure time.[85]

Of the other oxidants, the effects of PAN and PAN + CO have been evaluated during exercise stress.[20,31,86–88] During submaximal exercise (35% $\dot{V}_{O_2max}$) of 3 hours duration while breathing 0.24 ppm PAN or PANCO (50 ppm; COHb, 4 to 6%), no remarkable changes in cardiorespiratory function were observed in either younger (18 to 30 years) or older (40 to 55 years) subjects.[31,88] Forced vital capacity was reduced 4 to 7% in the younger subjects with PAN, but the significance is questionable. Also, no significant reductions in $\dot{V}_{O_2max}$ were reported while breathing these same concentrations of PAN or PANCO.[20,86,87] It seems premature, however, particularly regarding maximal exercise responses, to conclude that PAN or PANCO have no adverse effects on exercise performance. The concentration of PAN (0.24 ppm) in these few experiments may be at or slightly below the threshold level needed for demonstrable physiologic effects.

Even less is known about the exercise-related effects of another oxidant (NO_2) and the sulfur oxides, as represented by SO_2. Concentration levels of 0.62 ppm

NO_2 were evaluated after 2 hours of exposure at 40% $\dot{V}_{O_2max}$ with no significant alterations in cardiorespiratory function.[52] At a very low submaximal exercise intensity (only double the resting $\dot{V}_E$), exposure to 0.37 ppm pure SO_2 did not change ventilatory function after 2 hours of intermittent exercise exposure; no other physiologic responses were described.[47] Maximal exercise responses to these two pollutants have not been reported. A synergistic effect between SO_2 and O_3 has been described in terms of a greater reduction in ventilatory function during exercise, raising the question of possible synergism among other pollutants.[47] In addition, little information is currently available concerning the physiologic responses to chronic or prolonged exposure (> 4 hours) to any of these atmospheric air pollutants at various concentration levels during exercise.

CARDIOVASCULARLY IMPAIRED INDIVIDUALS. Of the various pollutants, only CO has been directly evaluated during exercise in cardiovascularly impaired individuals. It has been suggested that there is a relationship between CO and the advanced development of coronary arteriosclerosis, and that CO in the presence of significant CHD hastens myocardial infarction, angina pectoris, or sudden death.[41] In a study of 10 patients with documented CHD, exposure to heavy freeway traffic for 90 minutes increased COHb to an average level of 5.08%, causing a decrease in exercise time to angina onset and significant reductions in systolic blood pressure and HR at the onset of angina.[7] Ischemic ST segment depressions were also noted in 3 of 10 patients while breathing freeway air, in contrast to no abnormalities during freeway driving while breathing compressed, purified air. In two studies, each involving 10 patients with documented angina, exercise angina onset time was determined while breathing either 50 ppm CO (COHb, 2.7%) for 2 hours or 50 ppm CO (COHb, 2.9%) and 100 ppm CO (COHb, 4.5%) for 4 hours.[4,8] During both studies at either CO concentration, the average exercise times to onset of angina were reduced when compared to values while breathing compressed, purified air. Duration of angina was significantly prolonged after breathing 100 ppm CO, but not after breathing 50 ppm CO.[4] Generally, deeper and more prolonged ST segment depressions were noted after breathing CO.[4] Ischemic ST segment depressions of greater than 1 mm were also noted in 10% of a sample of clinically normal individuals during maximal treadmill exercise after inhalation of 100 ppm CO (COHb, 3.95%).[6] Thus, CHD patients are at significant risk during exercise at low levels of COHb (2.5 to 3.0%). Raven concludes that "the cardiac-impaired exercising patient will be placed at increased risk of incurring additional coronary events if ambient levels of CO in the inspired air are capable of causing a rise of blood COHb levels above 1.5 to 2.0%."[85]

Exercise performance responses to other atmospheric pollutants in cardiovascularly impaired individuals can only be inferred from evidence that exists from tests in normal, healthy individuals. Lower blood COHb levels in CHD patients produced significant reductions in exercise performance and more frequent electrocardiographic abnormalities when compared to no such impairment in healthy individuals. Therefore, similar or even lower concentrations of such pollutants as oxidants or sulfur oxides, which produce either questionable or no exercise performance effects in normal persons, may produce adverse cardiovascular effects in the cardiovascularly impaired individual (see Table 6–1). Certainly, individuals with cardiovascular or pulmonary disorders would be at greater risk during exercise while exposed to oxidants and sulfur oxides because of their limited cardiovascular or pulmonary reserve capacities.

Impact of Adverse Air Quality on Exercise Testing and Exercise Prescription

Submaximal exercise performance of individuals without cardiorespiratory disorders does not appear to be compromised within the limits of the particular concentration levels evaluated for the different atmospheric air pollutants. At near maximal or maximal exercise, performance appears limited for the same individuals when exposed to the same pollutants. In contrast, individuals with impaired cardiovascular systems are at even greater risk during submaximal exercise and exposure to CO; tissue hypoxia and myocardial ischemia may result from the binding of CO to hemoglobin. Evidence is limited concerning the adverse effects of the oxidants and sulfur oxides on the cardiovascular system of these compromised individuals during exercise. The oxidants (O_3, NO_2, and PAN) and sulfur oxides, which increase airway resistance because of reflex bronchoconstriction, place individuals with lung and respiratory tract disorders at particular risk during exercise. Obviously, the individual with disorders of both the cardiovascular and respiratory systems is at even greater risk during exercise when exposed to these pollutants.

The current primary U.S. government concentration standards for these common atmospheric air pollutants are: 9 ppm / 8 hours of CO exposure and 35 ppm / 1 hour CO exposure; 0.12 ppm / 1 hour O_3 exposure; 0.26 ppm / 1 hour NO_2 exposure, and 0.50 ppm / 1 hour SO_2 exposure. Exercise should not be done outdoors by individuals with cardiovascular or respiratory disorders when these first-alert levels of adverse air quality are reported.[85] As a general precaution for greatly industrialized or densely populated urban areas, exercise prescriptions for impaired individuals should focus on indoor exercise.

Most of the reported research concerning exercise performance and atmospheric air pollutants involves relatively acute exposure to the particular pollutant(s). Little is known about chronic exposure to adverse air quality and the impact on exercise performance. For many of the atmospheric air pollutants, such as CO, it takes 8 to 12 hours or longer to reach an equilibrium state between the inspired concentration and the level within the body.[4] Therefore, the cardiovascular or pulmonary burden should be even greater during exercise after prolonged exposure to adverse air quality. In addition, the possible synergism between various pollutants (in terms of added cardiorespiratory distress for acute or prolonged exposure) has not been evaluated during exercise and may further tax the cardiac or pulmonary reserves. Given the many unanswered questions concerning adverse air quality and those individuals specifically at risk during exercise, the supervising professionals who prescribe and lead exercise programs should act conservatively when this environmental stress is considered.[85]

EXPOSURE TO VARIOUS INTERSTRESSORS

Of the various environmental stressors discussed in this chapter, only the physiologic responses to the combined effects of environmental heat and adverse air quality, and the combined effects of environmental cold and high altitude, during exercise have been reported. The only other combination for practical consideration with possible detrimental consequences concerning exercise performance would appear to be altitude and adverse air quality. The combined effects of environmental heat stress and atmospheric air pollutants (specifically CO, O_3, PAN, and PANCO) have been evaluated. Only O_3, however, has been systematically studied at a variety of ambient temperatures. All pollutants (except for one series of experiments in which maximal exercise responses to CO, PAN, and PANCO were evaluated) have been studied only at low exercise intensities (35 to 40% $\dot{V}_{O_2max}$) in the heat. In contrast, much of the reported information concerning cold ambient temperatures and altitude is a result of the prevalence for these colder temperatures in the high mountains rather than by the specific experimental design per se. Generally, the physiologic responses during exercise to cold and altitude have been evaluated from brief exposures to the extremes for these two conditions. To date, there are no studies to assess the effects of any of these interstressors on individuals with specific cardiovascular or respiratory disorders.

Environmental Heat and Adverse Air Quality

Because the level of many air pollutants is high during periods of air stagnation and is often accompanied by elevated T_a, the individual with an impaired cardiovascular or respiratory system would be at even greater risk. Submaximal exercise performance (40% $\dot{V}_{O_2max}$) during O_3 exposure (0.50 ppm) has been evaluated at four different environmental conditions (25°C, 45% rh; 31°C, 85% rh; 35°C, 40% rh; and 40°C, 50% rh). A trend was found that indicated greater impairment in pulmonary function during combined exposure to O_3 and heat stress.[23] Decrements in pulmonary function after exposure to ozone and heat were greatest immediately after exercise. Reductions in vital capacity and maximal voluntary ventilation were significant during the most extreme heat exposure (40°C, 50% rh); exercise $\dot{V}_E$ was highest at this T_a (plus ozone). Because heat and ozone exposure were not related to additional reductions in any flow variables when compared to O_3 alone, these authors suggest that some other mechanism or mechanisms besides bronchoconstriction are related to the observed decrements in pulmonary function during exposure to the combined stresses; they do not speculate as to the mechanism(s) responsible, however.

Although other atmospheric air pollutants (CO, PAN, and PANCO) have been evaluated during exercise-heat stress, the environmental conditions were limited to 30% rh at 25°C and 35°C.[20,31,86–88] During these experiments, however, both maximal and submaximal (35% $\dot{V}_{O_2max}$) exercise intensities were evaluated. The $\dot{V}_{O_2max}$ was not altered during exposure to CO, PAN, or PANCO at 35°C. While breathing filtered air, exposure to this level of heat stress (35°C) was more effective in lowering $\dot{V}_{O_2max}$ (~4%) than exposure to either single pollutant or the two in combination at 25°C. During submaximal exercise, no significant changes in physiologic responses were reported while breathing CO, PAN, or PANCO at 35°C. Nevertheless, subjective complaints were greater at 35°C, particularly for PAN and PANCO. Drinkwater et al. speculate that the combination of CO and heat stress is important in the more pronounced respiratory disturbances seen at this elevated temperature.[20] As a final note, the effects of CO might well be enhanced at altitude due to the reduction in mean capillary oxygen pressure.[41]

Because each of these two environmental stressors (heat and pollution) pose additional risks when presented separately to the exercising individual with an impaired cardiovascular or respiratory system, it is not surprising that the risk is potentiated when these two stressors are combined. Information available seems to indicate that individuals with limited cardiac or pulmonary reserve capacities are at greater risk during combined exposure to environmental heat plus either CO or O_3. Because experimental evidence is limited, it is premature to conclude that the other pollutants do not adversely affect exercise performance at elevated T_a, particularly in those individuals at risk. Therefore, outdoor physical exercise should not be prescribed for individuals at risk when heat stress levels necessitate caution for healthy individuals or when the current primary federal standards for air pollutants are exceeded.[85]

Environmental Cold and High Altitude

As one ascends mountainous terrain, both T_a and humidity decrease, with corresponding increases in wind velocity and solar radiation. Although there is considerable variation, T_a decreases about 1°C for every 150 m of ascent.[102] The low humidity level seen at high altitude promotes increased heat loss through more effective evaporative cooling. Low humidity combined with the high pulmonary ventilation observed at altitude can result in a marked increase in heat loss with serious performance consequences.[10] The increased wind velocity seen in cold, mountainous terrain decreases the effective temperature at the skin surface. The effects of this wind-chill factor are of particular consequence in the prevention of peripheral freezing cold injuries due to local skin cooling of exposed surface areas. Increased wind velocity may hamper locomotion, elevate $\dot{V}_{O_2}$, and help to contribute to fatigue or exhaustion.[102] In addition, wind penetration of clothing disturbs the trapped dead air layer and decreases insulation. Although precautions must be taken to prevent sunburn damage, the solar radiation at altitude provides a necessary source of heat gain. In contrast to hot environments, it seems important to wear dark colors at altitude, because black clothing absorbs 88% of the solar radiation, khaki 57%, and white only 20%.[102]

In addition to the selection of dark clothing at altitude, three basic principles for clothing design are suggested to help reduce heat loss.[10] The first principle involves entrapment of air within the clothing ensemble and utilization of its insulative properties plus that of the fabric to reduce heat loss. The second principle involves the use of multiple-layered clothing systems that help to maximize the use of the entrapped air layer and allow for removal or addition of clothing layers as needed. The final clothing principle suggests layering more heavy and less permeable clothing over more coarsely woven clothing, as this also reduces dampness and heat transfer. The clothing must be kept as dry as possible; wet clothing (either from sweat production or environmental moisture) reduces its insulative properties and results in increased heat loss.

The interactive effects of cold and hypoxic stresses on exercise performance are not well understood, principally because of a lack of experimental information. Ward, however, suggests a number of factors that may decrease exercise performance during cold exposure at altitude.[102] Cold and hypoxic stresses combined may decrease mental function and could alter exercise performance. Because $\dot{V}_{O_2max}$ is reduced at altitude, heat production during exercise is limited at altitude and therefore is associated with a greater risk of cold injury. The increased $\dot{V}_E$ at altitude increases heat and water loss, both of which are an obvious disadvantage during cold exposure. Both cold and hypoxic stress are associated with hemoconcentration and a possible additive increase in blood viscosity, leading to decreased blood flow. Severe peripheral vasoconstriction (cold stress) and high blood viscosity (enhanced by dehydration at altitude) can lead to impairment of tissue perfusion and possible tissue necrosis. Because skin blood flow is reduced by hypoxic vasoconstriction at altitude in thermoneutral temperatures, this response may magnify the reduction in skin blood flow known to occur during cold exposure. Both cold and hypoxic stresses may increase the production of lactic acid for a given exercise intensity, possibly complicating exercise performance. Finally, because combined cold and hypoxic stress can produce a life-threatening situation for the normal, healthy individual during exercise, the added risks to those with disorders of the cardiovascular or pulmonary systems are obvious.

ACKNOWLEDGMENT. The author gratefully acknowledges the assistance of Drs. Ralph F. Goldman, John T. Maher, Michael N. Sawka, and Andrew J. Young for their critical review of this chapter, and Ms. Pat Basinger for her technical assistance in manuscript preparation.

REFERENCES

1. Adolph, E.F.: Physiology of Man in the Desert. New York, Interscience Publishers, 1947.
2. Alexander, J.K., Hartley, L.H., Modelski, M., and Grover, R.F.: Reduction of stroke volume during exercise in man following ascent to 3,100 m altitude. J. Appl. Physiol., 23:849, 1967.
3. American College of Sports Medicine: The prevention of thermal injuries during distance running. Med. Sci. Sports Exerc., 19:529, 1987.
4. Anderson, E.W., et al.: Effect of low-level carbon monoxide exposure on onset and duration of angina pectoris: a study in ten patients with ischemic heart disease. Ann. Intern. Med., 79:46, 1973.
5. Armstrong, L.E., and Pandolf, K.B.: Physical training, cardiorespiratory physical fitness and exercise-heat tolerance. In Human Performance Physiology and Environmental Medicine

6. at Terrestrial Extremes. Edited by K.B. Pandolf, M.N. Sawka, and R.R. Gonzalez. Indianapolis, Benchmark Press, 1988.
6. Aronow, W.S., and Cassidy, J.: Effect of carbon monoxide on maximal treadmill exercise: a study in normal persons. Ann. Intern. Med., 83:496, 1975.
7. Aronow, W.S., et al.: Effect of freeway travel on angina pectoris. Ann. Intern. Med., 77:669, 1972.
8. Aronow, W.S., and Isbell, M.W.: Carbon monoxide effect on exercise-induced angina pectoris. Ann. Intern. Med., 79:392, 1973.
9. Åstrand, P.-O., and Rodahl, K.: Textbook of Work Physiology. 3rd Ed. New York, McGraw-Hill, 1986.
10. Baker, P.T. (ed.): The Biology of High-Altitude Peoples. Cambridge, Cambridge University Press, 1978.
11. Balke, B.: Cardiac performance in relation to altitude. Am. J. Cardiol., 14:796, 1964.
12. Balke, B., Nagle, F.J., and Daniels, J.: Altitude and maximum performance in work and sports activity. JAMA, 194:646, 1965.
13. Boutelier, C.: Survival and Protection of Aircrew in the Event of Accidental Immersion in Cold Water. AGARD Report No. 211, 1979.
14. Buskirk, E.R.: Decrease in physical working capacity at high altitude. In Proceedings Symposium on Biomedical Problems of High Terrestrial Elevations. Edited by A.H. Hegnauer. Natick, MA, U.S. Army Research Institute of Environmental Medicine, 1969, p. 206.
15. Bynum, G.D., et al.: Induced hyperthermia in sedated humans and the concept of critical thermal maximum. Am. J. Physiol., 235:R228, 1978.
16. Carlson, L.D., Burns, H.L., Holmes, T.H., and Webb, P.P.: Adaptive changes during exposure to cold. J. Appl. Physiol., 5:672, 1953.
17. Cassin, S., Gilbert, R.D., and Johnson, E.M.: Capillary development during exposure to chronic hypoxia. Report SAM-TR-66-16, USAF School of Aviation Medicine, Randolph Field, TX, 1966.
18. Cruz, J.C., et al.: Ventilatory acclimatization to high altitude is prevented by CO_2 breathing. Respiration, 39:121, 1980.
19. Drinkwater, B.L., et al.: Aerobic power as a factor in women's response to work in hot environments. J. Appl. Physiol., 41:815, 1976.
20. Drinkwater, B.L., et al.: Air pollution, exercise, and heat stress. Arch. Environ. Health, 28:177, 1974.
21. Eagan, C.J.: Introduction and terminology. Fed. Proc., 22:930, 1963.
22. Epstein, S.E., et al.: Effects of a reduction in environmental temperature on the circulatory response to exercise in man. N. Engl. J. Med., 280:7, 1969.
23. Folinsbee, L.J., et al.: Influence of exercise and heat stress on pulmonary function during ozone exposure. J. Appl. Physiol., 43:409, 1977.
24. Folinsbee, L.J., Silverman, F., and Shephard, R.J.: Exercise responses following ozone exposure. J. Appl. Physiol., 38:996, 1975.
25. Folinsbee, L.J., Silverman, F., and Shephard, R.J.: Decrease of maximum oxygen uptake fol-

lowing exposure to ozone. Physiologist, *18*:215, 1975 (Abstract).

26. Gisolfi, C.V.: Work-heat tolerance derived from interval training. J. Appl. Physiol., *35*:349, 1973.
27. Gisolfi, C.V., and Cohen, J.S.: Relationships among training, heat acclimation, and heat tolerance in men and women: the controversy revisited. Med. Sci. Sports, 11:56, 1979.
28. Givoni, B., and Goldman, R.F.: Predicting effects of heat acclimatization on heart rate and rectal temperature. J. Appl. Physiol., *35*:875, 1973.
29. Givoni, B., and Goldman, R.F.: Predicting heart rate response to work, environment, and clothing. J. Appl. Physiol., *34*:201, 1973.
30. Givoni, B., and Goldman, R.F.: Predicting rectal temperature response to work, environment, and clothing. J. Appl. Physiol., *32*:812, 1972.
31. Gliner, J.A., et al.: Man's physiologic response to long-term work during thermal and pollutant stress. J. Appl. Physiol., *39*:628, 1975.
32. Goldman, R.F.: Protection against cold injury. Contemp. Orthop., *2*:263, 1980.
33. Goldman, R.F., Newman, R.W., and Wilson, O.: Effects of alcohol, hot drinks, or smoking on hand and foot heat loss. Acta Physiol. Scand., *87*:498, 1973.
34. Gonzalez, R.R.: Biophysical and physiological integration of proper clothing for exercise. *In* Exercise and Sport Sciences Reviews. Edited by K.B. Pandolf. New York, Macmillan, 1987.
35. Greenleaf, J.E., Castle, B.L., and Ruff, W.K.: Maximal oxygen uptake, sweating and tolerance to exercise in the heat. Int. J. Biometeorol., *16*:375, 1972.
36. Grover, R.F.: Future studies in adaptations to altitude. *In* Environmental Physiology: Aging, Heat and Altitude. Edited by S. Horvath, and M.K. Yousef. New York, Elsevier-North Holland, 1981.
37. Grover, R.F.: Performance at altitude. *In* Sports Medicine and Physiology. Edited by R.H. Strauss. Philadelphia, W.B. Saunders, 1979.
38. Grover, R.F., Reeves, J.T., Grover, E.B., and Leathers, J.E.: Muscular exercise in young men native to 3,100 m altitude. J. Appl. Physiol., *22*:555, 1967.
39. Grover, R.F., et al.: Maintained stroke volume but impaired arterial oxygenation in man at high altitude with supplemental CO_2. Circ. Res., *38*:391, 1976.
40. Grover, R.F., Weil, J.V., and Reeves, J.T.: Cardiovascular adaptation to exercise at high altitude. *In* Exercise and Sport Sciences Reviews. Edited by K.B. Pandolf. New York, Macmillan, 1986.
41. Hackney, J.D.: Relationship between air pollution and cardiovascular disease; a review. *In* Clinical Implications of Air Pollution Research. Edited by A.J. Finkel, and W.C. Duel. Acton, MA, Publishing Sciences Group, 1976.
42. Hannon, J.P., and Vogel, J.A.: Oxygen transport during early altitude acclimatization: a perspective study. Eur. J. Appl. Physiol., *36*:285, 1977.
43. Hardy, J.D. (ed.): Temperature: Its Measurement and Control in Science and Industry. Vol. 3, Part 3. New York, Reinhold Publishing, 1963.

44. Hardy, J.D., Gagge, A.P., and Stolwijk, J.A.J. (eds.): Physiological and Behavioral Temperature Regulation. Springfield, IL, Charles C Thomas, 1970.
45. Hartley, L.H.: Effects of high-altitude environment on the cardiovascular system of man. JAMA, *215*:241, 1971.
46. Hartley, L.H., Vogel, J.A., and Cruz, J.C.: Reduction of maximal exercise heart rate at altitude and its reversal with atropine. J. Appl. Physiol., *36*:362, 1974.
47. Hazucha, M., and Bates, D.V.: Combined effect of ozone and sulphur dioxide on human pulmonary function. Nature, *257*:50, 1975.
48. Henane, R., Flandrois, R., and Charbonnier, J.P.: Increase in sweating sensitivity by endurance conditioning in man. J. Appl. Physiol., *43*:822, 1977.
49. Herrington, L.P.: The range of physiological response to climatic heat and cold. *In* Physiology of Heat Regulation and the Science of Clothing. Edited by L.H. Newburgh. New York, Hafner Publishing, 1968.
50. Hines, E.A., Jr.: The significance of vascular hyperreaction as measured by the cold pressor test. Am. Heart J., *19*:408, 1940.
51. Horstman, D., Weiskopf, R., and Jackson, R.E.: Work capacity during 3-wk sojourn at 4,300 m: effects of relative polycythemia. J. Appl. Physiol., *49*:311, 1980.
52. Horvath, S.M., and Folinsbee, L.J.: The effect of nitrogen dioxide on lung function in normal subjects. Washington, DC, U.S. Department of Commerce, National Technical Information Service PB-277 671, 1978.
53. Horvath, S.M., Raven, P.B., Dahms, T.E., and Gray, D.J.: Maximal aerobic capacity at different levels of carboxyhemoglobin. J. Appl. Physiol., *38*:300, 1975.
54. Itoh, S.: Physiology of Cold-Adapted Man. Sapporo, Hokkaido University School of Medicine, 1974.
55. Keatinge, W.R.: The effect of repeated daily exposure to cold and of improved physical fitness on the metabolic and vascular response to cold air. J. Physiol. (Lond), *157*:209, 1961.
56. Kellogg, R.H.: Oxygen and carbon dioxide in the regulation of respiration. Fed. Proc., *36*:1658, 1977.
57. Khanna, P.K., Dham, S.K., and Hoon, R.S.: Exercise in an hypoxic environment as a screening test for ischaemic heart disease. Aviat. Space Environ. Med., *47*:1114, 1976.
58. Kollias, J., and Buskirk, E.R.: Exercise and altitude. *In* Science and Medicine of Exercise and Sport. 2nd Ed. Edited by W.R. Johnson, and E.R. Buskirk. New York, Harper & Row, 1974.
59. LeBlanc, J.: Man in the Cold. Springfield, IL, Charles C Thomas, 1975.
60. LeBlanc, J.: Evidence and meaning of acclimatization to cold in man. J. Appl. Physiol., *9*:395, 1956.
61. Leithead, C.S., and Lind, A.R.: Heat Stress and Heat Disorders. Philadelphia, F.A. Davis, 1964.
62. Leon, D.F., Amidi, M., and Leonard, J.J.: Left heart work and temperature responses to cold exposure in man. Am. J. Cardiol., *26*:38, 1970.

63. Lewis, T.: Observations upon the reactions of the vessels of the human skin to cold. Heart, *15*:177, 1930.
64. Lind, A.R.: Physiologic responses to heat. *In* Medical Climatology. Edited by S. Licht. New Haven, Elizabeth Licht, 1964.
65. Maher, J.T., Jones, L.G., and Hartley, L.H.: Effects of high-altitude exposure on submaximal endurance capacity of man. J. Appl. Physiol., *37*:895, 1974.
66. Maron, M.B., Wagner, J.A., and Horvath, S.M.: Thermoregulatory responses during competitive marathon running. J. Appl. Physiol., *42*:909, 1977.
67. Nadel, E.R. (ed.): Problems with Temperature Regulation during Exercise. New York, Academic Press, 1977.
68. Nadel, E.R., Pandolf, K.B., Roberts, M.F., and Stolwijk, J.A.J.: Mechanisms of thermal acclimation to exercise and heat. J. Appl. Physiol., *37*:515, 1974.
69. Neill, W.A., Duncan, D.A., Kloster, F., and Mahler, D.J.: Response of coronary circulation to cutaneous cold. Am. J. Med., *56*:471, 1974.
70. Newburgh, L.H. (ed.): Physiology of Heat Regulation and the Science of Clothing. New York, Hafner Publishing, 1968.
71. Newman, R.W.: Cold acclimation in Negro Americans. J. Appl. Physiol., *27*:316, 1969.
72. Newman, R.W.: Cold acclimation in Puerto Ricans. J. Appl. Physiol., *25*:277, 1968.
73. Nielsen, M.: Die Regulation der Körpertemperatur bei Muskelarbeit. Skand. Arch. Physiol., *79*:193, 1938.
74. Pandolf, K.B.: Air quality and human performance. *In* Human Performance Physiology and Environment Medicine at Terrestrial Extremes. Edited by K.B. Pandolf, M.N. Sawka, and R.R. Gonzalez. Indianapolis, Benchmark Press, 1988.
75. Pandolf, K.B.: Effects of physical training and cardiorespiratory physical fitness on exercise-heat tolerance: recent observations. Med. Sci. Sports, *11*:60, 1979.
76. Pandolf, K.B., Burse, R.L., and Goldman, R.F.: Role of physical fitness in heat acclimatisation, decay and reinduction. Ergonomics, *20*:399, 1977.
77. Pandolf, K.B., Cafarelli, E., Noble, B.J., and Metz, K.F.: Hyperthermia: effect on exercise prescription. Arch. Phys. Med. Rehabil., *56*:524, 1975.
78. Pandolf, K.B., Griffin, T.B., Munro, E.H., and Goldman, R.F.: Persistence of impaired heat tolerance from artificially induced miliaria rubra. Am. J. Physiol., *239*:R226, 1980.
79. Pandolf, K.B., Griffin, T.B., Munro, E.H., and Goldman, R.F.: Heat intolerance as a function of percent of body surface involved with miliaria rubra. Am. J. Physiol., *239*:R233, 1980.
80. Pandolf, K.B., Shapiro, Y., Breckenridge, J.R., and Goldman, R.F.: Effects of solar heat load on physiological performance at rest and work in the heat. Fed. Proc., *38*:1052, 1979 (Abstract).
81. Pandolf, K.B., et al.: Prediction modeling of physiological responses and human performance in the heat. Comput. Biol. Med., *16*:319, 1986.
82. Pirnay, F., Dujardin, J., Deroanne, R., and Petit, J.M.: Muscular exercise during intoxication by carbon monoxide. J. Appl. Physiol., *31*:573, 1971.
83. Politte, L.L., Almond, C.H., and Logue, J.T.: Dynamic electrocardiography with strenuous exertion at high altitudes. Am. Heart J., *75*:570, 1968.
84. Pugh, L.G.C.E.: Cardiac output in muscular exercise at 5,800 m (19,000 ft). J. Appl. Physiol., *19*:441, 1964.
85. Raven, P.B.: Heat and air pollution: the cardiac patient. *In* Heart Disease and Rehabilitation. Edited by M.L. Pollock, and D.H. Schmidt. Boston, Houghton and Mifflin, 1979.
86. Raven, P.B., et al.: Age, smoking habits, heat stress, and their interactive effects with carbon monoxide and peroxyacetylnitrate on man's aerobic power. Int. J. Biometeorol., *18*:222, 1974.
87. Raven, P.B., et al.: Effect of carbon monoxide and peroxyacetylnitrate on man's maximal aerobic capacity. J. Appl. Physiol., *36*:288, 1974.
88. Raven, P.B., Gliner, J.A., and Sutton, J.C.: Dynamic lung function changes following long-term work in polluted environments. Environ. Res., *12*:18, 1976.
89. Reynafarje, B.: Myoglobin content and enzymatic activity of muscle and altitude adaptation. J. Appl. Physiol., *17*:301, 1962.
90. Reynafarje, C.: The influence of high altitude on erythropoietic activity. Homeostatic mechanisms. Brookhaven Symp. Biol., *10*:132, 1957.
91. Roberts, M.F., Wenger, C.B., Stolwijk, J.A.J., and Nadel, E.R.: Skin blood flow and sweating changes following exercise training and heat acclimation. J. Appl. Physiol., *43*:133, 1977.
92. Rowell, L.B.: Human cardiovascular adjustments to exercise and thermal stress. Physiol. Rev., *54*:75, 1974.
93. Saltin, B.: Mexico City Olympic stad ett hojdfysiologiskt experiment. Stockholm, Framtiden, 1966.
94. Saltin, B., et al.: Maximal oxygen uptake and cardiac output after 2 weeks at 4,300 m. J. Appl. Physiol., *25*:400, 1968.
95. Savin, W.M., and Adams, W.C.: Effects of ozone inhalation on work performance and $V_{O_2 max}$. J. Appl. Physiol., *46*:309, 1979.
96. Sawka, M.N., and Pandolf, K.B.: Effects of body water loss on physiological function and exercise performance. *In* Perspectives in Exercise Science and Sports Medicine, Volume 3: Fluid Homeostasis During Exercise. Edited by C.V. Gisolfi and D.R. Lamb. Indianapolis, Benchmark Press, 1990.
97. Scholander, P.F., Hammel, H.T., Andersen, K.L., and Løyning, Y.: Metabolic acclimation to cold in man. J. Appl. Physiol., *12*:1, 1958.
98. Shvartz, E., Saar, E., Meyerstein, N., and Benor, D.: A comparison of three methods of acclimatization to dry heat. J. Appl. Physiol., *34*:214, 1973.
99. Shvartz, E., Shapiro, Y., Magazanik, A., et al.: Heat acclimation, physical fitness, and responses to exercise in temperate and hot environments. J. Appl. Physiol., *43*:678, 1977.
100. Strydom, N.B., and Holdsworth, L.D.: The effects of different levels of water deficit on physi-

ological responses during heat stress. Int. Z. Angew. Physiol., *26*:95, 1968.

101. Vogel, J.A., and Gleser, M.A.: Effect of carbon monoxide on oxygen transport during exercise. J. Appl. Physiol., *32*:234, 1972.

102. Ward, M.: Mountain Medicine: A Clinical Study of Cold and High Altitude. London, Crosby Lockwood Staples, 1975.

103. Wenger, C.B.: Human heat acclimatization. *In* Human Performance Physiology and Environmental Medicine at Terrestrial Extremes. Edited by K.B. Pandolf, M.N. Sawka, and R.R. Gonzalez. Indianapolis, Benchmark Press, 1988.

104. Williams, C.G., Wyndham, C.H., and Morrison, J.F.: Rate of loss of acclimatization in summer and winter. J. Appl. Physiol., *22*:21, 1967.

105. Wolf, S., and Hardy, J.D.: Studies on pain: observation on pain due to local cooling and on factors involved in the cold pressor effect. J. Clin. Invest., *20*:521, 1941.

106. Woodcock, A.H.: Clothing and climate. *In* Medical Climatology. Edited by S. Licht. New Haven, Elizabeth Licht, 1964.

107. Wyndham, C.H.: The physiology of exercise under heat stress. Annu. Rev. Physiol., *35*:193, 1973.

108. Wyndham, C.H., Strydom, N.B., Williams, C.G., and Heyns, A.: An examination of certain individual factors affecting the heat tolerance of mine workers. J.S. Afr. Inst. Mining Met., *68*:79, 1967.

109. Young, A.J.: Human adaptation to cold. *In* Human Performance Physiology and Environmental Medicine at Terrestrial Extremes. Edited by K.B. Pandolf, M.N. Sawka, and R.R. Gonzalez. Indianapolis, Benchmark Press, 1988.

110. Young, A.J., et al.: Human thermoregulatory responses to cold air are altered by repeated cold water immersion. J. Appl. Physiol., *60*:1542, 1986.

111. Zhongyuan, S., et al.: Comparison of physiological responses to hypoxia at high altitudes between highlanders and lowlanders. Sci. Sin. [B.], *22*:1455, 1979.

SPECIAL CASES

7

CHAPTER

Rheumatoid Arthritis

by
Björn Ekblom and Rolf Nordemar

GENERAL DESCRIPTION

Rheumatic diseases have been recognized since long before Christ, and the problems of pain, stiffness, weakness, and restricted mobility are probably as old as man himself. Rheumatoid arthritis (RA), however, was not described as a distinctive rheumatoid disease until about 100 years ago. Diagnostic criteria for RA have varied during the years and among different clinicians and traditions. During the past few decades, the diagnostic criteria of the American Rheumatism Association (see Table 7–1) have been most widely used.[1]

For classification purposes, a patient is said to have RA if he/she has satisfied at least 4 of the 7 criteria in Table 7–1. Criteria 1 through 4 must have been present for at least 6 weeks. Patients with two clinical diagnoses are not excluded. Designation as classic, definite, or probable rheumatoid arthritis should not be made.

Although the etiology of RA is not known, immunologic factors are considered to be of great importance.[39] The activation of the complement system by immune complexes in the joints is believed to cause the migration of polymorphonuclear leukocytes into the joints. These leukocytes phagocytose the immune complexes and release lysosomal enzymes, which cause synovitis.[7] The inflammatory synovial tissue then releases enzymes that cause destruction of the articular cartilage and subchondral bone. Prostaglandins are mediators of these inflammatory events.

There are as yet many unknown steps in this chain of events, and what initiates the whole reaction is still unknown. The study of histocompatibility antigens in RA has not provided any clear evidence of a disease-promoting genetic factor, although such is the case in ankylosing spondylitis.

RA usually has a gradual onset, with pain, swelling, and stiffness of small peripheral joints. Onset can be at any age, but most commonly occurs between 25 and 60 years of age and with a female preponderance of 3 to 1. RA usually has a slowly progressive course, with periods of remission and exacerbation. Individual patient outcome may be difficult to predict at the onset. The inflammatory process engages the joints, with gradual destruction of the joint surface and underlying bone structure; the joint capsule and ligaments are also weakened. Tendons and tendon sheaths might become inflamed, and local or generalized inflammatory changes often occur in the skeletal muscles.[4] It should also be remembered that the disease is systemic and might be associated with symptoms from the cardiovascular system (pericarditis and vasculitis), the pulmonary system (pleuritis and fibrosis), and the nervous system (neuropathy and mononeuritis).[30] Amyloidosis due to RA may involve the gastrointestinal tract, the liver, and the kidneys. Common ocular manifestations are episcleritis or scleritis and keratoconjunctivitis sicca. Most patients with RA have a therapy-resistant

113

TABLE 7–1. The 1987 Revised Criteria for the Classification of Rheumatoid Arthritis (RA)

Criterion	Definition
1. Morning stiffness	Morning stiffness in and around the joints, lasting at least 1 hour before maximal improvement.
2. Arthritis of 3 or more joint areas	At least three joint areas simultaneously have had soft tissue swelling or fluid (not bony overgrowth alone) observed by a physician. The 14 possible areas are right or left PIP, MCP, wrist, elbow, knee, ankle, and MTP joints.
3. Arthritis of hand joints	At least one area swollen (as defined above) in a wrist, MCP, or PIP joint.
4. Symmetric arthritis	Simultaneous involvement of the same joint areas (as defined in 2) on both sides of the body (bilateral involvement of PIP, MCP, or MTP is acceptable without absolute symmetry).
5. Rheumatoid nodules	Subcutaneous nodules over bony prominences or extensor surfaces, or in juxta-articular regions, observed by a physician.
6. Serum rheumatoid factor	Demonstration of abnormal amounts of serum rheumatoid factor by any method for which the result has been positive in < 5% of normal control subjects.
7. Radiographic changes	Radiographic changes typical of rheumatoid arthritis on posteroanterior hand and wrist radiograph, which must include erosions or unequivocal bony decalcification localized in or most marked adjacent to the involved joints (osteoarthritis changes alone do not qualify).

DIP = distal interphalangeal joints; PIP = proximal interphalangeal joints; MCP = metacarpophalangeal joints; MTP = metatarsophalangeal joints

anemia, and generalized or periarticular osteoporosis is common.

Pathologic changes of the synovial joints in RA are significant. Synovial tissue is infiltrated with lymphocytes and plasma cells. In the lining cells and in the synovial stroma, there might also be focal synovial necrosis. Exudation into the synovial tissue and into the synovial cavity occurs early in the progression of the disease and in connection with exacerbations (i.e., increased activity of the disease). There is a proliferation of vascular connective tissue in synovial tissue, with a multiplication of stromal cells. The articular cartilage is gradually destroyed, beginning in the zone where synovial tissue meets articular cartilage. In the synovial fluid, phagocytes, degrading enzymes (e.g., collagenases), antibodies, complement, lymphocytes, and chemical inflammatory mediators may be found. The partial pressure of oxygen in synovial fluid is usually below normal levels.

Immunopathologic investigation often reveals high levels of IgG and IgM (immunoglobulin, types G and M) in the lining cells of the synovial tissue and in the infiltrating plasma cells. Complement C3 and immune complex IgG/IgM are found in synovial tissue and within the synovial fluid phagocytes. Numbers of complement factors are usually below normal in synovial fluid during active phases of the disease.[33]

Rheumatoid synovitis often occurs in bursae and tendon sheaths. Under such circumstances, a large cyst might develop in the popliteal bursa causing reduced mobility of the knee joint. Inflammatory changes in tendons and tendon sheaths might lead to weakening and rupture or entrapment of the tendon within the sheath.

Pathologic changes in the skeletal muscles include interstitial lymphocyte infiltration and localized muscular degradation with lymphocytic infiltrates.[4,35] These pathologic findings are indistinguishable from those found in other inflammatory diseases.

Evaluating a patient with RA is a complex task and includes such factors as the individual's pain, feelings, and social functioning. Also included are laboratory tests to indicate the intensity of the inflammatory process and radiographic examination to show the degree of destruction. The clinical examination aims to record tenderness, mobility, deviation, and swelling of the joints, as well as muscular weakness and general functional capacity. Questions about the duration of the patient's morning stiffness and fatigue are also included in the evaluation.

Four classifications of a patient's general functional capacity are often made by using the criteria of the American Rheumatism Association:[33]

Class 1: complete ability to carry on all usual duties without handicaps.

Class 2: adequate ability for normal activities despite handicap, discomfort, or limited motion at one or more joints.

Class 3: ability limited to little or none of the duties of usual occupation or to self-care.

Class 4: incapacitated, largely or wholly. Bedridden or confined to a wheelchair; little or no self-care.

This classification has the obvious disadvantage of being too crude to be able to register minor improvements or deteriorations. Another more sensitive means to evaluate functional capacity is with a scoring system of 50 to 100 separate "activities of daily living" (ADL).[32] Each activity that a patient can manage is worth one point in the scale; full functional capacity yields the highest scale total. Although this scoring system has the disadvantage of being time-consuming, studies have shown that a patient-administered formula is both valid and reliable for assessing ADL functional capacity.[10,13]

In the clinical evaluation of joint status, a joint score is usually used, which is the sum of all the joints in the body (except the spine) that are tender with palpation or passive movement. Some joint scores are so constructed that they compensate for differences in joint size or differences in tenderness by palpation.[1,22] Newer ways of assessing individual joint inflammatory activity by using scintigraphy or thermography have generally been disappointing so far.

Clinical Effects

The cardinal symptom of RA is pain. Chronic pain can have a severe effect on the personality of RA patients, as depression, feelings of helplessness, and guilt or anxiety are common. The pain also demands attention, which means that patients have less ability to concentrate on other matters. In combination with a decreased functional capacity and general inactivity, these factors lead to isolation of the individual from his environment and from society. Most patients with RA have experienced some degree of isolation and regularly remark that they find it hard when they lose friends or cannot participate fully in work and hobbies.

Decreased functional capacity can lead to dependency for some persons; it is estimated that about 10% of RA patients are dependent on another person for daily activities. Muscular weakness and low endurance are common, and are caused by inactivity and such disease-related processes in the muscle as myositis and reduced blood flow.[4,15,30,35] Most patients also develop decalcification of the bones, with fragility and a tendency to fracture with moderate traumas. During periods of increased disease activity (more joint inflammation, higher erythrocyte sedimentation rate, and more pain), most patients have a reduced appetite. Even if appetite is unchanged, body weight is usually reduced because the body is in a catabolic state and has an increased turnover of amino acids and reduced plasma albumin.[38] Because muscles are the largest protein stores in the body, they are reduced during these catabolic periods associated with increased disease activity.

Modes of Treatment

Medical Therapy

There is no simple way to treat a patient with RA; the etiology of the disease is unknown and there are no reliable means to a cure. Therapy must be broad to arrest

115

the progress of the disease as much as possible and to help the patient adapt to a chronic, progressive, and function-reducing condition. It is important to inform the patient as early as possible about the disease prognosis and its consequences regarding life situation. At the onset of RA, many patients (especially young persons) deny its presence and are not ready to receive information about its prognosis or consequences. Most patients, however, are able to adapt to reality after a few months; readaptation and rehabilitation might begin at that time.

Pharmacologic therapy often starts with salicylic acid compounds; these are pain-reducing agents with an anti-inflammatory action that is adequate for many patients. By adding such drugs as indomethacin, naproxene, or ibuprofen, most patients receive satisfactory analgesic and anti-inflammatory therapy. Most patients, however, periodically have arthritic symptoms from one or many joints, and local cortisone injections may then be needed. All of the drugs mentioned have an effect on the symptoms of the disease but do not basically alter its course.

There are, however, drugs that might alter the course of RA; these agents are therefore called anti-rheumatic drugs. These drugs are all slow acting (i.e., their effects are not evident until 4 to 6 weeks of treatment) and might introduce a remission of RA for brief or prolonged periods. Examples of these drugs are gold, penicillamine, and levamisol, and such anti-malarial drugs as cloroquine and hydroxycloroquine. All of these slow-acting agents have multiple side-effects and are not used except with patients in whom activity is high and the disease progress is so rapid that the use of such hazardous drugs is justified.

Corticosteroids can alleviate rheumatic symptoms in patients with RA, but they must be used with care and only under special indications when given orally. When indicated, however, corticosteroids are the most effective anti-inflammatory drugs known. Nevertheless, these drugs have so many undesirable side-effects that

their oral use is justified only in patients with highly progressive disease and after a trial of general measures and anti-rheumatic drugs. Very few patients with RA are included in this group.

Physical therapy and rehabilitation are extremely important in the treatment of RA. Patients need periods of rest combined with regular periods of physical exercise. It is generally believed that rest therapy is the single most important factor in the treatment of active arthritis, even though longitudinal studies concerning its efficacy have not been conducted. On the other hand, it is well known that physical activity is essential to maintain the function of the locomotor system. As in many other clinical problems (e.g., myocardial infarction, recovery from surgery, and fractures), the trend today is toward less bed rest and more activity. Patients are taught how to rest in certain positions in which the risks of developing contractures in hip or knee joints are diminished. Splints for certain joints are often prescribed to reduce the stress on the joint, as well as to diminish pain and increase stability. Arthritis in the wrist may lead to an inability to use the hand, but hand function can improve markedly with a stabilizing splint on the wrist. Support in the shoe just behind the metatarsophalangeal joints might transfer weight away from the painful area in the forefoot.

Heat, either by local heating of the skin with hot packs or by deep heating (shortwave and microwave), might give symptomatic relief of pain, whereas local cooling might have the same effect in some patients. A new method for giving symptomatic pain relief is transcutaneous electric nerve stimulation (TENS); some patients with RA who do not have pain controlled satisfactorily with pharmacologic agents have reduced pain when using TENS.

The aim of physiotherapy for RA is to restore and maintain strength, mobility, and functional capacity of the locomotor system. Treatment of contractures and teaching patients to use movements that reduce excessive stress on joints and ligaments are essential. Therapy may consist of passive or active movements, with or without resistance. Training individuals to improve or regain functional capacity can be done very well in a pool with warm water, in which movements are lightly resisted and the body is supported.

The aim of occupational therapy is to restore and preserve functional capacity, especially the upper extremities. Therapy includes such functional training as knitting, sewing, and undertaking of ADL activities with and without technical aids. These aids are of special importance for patients with destructive changes in their hands, elbows, or arms so that they compensate for this loss of function. Examples of technical aids are adapted cutlery, keyholders, and faucet turners with a long lever.

Rehabilitative measures include counselling the patient and sometimes the entire family with information about the disease prognosis and adaptive measures. Because the disease has consequences that affect the patients, as well as their family, work, and hobbies, the adaptive process can be painful and time-consuming. Rearrangement of housing, work, and transportation may be necessary and a social worker, psychologist, and work counselor are needed in the rehabilitation team.

Surgical Therapy

Surgery is performed in the early phase of RA in an attempt to reduce symptoms and to arrest the disease process. In this respect, synovectomy might be done early on metatarsophalangeal, metacarpophalangeal, or knee joints. The inflamed synovial tissue is reduced with this procedure, but there is usually a regrowth of synovial tissue with synovitis thereafter.

When destructive changes in the joints have developed, arthrodesis, resection, or arthroplasty may be indicated. Arthrodesis (fusion) produces immobile and painfree joints and can be used for the subtarsal, ankle, knee, hip, and wrist joints. Provided that the joints surrounding the arthrodesis are rather mobile and stable, the operation may improve function and

reduce pain at the expense of mobility. Resection (removal) of some or all of the metatarsophalangeal joints is done to reduce pain in the forefoot during walking. The operation is usually successful; the return of symptoms in the forefoot usually indicates that the resection was not sufficiently radical. Arthroplasty (plastic surgery of the joints) is the most important surgical procedure used today in the treatment of RA. There have been good results reported in reducing pain and in improving function in the hips, knees, and metacarpophalangeal joints. The use of prostheses for the elbows have yielded some unsatisfactory results. Thus, these devices are not used regularly.

RHEUMATOID ARTHRITIS AND EXERCISE

RA and the Ability to Exercise

Because RA is a disease that involves both joints and muscles, its activity in the different functional classes influences the patient's ability to exercise. In high activity phases of RA, exercise capacity is generally low at all functional classes. This loss of function depends mainly on the pain from the joints and muscles during exercise, stiffness, and both muscular and psychologic fatigue. For these reasons, patients tend to avoid exercise during phases of high disease activity. Whether exercise in this situation increases joint destruction has not been clarified. RA may also affect the heart and lungs, as well as peripheral circulation and nerves, causing a further reduction in physical performance. Myocarditis, epicarditis, and endocarditis can modify the ability to exercise, e.g., due to arrhythmias. Pleuritis and lung fibrosis can reduce ventilation and may cause a perception of increased exertion during exercise. Neuritis and vasculitis may reduce peripheral sensitivity, motor function, and circulation.

A patient in Functional Class 1 may perform any type of exercise because the disease involvement has not yet reached major importance. Exceptions may include hard physical exercise, running, and individual racket sports, if hard, specific stress is placed on the knees and feet, especially if there are active processes in these joints. In almost all cases, bicycle exercise is possible.

Patients in Functional Class 2 and a few in Class 3 can perform most types of exercise (especially cycling, walking, heated pool exercise and even jogging) in low activity phases of RA.[2,6,8,16–18,20,21,24,25,29,31,36,37] In high activity phases, they can exercise only with "no load" or very low loads (e.g., 25 W on a cycle ergometer) due to the inflammatory process in the joints, muscles, and tendons. The ability to exercise returns fairly soon after the most acute phase of RA, and it is possible to exercise, even though all signs of active engagement in the joints have not fully disappeared.[29]

Although a few patients in Functional Class 3 can walk, jog, and perform similar types of exercise, most persons in this class can swim or exercise on a bicycle if the type of exercise, its intensity, and its range of motion are modified according to the patient's anatomic and pathologic conditions.[29] In this functional class, polyneuritis and vasculitis are common and may also modify the ability to exercise.

By definition, most patients in Functional Class 4 are not able to carry out complicated movements. Quite a few patients, however, may perform some physical activity, e.g., if they are supported in water or if they can do "free" exercise without preset levels of intensity or frequency.

Clinical Effects of Acute Exercise

Patients in low activity phases of RA (Functional Classes 1 and 2 and even most in Class 3) have a mechanical efficiency during exercise on a bicycle ergometer that is about the same as that found in comparable groups of healthy individuals. Thus, with increasing power outputs, oxygen consumption, blood lactate accumulation, and ratings of perceived exertion show the same pattern as that found in "normal" individuals of the same age and degree of training status.[3] In more complicated modes of exercise, such as fast walking, efficiency is often reduced because of limping. The degree of reduction depends on such factors as disease activity and the number and type of joints affected. Because hard exercise should be avoided during high activity phases, adaptation to graded exercise in this situation has not been evaluated.

Although most Functional Class 1 and 2 patients can perform common tests for measuring isometric and dynamic muscle strength during phases of low disease activity, many patients have difficulty performing rapid movements (e.g., knee extension). Furthermore, total range of "normal" movement is not always achieved. The latter two problems become more pronounced at the higher functional classes. These problems can also make any measurement of muscle strength impossible during acute phases because of pain in the involved joints, muscles, and tendons.

Acute exercise causes some discomfort in about 85% of patients with RA.[29] About 25% of these patients report that this discomfort lasts for several hours. Another 50% of affected individuals report that pain lasts for about 24 hours, and in the remaining 25%, discomfort lasts for several days. During a period of physical training, this joint and muscle discomfort is reduced in intensity, frequency, and duration. Even though most patients feel more discomfort after acute exercise, a majority (70%) also feel more brisk.[26,29] Clinically, there is evidence of more synovitis with increased heat and exudation (especially in joints where the mechanical forces have been high) in less than the majority of patients. Some individuals also experience myalgias, spontaneously or with palpation. In persons with RA who are not used to exercise, there is an increased risk of such injuries as sprain or dislocation. Because RA patients are osteopenic, the risk of fractures must also be kept in mind. Finally, patients with cardiac arrhythmias might demonstrate an increased frequency of occurrence during exercise.

Effects of Medication on the Ability to Exercise

Pain and stiffness are the main problems noted by RA patients and that reduce the capacity of the individual to perform ADL. Therefore, because most drugs used to treat RA reduce pain and inflammation, they also increase a patient's ability to exercise. It must be remembered, however, that analgesic therapy not only reduces unwanted pain but also reduces the pain that actually signals threatening or ongoing tissue damage. Analgesics should thus be used with caution in active stages of RA. Training activity must be modified according to the actual pain, instead of disregarding the pain with the aid of analgesics. The same consideration is true with the use of local cortisone injections. In the hands of an experienced rheumatologist and for patients who are aware of the symptom-reducing effect of cortisone, training activity may proceed with certain modifications after local injections. It must then be emphasized that if arthritic symptoms in a joint return soon after local injection, the training must be temporarily discontinued. Our experience indicates that a few days or weeks of rest from a certain training activity might be enough to cause the increased symptoms to disappear. After such a rest period, training can begin again at a slightly lower intensity.[29]

Gold, penicillamine, and cytostatics are toxic drugs with many side-effects. Some of the patients we have trained have taken gold or penicillamine, and we have not found that these drugs negatively influence the patient's ability to train or that training increases the risk of side-effects. We have, however, had only a few patients who were taking these drugs, and thus any general conclusions cannot be drawn. There are reports of myopathy occurring after treatment with cortisone and cloroquine.[11,34] Penicillamine might induce a myasthenia gravis-like syndrome.[5] It is probably wise to be cautious with the use of high intensity training in patients during phases of high activity, regardless of whether they are treated with gold, penicillamine, or cloroquine.

Exercise Testing

Cardiovascular and locomotor factors can limit physical performance in persons with RA. Furthermore, inflammatory processes in the heart, lungs, and peripheral arteries and nerves may modify an individual's ability to exercise. The aim of a bicycle test is to establish the status of the cardiovascular system and to evaluate the patient's level of physical fitness. Current bicycle protocols are adequate for these patients. This statement is supported by the fact that maximal oxygen intake (using the criterion of a plateau with increasing exercise) on the bicycle ergometer can be obtained with many RA patients in Functional Classes 1 to 3.

Muscle strength tests can be effectively performed by using isokinetic and strain gauge techniques for most patients in Functional Classes 1 and 2, as well as many in Class 3. In any of these patients, however, there may be angles within the range of motion that should be avoided due to stiffness, muscle or joint pain, or other anatomic considerations. Furthermore, it is of value if the patient can be given some kind of prior active or passive "warm-up" of the joints and muscles that are to be tested. The range of mobility will probably then be increased and patients will be able to move at higher angular velocities. Because inhibition resulting from pain may occur in some patients, the values obtained will be more valid. Range of motion tests can be applied to these patients in the same way as they are given to healthy persons. However, because muscle contractures, joint destruction, and other components can cause reduced mobility, a distinction must be made between reduced muscle stretching due to muscle pain or contractures and joint engagements due to joint pain, contractures, or anatomic destructions. In these types of tests, it is especially important to standardize the pretest procedures (e.g., warm-up) and information to patients who are often afraid of being tested.

Exercise Prescription

Before prescribing exercise, the medical and psychologic state of the patient must be properly evaluated with specific regard to the activity of the inflammatory process and range of mobility in different joints. Cardiovascular function, lung function, muscle strength, muscle endurance, and the patient's earlier experiences with exercise must be considered. It is also important to examine the patient's attitude toward exercise and toward the disease process in general. Some patients have a very optimistic attitude and are determined to do something that might improve their functional capacity. Other patients are less optimistic or have lost faith in their own ability to do anything about their situation. This latter group needs information and encouragement to become motivated enough to start exercising. The first group of patients may need to be cautioned not to disregard increasing symptoms from the locomotor system after exercise. In our experience, individually modified exercise prescriptions are an important part of rehabilitation in RA. Many patients are unjustifiably afraid of exercise, and many have been inactive for a long time or have had very little experience with exercise. Although some individuals have experienced various forms of high intensity training, these programs are not recommended for most RA patients.

When prescribing exercise, the stage and activity of disease are important considerations.[16,17,29] When the disease activity level is high, exercise that puts a high load on the affected joints must be avoided. In contrast, "low load" exercise for 12 to 15 minutes on a bicycle ergometer and swimming in warm water (30 to 32°C) may be performed (even in RA patients with arthritic symptoms in the hips and knee joints) and are often well accepted. Patients with much pain can move freely in the water for 15 to 25 minutes without need for a specific prescription for swimming speed or distance. Mobility training is recommended, when done under the supervision of a physiotherapist, to avoid contractures. According to our experiences, both types of exercise are important ways to keep patients active and to maintain their training habits during periods of high disease activity.

After a period of high disease activity, most Class 1 and 2 and some Class 3 patients can train by cycling and walking for cardiovascular fitness. They can also perform some isometric and dynamic exercises for improving muscular strength, plus different types of gymnastics to increase joint mobility. It is important to prevent the development of contractures, especially in the shoulders, elbows, hips, and knees. Lying prone for 30 minutes daily might prevent contractures in the hips and knees.

Bicycle training should begin with continuous exercise at low loads (e.g., 25 minutes at 25 to 75 W, three times per week). After a few weeks, higher loads with more interval-type training might be used for rehabilitation. From our experience, most patients prefer training three to five times per session at a load of 75 to 150 W for 3 to 5 minutes. Bicycle training can also be performed at home, but most of our patients have put the bicycle aside after several months and have preferred to walk; they might use the bicycle sporadically during periods of higher disease activity, but they then return to walking. We have found that walking is very suitable for RA patients and have therefore introduced it into the rehabilitation process as soon as possible. Patients are initially encouraged to walk 15 to 30 minutes at a comfortable pace. Duration is later extended and the speed is increased to fast walking. Many of our patients walk fast or jog for 30 to 60 minutes, three to five times per week. After several months of training, many patients in Classes 1 and 2 may transfer to jogging programs; even fairly advanced jogging programs can be done by some patients. There are even RA patients who have run marathons.

Swimming and rowing, as well as bicycling, are good types of exercise for persons affected with RA because body weight does not completely load the joints or lower extremities. This fact accounts in part for why the performance of these exercises at a low intensity are recommended during periods of exacerbation. To recommend total bed rest is not only unnecessary for most patients, but also it might increase the risk of developing contractures and immobility. After 3 or 4 months of training, most patients choose their own mode of exercise, with many realizing benefits from a home program of gymnastics combined with walking, swimming, or skiing.

In our long-term follow-up study of as many as 8 years, 80 to 85% of the patients who started training have continued to do so regularly (see Tables 7–2 and 7–3).[26,29] We have offered these individuals group training for 1 hour once every second week. On that occasion, there is training for general mobility, as well as cycling for cardiovascular fitness. Some patients also had knee or hip extension training to increase the mobility of their affected joints and to strengthen their muscles.

Depending on the state of pain, training may be dynamic or isometric. For those persons with a great deal of pain, we have found that isometric training is preferred because joint movement is restricted. Although isometric training does not prevent the development of contractures, it can preserve muscle strength. With some patients, we have used dynamic training within the limited range of the total mobility of a joint. It is often possible to find a range in which joint pain is tolerable during training.

Group training was led by a physiotherapist, which gave patients the opportunity to talk about their present problems with the group leader and, just as importantly, with each other. Group training was appreciated by the patients, and 80% of those persons in the follow-up study wanted to continue with a group. For most patients, we regard group training as necessary, because it encourages them to continue to exercise regularly. Training in a group does not have to occur more than every second week if patients train on their own between sessions. Every second week, they can consult the physiotherapist and the program can be modified for their present joint problems. To work properly, this program must involve close cooperation between the physician and the physiotherapist, and both health professionals must have had experience training patients with RA.

Because affected joints are sore and muscles are often weak in the acute phases of RA, exercises that involve a heavy load on the affected joints and muscles must be avoided. This restriction applies especially to high intensity training. Furthermore, eccentric muscle contractions (such as occurs when a movement is resisted, as in walking or running downhill and in most racket sports), as well as exercises involving high angular velocities are often not accepted by patients. All of these activities should be avoided because of an increased risk of accidents. Low body temperatures may also increase the risk of injury. After institution or completion of proper training programs that produce increased strength and mobility, however, these types of activities can be easily performed by many patients during the low activity phases of RA. In fact, some patients with RA run long distance races and play tennis.

The types of activity that almost all patients can do, even in close proximity to their high activity phases, include swimming (especially in warm water), cycling, and other modes of exercise that avoid the aforementioned physiologic stresses. Patients must be well informed about the acute effects of exercise and that a warm-up period should be given. They should also know that if an activity causes pain in the muscles or joints, they should analyze and modify the type of exercise.

Effects of Training

As has been noted, RA patients generally have a low exercise capacity. Thus, there are fairly rapid improvements in subjective performance indices and in different measured physiologic parameters, even after a short period and a moderate amount of training.[14,16,17,19]

TABLE 7-2. Selected Observations in a Training (n = 23) and a Control (n = 23) Group Before and After an Average Period of 5.5 Years (range 4 to 8 years)

	Training Group			Control Group			Significant Difference Between Groups Before and After
	Before	After	% Difference	Before	After	% Difference	
Sick leave/sick pension (%)	35	36	+1	52	81	+29	p < 0.001
Stair test (sec)	13.4 ± 3.6	12.6 ± 7.5	−6	16.0 ± 10.1	19.3 ± 16.6	+21	p < 0.05
Radiographic index*	6.2 ± 5.9	10.2 ± 7.2	+65	6.7 ± 5.4	13.6 ± 5.8	+103	p < 0.025
Joint index†	93 ± 37	59 ± 51	−37	85 ± 30	76 ± 51	−11	p < 0.05
Quadriceps torque (nM)	17.4 + 4.7	19.6 ± 5.9	+13	17.2 ± 7.6	15.7 ± 8.4	−9	p < 0.05
Oxygen pulse, submaximal exercise (ml · beat^{-1})	8.7 ± 1.4	8.5 ± 1.9	−2	7.8 ± 2.4	8.0 ± 2.2	+3	p > 0.05

* From Larsen.[23]
† From Lansbury.[22]

TABLE 7-3. Ability to Perform ADL Functions*

Function	Training Group		Control Group		Significant Difference
	Able	Unable†	Able	Unable†	
Wash hair	22	1	19	4	ns‡
Wash face	23	0	22	1	ns
Intimate hygiene	23	0	21	2	ns
Wash feet	21	2	17	6	ns
Toilet	23	0	22	1	ns
Socks, on and off	23	0	20	3	ns
Shirt, on and off	21	2	16	3	ns
Trousers/shirt, on and off	23	0	18	2	ns
Do buttons	21	2	18	5	ns
Raise from lying to standing	22	1	19	3	ns
Walk on even ground	22	1	21	2	ns
Walk upstairs and downstairs	22	1	13	8	$p = 0.007$
Eat with knife and fork	22	1	22	1	ns
Cook	21	1	20	3	ns
Wash dishes	22	1	20	3	ns
Go shopping	17	3	13	9	$p = 0.06$
Clean house	18	3	9	13	$p = 0.003$
Wash laundry	19	2	12	10	$p = 0.009$
Make bed	18	3	18	5	ns
Use pair of scissors	21	2	20	3	ns
Use public transportation	17	5	11	12	$p = 0.04$
Pick up object from floor	22	1	21	2	ns
Take object from shelf§	23	0	16	6	$p = 0.009$
Write a letter	21	1	22	1	ns
Σ of different ADL functions					$p < 0.01$

* Comparison of same groups as described in Table 7-1.
† Without help from another person.
‡ Not significant.
§ Above shoulder height.

We have studied the effects of short and long-term training programs on RA patients, with special reference to the effects on physical performance and related physiologic, medical, and sociopsychologic factors.[26-29] After 6 weeks of rehabilitation in a hospital ward, performance in a group of 23 patients increased 14% while walking on level ground, 25% while walking up stairs, and 15 to 20% while stepping up on foot stools (the tallest possible). In addition to ordinary physiotherapy, the program consisted of bicycle and strength training, as described, once per day for 5 days per week. Maximal oxygen intake increased from 1.22 to 1.47 $L \cdot min^{-1}$, and average dynamic and isometric strength improved 23 to 73%. Thus, rehabilitative exercise programs will produce a good training response. Although there is muscular hypotrophy in patients with RA (mainly selective fast-twitch or Type II fibers), this type of training increases muscle fiber area, as evaluated from muscle biopsies.[12,28]

Some of the effects of this short-term training program are illustrated in Figure 7-1. It is of interest to observe that both "central" and "local" ratings of perceived fatigue were markedly reduced. This finding indicates that not only can patients perform a given work task with less exertion, but also that they can perform exercise at a higher intensity. This finding is also confirmed in the questionnaires about their ADL performances after training.

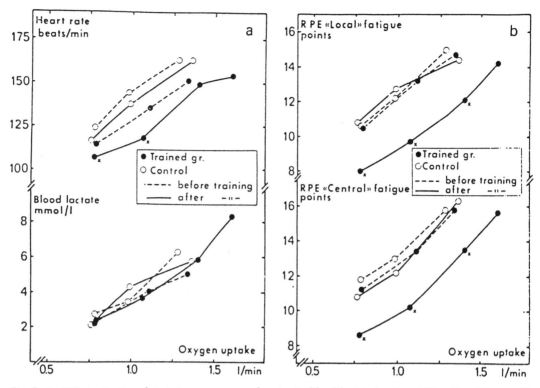

Fig. 7-1. *Effects of a 6-week training program on heart rate, blood lactate level, and "local" and "central" ratings of perceived exertion (RPE).*

Long-term training not only restores physiologic parameters toward or above the normal range for respective age groups, but also there are positive clinical, psychologic, sociologic and other effects, some of which are listed in Table 7–2.[9,26,29] During an average observation period of 5.5 years, patients who trained had a total hospital stay of 16.4 days, compared to 35.6 days in the control group (p < 0.05). In comparison with the control group, trained patients arrested the progress of their disease. Radiography demonstrated that the speed of reduction in joint cartilage and bone was significantly diminished.[23,29] Clinical examination revealed a better joint state, and the patients reported significantly better ADL functional capacity (Table 7–3).[26,29] Concerning the social situation, it can be concluded that trained patients had significantly less sick leave, less sick pension, and stayed in the hospital for less than one half as many days as the persons in the control group.

It is obvious that physical training is one of the few means by which patients can influence their situation. There are many indications that there are beneficial psychologic consequences for the whole rehabilitation process. When taking part in group training, patients also get together and have opportunities to talk about their situation and to get ideas about how to solve certain problems within the family, at work, and the like. Many patients spontaneously state that this contact is important. Unfortunately, it is a forgotten part of RA management in many hospitals. A feeling of isolation occurred almost twice as often in the control group members (36%) as in the trained patients (20%).

Finally, it is of great interest to note that all patients in our training study wished to take part in some form of training in the future. We conclude that physical training for persons with RA has physical, psychologic, and social consequences that are clearly beneficial. We recommend training be one part of the many involved in the complicated treatment of RA.

REFERENCES

1. Arnett, F.C., Edworthy, S.M., Bloch, D.A., et al.: The American Rheumatism Association 1987 Revised criteria for the classification of rheumatoid arthritis. Arthritis Rheum., *31*:315–324, 1988.
2. Boström, C., and Ljungquist, T.: Active dynamic training—something for rheumatics with shoulder pain. Sjukgymnasten, *14*:25–29, 1984.
3. Borg, G.: Physical Performance and Perceived Exertion. Lund, Sweden, Gleerup, 1962.
4. Brooke, M.H., and Kaplan, H.: Muscle pathology in rheumatoid arthritis, polymyalgia rheumatica, and polymyositis. Arch. Pathol. Lab. Med., *94*:101, 1973.
5. Bucknall, R.C., et al.: Myasthenia gravis associated with penicillamine treatment for rheumatoid arthritis. Br. Med. J., *1*:600, 1975.
6. Byers, P.H.: Effect of exercise on morning stiffness and mobility in patients with rheumatoid arthritis. Res. Nurs. Health, *8*:275–281, 1985.
7. Chayen, J., and Bitensky, L.: Occasional survey: lysosomal enzymes and inflammation with particular reference to rheumatoid diseases. Ann. Rheum. Dis., *30*:522, 1971.
8. Danneskiold-Samsöe, B., Lyngberg, K., Risum, T., and Telling, M.: The effect of water exercise therapy given to patients with rheumatoid arthritis. Scand. J. Rehab. Med., *19*:31–35, 1987.
9. De Haas, W.H.D., et al.: Rheumatoid arthritis of the robust reaction type. Ann. Rheum. Dis., *33*:81, 1974.
10. Donaldson, S.W., Wagner, C.C., and Gresham, T.: A unified ADL evaluation form. Arch. Phys. Med. Rehabil., *54*:175, 1973.
11. Eadie, M.J., and Ferrier, T.M.: Chloriquine myopathy. J. Neurol. Neurosurg. Psychiatry, *19*:331, 1966.
12. Edstrom, L., and Nordemar, R.: Differential changes in Type I and Type II muscle fibres in rheumatoid arthritis. Scand. J. Rheumatol., *3*:155, 1974.
13. Eggert, G.M., et al.: Caring for the patient with long-term disability. Geriatrics, *32*:102, 1977.
14. Ekblom, B., and Goldberg, A.: The influence of physical training and other factors on the subjective rating of perceived exertion. Acta Physiol. Scand., *83*:399, 1971.
15. Ekblom, B., et al.: Physical performance in patients with rheumatoid arthritis. Scand. J. Rheumatol., *3*:121, 1974.
16. Ekblom, B., et al.: Effect of short-term physical training on patients with rheumatoid arthritis I. Scand. J. Rheumatol., *4*:80, 1975.
17. Ekblom, B., et al.: Effect of short-term physical training on patients with rheumatoid arthritis—a six-month follow-up study. Scand. J. Rheumatol., *4*:87, 1975.
18. Ekdahl, C., Andersson, S.I., Moritz, U., and Svensson, B.: Dynamic versus static training in patients with rheumatoid arthritis. Scand. J. Rheumatol., *19*:17–26, 1990.
19. Harkcom, T.M., et al.: Therapeutic value of graded aerobic exercise training in rheumatoid arthritis. Arthritis Rheum., *28*:32, 1985.
20. Karper, W.B., and Evans, B.W.: Cycling program effects on one rheumatoid arthritic. Am. J. Phys. Med., *65*:167–172, 1986.
21. King, A.C., Ahles, T.A., Martin, J.E., and White, R.: EMG biofeedback-controlled exercise in chronic arthritic knee pain. Arch. Phys. Med. Rehabil., *65*:341–343, 1984.
22. Lansbury, J.: Report of a three-year study on the systemic and articular indexes in rheumatoid arthritis. Arthritis Rheum., *1*:505, 1958.
23. Larsen, A.: Radiological grading of rheumatoid arthritis. An interobserver study. Scand. J. Rheumatol., *2*:136, 1973.
24. Lyngberg, K., Danneskiold-Samsöe, B., and Halskov, O.: The effect of physical training on patients with rheumatoid arthritis: changes in disease activity, muscle strength and aerobic capacity: a clinically controlled minimized crossover study. Clin. Exp. Rheumatol., *6*:253–260, 1988.
25. Minor, M.A., Hewett, J.E., Webel, R.R., et al.: Efficacy of physical conditioning exercise in patients with rheumatoid arthritis and osteoarthritis. Arthritis Rheum., *32*:1396–1405, 1989.
26. Nordemar, R.: Physical training in rheumatoid arthritis—a controlled long-term study. 2. Functional capacity and general attitudes. Scand. J. Rheumatol., *10*:24, 1981.
27. Nordemar, R., et al.: Changes in muscle performance in patients with rheumatoid arthritis after 7 months' physical training. Scand. J. Rheumatol., *5*:233, 1976.
28. Nordemar, R., Edstrom, L., and Ekblom, B.: Changes in muscle fibre size and performance in patients with rheumatoid arthritis after short-term physical training. Scand. J. Rheumatol., *5*:70, 1976.
29. Nordemar, R., et al.: Physical training in rheumatoid arthritis—a controlled long-term study. Scand. J. Rheumatol., *10*:17, 1981.
30. Oka, M., Rekonen, A., and Elomaa, L.: Muscle blood flow in rheumatoid arthritis. Acta Rheumatol. Scand., *17*:203, 1971.
31. Schaufler, J., Sverdlik, S.S., Baker, A., and Krewer, S.E.: "Hand gym" for patients with arthritic hand disabilities: preliminary report. Arch. Phys. Med. Rehabil., *59*:221–226, 1978.
32. Schoening, H.A., and Iverson, J.A.: Numerical scoring of self-care status: study of Kenney self-care evaluation. Arch. Phys. Med. Rehabil., *49*:221, 1968.
33. Scott, J.T. (ed.): Copeman's Textbook of the Rheumatic Diseases. 5th Ed. London, Churchill Livingstone, 1978.
34. Smith, B.: Histological and histochemical changes in the muscles of rabbits given the corticosteroid triamcinolone. Neurology, *14*:857, 1964.
35. Steiner, G., et al.: Lesions of skeletal muscles in rheumatoid arthritis. Nodular polymyositis. Am. J. Pathol., *22*:103, 1946.
36. Tegelberg, A., and Kopp, S.: Short-term effect of physical training on temporomandibular joint disorder in individuals with rheumatoid arthritis and ankylosing spondylitis. Acta Odontol. Scand., *46*:49–56, 1988.
37. Van Deusen, J., and Harlowe, D.: The efficacy of the ROM Dance Program for adults with rheu-

matoid arthritis. Am. J. Occup. Ther., *41*:90–95, 1987.

38. Wilkinson, P., et al.: The mechanism of hypoalbuminemia in rheumatoid arthritis. Ann. Intern. Med., *63*:109, 1965.

39. Zvaifler, N.J. (ed.): Clinics in Rheumatic Diseases. Vol. 4. Immunology. London, W.B. Saunders, 1978.

8
CHAPTER

Osteoporosis

by
Catherine Gilligan, Mary M. Checovich and Everett L. Smith

Osteoporosis is the clinical manifestation of bone atrophy resulting in low-trauma fractures. Most common are wedge or crush fractures of the spine, Colles' (wrist) fractures, and hip fractures. Frequently, diminished bone mineral density (BMD), or osteopenia, is also referred to as osteoporosis because of the increased risk of fracture, with as little as a 10% reduction in BMD.[53]

Osteoporosis has been divided into two syndromes that represent different pathogenetic mechanisms.[63] Type I osteoporosis is related to menopause, associated with accelerated trabecular bone loss, and characterized by Colles' fractures and crush fractures of the spine within 15 to 20 years after menopause. Type II osteoporosis is age-related, generally occurring after age 70, and is characterized by hip fractures and multiple wedge fractures of the vertebrae. Other causes of osteoporosis include disorders of bone marrow and connective tissue, immobilization, and drug-related effects (e.g., corticosteroids or anticonvulsants).

At least 1.3 million fractures annually in the United States are attributed to osteoporosis.[20,54,57] By age 80, the majority of women have at least one partial vertebral fracture.[20] Vertebral crush fractures typically affect T8–L3 and can occur during routine activities of daily living. Vertebral fractures are not always accompanied by pain and may be detected only if a radiograph is taken. Height loss or the development of kyphosis may be the only signs of multiple vertebral fractures. In the United States, about 250,000 adults over age 45 fracture a hip each year.[88] Hip fractures are associated with a 12 to 20% excess mortality,[42] and only one-quarter of hip fracture patients regain full independence.[21] Because there is no real cure for osteoporosis, strategies to reduce bone loss and enhance bone mass have been the focus of much research.

FACTORS ASSOCIATED WITH FRACTURES

Low BMD is a major determinant of fracture incidence, but there is a large overlap in BMD between subjects with and without fractures.[64] The only known measurable risk factor for spine fractures is low spine BMD. Hip and wrist fractures, however, frequently are pursuant to falls (Fig. 8–1).[21] Risk factors for falls include neurologic deficits, impaired vision, medication-induced sedation, and impaired balance, reaction time, gait, and strength.[86] Exercise can reduce the risk of fractures not only by countering bone loss, but by enhancing neuromuscular abilities that can aid in averting falls and reducing the impact if a fall occurs. Cross-sectional and prospective studies have indicated that more-active subjects have a lower risk of falls and fractures.[9,14,15,92]

BONE PHYSIOLOGY

Complex cellular, metabolic, and physiologic factors underlie the pathogenesis of osteoporosis. It is imperative to remember

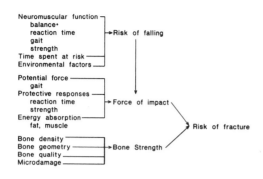

Neuromuscular function
  balance*
  reaction time
  gait
  strength
Time spent at risk
Environmental factors → Risk of falling

Potential force
  gait
Protective responses
  reaction time
  strength
Energy absorption
  fat, muscle → Force of impact

Bone density
Bone geometry
Bone quality
Microdamage → Bone Strength

→ Risk of fracture

*Subheadings list only factors that may be affected by exercise

Fig. 8–1. *Determinants of hip and wrist fractures. (Adapted from Cummings, S.E., Kelsey, J.L., McNevitt, M.C., and O'Dowd, K.J.: Epidemiology of osteoporosis and osteoporotic fractures. Epidemiol. Rev., 7:178–208, 1985.)*

that the skeleton is not a static system, but undergoes a continual process of resorption and formation. The skeleton has three basic functions. It provides 1) protection for vital organs, 2) structural support and a system of levers to which muscles attach for movement, and 3) a repository for calcium and phosphorus. Control of bone formation and resorption is related to the latter two functions.

Cell Function

Skeletal balance involves three types of cells: osteoblasts, osteocytes, and osteoclasts. The osteoblasts arise from preosteoblasts produced by differentiation of local mesenchymal stem cells. Bone formation occurs in two phases. The osteoblast first secretes collagen into the extracellular space forming a network of fibers; this uncalcified matrix (osteoid tissue) is present for about 10 days. In the second phase, the matrix becomes calcified. Once encased by calcified matrix, the osteoblast is called an osteocyte, which maintains the bone matrix. Osteocytes and periosteal and endosteal lining cells are interconnected by gap junctions. Once the matrix is calcified, its structure can be changed only by adding to the existing structure (modeling) or by osteoclastic resorption and the formation of a new matrix (remodeling). Osteo-

clasts are derived from bone marrow and are thought to arise from mononuclear phagocytes. They are carried to the site of remodeling by the blood stream. When activated, the multinucleated osteoclast is found in contact with the bone surface where it acidifies and resorbs the bone matrix. Each bone cell is influenced by chemical intermediaries initiated by the hormonal system, local growth factors, and mechanical strain.

Gross Integrity

In the normal adult, bone formation and resorption are closely coupled, and the bone matrix removed by osteoclastic activity is replaced by osteoblastic activity. Bone cells organize and maintain an extracellular matrix that provides the structural and functional properties of skeletal tissue. These properties depend on the interrelationship of collagen and mineral quantity, quality, and architectural organization. The mineralized matrix provides bone with a strength and stiffness that enable it to resist deformation and maintain its integrity, even under large loads.

Cellular Response to Hormonal and Mechanical Stimuli

Bone formation and resorption are controlled by the interaction of two homeostatic mechanisms: hormonal and mechanical. Bone remodeling is regulated by hormones and local factors that affect osteoclasts and osteoblasts. The end-product of remodeling is the formation of a new mineralized bone matrix. Hormones (e.g., parathyroid hormone, calcitonin, and vitamin D) are involved with maintaining serum calcium, which is necessary to the physiologic function of such body tissues as muscles and nerves. Other hormones (e.g., estrogen, testosterone, growth hormone, and glucocorticoids) affect bone but are less specifically involved with maintaining serum calcium levels. Regulation of serum calcium levels modulates activity of specific cells in bone.

Although the hormonal system is necessary to maintain serum calcium, skeletal integrity also depends on mechanical loading. In the absence of mechanical loads, bone atrophies. In the presence of mechanical loading, bone hypertrophies. Lanyon has proposed that the osteocyte is the cell that monitors changes in strain induced by mechanical loading.[47] With over 25,000 cells per cubic millimeter, osteocytes can be precise indicators of strain. Although the hormonal stimuli produce an overall skeletal response, it appears that mechanical loading produces a local response in conjunction with such local growth factors as insulin-like growth factor (IGF-1), transforming growth factors (TGF-β), and platelet-derived growth factor (PDGF).

Although hormonal and mechanical stimuli both affect bone, the interactions of these two homeostatic mechanisms are still unclear. If an organism is completely deprived of calcium, skeletal calcium mobilization is increased in order to meet the demands of the serum calcium requirements. If increased mechanical load is placed on the bone, as observed in osteotomies, bone hypertrophies as much as 100% within 6 months in response to the high overload.[17]

Bone Loss with Age

With age, the efficiency of osteoblasts declines, resulting in the inability to completely replace the volume of bone resorbed. This net deficit leads to the loss of bone seen with aging in both men and women, with women having a higher rate of loss starting at an earlier age (30 to 35 years of age). Natural or surgical menopause, leading to estrogen deficiency, is a critical turning point in which turnover and bone loss may double.

In most cases, there are no discernible abnormalities in bone tissue of subjects with osteoporotic fractures, except for reduced BMD. However, accompanying structural changes are also important determinants of bone strength. Osteoporotic bone may differ in geometry (increased medullary cavity, decreased wall thickness, greater cortical porosity and increased distance between trabeculae), which affects strain distribution, bone quality (increased cell death), and the accumulation of microdamage. Bone loss through trabecular thinning and removal of trabeculae disrupts normal bony architecture, which leads to a reduction in bone strength and an increased risk of fracture.[61]

TESTING AND EVALUATION

General Exercise and Testing Guidelines

Exercise testing should follow the guidelines of the American College of Sports Medicine.[7] For most older subjects, this requires a 12-lead electrocardiogram and physical examination, followed by an aerobic work capacity test.

Subjects recovering from a hip fracture or with severe back pain from vertebral fractures may not be able to perform an aerobic work capacity test on a treadmill or bicycle ergometer but may be able to perform the Chair Step Test.[81] Subjects with hip fractures also might perform an arm ergometry test to provide an estimate of aerobic fitness and cardiovascular response to exercise. For subjects who cannot perform an aerobic work capacity test, any exercise program must be kept at low intensity and focus on flexibility and regaining mobility.

A maximal work capacity test is not necessary, with the understanding that aerobic training levels should never exceed the heart rate (HR) attained on the individual's work capacity test. Because individual maximal HRs range approximately 20% above and below the age-predicted maximal HR,[75] target HR prescriptions are more accurate if a maximal work capacity test is performed and the HR reserve is calculated for each individual.

Evaluation of Osteoporosis Risk Factors

In evaluating subjects for a fracture prevention program, several additions to the standard medical examination should be considered. If a subject has a history of falls, a careful review of medications and a vision examination including contrast sensitivity and visual field are strongly recommended. An evaluation of nutritional intake is also important for subjects at risk for osteoporosis.

Most of the sophisticated equipment to test the exercise-related risk factors for fracture will not be available to the general practitioner or physical therapist. However, some clinical methods are available to assess strength, balance, and gait. These will be discussed in the following sections. Flexibility measures are easily achieved using a goniometer.[6]

The evaluations of strength, balance, gait, and flexibility are recommended to determine the subject's level of ability and to aid in planning an exercise program and in making individualized recommendations. Re-evaluations after participation in exercise training can provide feedback to the subjects and to the instructor on the effectiveness of the program.

The type of exercise and the amount of supervision can be based on evaluations of the subject's fitness. For example, a 5-point rating scale for subjects with osteoporotic fractures could be used for each of aerobic work capacity, strength, balance, and gait. The type of program to be assigned would then be based on the average rating as follows:

1. Individual physical therapy
2. Small group (four to six) pool or chair exercises supervised by exercise specialists
3. Small group exercise, including weight-bearing activities supervised by exercise specialists
4. Group exercise supervised by exercise specialists or
5. Individual unsupervised exercise or community programs

It is expected that individuals would increase in fitness and progress from one program to the next. Each exercise program should have elements to improve the subject's weak areas.

BONE MINERAL DENSITY. The difference in absorption characteristics of bone and soft tissue is the basis of all methods used to identify or quantify bone changes with age or fracture. Historically, radiographs have been used to evaluate collapse, wedging, and ballooning of the spine, but they are insensitive for quantifying and monitoring BMD. Currently, the most common methods for measuring BMD are single-photon absorptiometry (SPA)[89] for the wrist (15 mRem), and dual-photon absorptiometry (DPA)[89] for the spine and femur (5 mRem per site). Recently, dual-energy x-ray absorptiometry (<5 mRem) was introduced. This method has increased precision and reduced radiation compared to DPA.[51] Other methods currently used include quantitative computed tomography (100 to 1000 mRem) and neutron activation analysis.[89] Fracture risk indices have been constructed from values of BMD at various single sites (axial and appendicular), but the predictability of BMD at one site from BMD at another is poor; correlation coefficients are about 0.36 to 0.65 for BMD in different bones and about 0.84 for BMD at different sites in the same bone.[38]

Factors that can contribute to low bone mass include female gender, Northern European heritage, small or light build, early menopause, a family history of osteoporosis, and excessive alcohol and tobacco use.[24,39,74,78] For subjects with multiple risk factors, BMD measurements should be considered. If the BMD is below the fracture threshold (e.g., 0.75 for the femur and 0.92 for the spine[52]) and if pathologic conditions other than osteoporosis have been ruled out, aggressive treatment may be indicated. This treatment may include calcium supplements to bring total intake to 1500 mg/day, medications (e.g., estrogen replacement therapy, biphosphonates, calcitonin, or fluoride*), and individualized exercise programs. If a subject complains of back pain or has the dowager's hump typical of spine fractures, it is appropriate to obtain anteroposterior and lateral spine radiographs to determine the

---

* Fluoride therapy is still in the research stage and should be prescribed only by experienced specialists. It has numerous side effects, including gastrointestinal upset and joint pain.

location, extent, and type of vertebral fractures. Again, the therapy chosen must be based on a careful evaluation of all available data and an individual program must be initiated.

Although SPA and DPA have high precision, accurately assessing bone loss rate or response to treatment for an individual requires multiple measures and long-term follow-up.[22,71] It is therefore not practical to monitor bone loss for most subjects who enroll in an exercise program, unless the severity of the disease requires close and routine monitoring.

BALANCE. In research settings, balance is often assessed by measurements on a balance platform of area and velocity of sway while standing and in response to perturbations. Clinical measures include observation scales, such as that developed by Tinetti,[87] and timed-single-leg stance.[65]

REACTION TIME. Reaction time consists of both central (premotor) and peripheral (motor) components of response. Reaction time can be discriminated into premotor and contractile components with the use of electromyography.[10] Total reaction time including speed of movement is easily measured, although the equipment is not routinely available. Multiple trials are advised to ensure precision.[10] Reaction time may differ depending on whether the stimulus is visual, auditory, or proprioceptive. Most research on the effects of exercise has used visual stimuli.

GAIT. In research settings, gait is often measured using force platforms and video cameras to determine force, cadence, stride length, velocity, and joint ranges of motion. Clinical measures of gait velocity and stride length can be accomplished by trained observers almost anywhere with the use of a stopwatch and by chalking or inking shoe heels. Gait abnormalities can be assessed by observation using a scale such as that developed by Tinetti.[87]

STRENGTH. Many research studies have used dynamometers to assess strength. There has been some question about the applicability of these measures to strength gains made with resistance training, because of the specificity of training effects. If resistance training using general weight-training equipment is a mode of exercise, the best measure of strength gains is the one-repetition maximum (1-RM) test for each of the movements trained. Dynamometers, strain gauges, or resistance-training equipment could be used to test strength for other programs.

In a 1-RM test, or any time a maximal motor effort is performed, recruitment of nontarget motor groups and altered body mechanics may occur. Guidelines to minimize this for each muscle group need to be developed and used, especially in testing older persons. For example, in standing hip-strength evaluations, the equipment should be modified to provide external upper trunk and pelvic stabilization and to limit the available joint excursion.

EXERCISE BASED ON AFFECTING OSTEOPOROSIS RISK FACTORS

The general principles of exercise programming (see Chapter 2 by Skinner) apply to subjects at risk for fracture. Each session should include warm-up and cool-down periods with flexibility training. Aerobic training requires at least 20 min, 3 days/week, at 40 to 70% of HR reserve.[8,45] Many older people will not be able to complete 20 min of continuous aerobic exercise at the start of their exercise program. Beginning with 3 to 5 min of aerobic exercise and gradually adding minutes is one method. Another is to intersperse aerobic activity with resistance-training exercises, gradually reducing the time for the resistance exercises. If the form of exercise is aerobic dance, such simple movements as walking should be used first, with more complicated movements added gradually as the participants become more accustomed to moving to music. For most elderly subjects, a 60-min total training period (including warm-up, cool-down, and aerobic and/or resistance training) is recommended. It may take 4 to 12 weeks for elderly subjects with low fitness to build up to 20 min of training at the target HR or to a 60-min program.

The following sections review the research on the effects of exercise on fracture risk factors and give recommendations for exercise activities to affect each factor. It should be noted that research on the specific type of exercise for maximal improvement in BMD, balance, gait, and reaction time is sparse and that these areas require further study.

Bone Mineral Density

Exercise intervention programs have reduced bone loss or increased bone mass in both men and women of various ages and initial bone status. These benefits have been shown for arm bone mineral content (BMC),[67,76,79,80,91] total body calcium,[3] spine BMD,[23,35,46] calcium bone index (CaBI, a measurement of calcium content by neutron activation analysis of the central third of the body),[18,19] and tibia BMC.[50] Few intervention studies have measured femur BMD, and these studies did not report a significant exercise effect.[56,69] Cross-sectional studies indicate that femur BMD is higher in athletes than in controls.[13,40]

Although it is known that bone responds to exercise, the type of exercise most effective for enhancing bone density and quality has not been determined. Most exercise programs that have affected spine or lower-body BMD used walking or weight-bearing aerobic training as a major part of the exercise sessions.[3,18,19,23,46,50,72] Wrist BMD was affected in studies incorporating some form of upper-body resistance training[67,76,79,80] but not in programs using weight-bearing activity alone.[3,73] Several recent studies have investigated other forms of training, such as squeezing tennis balls,[12] forearm loading,[76] and bicycle ergometer training.[44,56] Differences between exercise and control subjects in these studies has tended to be small. Resistance training effects on BMD have only recently been investigated. Chow et al. reported that the addition of strength training to aerobic training tended to increase CaBI more than aerobic training alone, but the difference was not significant.[19] Similarly, Rikli and McManis reported that

the addition of upper-body weight training to general aerobic training tended to increase radius bone mass more than general aerobic training alone.[67] Other intervention studies of resistance training alone reported nonsignificant effects of resistance training on BMD of the spine,[56,77] radius,[56] and femur.[56] Rockwell et al. reported that a 9-month weight training program had a significant negative effect on spine BMD in premenopausal women.[69] In contrast, Gleeson et al. reported that a 12-month weight lifting program improved spine BMD in exercisers relative to matched-pair controls.[35] Femur BMD appears to be greater in bodybuilders than in other athletes or sedentary individuals.[13,40]

Until further information is available, it is conservative to recommend a general weight-bearing exercise program for spine BMD and upper-body resistance-training for wrist BMD. Resistance training of all the major muscle groups that load the proximal femur may be necessary to increase femur BMD.

Balance

Balance is a complex behavior incorporating a wide variety of factors, including vision, proprioception, flexibility, and muscular strength. Few studies have evaluated the effect of exercise on balance. In a cross-sectional study, active elderly women had significantly better balance (measured by a timed single-stance test) than inactive elderly women.[65] Lichtenstein et al., using a biomechanics platform, reported conflicting results of balance training on area of sway.[49] The training program consisted of 10 min stretching, 10 min static balance (e.g., standing on one leg), 15 min active balance (e.g., tandem heel/toe gait), 10 min response exercise (performing maneuvers in response to signals), 10 min walking, and 5 min cool-down and relaxation. Classes were held 4 days/week for 16 weeks. Trained subjects improved compared to controls in the eyes-open, single-stance condition, but controls improved compared to exercisers in the eyes-closed, single-stance condition. In contrast, Roberts reported that a 6-week walking program significantly improved balance (average time for eight stances) in elderly women and men.[68] Exercise subjects walked 30 min, 3 days/week for 6 weeks at 60 to 70% of HR reserve. Similarly, women (mean age 70) in a 3-year exercise program improved significantly in single-stance (eyes open) time.[66] Change in balance differed significantly between the exercisers and controls (whose balance decreased).

Balance and the likelihood of falls are associated with muscular weakness of the lower limbs.[33,85,90] Muscle weakness in the lower extremities makes it difficult to steadily perform such everyday tasks as standing on one foot or rising from a chair. Consequently, programs that improve lower-body muscular strength should convey better balance.

Reaction Time

Various studies have reported that reaction time is faster in active subjects than in inactive subjects.[8,83] Spirduso et al. reported that young and old men with long-term regular participation in racket sports had a faster reaction time than inactive subjects of similar age.[83] Baylor and Spirduso found that aerobically active older persons had significantly faster reaction time (both central and peripheral components) than sedentary subjects.[8] Rikli and Edwards reported that simple ($p = 0.027$) and choice ($p < 0.01$) reaction times improved in subjects in a 3-year aerobics and calisthenics program.[66] Reaction time worsened in the control group, and there was a significant group $\times$ time interaction term for simple ($p = 0.014$) but not choice ($p = 0.034$) reaction time. In another intervention study, Dustman et al. reported that reaction time improved significantly in subjects 50 years old and older who participated in a 16-week aerobic training program, but did not change significantly in control subjects or subjects participating in a relaxation program.[27] Panton et al., however, did not find significant differences between control, aerobic training,

and strength training groups, although reaction time tended to improve in both exercise groups.[58]

Tentatively, aerobic training is recommended for increasing reaction time. An improved reaction time could facilitate responses to unsteady conditions and aid in performing protective movements to reduce impact if a fall occurs.

Strength

The principle of overload to increase muscular strength is well accepted. Gains in strength can be accomplished only by overload, that is, muscular force exceeding that required by activities of daily living. The highest strength gains are accomplished with few repetitions and a high resistance.

Various studies have demonstrated that elderly subjects can improve their strength with resistance training. In an uncontrolled study recently reported by Frontera et al., older men (aged 60 to 72 years) significantly increased quadriceps strength and developed muscle fiber hypertrophy as a result of a knee-extension resistance-training program.[32] Similarly, Fiatarone et al. reported that high-intensity resistance training significantly improved strength and muscle mass in elderly men and women (mean age 90).[29]

It may not be necessary, or appropriate, to use resistance-training equipment for frail subjects or subjects with arthritis. These subjects, however, can enjoy strength gains from less-rigorous strength training. Strength of elderly subjects improved in studies using light wrist and ankle weights,[2] elastic tubing, and/or body weight to provide resistance.[4,5,26]

An alternative way to provide resistance is through water exercise. Water exercise improved strength in young women,[84] and in subjects with multiple sclerosis[34] and rheumatoid arthritis.[25] It has been recommended for patients recovering from hip fracture.[36]

Both lower- and upper-body strength may help in avoiding falls and fractures. Ideally, resistance training for fracture prevention or fracture recovery should include all the major muscle groups.

Gait

The effect of exercise on gait has not been addressed in the research literature. Deficits in aerobic capacity, muscular strength, and flexibility can all place limitations on gait. The principles for training to improve these factors are well known. Removal of these limitations may not automatically improve a subject's gait. The gait of exercise participants should be carefully observed and participants should be instructed on correct posture and gait and frequently reminded to use them. Note that some gait abnormalities may be adaptations based on the subject's fear of falling (e.g., shortened stride length, reduced velocity, and increased double support time). These gait adaptations, however, may exacerbate deficiencies in leg strength and flexibility and in aerobic work capacity.

ADDITIONAL CONSIDERATIONS IN PROGRAMMING FOR SUBJECTS WITH FRACTURES

For anyone, but particularly for someone who has already experienced osteoporotic fracture, the physiologic benefits of exercise must be balanced against the possibility that certain activities may produce injuries, falls, or fractures. Such high-impact activities as jogging or tennis are not recommended for subjects with osteoporotic fractures. Exercise training programs must be established on an individual basis. Water or chair exercise programs are considered safe alternatives for high-risk populations, because the individual is able to concentrate on moving without fear or risk of falling. For people with low levels of fitness, aerobic workouts at a 2 to 4-MET level can be achieved in a chair.

The progression in intensity and movement complexity of exercise programs for high-risk populations should be gradual. People with poor fitness and a historically sedentary lifestyle often are uncomfortable with exercise. In our experience, they tend to have more difficulty learning exercise routines and express discomfort as a result of exercise more frequently. It is important not to discourage participation by making the program too difficult.

For subjects with impaired balance, weight-bearing activities should be kept simple at first. Complex movement patterns and walking backwards should be used with caution. Participants who have a history of falls may feel uncomfortable with these movements and could fall as a result of the combination of poor balance and unusual movement pattern.

In resistance training or flexibility portions of an exercise class, trunk flexion is contraindicated for subjects with spine fractures. Subjects with a hip prosthesis will have limited range of motion and strength of the hip and may not be able to perform some forms of hip resistance training. Hip abduction and internal rotation are contraindicated for these subjects. Unilateral training is not recommended. Special care must be taken that subjects with fractured hips do not apply torsion to the hip.

Subjects with hip or spine fractures may initially find it difficult to participate in weight-bearing exercise. Chair exercises or water exercise may be used to build up strength and aerobic fitness. Canes and walkers pose another limit to participation in weight-bearing exercise. Although these devices may be necessary to provide stability and reduce falls and the fear of falls, incorrect use can further disable the subject. Subjects may become dependent on these devices and be unwilling to give them up, even when they have adequately recovered. Special care must be taken that subjects using these devices maintain good posture and gait.

Because low body weight is often associated with osteoporosis, subjects with low to normal body weight should be encouraged to maintain their body weight by increasing their caloric intake to balance the energy expenditure of exercise.

In group exercise classes, participant-to-instructor ratios should be kept small, so that individual instruction can be given as needed. A noncompetitive atmosphere should be fostered so that participants work at their own levels. In choosing an exercise facility, floor surfaces should be kept in mind. Cement surfaces create hazards for joint injuries and stress fractures. The ideal surface is a sprung wood floor.

CONCLUSIONS

To our knowledge, no exercise programs for fracture prevention have been published. Publications regarding exercise programs for seniors,[1,11,16,30,48,55,59,60] chair exercises,[31,70,82] water exercise,[37,43,62] or resistance training using elastic tubing[28,41] are available.

Exercise programs to prevent or treat osteoporosis must first follow basic guidelines for exercise programs. A program that encompasses weight-bearing aerobic training, strength training, and flexibility training is recommended (Table 8–1). The time required to effectively train aerobic capacity plus upper- and lower-body strength in one session is likely to be excessive for this population. Aerobic and strength training could be accomplished on alternate days, or one component of strength training could be combined with aerobic training each session. Many subjects may find the time and energy commitment of this "ideal" program daunting. Two to three days per week of exercise, leaving out some of the components recommended, is better than no exercise.

Accumulated evidence indicates that a carefully planned exercise program executed on a regular basis can slow or prevent age-related bone loss and possibly increase bone mass. A regular exercise program is also beneficial in enhancing factors that aid in preventing falls and reducing their impact: gait, balance, strength, and reaction time. Because there is no cure for osteoporosis, reducing the risks of fractures is the only sensible strategy.

REFERENCES

1. Addison, C., and Humphrey, E.: Fifty "Positive Vigor" Exercises for Senior Citizens. Waldorf, MD, AAHPERD Publications, 1979.
2. Agre, J.C., et al.: Light resistance and stretching exercise in elderly women: effect upon strength. Arch. Phys. Med. Rehabil., 69:273, 1988.
3. Aloia, J.F., et al.: Prevention of involutional bone loss by exercise. Ann. Intern. Med., 89:356, 1978.
4. Aniansson, A., and Gustafsson, E.: Physical training in elderly men with special reference to quadriceps muscle strength and morphology. Clin. Physiol., 1:87, 1981.
5. Aniansson, A., Ljungberg, P., Rundgren, A., and Wetterqvist, H.: Effect of a training programme for pensioners on condition and muscular strength. Arch. Gerontol. Geriatr., 3:229, 1984.
6. American Academy of Orthopedic Surgeons. Joint Motion. Method of Measuring and Recording. Edinburgh, Churchill Livingstone, 1966.
7. American College of Sports Medicine: Guidelines for Exercise Testing and Prescription. 4th Ed. Philadelphia, Lea & Febiger, 1990.
8. Åstrand, P.-O., and Rodahl, K.: Textbook of Work Physiology. New York, McGraw Hill, 1970.
9. Astrom, J., Ahnqvist, S., Beertema, J., and Jonsson, B.: Physical activity in women sustaining fracture of the neck of the femur. J. Bone Joint Surg., 69B:381, 1987.
10. Baylor, A.M., and Spirduso, W.W.: Systematic aerobic exercise and components of reaction time in older women. J. Gerontol., 43:121, 1988.
11. Berland, T.: Fitness for Life. Washington, D.C., American Association of Retired Persons, 1986.
12. Beverly, M.C., Rider, T.A., Evans, M.J., and Smith, R.: Local bone mineral response to brief exercise that stresses the skeleton. Br. Med. J., 299:233, 1989.
13. Block, J.E., et al.: Determinants of bone density among athletes engaged in weight-bearing and

TABLE 8–1. **Type of Exercise for Reducing Risk of Fracture**

	Weight-Bearing	Resistance Training	Aerobic Training	Flexibility Exercises
Spine BMD	X	?		
Wrist BMD		X		
Femur BMD	?	?		
Balance	?	?	?	?
Reaction time		?	?	
Strength		X		
Gait	X	?	?	?

non-weight-bearing activity. J. Appl. Physiol., 67:1100, 1989.

14. Boyce, W.J., and Vessey, M.P.: Habitual physical inertia and other factors in relation to risk of fracture of the proximal femur. Age Ageing, 17:319, 1988.

15. Campbell, A.J., Borrie, M.J., and Spears, G.F.: Risk factors for falls in a community-based prospective study of people 70 years and older. J. Gerontol., 44:M112, 1989.

16. Caplow-Linder, E., Harpas, L., and Samberg, S.: Therapeutic Dance Movement: Expressive Activities for Older Adults. New York, Human Sciences Press, 1979.

17. Chamay, A., and Tschantz, P.: Mechanical influences in bone remodeling. Experimental research on Wolff's law. J. Biomech., 5:173–180, 1972.

18. Chow, R.K., et al.: The effect of exercise on bone mass of osteoporotic patients on fluoride treatment. Clin. Invest. Med., 10:59–63, 1987.

19. Chow, R.K., Harrison, J.E., and Notarius, C.: Effect of two randomised exercise programmes on bone mass of healthy postmenopausal women. Br. Med. J., 292:607, 1987.

20. Cummings, S.R., Kelsey, J.L., McNevitt, M.C., and O'Dowd, K.J.: Epidemiology of osteoporosis and osteoporotic fractures. Epidemiol. Rev., 7:178–208, 1985.

21. Cummings, S.R.: Epidemiology of osteoporotic fractures. In Osteoporosis Update 1987. Edited by H.K. Genant. San Francisco, Radiology Research and Education Foundation, 1987, pp. 7–12.

22. Cummings, S.R.: Use of bone density measurements. In Osteoporosis Update 1987. Edited by H.K. Genant. San Francisco, Radiology Research and Education Foundation, 1987.

23. Dalsky, G.P., et al.: Weight-bearing exercise training and lumbar bone mineral content in postmenopausal women. Ann. Intern. Med., 108:824, 1988.

24. Daniell, H.W.: Osteoporosis and the slender smoker. Arch. Intern. Med., 136:298, 1976.

25. Danneskiold-Samsöe, B., Lyngberg, K., Risum, T., and Telling, M.: The effect of water exercise therapy given to patients with rheumatoid arthritis. Scand. J. Rehab. Med., 19:31, 1987.

26. deVries, H.A.: Physiological effects of an exercise training regimen upon men aged 52 to 88. J. Gerontol., 25:325, 1970.

27. Dustman, R.E., et al.: Aerobic exercise training and improved neuropsychological function of older adults. Neurobiol. Aging, 5:35, 1984.

28. Ensign, C., McAdam, M., and Smith, E.L.: Healthline. Madison, WI, Healthline, Inc., 1988.

29. Fiatarone, M.A., et al.: High-intensity strength training in nonagenarians. JAMA, 263:3029, 1990.

30. Frankel, L.J., and Richard, B.B. Be Alive as Long As You Live. Charleston, WV, Preventicare Publications, 1977.

31. Frankel, L.J., and Richard, B.B.: Age and Mobility: Exercises for the Homebound and Chairbound. Charleston, WV, Preventicare Publications, 1979.

32. Frontera, W.R., et al.: Strength conditioning in older men: skeletal muscle hypertrophy and improved function. J. Appl. Physiol., 64:1038, 1988.

33. Gehlsen, G.M., and Whaley, M.H.: Falls in the elderly. Part II. Balance, strength, and flexibility. Arch. Phys. Med. Rehabil., 71:739, 1990.

34. Gehlsen, G.M., Grigsby, S.A., and Winant, D.M.: Effects of an aquatic fitness program on the muscular strength and endurance of patients with multiple sclerosis. Phys. Ther., 64:653, 1984.

35. Gleeson, P.B., et al.: Effects of weight lifting on bone mineral density in premenopausal women. J. Bone Min. Res., 5:153, 1990.

36. Golland, A.: Basic hydrotherapy. Physiotherapy, 67:258, 1981.

37. Grimes, D.C., and Krasevec, J.A.: HydroRobics. Champaign, IL, Leisure Press, 1983.

38. Guesens, P., Dequeker, J., Verstraeten, A., and Niis, J.: Age, sex, and menopause-related changes of vertebral and peripheral bone: population study with dual and single photon absorptiometry and radiogrammetry. J. Nucl. Med., 27:1540, 1987.

39. Heaney, R.P., and Recker, R.R.: Effects of nitrogen, phosphorus and caffeine on calcium balance in women. J. Lab. Clin. Med., 99:46, 1982.

40. Heinrich, C.H., et al.: Bone mineral content of cyclically menstruating female resistance and endurance trained athletes. Med. Sci. Sports Exerc., 22:558, 1990.

41. Herndon, B.: Tubex. New York, Vintage Books, 1986.

42. Holbrook, T.L., Grazier, K., Kelsey, J.L., and Stauffer, R.N.: The Frequency of Occurrence, Impact, and Cost of Musculoskeletal Conditions in the United States. Chicago, American Academy of Orthopedic Surgeons, 1984.

43. Huey, L., and Knudson, R.R.: The Waterpower Workout. New York, New American Library, 1986.

44. Ismail, F., et al.: The influence of exercise on bone mineral metabolism in the elderly [abstract]. J. Bone Min. Res., 4:S231, 1989.

45. Karvonen, M.J.: The effects of training on heart rate. A longitudinal study. Ann. Med. Exper. Biol. Fenn., 35:307–315, 1957.

46. Krolner, B., Toft, B., Nielson, S.P., and Tondevold, E.: Physical exercise as prophylaxis against involutional vertebral bone loss: a controlled trial. Clin. Sci., 64:541, 1983.

47. Lanyon, L.E.: Strain-related bone modeling and remodeling. Top. Geriatr. Rehabil., 4:13, 1989.

48. Leslie, D.K., and McLure, J.W.: Exercises for the Elderly. Iowa City, IA, Dept. of Physical Education-University of Iowa, 1977.

49. Lichtenstein, M.J., Shields, S.L., Shiavi, R.G., and Burger, C.: Exercise and balance in aged women: a pilot controlled clinical trial. Arch. Phys. Med. Rehabil., 70:138, 1989.

50. Margulies, J.Y., et al.: Effect of intense physical activity on the bone-mineral content in the lower limbs of young adults. J. Bone Joint Surg., 68A:1090, 1986.

51. Mazess, R., et al.: Performance evaluation of a dual energy x-ray bone densitometer. Calcif. Tissue Int., 44:228, 1989.

52. Mazess, R.B.: Bone densitometry for clinical diagnosis and monitoring. In Osteoporosis: Physiological Basis, Assessment, and Treatment. Edited by H.F. DeLuca and R. Mazess. Amsterdam, Elsevier, 1990.

53. Melton, L.J., et al.: Bone density specific fracture risk: a population based study of the relationship between osteoporoses and vertebral fractures. J. Nucl. Med., 26:24, 1985.
54. Melton, L.J., Eddy, D.M., and Johnston, C.C.: Screening for osteoporosis. Ann. Intern. Med., 112:516, 1990.
55. Moran, J.M.: Leisure Activities for the Mature Adult. Minneapolis, Burgess Publishing, 1979.
56. Moroz, D., Sale, D., and Webber, C.: The effect of intensive training on axial and appendicular bone mineral in normal postmenopausal women [abstract]. J. Bone Min. Res., 4:S233, 1989.
57. Osteoporosis. Consensus Conference. JAMA, 252:799, 1984.
58. Panton, L.B., et al.: Effect of aerobic and resistance training on fractionated reaction time and speed of movement. J. Gerontol., 45:M26, 1990.
59. Peery, J.: Exercises for Retirees. Oregon City, OR, Clackamas Community College, 1976.
60. Piscopo, J.: Fitness and Aging. New York, John Wiley and Sons, 1985.
61. Podenphant, J., et al.: Bone mass, bone structure and vertebral fractures in osteoporotic patients. Bone, 8:127, 1987.
62. President's Council on Physical Fitness and Sports: Aqua Dynamics: Physical Conditioning through Water Exercises. Washington, D.C., U.S. Government Printing Office, 1977.
63. Riggs, B.L., and Melton, L.J.: Evidence of two distinct syndromes of involutional osteoporosis. Am. J. Med., 314:1676, 1983.
64. Riggs, B.L., et al.: Changes in bone mineral density of the proximal femur and spine with aging. J. Clin. Invest., 70:716, 1982.
65. Rikli, R., and Busch, S.: Motor performance of women as a function of age and physical activity level. J. Gerontol., 41:645, 1986.
66. Rikli, R.E., and Edwards, D.J.: Effects of a three-year exercise program on motor function and cognitive processing speed in older women. Res. Quart. Exerc. Sports, 62:61, 1991.
67. Rikli, R.E., and McManis, B.G.: Effects of exercise on bone mineral content in postmenopausal women. Res. Quart. Exerc. Sport, 61:243, 1990.
68. Roberts, B.L.: Effects of walking on balance among elders. Nurs. Res., 38:180, 1989.
69. Rockwell, J.C., et al.: Weight training decreases vertebral bone density in premenopausal women: a prospective study. J. Clin. Endocrin. Metab., 71:988, 1990.
70. Rosenberg, M.: Sixty-Plus and Fit Again. New York, M. Evans and Company, 1977.
71. Ross, P.D., Davis, J.W., Washnich, R.D., and Vogel, J.M.: The clinical application of serial bone mass measurements. Bone Min., 12:189, 1991.
72. Rundgren, A., Aniansson, A., Ljungberg, P., and Wetterqvist, H.: Effects of a training programme for elderly people on mineral content of the heel bone. Arch. Gerontol. Geriatr., 3:243, 1984.
73. Sandler, R.B., et al.: The effects of walking on the cross-sectional dimensions of the radius in postmenopausal women. Calcif. Tissue Int., 41:65, 1987.
74. Saville, P.D.: Changes in bone mass with age and alcoholism. J. Bone Joint Surg., 47A:492, 1965.
75. Shephard, R.J.: Physical Activity and Aging. London, Croom Helm, 1978.
76. Simkin, A., Ayalon, J., and Leichter, I.: Increased trabecular bone density due to bone-loading exercises in postmenopausal osteoporotic women. Calcif. Tissue Int., 40:59, 1986.
77. Sinaki, M., Wahner, H.W., Offord, K.P., and Hodgson, S.F.: Efficacy of nonloading exercises in prevention of vertebral bone loss in postmenopausal women: a controlled trial. Clin. Proc., 64:762, 1989.
78. Slemenda, C.W., Hui, S.L., Longcope, C., and Johnston, C.C.: Cigarette smoking, obesity, and bone mass. J. Bone Min. Res., 4:737, 1989.
79. Smith, E.L., et al.: Exercise reduces bone involution in middle-aged women. Calcif. Tissue Int., 44:312, 1989.
80. Smith, E.L., Reddan, W., and Smith, P.E.: Physical activity and calcium modalities for bone mineral increase in aged women. Med. Sci. Sports Exerc., 13:60, 1981.
81. Smith, E.L., and Gilligan, C.: Physical activity prescription for the older adult. Phys. Sportsmed., 11:91, 1983.
82. Smith, E.L., and Stoedefalke, K.G.: Aging and Exercise. Madison, WI, Dept. of Preventive Medicine-University of Wisconsin, 1978.
83. Spirduso, W.W.: Reaction and movement time as a function of age and physical activity level. J. Gerontol., 30:435, 1975.
84. Spitzer, T.A., Moore, J.R., Hopkins, D.R., and Hoeger, W.W.K.: Aquatic exercise research: a comparison of selected training responses to water aerobics and low-impact aerobics. AKWA Lett., 4:5, 1991.
85. Studenski, S., Duncan, P., and Chandler, J.: Platform perturbation and clinical correlates in unexplained falls. Am. Geront. Soc. [Abstract A26], 1989.
86. Tinetti, M.E., Speechley, M., and Ginter, S.F.: Risk factors for falls among elderly persons living in the community. N. Engl. J. Med., 319:1701, 1988.
87. Tinetti, M.E.: Performance-oriented assessment of mobility problems in elderly patients. J. Am. Geriat. Soc., 34:119, 1986.
88. U.S. Department of Health and Human Services, Public Health Service: Healthy People 2000—National Health Promotion and Disease Prevention Objectives. Washington, D.C., U.S. Government Printing Office, 1990.
89. Wahner, H.W., Dunn, W.L., and Riggs, B.L.: Assessment of bone mineral, part 2. J. Nucl. Med., 25:1241, 1984.
90. Whipple, R.H., Wolfson, L.I., and Amerman, P.M.: The relationship of knee and ankle weakness to falls in nursing home residents: an isokinetic study. J. Am. Geriat. Soc., 35:13, 1987.
91. White, M.K., et al.: The effects of exercise on the bones of postmenopausal women. Int. Orthop., 7:209, 1984.
92. Wickham, C.A.C., et al.: Dietary calcium, physical activity, and risk of hip fracture: a prospective study. Br. Med. J., 299:889, 1989.

9
CHAPTER

Spinal Disorders and Low Back Pain

by
Neil B. Oldridge and James E. Stoll

Low back pain occurs in the majority of adults during their lives and is the most frequent cause of limitation to activities of daily living, including work, housekeeping, school, and recreation in persons under the age of 45 years. Low back pain frequently occurs as a result of activity-related spinal disorders. Typically, non-operative, conservative therapy for low back pain will be prescribed before such invasive intervention as spinal surgery is attempted. These conservative therapies include oral and injected drugs, physical measures (e.g., bed rest, manipulation, weight loss, and exercise), counter-stimulation measures (e.g., transcutaneous electrical nerve stimulation, cold massage, and acupuncture), and other measures (e.g., biofeedback, behavioral therapy, and patient education).

Careful evaluation of these modalities for activity-related spinal disorders suggests that in the majority of cases, symptoms of acute spinal pain tend to resolve spontaneously. Prolonged bed rest may be counterproductive. Although biologic effects provide the rationale for the majority of treatments and therapies, few of the effects have been validated in scientifically admissible investigations.[24,76] Treatment and rehabilitation goals for activity-related spinal disorders increasingly include the restoration and preservation of functional capacity and exercise tolerance.

This work was partially supported by NIA grant #1 R15 AGO9059-01.

"Physical inactivity dictated by the pain leads to a bodily deconditioning that aggravates the organic foundation of the problem."[76] The wide range of factors (physiologic, psychological, socio-economic, and emotional) that impact on outcome in patients with activity-related spinal disorders and low back pain demands an interdisciplinary team approach for optimal resolution in most cases, but especially in those that do not resolve spontaneously.[31,32]

As reported during 1986 by one large insurance company,[87] compensable low back pain (LBP) amounted to a mean cost of $6807 per case (median = $391, because 95% of the costs were accounted for by 25% of the cases). When extrapolated to the U.S. adult population, this amounted to an estimated $11.1 billion during 1986, not including indirect costs,[87] which significantly increase the total costs of LBP by as much as an additional $3 billion.[72] These estimates represent an increase of 241% for compensable LBP costs since 1980 and should be compared to the 184% increase in total worker's compensation costs over the same period.[87] These statistics for compensable LBP reflect only a small component of the total cost of LBP to society. Physician visits for LBP are second only to visits for the common cold. The annual incidence of LBP in the United States is approximately 5 to 7%; the lifetime prevalence is between 60% and 90%, with males and females approximately equally affected below the age of

60 years, after which age females report more LBP. Slightly more than 50% of the events occur between the ages of 20 and 39 years, and LBP occurs most frequently among whites and those with elementary school education or less.[26,29] The data suggest that, in the United States, LBP is the most significant cause of premature disability and limitation of normal activities,[72,76,87] even though approximately 75% of patients return to work within 30 days.[29,76] Further, there is considerable economic evidence from industrialized countries that the less than 10% of patients with LBP who were absent from work for more than 6 months account for more than 75% of the total compensation costs for spinal disorders and about 25 to 30% of total compensation costs.[76]

The purposes of this chapter are threefold. We will first outline 1) the epidemiology of activity-related spinal disorders and LBP. We will then present epidemiologic and experimental data on the role of physical capacity evaluation and exercise 2) in the prediction and prevention of activity-related spinal disorders and LBP and 3) on the treatment and rehabilitation of activity-related spinal disorders and LBP.

EPIDEMIOLOGY OF ACTIVITY-RELATED SPINAL DISORDERS

Although previous LBP is a risk factor for repeated episodes of LBP, epidemiologic studies have been integral in identifying many of the risk factors that may help predict both the initial development and the prolongation of LBP. Probably the most extensive examination of the predictive value of cardiovascular fitness, strength, and flexibility for subsequent LBP is the series of four articles[6-9] recently published on 3020 employees (mean age = 36.2 years, range = 21 to 67 years; 78% male) at a Boeing aircraft plant in the Pacific Northwest who volunteered to participate in a prospective study of risk factors associated with report of back pain. All hourly-wage employees were given the opportunity to participate, and 75% did.[7]

Although there may be some familial predisposition to discogenic LBP, the majority of the risk factors are demographic or environmental in nature[36]; those risk factors that are amenable to intervention are particularly important. The demographic risk factors (e.g., younger age, female gender at older ages, height, and white race) are not modifiable, and having elementary school or less education generally is not modified after the fact.[26,29,36,37] Certain occupations and occupational tasks are associated with increased reports of LBP. These involve a number of tasks that are considered to be modifiable (e.g., repetitive lifting in the forward bent and twisted position, lifting loads greater than the individual's physical capacity, exposure to vibrations caused by industrial machinery or driving motor vehicles, sudden starting and stopping, and lack of proper seating support and position of the legs while seated in motor vehicles).[29,36,40,67] These associations with LBP, particularly for driving, appear to be strong, relevant in time sequence, dose-related, and biologically plausible.[36] Patient characteristics associated with occupational and psychological profiles may help further identify persons at high risk for LBP; these include negative perceptions about work (boring, repetitious, dissatisfying), psychological distress (depression, anxiety), alcoholism, and poor health.[26,29,36,41] Recent work has been published suggesting that the factors most predictive of acute back pain at work are work perceptions and certain psychosocial responses on the Minnesota Multiphasic Personality Inventory. For example, people who responded that they "hardly ever" enjoyed their job tasks were 2.5 times more likely to report a back injury than those who "almost always" enjoyed their job tasks.[13] Stress associated with life events, but not psychiatric illness, has recently been suggested as a factor in the onset of LBP.[22] Other modifiable patient characteristics that may be associated with the incidence of LBP include smoking and overweight.[25] Although a positive association between smoking and LBP has been demonstrated in some studies and the rationale for smoking meets the time sequence, consistency, and biologic plausibility criteria,[29,36,41] the reported associations are not strong and are associated with such potential confounders as occupation. Overweight may be considered a logical potential risk factor for LBP but the scientific evidence is not strong enough to demonstrate that weight reduction is an effective intervention in LBP.[36] Physical fitness and muscle strength may be risk factors[29,30,36,37] but the association between leisure-time activities and the occurrence of LBP is generally weak.[11,26,37,70]

Physical activity, which is a modifiable risk factor, can have both beneficial and negative effects for the lower back. Regular and appropriate exercise has beneficial effects on strength of bone, joints, tendons, ligaments, muscle, and connective tissue, although the effects on joint cartilage and the intervertebral discs are not as clear, even though there is enhanced nutrition with exercise.[59] However, physical inactivity may also have detrimental effects on each of the above.[59] Our understanding is that the balance between regular physical activity and inactivity as they relate to LBP is unclear. Both acute and chronic LBP frequently interfere with leisure-time activities.[82] In a recent Finnish study, approximately 40% of patients reported that they needed to reduce their leisure-time activities as a result of LBP.[37] Although there is little evidence to suggest a protective effect of regular physical exercise for LBP in a study of nurses,[23,83] there is evidence to suggest that when occupational handicap was assessed before and after surgery and correlated with preoperative leisure-time activities, there appears to be an inverted U-shaped response curve, with a better occupational handicap prognosis most likely to be associated with moderate leisure-time activity levels.[2]

Although the overall incidence of LBP in sports is low,[41,73] the incidence is considerably higher in certain sports with a combination of repetitive high-velocity twisting, bending, and body contact. The incidence of LBP is particularly high in gymnastics,[43,50,61] both men's and women's,[73] although at least one group of investigators report more frequent LBP in male gymnasts,[78] racquet sports,[40,45] and wrestling and heavy lifting.[33,51] The incidence of LBP may be exaggerated by competition in growing children.[4,62] There appear to be conflicting data about the association between anthropometric characteristics of athletes and the prediction of LBP.[77] Following lumbar discectomy, a good prognosis has been reported in both athletes[74] and nonathletes with high preoperative levels of leisure-time activities.[84]

PHYSICAL CAPACITY EVALUATION AND EXERCISE

Prediction and Prevention of LBP

Physical exercise has long been postulated as an integral part of a healthy lifestyle, particularly in populations in which regular physical activity is no longer the norm and important outcomes of regular physical exercise include better health and improved physical fitness.[14] Three major components of physical fitness include cardiovascular fitness (aerobic power or exercise tolerance), strength, and flexibility. The evidence for many of the other claims for exercise and health maintenance are inconclusive, but LBP was not one of the chronic conditions considered in the review by Phelps.[66] For the patient with LBP, the potential benefits of regular exercise include greater cardiovascular fitness, strength, and flexibility.[47]

Evidence for the role of physical exercise, with its associated cardiovascular fitness, strength, and flexibility, and the likelihood of LBP (or alternatively, the prevention of LBP), is generally weak and inconclusive. In 1979, Cady and co-workers reported an association between higher fitness levels and a lower incidence of LBP in a prospective investigation of the hypothesis of a protective effect of physical fitness against back injury in Los Angeles firefighters.[20] The specific objective of the study was to "relate prior ratings of physical activity and prior mea-

141

sures of physical conditioning to the frequency of subsequent back injuries and costs per back injury in a group of 1652 firefighters aged 20 to 55 years."[20] Measurement of physical fitness included tests of flexibility, isometric lifting strength, the 2-min recovery heart rate (HR) following cycle ergometer exercise, diastolic blood pressure at a HR of 160 bpm, and the power output required to sustain a HR of 160 bpm. Based on the results, firefighters were allocated to one of three fitness groups (low = bottom 16% of the sample, moderate = mid 66%, and high = top 16%). The number of back injuries incurred during the subsequent 3 years were then tabulated and analyzed with respect to the fitness groups. The results demonstrated an injury rate of 7.7% in the low-fit group, decreasing to 3.19% in the moderate-fit group, and to 0.77% in the high-fit firefighters. Although the number of injuries in the high-fit group were too low for an accurate estimate of costs per injury, the costs in the middle and low groups were similar and considerably greater. There was a subgroup analysis of those with previous back injury who were ineligible for the main study. The results essentially supported the observations in those without prior back injury—that is, during the 3 years, 30% of the low-fit group and none in the high-fit group sustained back injuries.[20] Although the authors do appear justified in their conclusions that physical fitness and conditioning in these firefighters prevented back injuries, the fitness scale used was a composite of cardiovascular fitness, strength, and flexibility, and the independent roles of the three components of fitness could not be identified. These initial observations of a potential protective effect of physical fitness have been indirectly substantiated in a follow-up report, which provided suggestive evidence for the benefits of an employee fitness program to reduce LBP disability and disability costs.[21]

More recently, there have been a number of studies that have attempted to clarify the roles of cardiovascular fitness, strength, and flexibility in the occurrence of LBP. In the Boeing study, 2434 of the 3020 employees underwent treadmill testing, with 28.4% (no difference between genders) reporting a history of back pain.[7] Future back-injury reports were not associated with cardiovascular fitness (measured as maximal oxygen uptake or $\dot{V}_{O_2max}$) in employees when controlling for age and gender. The mean $\dot{V}_{O_2max}$ among women with no subsequent LBP was approximately 37 ml $\cdot$ kg^{-1} $\cdot$ min^{-1} compared to 39 ml $\cdot$ kg^{-1} $\cdot$ min^{-1} among those with LBP. The respective figures for males were 41.8 and 41.5 ml^{-1} $\cdot$ kg^{-1} $\cdot$ min^{-1}.[7] Although the approach to the use of aerobic exercise in patient care is gaining popularity,[47,57] the observations reported by Battie et al. are not consistent with those of Cady and colleagues[20,21] and others.[19] Although there very well may be lower cardiovascular fitness in patients with recent LBP, this more likely is associated with the pain and consequent inactivity following the acute event and not necessarily with chronically poor cardiovascular fitness. The associations between prevention of LBP and cardiovascular fitness need further investigation, particularly because cardiovascular fitness is associated with other health benefits[14] and may also affect an individual's response to and recovery from an acute event and the associated rehabilitation costs.[15,19,20]

The back muscles maintain the correct posture of the spine. It has been demonstrated that good isometric endurance of the back muscles may prevent the first occurrence of LBP in men.[12] Results from Troup and colleagues,[81] as well as the evidence from the Boeing study described in greater detail above, suggest that there is little effect of isometric strength on future back injury.[6] Of the 3020 Boeing employees, 2178 underwent strength testing in three upright positions to measure torso, arm, and leg lift strength. Contrary to predictions, greater strength was associated with a higher, and not a lower, risk of industrial back claims. However, when age was controlled for, the significant association between greater strength and back injury disappeared; this can be accounted for by the negative associations between increasing age and both strength and back injury. Importantly, the observation of a poor prediction for injury based on general isometric lifting strength held for blue collar workers, among whom strength screening would not have reduced subsequent back injury reports.[6] In another report, the same team of investigators demonstrated that pain elicited on straight leg raising was significantly associated with subsequent LBP, and only age added to its predictive power in both females and males.[9] However, McQuade and colleagues have reported that poor strength and not flexibility or cardiovascular fitness was the fitness variable most closely associated with negative outcomes of LBP.[52] Consistent with this observation, in a prospective study of conservative treatment for LBP in males aged 54 to 63 years, Mellin reported a significant association between pretreatment LBP and strength, as well as a capacity for such "dynamic exercise" as situps, trunk raising, and straight leg raising.[54]

Flexibility examinations are routinely used to evaluate impairment and disability, although the association between past back problems and future back injury is not clear.[8,18,80] In a prospective study of males aged 54 to 63 years, Mellin reported a significant association between pretreatment LBP and flexibility.[54] On the other hand, in the Boeing study, with all 3020 employees undergoing flexibility assessment in the sagittal and frontal planes, the conclusion drawn by the authors was that flexibility in these two planes was not predictive of future back injury, even though flexibility was associated with prior back problems.[8] The results of the modified Schober test for flexion of the lumbosacral spine are presented in Figure 9–1 and demonstrate that there was no predictive power for flexibility in males; the same observations held true for females.[8]

Thus, although back injury may be associated with certain physical measures of body mechanics in the acute phase,[54] evaluation of cardiovascular fitness, strength, and flexibility (except perhaps for straight

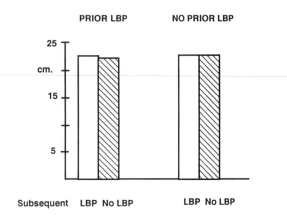

Fig. 9–1. *Modified Schober test used to measure flexion of the lumbosacral spine in 1788 males in the Boeing study, and subsequent LBP in the next 4 years.*[7]

leg raising in the large cohort of Boeing employees followed up for at least 3 to 4 years) generally were not useful in predicting future back injury.[6–9] Whether physical fitness prevents the occurrence or recurrence of LBP is still uncertain, but there is increasing evidence that the evaluation of physical capacity, the prescription of exercise, and improved fitness may be important in the treatment and rehabilitation of patients with LBP.

Treatment and Rehabilitation of LBP

In an extensive monograph on the scientific approach to the assessment and management of activity-related spinal disorders published by the Quebec Task Force in 1987,[76] the following categories were used to classify studies according to their strength of scientific evidence for support or rejection of the intervention: 1) randomized controlled trial, 2) well-conducted cohort or case-control study, 3) descriptive studies without control group, case series, or opinion of experts, and 4) literature review and other studies not otherwise classified. After reviewing 721 articles on LBP, the task force rejected 252 studies and classified only 50 (10.7%) of the remaining studies as very good (interestingly, only 16.7% of the 84 randomized trials were classified as very good). Although they did stipulate that a lack of scientific evidence does not demonstrate that interventions are useless, they concluded that "while biologic effects provide the rationale for the use of most treatments . . . few have been validated in scientifically admissible clinical or epidemiologic investigations . . . and that of those that have been studied, few have been shown to facilitate healing of non-specific spinal disorders."[76] Some of the treatments considered by the task force for chronic LBP and a summary statement of their interpretation of the literature are presented in Table 9–1. They also presented certain therapeutic guidelines, including the following: symptoms of acute lumbar, dorsal, and cervical pain tend to resolve spontaneously; bed rest is unnecessary for LBP without radiation; prolonged bed rest may be counterproductive; and surgery is not a proven remedy for back pain alone, is generally contraindicated in the absence of hard neurologic signs or demonstrated anatomic distortion, and is indicated only after conservative treatment has failed.[76]

Since publication of the Quebec Task Force monograph,[76] a number of randomized trials of treatments for LBP and activity-related spinal disorders have been published. Generic pain clinics have un-fortunately not been successful in addressing such major issues as return to work, and their value has been challenged.[75] For example, as the content of the educationally based "back schools" varies considerably, demonstration of their potential value is limited.[10,38] However, when carefully controlled, back school has been shown to be effective.[34,55] A recent trial of chiropractic and hospital outpatient treatment suggests significant positive benefits in favor of chiropractic treatment.[53] The Quebec Task Force specifically stated that the goals of therapy should be to maximize the number of patients returning to productive lives within 1 month and to minimize the number who are idle for 6 months or more.[76] There is little doubt that as time following the acute event increases, the rehabilitation process becomes increasingly difficult. A number of studies (including randomized clinical trials) of physical capacity evaluation, endurance conditioning, and strength training included as integral components of the treatment modality for patients with LBP have been published since the Quebec Task Force report.[76] The results of some of these will be discussed in greater detail in the next section.

TABLE 9–1. **Treatments for Chronic Low Back Pain, as Summarized in the 1987 Quebec Task Force Monograph on the Assessment and Management of Activity-Related Spinal Disorders**

Treatments	Assessment of their value
Acupuncture	No scientific study demonstrating superiority over other modalities
Back school	Content of courses varies considerably
Biofeedback	Has not been demonstrated to be effective
Cryotherapy	No precise in-depth study
Exercise (endurance, strength, flexibility)	No controlled study has demonstrated efficacy
Functional training	Treated group had better return-to-work rate than control group
Manipulation	Temporary relief of pain, with no reduction in duration of work absence
Medication	Utility of antidepressant, nonsteroid antiinflammatory drug, and muscle relaxant drugs in chronic phase not clearly demonstrated
Pain clinic	Controlled studies have shown various results
Postural information	Inconsistent results
Thermotherapy	No specific study to support reduction of edema and pain
Traction	No controlled study has demonstrated efficacy

Exercise Conditioning

Identification of physical capacity and the appropriate prescription of exercise as an adjunctive therapeutic modality to improve functional capacity is an approach routinely used in the rehabilitation of cardiac patients.[63] Nachemson, in the proceedings of a recent workshop on new perspectives on LBP, stated that "there must be a reappraisal of activity instead of rest in the treatment of low back disorders ... [but, that while] immobilization by bed rest for more than one or two days seems contraindicated in acute LBP, ... there is little evidence that general fitness and exercise play a major role ... however, as the duration of the attack increases, some activation programs intended to increase endurance have beneficial effects (in chronic LBP)."[58] Objective assessment of physical functional capacity is now possible for most body systems, and it is known that most, if not all, tissues can benefit from regular physical activity, particularly with increasing age.[16]

Physical function, whether strength, flexibility, or aerobic power, is increasingly being used as an outcome measure in the treatment and rehabilitation of patients with activity-related spinal disorders and LBP. In a non-randomized sample of 151 men ranging from 54-63 years, Mellin observed that progress 12 months after back school was significantly associated with increases in flexibility and trunk strength.[54] Although there was relatively little emphasis on exercise (<20% of treatments) in the back school treatment, it is important to note that the author reported that dynamic exercises were the best indicators of LBP and that trunk extensor strength was the best indicator of progress.[54] More recently, the observation of the importance of strength in the treatment of LBP has been substantiated in randomized controlled trials. In a trial of the efficacy of inpatient and outpatient treatment of LBP, both interventions consisted of modified Swedish back school (four sessions), back exercises (15 sessions),

and relaxation exercises (nine sessions). Patients carried out physical exercises and strength exercises, and all were taught a back exercise program to be carried out after treatment.[34,55] The inpatient program was available for a 3-week period at a rehabilitation center, whereas the outpatient program was held at work or the local health center. Control patients attended examinations and completed questionnaire surveys but were given no systematic treatment. At the 3-month follow-up, inpatients had improved their strength and flexibility significantly more than outpatients or controls, neither of whom improved or differed from each other.[55] On the other hand, both treatment groups reported less pain and disability than the control group, with the inpatients reporting significantly less pain and estimating overall treatment benefits to be greater than the outpatients.[34] The use of EMG biofeedback in back-muscle strengthening has been reported recently to be effective. This technique resulted in greater increases in strength than standard therapy, but the investigators point out that it was not clear whether their observations were the result of increased muscle strength or a reduced fear of muscle contraction.[3]

In an attempt to evaluate the effectiveness of exercise treatment programs, 142 employees with at least three reported annual episodes of LBP were randomly allocated to two treatment conditions or to a control group. Patients participated in either a back school (four 90-min sessions of body mechanics, back and abdominal exercises over a 2-week period, with encouragement to do these at home plus one session 2 months later) or in exercise sessions that were aimed at strengthening abdominal muscles, increasing flexibility, and improving general posture (run biweekly for 3 months by a trained instructor).[28] Over the next year, there were significantly fewer LBP episodes in the exercise group than in the back-school group. The authors attribute this benefit partly to the significant increases in flexibility and abdominal muscle strength seen in the exercising group, but they also comment that the short duration of the back school may have attributed to its lack of success.[28] In another of these trials, 105 men without clinical signs of lumbar nerve root compression or radiologic evidence of spondylolysis or osteomalacia were randomized to either 1) 30 sessions of intensive dynamic back-extensor exercises over 3 months, 2) a similar program at 20% of the exercise intensity, or 3) a control group.[44] There were no adverse outcomes in the intensive exercise group, whereas there were significant treatment differences in LBP ratings in favor of the intensive exercise group at the conclusion of treatment and 3 months later. The improvements may be partially explained by the treatment intensity and duration, but because the treatment included both muscle training and flexibility hyperextension back exercises, the benefits cannot be attributed to one or the other exercise.[44]

Flexion and extension back strengthening programs were compared in 48 patients with symptomatic back pain secondary to lumbar spondylolisthesis randomly assigned to one or the other program.[71] Considerably more patients in the extension program had moderate or severe pain after both 3 months and 3 years (67% at both times) than those in the flexion program (27% and 19%, respectively). Further, more patients in the extension program (61% at both times) were unable to work or were restricted in their work when compared to those in the flexion program (32% and 24%). The overall recovery rates at 3 months for the extension group were 6% versus 58% for flexion group. At 3 years, the rates were 0% for the extension program, compared to 62% for the flexion program. From these data, back flexion exercises appear to be favored for the rehabilitation of patients with spondylolisthesis.[71] This reinforces the importance of prescribing different exercise programs for different subgroups of patients with LBP.

In further investigating the importance of exercise in the rehabilitation of back pain, 40 male and female subjects with a primary diagnosis of "chronic lumbosacral strain" were randomly assigned to either a supervised experimental group or to an unsupervised control group.[68] Each group was given the same exercise prescription comprising flexibility, strength, and aerobic exercises. The experimental group patients were assigned to a specialist at each of the health clubs and completed their programs under that person's supervision, whereas the control group patients were given the names of health clubs they could attend and compliance was monitored by the staff. Aerobic endurance, strength, and self-reported pain were all significantly improved in the supervised group. The authors state that "since the experimental group completed 91% of their sessions, compared to 32% for the control group, it could be concluded that supervision increases the chances for compliance and success. . . ."[68] This observation about success and compliance has been reported in cardiac rehabilitation[64] and may partially explain the results reported by Donchin et al.[28] and Mellin et al.,[56] as well as the long-term results in the recently published controlled trial of transcutaneous electrical nerve stimulation (TENS) reported by Deyo and colleagues.[27] They randomly assigned subjects to one of four groups: TENS alone, TENS plus exercise, sham TENS and exercise, and sham TENS. The exercise regime consisted of a uniform set of three relaxation exercises and nine exercises to improve flexibility of the spine, hip, and lower extremities, carried out under supervision twice-weekly for 4 weeks. The 95% confidence intervals excluded a major clinical benefit for TENS. On the other hand, subjects in the exercise groups, with and without TENS, demonstrated significantly improved self-rated pain scores (52%) at 1 month compared to 37% in the nonexercise groups, with or without TENS. The exercise groups also reported a significant reduction in pain frequency and increased levels of activity. However, these improvements were not apparent at 3 months when more than 50% of the subjects in the exercise groups had discontinued their exercises. There was no placebo group for exercise, however, so the authors could not rule out the possibility that the effects seen with exercise might have been due to the "Hawthorne effect." They do state that the "data support a trend favoring active over passive therapy" and suggest that TENS adds no apparent benefit to that of exercise alone.[27]

In all of these studies of aerobic exercise conditioning, strength training, and flexibility in the treatment of LBP, there was a consistent reduction in pain levels concomitant with the improvements in return to work and fitness. This suggests that Nachemson's comment that "some activation programs intended to increase endurance have beneficial effects"[58] increasingly is being substantiated.

Functional Restoration

Perhaps the most exciting clinical experimental evidence of the positive adjunctive effect of physical function evaluation and appropriately prescribed physical exercise for patients with spinal disorders and LBP is the "functional restoration" approach,[5,42,47–49] similar to the approach routinely used in cardiac rehabilitation.[65] The basic premise underlying functional restoration is that dysfunction and persistent LBP may be substantially affected by deficits in physical functional capacity and that correction of these by objective assessment and physical conditioning, together with aggressive disability management, may minimize the number of long-term disabled patients and maximize the number of patients returning to work. The sports medicine approach involves assessment and quantification of dysfunction with comparisons to published norms. On the basis of the assessments, programs of physical conditioning are prescribed to counter muscle atrophy, to increase strength and joint range of motion, and to improve aerobic capacity. In summary, functional restoration is a composite of validated sports medicine technologies with an emphasis on flexibility, muscle strengthening, progressive aerobic endurance conditioning, aggressive pain management,

and education to better identify and cope with the socioeconomic issues of LBP.[47,57]

Initial reports on 1-year outcomes of the functional restoration approach in 66 carefully selected patients with chronic LBP for whom objective functional capacity measurements were used to develop a treatment program, compared to 38 control patients denied entry by the insurance carrier (based almost exclusively on a negative attitude to "pain clinics"), reinforced the importance of the objective functional capacity data in effective treatment program design.[48] Phase I of the treatment program consisted of an intensive 3-week rehabilitation program requiring 57 hours/week, with extensive objective assessments of physical capacity and psychological function, specific endurance and strength exercises, training in functional tasks, education, and work simulation/hardening, as well as a multimodal pain management program. Phase II consisted of follow-up at the clinic for 2 hours/day, 0 to 4 times/week for a mean of 5 weeks. Phase III was a 6-hour post-program evaluation. The cost of the program ranged from $5000 to $8000 per patient. Although this was not a randomized trial in the usual sense of the term, the authors did assign patients to the control and treatment groups based on random selection of the employer's insurance company. Functional capacity increased in approximately 80% of the patients for whom functional restoration strategies were used. Further, the rate of return to work in the treated patients was twice that of the controls, and health care visits took place substantially less often.[48] A 2-year follow-up survey of 116 patients in the functional restoration program and of 72 patients for whom the treatment program was not prescribed because of insurance denial substantiated the initial report. Compared to 41% of those not receiving treatment, 87% of the treated patients were actively working. Subsequent surgery in the treated patients occurred at a rate of approximately 50%, and health care visits took place approximately 20% of the time for those not treated.[49] The observation that the treatment dropouts had outcomes that were worse than those of the control patients substantiates the importance of compliance in rehabilitation, not only of patients with spinal disorders[66] but also observations on patients with coronary heart disease undergoing exercise rehabilitation programs.[63,64] In a recent publication, comparing the more aggressive functional restoration rehabilitation strategies that have evolved since the earlier efforts, Mayer and his colleagues have demonstrated considerably greater gains in improving physical capacity (specifically strength and range of motion), whereas return to work rates have remained constant at approximately 85%.[42] This group of investigators has also shown that psychological measures, pain intensity ratings, prior surgical history, and level of a worker's compensation are predictors of success in their functional restoration programs.[5]

Important questions have been raised about the patient selection criteria used and the costs of the functional restoration program as described by Mayer,[47,48] as well as about the transposition of the model to other sites. Results of a prospective investigation of treatment programs modeled on the functional restoration approach have been reported recently. Hazard and his colleagues[35] demonstrated return to work rates similar to those reported by Mayer[48,49]: i.e., 81% of treatment graduates, 41% of dropouts, and 29% of those denied the program had returned to work by 12 months.[35] They also reported improved pain levels, disability, depression, and physical capacity after 3 weeks of treatment and suggested that the use of repeated objective measures in monitoring physical conditioning was one of the most effective features of the treatment program.[35] In terms of the measures of physical capacity, highly significant increases were seen in trunk flexibility, lifting, isokinetic trunk extension strength, and cycling endurance at discharge. Even though only flexibility and isokinetic strength had been maintained, all mea-

sures were still greater than pretreatment levels at the 12-month evaluation.[35]

A retrospective analysis of patients referred to a modified functional restoration work tolerance program and addressed issues of functional work tolerance, return to work, pain, and disability in nonselected patients with LBP.[69] The program consisted of functional capacity testing, strength and endurance exercise, didactic sessions about LBP, behavioral modification, and psychosocial counseling strategies requiring 12 4-hour work sessions for 3 days per week and costing a mean of $1440 per patient. As with many noncontrolled studies, there were problems with patient follow-up that might have led to potential bias. Bearing in mind the limitations of the lack of control group data, the clinical approach they describe did enhance return to work, may be more cost-effective than the program described by Mayer,[48,49] and is significantly more effective than physical capacity tolerance testing without the functional physical rehabilitation program.

Because the return-to-work rates of 80 to 85% are already higher than those observed in other treatment modalities and probably are as high as can be expected, the question arises as to whether the additional gains in physical capacity with the functional restoration approach will make a difference in future low-back injury rates. This and other questions on the efficacy of the functional restoration approach following spinal surgery are under investigation. At this time, however, the promising results of this functional physical rehabilitation approach with the use of exercise as an assessment tool, as an intervention, and as an outcome measure would have to be categorized as "usefullness demonstrated by non-randomized controlled trial" using the Quebec Task Force classification schema.[76] Nevertheless, although substantiation by randomized controlled trial for the functional restoration approach to LBP is not yet available, this approach to rehabilitation has antecedents in such other conditions as heart disease,[65] appears to be conceptually safe and sound for selected LBP patients, and has demonstrated effectiveness in improving physical functional capacity, increasing rates of return to work, and reducing health care costs in these patients.

DISCUSSION

Is there a role for exercise in the prevention of LBP? The evidence suggests that a healthy lifestyle that includes regular exercise has an indirect preventive role in LBP.[59] However, this role is probably secondary to other well-documented effects that include improved overall health and physical fitness, as well as positive psychological benefits associated with being more active.[14,17,65,66]

Is there a role for exercise in the treatment and rehabilitation of LBP? Jackson and Brown take the position that further investigation is needed and that although aerobic conditioning exercise may offer the greatest benefits, "the value of these exercises is often overstated."[39] However, the more-recent studies, including a number of randomized controlled trials reviewed in this chapter, clearly demonstrate that increased regular exercise should be considered an integral component of rehabilitation for patients with LBP.

Experimental studies show a reduced level of pain, an improved function, a reduced illness behavior, and an increased rate of return to work with carefully prescribed progressive exercise rehabilitation regimens. Adequate trunk strength appears to be necessary for employment, and aerobic conditioning may be associated with decreased pain and is associated with improved aerobic fitness. Chronic LBP reinforces fear of injury, which in turn reinforces physical inactivity and further exaggerates such psychosocial factors as anxiety and depression.[46] Therefore, it seems that the benefits of regular and appropriate physical exercise in the rehabilitation of LBP may be as much the result of a holistic effect as a specific conditioning one. Nevertheless, substantiating the position taken by Jackson and Brown[39] and others,[46,58,59,79] we emphasize that the role

of exercise and its prescription in the rehabilitation of LBP is not well understood, needs considerable further investigation, and is only one modality in a comprehensive approach, as is the case in other conditions such as the rehabilitation of coronary heart disease.[65]

Waddell has introduced a biopsychosocial conceptual model for the rehabilitation of LBP that focuses on the need to treat patients rather than spines and on illness rather than disease.[85,86] It is based on observations that LBP may be regarded as normal, that disability from LBP appears to be a recent Western epidemic, and that conventional medical treatment for LBP has failed.[85,86] It appears that the outcome of treatment is largely determined by an interaction between physical and psychological factors, with return to work often determined more by psychosocial factors than physical disease.[79,80] The experimental evidence discussed in this chapter demonstrates a strong relationship between controlled physical exercise and improved function and reduced pain. The biopsychosocial model that Waddell has described clearly reinforces the importance of management for LBP changing "from a negative philosophy of rest for pain to more active restoration of function."[85]

In an earlier paper, Alaranta and Kallio suggested that the close relationship between disability (functional status) and occupational handicap reinforces the need "not to forget the integrated activities of the body or the person as a whole . . . [and] more important than to increase strength on its own is to train muscle coordination and achieve a reasonable muscle balance in order to ensure rational integration of the activities of the body."[1] Although there probably will not ever be a cure for all LBP, there are ways to help patients with LBP to cope with their problems, and patients must be counseled to take a larger portion of the responsibility for their own progress. The 1964 World Health Organization definition of cardiac rehabilitation as "the sum of activity required to ensure patients the best possible physical, mental and social conditions so that *they may by their own efforts regain* as normal as possible a place in the community and lead an active productive life"[88] applies equally well to patients with LBP. Whether the practice of physical capacity evaluation and exercise prescription in the rehabilitation of patients with LBP will be generally accepted or not, the "main theme of management must change from rest to rehabilitation and restoration of function . . . [because] there is clear evidence that, despite general belief, activity is not harmful, and active rehabilitation not only restores function but also reduces pain."[85] If exercise results in an improved quality of life (i.e., an active and productive life), return to work, reduced pain, and increased control in even a relatively small percentage of patients, the cost-effectiveness of exercise as a therapeutic modality for patients with LBP would be considerable.

Many questions remain unanswered. How best to measure physical function? Should we measure cardiovascular endurance, muscle strength, muscle endurance, and flexibility? Should these be measured for both preventive and rehabilitative purposes? How should the exercise prescription be developed? What is the intensity, frequency, and duration of exercise? What type of exercise? How does the type of spinal disorder affect the exercise evaluation and prescription? How does the psychological status of the patient affect the evaluation and prescription? What is the likelihood of adequate compliance with exercise prescription? Is this likely to be the same for different exercise prescriptions? There is a need for continued demonstration of the efficacy and effectiveness of physical capacity evaluation and exercise prescription in the rehabilitation of patients with spinal disorders and LBP. A recent editorial in the journal *Spine* outlined the criteria for planning studies of intervention that should be of much value for researchers who wish to examine the potential role of exercise in the rehabilitation of patients with spinal disorders and LBP.[60] As Waddell has stated, "The following questions can no longer be avoided:

Rest or rehabilitation? Rest or restoration of function? Rest or recovery?"[85]

REFERENCES

1. Alaranta, H., and Kallio, V.: The concept of consequences of disease in patients with low back pain. Int. Rehabil. Med., 8:8, 1986.
2. Alaranta, H., Hurme, M., and Karppi, S.: Leisure time physical activities and the results of surgery of lumbar disc herniation. Scand. J. Rehab. Med., 19:105, 1987.
3. Asfour, S.S., et al.: Biofeedback in back muscle strengthening. Spine, 15:510, 1990.
4. Balague, F., Dutoit, G., and Waldburger, M.: Low back pain in schoolchildren. Scand. J. Rehab. Med., 20:175, 1988.
5. Barnes, D., et al.: Psychosocioeconomic predictors of treatment success/failure in chronic low-back pain patients. Spine, 14:427,1989.
6. Battie, M., et al.: Isometric lifting strength as a predictor of industrial back pain reports. Spine, 14:851, 1989.
7. Battie, M., et al.: A prospective study of the role of cardiovascular risk factors and fitness in industrial back pain complaints. Spine, 14:141, 1989.
8. Battie, M., et al.: The role of spinal flexibility in back pain complaints within industry. Spine, 15:768, 1990.
9. Battie, M., et al.: Anthropometric and clinical measures as predictors of back pain complaints in industry: a prospective study. J. Spine Disorders, 3:195, 1990.
10. Berwick, D.M., Budman, S., and Feldstein, M.: No clinical effect of back schools in an HMO. Spine, 14:338, 1989.
11. Biering-Sorensen, F.: A prospective study of low back pain in a general population. Scand. J. Rehab. Med., 15:71, 1983.
12. Biering-Sorensen, F.: Physical measurements as risk indicators for low back trouble over a one-year period. Spine, 9:106, 1984.
13. Bigos, S., et al.: A prospective study of work perceptions and psychosocial factors affecting the report of back injury. Spine, 16:1, 1991.
14. Blair, S.N., et al.: Physical fitness and all-cause mortality. A prospective study of healthy men and women. JAMA, 262:2395, 1989.
15. Bowne, D.W., et al.: Reduced disability and health care costs in an industrial fitness program. J. Occup. Ther. Med., 26:809, 1984.
16. Bortz, W.M.: Disuse and aging. JAMA, 248:1203, 1982.
17. Bouchard, C., et al. (eds.): Exercise, Fitness, and Health. Champaign, IL, Human Kinetics, 1990.
18. Brand, R.A., and Lehmann, T.R.: Low-back impairment rating practices of orthopedic surgeons. Spine, 8:75, 1983.
19. Brennan, G.P., Ruhling, R.O., Hood, R.S., et al.: Physical characteristics of patients with herniated discs. Spine, 12:699, 1987.
20. Cady, L.D., et al.: Strength and fitness and subsequent back injuries in firefighters. J. Occup. Ther. Med., 21:269, 1979.
21. Cady, L.D., Thomas, P.C., and Karwasky, R.J.: Program for increasing health and physical fitness of firefighters. J. Occup. Med., 27:111, 1985.

22. Crauford, D.I.O., Creed, F., and Jayson, M.I.V.: Life events and psychological disturbances in patients with low back pain. Spine, 15:490, 1990.
23. Dehlin, O., et al.: Effect of physical training and ergonomic counseling on the physiological perception of work and on the subjective assessment of low-back insufficiency. Scand. J. Rehabil. Med., 13:1, 1981.
24. Deyo, R.A.: Conservative therapy for low back pain. JAMA, 250:1057, 1983.
25. Deyo, R.A., and Bass, J.E.: Lifestyle and low-back pain. Spine, 14:501, 1989.
26. Deyo, R.A., and Tsui-Wu, Y.: Descriptive epidemiology of low-back pain and its related medical care in the United States. Spine, 12:264, 1987.
27. Deyo, R.A., et al.: A controlled trial of transcutaneous electrical nerve stimulation (TENS) and exercise for chronic low back pain. N. Engl. J. Med., 322:1627, 1990.
28. Donchin, M., et al.: Secondary prevention of low-back pain. Spine, 15:1317, 1990.
29. Frymoyer, J.W.: Back pain and sciatica. N. Engl. J. Med, 318:291, 1988.
30. Frymoyer, J.W., and Cats-Baril, W.: Predictors of low back pain disability. Clin. Orthop., 221:89, 1987.
31. Frymoyer, J.W., and Gordon, S.L.: Research perspectives in low-back pain. Spine, 14:1384, 1989.
32. Frymoyer, J.W., and Gordon, S.L., eds.: New Perspectives on Low Back Pain. Park Ridge, IL, American Academy of Orthopedic Surgeons, 1989.
33. Granhed, H., and Morelli, B.: Low back pain among retired wrestlers and heavyweight lifters. Am. J. Sports Med., 16:530, 1988.
34. Harkapaa, K., et al.: A controlled study on the outcome of inpatient and outpatient treatment of low back pain. Scand. J. Rehab. Med., 21:81, 1989.
35. Hazard, R.G., et al.: Functional restoration with behavior support. Spine, 14:157, 1989.
36. Heliovaara, M.: Risk factors for low back pain and sciatica. Ann. Med., 21:257, 1989.
37. Heliovaara, M., et al.: Descriptive epidemiology and public health aspects of low back pain. Ann. Med., 21:327, 1989.
38. Hurri, H.: The Swedish back school in chronic low back pain. Scand. J. Rehab. Med., 21:33, 1989.
39. Jackson, C.P., and Brown, M.D.: Is there a role for exercise in the treatment of patients with low back pain? Clin. Orthop., 179:39, 1983.
40. Jorgensen, U., and Winge, S.: Injuries in badminton. Sports Med., 10:59, 1990.
41. Kelsey, J.L., and Golden, A.L.: Occupational and workplace factors associated with low back pain. Occup. Med. State Art Rev., 3:7, 1988.
42. Kohles, S., et al.: Improved physical performance outcomes after functional restoration treatment in patients with chronic low-back pain. Spine, 15:1321, 1990.
43. Lanese, R.R., et al.: Injury and disability in matched men's and women's intercollegiate sports. Am. J. Pub. Health, 80:1459, 1990.
44. Manniche, C., et al.: Clinical trial of intensive muscle training for chronic low back pain. Lancet, 2:1473, 1988.
45. Marks, M.R., and Haas, S.S.: Low back pain in the competitive tennis player. Clin. Sports Med., 7:277, 1988.
46. Mayer, T.G.: Discussion: exercise, fitness, and back pain. In Exercise, Fitness and Health. Edited by C. Bouchard, et al. Champaign, IL, Human Kinetics, 1990.
47. Mayer, T.G., and Gatchel, R.J.: Functional Restoration for Spinal Disorders: The Sports Medicine Approach. Philadelphia, Lea & Febiger, 1988.
48. Mayer, T.G., et al.: Objective assessment of spine function following industrial injury. Spine, 10:482, 1985.
49. Mayer, T.G., et al.: A prospective two-year study of functional restoration in industrial low back injury. JAMA, 258:1763, 1987.
50. McCauley, E., et al.: Injuries in women's gymnastics. The state of the art. Am. J. Sports Med., 15:558, 1987.
51. McLennan, J.G., and McLennan, J.E.: Injury patterns in Scottish heavy athletes Am. J. Sports Med., 18:529, 1990.
52. McQuade, K.J., Turner, J.A., and Buchner, D.M.: Physical fitness and chronic low back pain. Clin. Orthop., 233:198, 1988.
53. Meade, T.W., et al.: Low back pain of mechanical origin: randomised comparison of chiropractic and hospital outpatient treatment. Br. Med. J., 300:1431, 1990.
54. Mellin, G.: Chronic low back pain in men 54–63 years of age. Spine, 11:421, 1986.
55. Mellin, G., et al.: A controlled study on the outcome of inpatient and outpatient treatment of low back pain. Scand. J. Rehab. Med., 21:91, 1989.
56. Mellin, G., Jarvikoski, A., and Verkasalo, M.: Treatment of patients with chronic low back pain. Scand. J. Rehab. Med., 16:77, 1984.
57. Mooney, V.: The failed back—an orthopaedic view. Int. Disabil. Studies, 10:32, 1988.
58. Nachemson, A.: The future of low back pain research. In New Perspectives on Low Back Pain, Edited by J.W. Frymoyer and S.L. Gordon. Park Ridge, IL, American Academy of Orthopedic Surgeons, 1989.
59. Nachemson, A.L.: Exercise, fitness, and back pain. In Exercise, Fitness, and Health. Edited by C. Bouchard, et al. Champaign, IL, Human Kinetics, 1990.
60. Nachemson, A.L., and LaRocca, H.: (Editorial). Spine, 12:427, 1987.
61. Ohlen, G., Wredmark, T., and Spangfort, E.: Spinal sagittal configuration and mobility related to low-back pain in the female gymnast. Spine, 14:847, 1989.
62. O'Neil, D.B., and Micheli, L.J.: Overuse injury in the young athlete. Clin. Sports Med., 7:591, 1988.
63. Oldridge, N.B.: Cardiac rehabilitation exercise programme: compliance and compliance-enhancing strategies. Sports Med., 4:784, 1988.
64. Oldridge, N.B.: Compliance with cardiac rehabilitation services. J. Cardiopulm. Rehabil., 11:115, 1991.
65. Oldridge, N.B., Foster, C., and Schmidt, D.H. (eds.): Cardiac Rehabilitation & Clinical Exercise Programs: Theory & Practice. Ithaca, NY, Movement Publications Inc., 1988.

151

66. Phelps, J.R.: Physical activity and health maintenance—exactly what is known? West. J. Med., *146*:200, 1987.
67. Pope, M.H.: Risk indicators in low back pain. Ann. Med., *21*:387, 1989.
68. Reilly, K., et al.: Differences between a supervised and independent strength and conditioning program with chronic low back syndromes. J. Occup. Med., *31*:547, 1989.
69. Sachs, B.L., et al.: Spinal rehabilitation by work tolerance based on objective physical capacity assessment of dysfunction. Spine, *15*:1325, 1990.
70. Saraste, H., and Hultman, G.: Life conditions of persons with and without low-back pain. Scand. J. Rehab. Med., *19*:109, 1987.
71. Sinaki, M., et al.: Lumbar spondylolisthesis: retrospective comparison and three-year follow-up of two conservative treatment programs. Arch. Phys. Med. Rehabil., *70*:594, 1989.
72. Snook, S.H., and Webster, B.S.: The costs of back pain in industry. Occup. Med. State Art Rev., *3*:7, 1988.
73. Spencer, C.W., and Jackson, D.W.: Back injuries in the athlete. Clin. Sports Med., *2*:191, 1983.
74. Spengler, D.M.: Lumbar discectomy—results with limited disc excision and selective foraminotomy. Spine, *7*:203, 1982.
75. Sturgess, E., Schaefer, C., and Sikora, T.: Pain center follow-up study of treated and untreated patients. Arch. Phys. Med. Rehabil., *65*:301, 1984.
76. Spitzer, W.O., LeBlanc, F.E., and DuPuis, M.: Scientific approach to the assessment and management of activity-related spinal disorders. Spine, *12*:S1, 1987.
77. Sward, L., Eriksson, B., and Peterson, L.: Anthropometric characteristics, passive hip flexion, and spinal mobility in relation to back pain in athletes. Spine, *15*:376, 1990.
78. Sward, L., et al.: Back pain and radiologic changes in the thoraco-lumbar spine of athletes. Spine, *15*:124, 1990.
79. Tollison, C.D., and Kriegel, M.L.: Physical exercise in the treatment of low back pain. Orthop. Rev., *17*:724, 1988.
80. Triano, J.L., and Schultz, A.B.: Correlation of objective measure of trunk motion and muscle function with low-back disability ratings. Spine, *12*:561, 1987.
81. Troup, J.D.G., et al.: The perception of back pain and the role of psychophysical tests of lifting capacity. Spine, *12*:645, 1987.
82. Vallfors, B.: Acute, subacute and chronic low back pain: clinical symptoms, absenteeism and working environment. Scand. J. Rehab. Med., *11*:1, 1985.
83. Videman, T., et al.: Low-back pain in nurses and some loading factors of work. Spine, *9*:400, 1984.
84. Videman, T., et al.: Patient-handling skill, back injuries, and back pain. Spine, *14*:148, 1989.
85. Waddell, G.: A new clinical model for the treatment of low-back pain. Spine, *12*:632, 1987.
86. Waddell, G., et al.: A concept of illness tested as an improved basis for surgical decisions in low-back disorders. Spine, *11*:712, 1986.
87. Webster, B.S., and Snook, S.H.: The cost of compensable low back pain. J. Occup. Med., *32*:13, 1990.
88. World Health Organization. Rehabilitation of patients with cardiovascular disease: Report of a WHO expert committee. WHO Tech. Rep. Ser., 1964.

10
CHAPTER

Diabetes

by
Arthur S. Leon

The tragic premature death of the great athlete Jackie Robinson in 1972 at the age of 53 dramatizes that diabetes mellitus (DM) remains an untamed killer disease. Robinson's DM was first diagnosed 20 years earlier, while he was a star infielder with the Brooklyn Dodgers. He subsequently developed most of the late complications associated with this condition, including progressive loss of vision, peripheral vascular and neurologic changes in the lower extremities limiting his ability to walk, and coronary heart disease (CHD). The immediate cause of his death was his third heart attack (a common cause of death in diabetic individuals). This chapter describes this disease, its cause, its early and late complications, and its management through diet, medications, and exercise.

EPIDEMIOLOGY

DM is one of the major health problems facing our nation, as well as other industrialized Western countries.[12,23,88,130] It is a common disorder whose prevalence is steadily increasing. About 15 million Americans, or about 5% of the population, are estimated to have DM. The incidence rate of DM increases with age. The rates are higher in nonwhite populations than in white populations, with the prevalence reaching a peak level of 10.5% among nonwhite individuals aged 65 and over.

The disease ranks as the sixth or seventh leading cause of mortality in the United States (depending on the mortality classifi-

cation system used) and is the direct underlying cause of at least 40,000 deaths annually. However, this mortality figure grossly underestimates the contribution of DM to mortality because many persons with this disease die as a result of associated cardiovascular complications (particularly heart attacks and strokes). In addition to vascular complications, DM is an important contributor to visual impairment, blindness, and renal failure.

DESCRIPTION

DM is one of the oldest diseases known to man. It was described in India in 400 B.C. and again in the fourth century B.C. in the Egyptian Ebers Papyrus.[66] Ancient Greek physicians first coined the term "diabetes," meaning to run through a siphon. The Latin word "mellitus," meaning honey, was added much later. In fact, for centuries after the discovery of "honey urine," DM was diagnosed by tasting the patient's urine for sweetness, a forerunner of the modern laboratory analysis for sugar (glucose) in the urine.

DM is actually a heterogenous group of metabolic disorders having in common an *actual or relative insufficiency of insulin secretion.* The best known actions of this peptide hormone synthesized in the beta (β) cells of the pancreatic islets are its ability to promote the transport of glucose across cell membranes in insulin-responsive tissues and subsequent glucose oxidation for energy production. Thus, insulin insufficiency reduces the ability of tissues, including skeletal muscle, to utilize glucose as a fuel. The ability of muscle to synthesize glycogen also is defective,[116] the end-result of which is an elevated level of glucose in the blood (hyperglycemia), the clinical hallmark of this disease. When the level of plasma glucose circulating through the kidney exceeds 160 to 180 mg/dl, glucose usually spills over into the urine (glycosuria). This is accompanied by increased frequency of urination and volume of urine excreted (polyuria). The associated loss of large amounts of body water increases sensation of thirst and water intake (polydipsia). However, dehydration may still result because of excess fluid loss due to hyperosmolarity of the glucose-containing urine. The major acute symptoms and signs of DM are summarized in Table 10–1.

In addition to its effect on glucose uptake and its utilization and storage as a fuel by muscle and the liver, other anabolic and metabolic actions of insulin include inhibition of hepatic glycogen breakdown and glucose release by the liver; increased triglyceride (TG) synthesis by the liver; TG synthesis, storage, and inhibition of its breakdown (antilipolytic effect) in adipose tissue; and increased cell amino acid uptake and protein synthesis throughout the body. Thus, an insufficiency of insulin leads to a host of wide-ranging metabolic derangements, as outlined below.

Increased lipolysis of TGs in adipose tissue raises the concentration of free fatty acids (FFAs) in the serum, promoting their use for fuel. Because the liver has a limited capacity to utilize acetyl-coenzyme A generated from FFA metabolism, this results in increased formation of the so-called ketone bodies (acetoacetate, beta-hydroxybutyrate, and acetone). Accumulation of ketone bodies in the blood and their excretion in the urine causes metabolic acidosis (ketoacidosis), excess fluid loss, and dehydration, which can terminate in coma. Before the discovery of insulin, severe ketoacidosis was the most common cause of premature mortality related to DM. Insulin replacement therapy now helps correct the metabolic deficiency state, controls the symptoms and signs of DM, prevents ketoacidosis, and improves long-term survival of insulin-dependent diabetic patients.

TYPES OF DIABETES MELLITUS

Evidence of Heterogeneity

Evidence that DM is a heterogeneous syndrome is derived from a variety of sources[98]:

1. Clinical and experimental data indicating that DM can be increased by a variety of pathophysiologic mechanisms, which include the following:
   a. Physical destruction by various mechanisms of the insulin-producing β cells of the pancreas (e.g., autoimmune reactions, chemical poisoning, viral infections, or malignancies).
   b. Defective β-cell synthesis of insulin.
   c. Defective release of insulin by β cells.
   d. Impaired glucose transport in β cells.[131]
   e. Tissue (cellular) insensitivity to insulin.
2. Heterogeneity of animal models of DM.
3. Association of DM with a variety of other endocrine diseases and genetic disorders.
4. Absence of typical late complications of DM in 20 to 30% of patients with "classic" disease.
5. Differences in patterns of inheritance.

TABLE 10–1. **Common Symptoms and Signs of Diabetes Mellitus**

Fatigue
Weakness
Weight loss
Hunger (polyphagia)
Thirst (polydipsia)
Frequent urination (polyuria)
Elevated blood sugar (hyperglycemia)
Sugar in the urine (glycosuria)
Acetone in the blood and urine (ketosis)

Classification

In the past, many systems were used to classify DM. The World Health Organization (WHO) classification is now commonly used to differentiate the major types of DM.[145] In this classification scheme, DM is divided into four major clinical types as follows: insulin-dependent or type I diabetes mellitus (IDDM); non–insulin-dependent or type II diabetes mellitus (NIDDM); malnutrition-related DM; and other secondary types of DM associated with various medical conditions or syndromes. In addition, DM first recognized during pregnancy is termed *gestational DM* and is subsequently reclassified if it persists after pregnancy. Further, the term "impaired glucose tolerance" (IGT) is used to describe the condition of individuals who have elevated levels of plasma glucose in the fasting, postprandial state, or after a glucose challenge, but whose glucose levels are not high enough to be diagnosed as DM. Like DM, IGT is associated with increased risk of future NIDDM and cardiovascular complications.

Table 10–2 compares the characteristics of the two most common forms of diabetes, IDDM and NIDDM. It should be noted that although the primary defect in IDDM is an absolute deficiency of insulin due to β islet cell damage; this generally is associated with some degree of peripheral insulin resistance, perhaps related to hyperglycemia or excess secretion of counterregulatory hormones.[34] On the other hand, in NIDDM, in which the primary defect is peripheral insulin resistance, it is usually accompanied by a relative deficiency in insulin release from the β islet cells.[103]

CAUSES

Predisposing Diabetogenic Factors

An inherited predisposition for both type I and II DM is well established.[6,7,12,66] Identical twins show a fourfold higher concordance for DM than nonidentical twins. If both parents have DM, their children have a 30% chance of eventually developing DM.[66] Twelve percent of individuals with newly diagnosed DM have close relatives with DM, as compared to only 2% of nondiabetic individuals. The presence of genetic etiologic factors is confirmed by the increased frequency of certain inherited blood group and human leukocyte histocompatibility antigen (HLA) types in IDDM and the documentation of genetically linked DM in animals.[34] The bulk of the present genetic evidence suggests a multifactoral mode of inheritance for both forms of DM.

Viruses and Autoimmune Mechanisms

In animal experiments, it has been possible to induce DM by infection with certain viruses that destroy pancreatic β islet cells.

TABLE 10–2. **Comparisons of Type I, Insulin-Dependent Diabetes Mellitus and Type II, Non–Insulin-Dependent Diabetes Mellitus**

Characteristics	Type I, IDDM	Type II, NIDDM
Former designation	Juvenile-onset	Maturity-onset
Age of onset	Usually < 35 years	Usually > 40 years
Clinical onset	Abrupt	Gradual
Family history	Yes	Yes
HLA association*	Yes	No
Body composition	Normal or thin	Usually obese (central-type)
Blood insulin levels	Reduced or absent	Normal or increased
Cell insulin resistance	Absent or minor	Present
Tendency for ketoacidosis (without replacement insulin)	Yes	No
Treatment for control of hyperglycemia	Insulin, diet, ± exercise	Weight loss, diet, exercise, oral hyperglycemic drugs, or insulin

* Association with specific genetically determined histocompatability leukocyte antigen (HLA) types.

In humans, although there is suggestive evidence that mumps and Coxsackie B viruses can induce DM in a similar manner, the relative contribution of viruses to IDDM remains an open question.[12] A possibility also exists that viral-damaged islet cells may act as antigens. Antibodies are then produced in susceptible individuals that can destroy remaining β cells through an autoimmune process.

There is, in fact, considerable evidence to support the hypothesis that IDDM is commonly caused by an autoimmune process.[34,140] This is believed to result in a gradual destruction of insulin-producing β islet cells, with eventual β cell failure. An asymptomatic phase of this process is thought to last for months or years based on findings of a high prevalence of circulating antibodies to islet β cells and to insulin itself (insulin autoimmune antibodies or IAA) in patients initially diagnosed with IDDM.[144] Moreover, the HLA types commonly associated with IDDM are known to be linked to immune response genes. Additional supporting evidence for the autoimmune cause hypothesis is the occasional association of IDDM with autoimmune disorders affecting other organs such as the thyroid, adrenals, or gastric parietal cells, as demonstrated by circulating antibodies to these tissues. Although circulating IAA and islet cell antibodies have been observed in patients prior to their developing IDDM, it has not been established whether these circulating antibodies are good markers for ultimate development of the disease.[140] The use of immunosuppressant drugs in the early management of IDDM is currently under experimental investigation.

Obesity

Epidemiologic studies have consistently shown that obesity is the principal risk factor for developing NIDDM; about 80% of people with this disease are obese.[139] In populations in which obesity is rare, the prevalence of DM is low despite the presence of genetic susceptibility. DM is more prevalent among women in populations in which middle-aged women are generally fatter than men and more prevalent among men in cultures in which the reverse is true.[66] Incidence rates in the very obese are more than 20 times greater than in the nonobese.[139] In contrast, the incidence rate of NIDDM is exceedingly low in lean individuals.

Additional supporting evidence of the role of obesity in causing NIDDM is the demonstration that weight gain and overweight may result in decreased peripheral activity of insulin through cellular resistance, probably related to a loss of insulin receptors, particularly in distended adipose cells.[66,139] This insulin resistance can be reversed by loss of excess weight and body fat. Furthermore, central or abdominal predominance of body fat distribution (as reflected by a waist-hip ratio > 1.0 in men and > 0.9 in women) has been shown to predict future DM in prospective studies, independent of relative weight.[26,91]

Physical Inactivity

Epidemiologic studies also indicate that sedentary lifestyle is an important risk factor for developing IDDM.[139] Although this is probably partially related to the common association of physical inactivity with obesity, experimental evidence also suggests a direct relationship. Inactivity, as provided by enforced bed rest, leads to glucose intolerance and oversecretion of insulin within a few days because of increased of cellular resistance to insulin.[82,83] In addition, in vitro studies have revealed decreased numbers of insulin receptors in white blood cells from physically inactive as compared to active people in both diabetic and nondiabetic individuals.[65,97,120]

Diet

A commonly held misconception is that DM results from excess sugar ingestion. It is now generally accepted that the principal diet-related contribution to NIDDM is an excess energy intake relative to physical activity.[12,139] A deficiency of dietary fiber in a Western-type diet also is postulated to play a role. In fact, it has been demonstrated that a diet high in complex carbohydrates improves glucose tolerance with either a decrease or no change in insulin requirements.[7,15,66] A Western-type diet high in saturated animal fat and cholesterol also is considered an important contributor to macrovascular complications of DM because of its blood cholesterol raising effect.[66,139] This helps explain why Oriental people with DM on a diet low in animal fat and high in starch (rice) have a much lower incidence of atherosclerotic complications than white people with DM.

Aging

The incidence of NIDDM increases with age, and the majority of diabetic people in our society (90% of whom have NIDDM) are over 40 years of age.[12,23,139] Glucose tolerance also is reported to decrease with age, but this may primarily reflect the increased proportion of the population with NIDDM.[23] The usual age-associated increase in adiposity and decrease in physical activity most likely contribute significantly to the age-related increased rate of NIDDM and glucose intolerance in North America.

Endocrine Disorders

Many hormones have metabolic actions that are counter-regulatory to those of insulin and that increase endogenous or exogenous insulin requirements,[127] such as thyroid hormones, epinephrine, cortisone, glucagon, growth hormone, and the sex hormones. An excess of any of these anti-insulin hormones can cause a "diabetic-like" metabolic state in susceptible individuals. Examples of endocrine conditions that commonly precipitate DM include hyperthyroidism, Cushing's disease (hyper corticosteroidism), primary hyperaldosteronism, acromegaly (excess growth hormone), and pheochromocytoma (excess catecholamines). Pregnancy may also convert a prediabetic state to a temporary or permanent subclinical or manifest diabetes.[139] Gestational DM affects up to 59% of all pregnant women, making it one of the most common complications of pregnancy.[49] The incidence of DM also increases with multiple pregnancies.

Drugs

Medications that may produce manifest DM in susceptible individuals include long-term glucocorticoid steroid therapy ("steroid diabetes"), thyroid hormones, oral contraceptive agents, and thiazide or related diuretics.[12]

Pancreatic and Liver Disease

Acute and chronic pancreatitis, carcinoma of the pancreas, hemochromatosis, mucovisidosis, and other diseases involving the pancreas can lead to diabetes if a significant proportion of the islet β cells are destroyed.[12] Cirrhosis of the liver is associated with an increased incidence of DM characterized by a poor response to insulin (hepatogenic DM).

Stress

It has been postulated that acute or chronic emotional stress can cause DM through increased sympathetic nervous system stimulation and associated increased epinephrine and glucocorticoid secretions from the adrenals, but evidence for this is inconclusive.[139] Although a transient increase in blood sugar can result from acute stress, it usually is self-limited. If stress continues, the glycemic response lessens because of adaptations.

CLINICAL ASPECTS OF DIABETES

Symptoms Associated with DM

Usual presenting symptoms of DM were previously discussed and summarized in Table 10–1.

Laboratory Diagnosis

A good laboratory is essential for diagnosis, control, and surveillance of DM. Commonly used tests for detecting and monitoring of DM are listed below.[5,6,11,66]

URINE SUGAR. Commercial test paper (e.g., Tes-Tape, Eli Lilly, Indianapolis) is currently the method of choice for detection and quantification of urinary glucose. This method depends on the specific enzymatic reaction of glucose with glucose oxidase and peroxidase. The shade of color on the paper strip gives an estimate of sugar concentration. Despite the relatively high sensitivity of paper strips, laboratory quantitative 24-hour assay of urine glucose is recommended for precise control of DM. A negative urine glucose test does not exclude diabetes because hyperglycemia may occur without glycosuria in the presence of a high renal threshold for sugar or vascular disease.

EXAMINATION OF URINE FOR KETONE BODIES. Qualitative testing of urine for ketone bodies can be carried out by test strips or tablets and is of special importance in IDDM management.

BLOOD GLUCOSE LEVEL. The most common methods for a definitive determination of plasma or serum glucose level are automated procedures. A self-administered, reasonably simple method (Dextrostix, Ames Co., Elkhart, IN) is now available for estimation of "true glucose" content of blood and requires only a single drop of capillary blood obtained by a spring-propelled lance. A fasting plasma glucose level of > 140 mg/dl or a random plasma glucose level of 200 mg/dl or more is diagnostic for DM. Levels of glucose in plasma or serum are 15% (not 15 mg/dl) higher than in whole or capillary blood. If the patient's hematocrit is normal, conversion can be made to plasma concentration by multiplying the whole blood value by 1.15. In mild cases of DM, the fasting plasma glucose level may be < 140 mg/dl. The diagnosis of DM may then be established by an oral glucose tolerance test (OGTT), as described below.

ORAL GLUCOSE TOLERANCE TEST. If subclinical diabetes is suspected, a provocative or tolerance test is required for confirmation. The most commonly used of such tests is the OGTT. For the results of this test to be meaningful, the patient should discontinue drugs that affect glucose tolerance and consume a carbohydrate-rich diet containing at least 250 g of carbohydrate daily for at least 3 days prior to the test. If dietary carbohydrates are restricted, a falsely positive OGGT may result. After a sample of blood is taken for fasting blood sugar, usually 75 g of glucose is administered in a commercial test drink. Blood samples for glucose values are then collected every 30 min for at least 120 min. Diagnosis of DM in a nonpregnant person requires a plasma glucose level of > 200 mg/dl at 120 min and at one other time during the test. A 2-hour plasma glucose level of 140 to 180 mg/dl is considered a positive result for impaired glucose tolerance.

GLYCOSYLATED HEMOGLOBIN. A laboratory test for evaluating long-term blood sugar control measures the level of glucose binding to the hemoglobin HbA_1 fraction and is based on the observation that chronically high serum glucose levels are associated with increased nonenzymatic glucose binding to proteins.[18] The concentration of glycosylated hemoglobin in percentage of total hemoglobin glycosylated into HbA_1 reflects the individual's usual serum glucose over a period of 2 to 3 months prior to the test. This technique has proven to be a useful tool in the evaluation of diabetic control. Glucose-protein binding also has been postulated to contribute to degenerative changes associated with DM in nerve fibers, the lens of the eye, capillary membranes, kidney glomeruli, and arterial wall linings.[22]

PLASMA INSULIN RADIOIMMUNOASSAY. Determination of plasma insulin levels by radioimmunoassay (RIA) before and after a glucose challenge is of value in distinguishing DM due to insulin deficiency from a primary insulin resistance syndrome.[45] In an 18-year longitudinal study using this technique, Turkington and Weindling demonstrated that individuals with a true hormonal secretory deficiency were more likely to develop complications specific for DM (i.e., diabetic retinopathy, neuropathy, and renal disease) than those with normal RIA levels.[130]

PLASMA C-PEPTIDE DETERMINATION. C-peptide is part of the proinsulin molecule, connecting the A and B chains of the insulin molecule. It is released along with insulin from the granules of the β islet cells. Measurement of serum levels of the C-peptide concentration serves as an indirect measure of insulin secretion, and is a useful tool to evaluate whether β cells of IDDM patients are still capable of producing insulin.[66] DM patients still capable of producing some of their own insulin, as evidenced by normal C-peptide levels, usually respond more easily to treatment.

ACUTE DIABETIC COMPLICATIONS

The natural history or course of DM is extremely variable, making it difficult to predict the specific outcome for any given person.[25] Many diabetic individuals from all socioeconomic strata remain free of significant complications and carry on active productive lives despite severe IDDM for many decades. These include such outstanding athletes as Wade Wilson (currently starting quarterback for the Minnesota Vikings National Football League team), Bobby Clarke (formerly of the Philadelphia Flyers National Hockey League team), and Bill Talbert and Hamilton Richardson (former world-class tennis players). Despite good control of their DM, others (e.g., Jackie Robinson) are plagued with acute and chronic complications. Acute situations that may occur any time in the course of DM and that are usually temporary and remediable include the following:

DIABETIC KETOACIDOSIS. As previously mentioned, this was a common life-threatening complication prior to the discovery of insulin; about two-thirds of those with IDDM died in ketoacidosis or so-called "diabetic coma." Currently, only about 1% of IDDM patients die of this complication.[25]

HYPOGLYCEMIA ("INSULIN REACTION"). Hypoglycemia or "low blood sugar" is one of the most common complications for diabetic patients receiving insulin or an oral hypoglycemic agent. It results from an overdosage of a glucose-lowering drug relative to dietary and physical activity status. Usual precipitating factors are either an insufficient food intake to cover the blood glucose-lowering effect of the hypoglycemic drug dosage or more physical activity than is customary for the individual.[66]

Although symptoms of hypoglycemia usually develop when the plasma glucose level drops below 50 mg/dl, they also may occur at much higher blood glucose levels in response to a rapid drop in glucose concentration. Resulting symptoms are of both sympathetic and central nervous system origin and include hunger, weakness, trembling, sweating, confusion, and headaches. If the diabetic individual fails to respond to these prodromal symptoms by consuming a carbohydrate-rich food or beverage, symptoms can progress to drowsiness or unconsciousness. Occasionally, a patient with subclinical DM develops hypoglycemia as an initial presenting symptom because of inappropriate timing and amounts of insulin released following meals.

SKIN AND MUCOSAL PROBLEMS. A multiplicity of skin and mucosal problems may occur in DM.[66] Such skin infections as furuncles and carbuncles (abscesses) may initially prompt an individual with type II DM to seek medical attention and lead to the discovery of the underlying disease. Abscesses and infections may also occur at insulin injection sites because of careless technique. Pruritus vulvae due to a yeast infection (monilia) is another frequent skin problem in diabetic women. Other common sites of infection are the gums and urinary tract. Necrobiosis lipoidica, consisting of reddish to yellow ulcerating papules usually on the exterior side of the legs, may occur during any stage of DM. A loss of fatty tissue just beneath the skin is not uncommon at the sites of insulin injection, resulting in unsightly hollowed-out areas (insulin atrophy), which may improve spontaneously over a period of a year.

LATE CHRONIC COMPLICATIONS

Late complications of DM are unlikely to occur until the disease has been present at least a year, with the incidence increasing with duration of the disease.[25,66,139] The late complications are the main contributors to premature mortality with DM.

These complications may be classified as *microvascular* complications, *macrovascular* or atherosclerotic complications, and *neuropathies*. The microvascular disorders and neuropathies are specific for DM, with a higher prevalence with IDDM than with NIDDM. Principal sites of microvascular complications are the retinae of the eyes and the kidneys.

Microvascular Disease

DIABETIC RETINOPATHY. This is the most common late complication of DM and is found in one-quarter to one-half of all diabetic patients.[25,85] Microaneurysms in the area of the retinal capillaries are the characteristic initial lesions. These lesions may be benign and not interfere with vision or can result in retinal hemorrhage followed by scarring and new vessel formation (proliferative retinopathy), which can lead to retinal detachment, progressive visual impairment, and blindness. Diabetic individuals also have an increased incidence of glaucoma and cataracts, which can impair vision. Although many long-term diabetics have some degree of visual impairment, relatively few (2%) become completely blind.[25] Nevertheless, despite recent therapeutic advances (including the use of laser beam photocoagulation and vitroectomy), diabetic retinopathy remains the leading cause of blindness in North America and Europe, contributing 5000 new cases of blindness each year in the United States and probably 30,000 to 40,000 worldwide.[85] Ocular complications also are important risk indications for premature mortality.[62]

DIABETIC NEPHROPATHY (DIABETIC GLOMERULOSCLEROSIS OR KIMMELSTIEL-WILSON'S DISEASE). Nephropathy may be a late complication of either NIDDM or IDDM but appears to be much more common in IDDM.[87] However, these data may be misleading because the distinction between the two types of DM is blurred because of the common practice of referring to all insulin-treated diabetic patients as having IDDM: this confounds efforts to structure the national history of DM by type. Nevertheless, about 40 to 50% of IDDM patients develop overt manifestations of renal disease within several decades of diagnosis. About two-thirds of these patients with evidence of renal involvement eventually develop renal failure and require renal dialysis and/or a renal transplant.[87] This makes DM the third leading cause of renal failure in the United States and Europe, behind only glomerulonephritis and hypertensive renal disease.[30] Renal failure also is a common cause of death in people under age 40 years with IDDM, accounting for up to 50% of deaths in this age group. Renal failure is a much less common cause of death in individuals with NIDDM as compared to IDDM, accounting for 6% of deaths in this population.

A significant racial difference exists in the incidence of diabetic end-stage renal disease, being 2.6 times higher in blacks than in whites, with the excess risk surprisingly occurring predominantly among blacks with NIDDM.[24] The reason for these racial differences is obscure, although the higher incidence of hypertension in blacks may be a contributing factor.[61,87]

A close pathophysiologic association exists between diabetic retinopathy and nephropathy.[85] The initial manifestation of diabetic nephropathy usually is the finding of albumin in the urine (proteinuria).[87] As the nephropathy progresses, serum albumin levels fall, which can lead to peripheral edema. The renal lesions are associated with increases in blood pressure level, blood cells and casts in the urine, a progressive rise in blood urea nitrogen and serum creatinine levels, and finally uremia due to kidney failure. Atherosclerosis of the renal vessels, chronic pyelonephritis, and uncontrolled high blood pressure can all contribute to the progressive loss of renal function. Preliminary data suggest that dietary protein restriction and administration of an angiotensin-converting enzyme (ACE) inhibitor drug can attenuate the underlying microvascular damage and help prevent renal failure.[9]

160

Macrovascular Disease (Atherosclerosis)

ETIOLOGICAL FACTORS. An accelerated form of atherosclerosis leading to cardiovascular complications is common in both major types of DM, as well as with IGT.[56] Typically, atherosclerotic complications appear only after many years of IDDM, usually after microvascular disease already is apparent. However, older individuals with NIDDM (or IGT) may present with atherosclerosis of the coronary and peripheral vessels relatively early in the course of known DM; this probably reflects atherosclerotic changes beginning during the subclinical phase of DM. In the Framingham study, the incidence of cardiovascular disease among diabetic men was about twice that of nondiabetic men.[60] Among diabetic women, the incidence was about three times that of nondiabetic women. About two-thirds to three-quarters of all deaths in diabetics in Western societies are attributed to cardiovascular disease.[56,60,66,139]

An increased understanding of some of the reasons for accelerated atherosclerosis with DM is now emerging and has been extensively reviewed.[56] An interaction of multiple factors appears to be involved, particularly artery endothelial lining abnormalities, hemostatic abnormalities due to blood platelet malfunctioning, lipid-lipoprotein disturbances, hyperinsulinemia, and blood pressure elevation.[25,56,61,72,108,117] Possible endothelial abnormalities include premature cell aging, altered permeability to plasma proteins, and osmotic damage. The last abnormality may be due to accumulation in endothelial cells of an abnormal metabolite, the sugar alcohol sorbitol. Sorbitol accumulation also has been implicated in cataract formation[85] and diabetic neuropathy.[99] Endothelial damage may be accelerated by elevated blood pressure frequently found associated with DM.[56,61,72,108,117] Platelet hyperaggregability and an associated diminished capacity of the body to counterregulate against platelet deposition on damaged endothelium also have been associated with DM.[3]

Abnormalities in the blood lipid-lipoprotein profile may accelerate the atherosclerotic process much as they do in nondiabetic individuals. There are many excellent extensive reviews on this topic.[17,33,56,72,73,105,148] A great deal of variability exists among diabetic individuals in plasma lipid and lipoprotein concentrations. Factors contributing to this variability include the heterogeneity of DM, the extent of diabetic control, and a wide variety of host factors that potentially influence lipid metabolism. Host factors include body fatness and fat distribution, physical activity status, dietary habits, alcohol use, drug and oral contraceptive use, and cigarette smoking.

It has long been recognized that poorly controlled IDDM with severe insulin deficiency and ketoacidosis commonly is associated with moderate to severe hypertriglyceridemia. This is principally due to an elevation of the principal lipoprotein TG carrier in the fasting state (very low-density lipoprotein, or VLDL) resulting from an overproduction of TG and VLDL by the liver. In turn, this is related to elevated FFA levels associated with the basic metabolic disturbances due to insulin deficiency and increased activity of adipocyte hormone-sensitive lipase. In addition, TG-rich chylomicrons may be present in significant amounts in fasting plasma, giving it a lactescent appearance.

Usually accompanying hypertriglyceridemia is a reciprocal reduction in levels of the antiatherogenic, plasma high-density lipoproteins (HDLs). Reduced HDL levels appear to be related to deficient activity of capillary lipoprotein lipase, an enzyme usually activated by insulin and required for catabolic conversion of TG-rich lipoproteins into HDL in the peripheral blood. Reduced HDL formation in the liver also may contribute to reduced levels in uncontrolled IDDM. There usually are normal or even reduced plasma levels of the atherogenic LDL, which is a catabolic product of VLDL. However, in the presence of elevated plasma glucose levels, glucose binding to LDL's apoprotein B is increased. Glycosylated LDL is cleared from the plasma at a slower rate than normal LDL because of altered binding to cell LDL receptors, which is believed to increase its atherogenicity.[17] Plasma total cholesterol level may be in the normal range in diabetic compared to matched nondiabetic people or may be slightly elevated because of the usual increase in VLDL cholesterol levels.

Upon initiation of insulin therapy, plasma TG and VLDL concentrations generally decrease rapidly to within their normal ranges. However, HDL cholesterol levels may temporarily decrease further upon initiation of insulin therapy and remain subnormal for several days or weeks after the correction of insulin deficiency. After a few weeks of intensive treatment, HDL cholesterol levels generally increase significantly, and the changes persist on long-term follow-up.[20,108] Thus, adequately treated patients with uncomplicated IDDM often have a normal blood lipid-lipoprotein profile. The situation is different in patients who develop diabetic nephropathy and renal failure in that their plasma lipoprotein profile often becomes extremely atherogenic because of elevation in levels of plasma total, VLDL and LDL cholesterol, and TG, plus the associated lower levels of HDL cholesterol.

Plasma lipid and lipoprotein concentrations in NIDDM are highly variable and strongly influenced by factors similar to those in IDDM, particularly severity of DM, degree of glycemic control, and the amount and distribution of body fat. As with uncontrolled IDDM, the most common lipid-lipoprotein abnormalities are elevated plasma TG and VLDL concentrations, particularly in patients with associated endogenous hyperinsulinemia. An increased hepatic secretion of VLDL appears to be the basis for these lipid abnormalities. In the majority of type II diabetic patients, hypertriglyceridemia is mild to moderate in severity, but occasionally is severe and associated with chylomicron accumulation in fasting plasma. Plasma HDL cholesterol concentrations vary inversely with TG and VLDL levels. Total and LDL cholesterol levels may either be normal or increased. Treatment of NIDDM with diet, weight reduction, exercise, and/or an oral hypoglycemic agent usually is accompanied by a decline in plasma TG and VLDL levels. The low HDL cholesterol levels are often less responsive to treatment.

There is growing awareness that high blood insulin levels (*hyperinsulinemia*) common in obese NIDDM patients promote the atherosclerotic process. Epidemiologic studies have consistently shown a positive relationship of plasma insulin levels to CHD risk.[102] In addition, experimental studies reveal that hyperinsulinemia increases the rate of lipid synthesis and deposition in the arterial wall and proliferation of arterial smooth muscle cells involved in the atherosclerotic lesions.[102] As previously indicated, elevated levels of circulating insulin promote liver synthesis of TGs and VLDLs. In addition, hyperinsulinemia may contribute to higher blood pressures through enhanced sodium reabsorption by the distal renal tubules.[105]

HEART DISEASE. As previously indicated, people with DM clearly are at excess risk for atherosclerotic CHD compared to matched nondiabetic individuals. They also are prone to other forms of cardiac problems, including cardiac enlargement due to hypertension and a specific diabetic cardiomyopathy, both of which may cause congestive heart failure.[27,56,119] Diabetic cardiomyopathy appears to result from microvascular change involving smaller intramural coronary vessels and capillaries. About one-quarter of patients with type I DM and one-half of those with type II DM die of heart problems.[25,139]

CEREBROVASCULAR DISEASE. The cerebral arteries are another common site of atherosclerosis associated with DM. Resulting cerebrovascular accidents (strokes) cause 6% and 15% of deaths in IDDM and NIDDM, respectively.[25]

PERIPHERAL VASCULAR DISEASE (PVD). Atherosclerosis of peripheral arteries is frequently found in diabetic individuals, particularly older ones.[10,149] Associated circulatory impairment may lead to gangrene and amputation of parts of the lower extremities. The prevalence of occlusive PVD in DM groups has been reported to range from 16 to 58% and appears to be at least 20 times more common in diabetics than in comparable nondiabetics. Half of all lower-extremity amputations in the United States performed for reasons other than traumatic accidents involve patients with DM.

The peripheral atherosclerotic lesions in diabetic individuals are similar to those in nondiabetics, but the distribution of lesions and extent of involvement are different. Although there is a similar prevalence of atherosclerotic lesions in the femoral artery, diabetic individuals have a higher prevalence of lesions in the tibial and peroneal arteries as compared to nondiabetic individuals. Risk factors associated with the development of PVD in diabetic patients are similar to those in nondiabetic individuals, raising the hope that controlling other risk factors responsible for atherogenesis (particularly cigarette smoking) can prevent PVD or at least attenuate its progression.

Diabetic Neuropathy (Nerve Damage)

Almost any nerve pathway in the body (peripheral motor or sensory, central, or autonomic) can be affected by DM.[41,99] Symptoms range in severity from mild to incapacitating. Common symptoms include numbness, tingling, or pain in the lower extremities; muscle wasting and weakness; foot drop; absent ankle jerk reflex; postural hypotension; abnormal cardiovascular responses to exercise; gastrointestinal symptoms; difficulty in bladder emptying (neurogenic bladder); and impotence.[66]

Blunting of sympathetic nervous system activity also may make it difficult for the diabetic individual to recognize hyperglycemic reactions. Silent myocardial ischemia or silent myocardial infarction also may be related to diabetic autonomic system neuropathy.

The prevalence of neuropathy is highest in long-term IDDM but is extremely vari-

able. Both microangiopathy of blood vessels supplying the nerves and metabolic derangements are postulated to contribute to nerve damage. As previously indicated, intracellular sorbitol, as well as fructose accumulation, are suspected of playing a role similar to that of mechanisms causing damage to artery linings and the lenses of the eye.[99]

DIABETIC MANAGEMENT

The treatment of DM is a lifetime affair. With modern treatment, the metabolic effects of the disease can be well regulated. The ultimate goal of treatment is to restore the patient's metabolism and lifestyle to as normal a state as possible. The therapeutic optimum is for the diabetic individual to have normal blood glucose levels, the urine free of sugar at least most of the time, and to remain free of significant late complications of DM.

Although many thousands of individuals with IDDM have been able to lead productive lives since the discovery of insulin about 70 years ago, relatively few have remained free of late complications over many decades.[66] Aside from the particular course of the disease, contributing factors to late complications may lie with failure to adhere to therapy by the patient, inadequate instruction on the part of the physician and staff, or inadequacies in the conventional therapeutic regime. This has led to recent changes in the therapeutic approach, especially as it relates to traditional dietary advice.

Preliminary data suggest that "tight diabetic control" appears to be more effective in prevention of microvascular and neurologic complications than those of macrovascular origin.[115] A multicenter clinical trial (the Diabetes Control and Complications Trial) is currently underway to test the prognostic value of "tight control."[1] It is hoped that application of recent advances in understanding of the atherosclerotic process also will eventually reduce the toll of cardiovascular complications.

A previous logo of the American Diabetic Association (ADA) consisted of a triangle to represent the symbolic balance between the three essential elements of diabetic control—diet, medication, and exercise. Even though the ADA has a new logo, these three modalities remain the bases for diabetic management, and each will be discussed below. Current preventive strategy also focuses on control or correction of other atherogenic risk factors, particularly cigarette smoking, abnormal blood lipid levels, hypertension, obesity, and physical inactivity.

Dietary Approaches

GENERAL PRINCIPLES. Diet has traditionally been considered the cornerstone in the management of both IDDM and NIDDM. Dietary guidelines have previously been published[4–8,11,66,105,132,147] and are summarized in Table 10–3. These include correction of obesity to improve glycemic control and reduce other CHD risk factors; substitution of complex carbohydrates for fat in the diet while minimizing the use of simple sugars, salt, and alcohol; eating nutritionally sound meals; and in IDDM, spreading food intake throughout the 24-hour period to cover insulin administration.

WEIGHT MANAGEMENT. Because a large proportion of individuals with NIDDM are obese, metabolic improvement or satisfactory glycemic control may result from a reduction in excess weight, with an associated improvement in peripheral insulin sensitivity. Thus, a reduction in total energy intake and increased physical activity to achieve and maintain proper body weight are important goals in the management of DM. These are not new observations. Caloric restriction and exercise were the primary basis of therapy of DM even in the pre-insulin era. The importance of total energy intake in determining insulin requirements also has been known since the advent of insulin therapy.

DIET COMPOSITION. The amount of carbohydrates to recommend for patients with DM has long been a subject of much debate. Thomas Willis in 1674 first proposed a high-carbohydrate, low-calorie regimen. However, until recent years, the prevailing view on dietary management of DM was to restrict carbohydrates and increase energy provided by protein and fat, especially for individuals with elevated blood sugar levels and sugar spilling over into the urine. However, evidence has been accumulating since the 1930s that improved carbohydrate tolerance and diminished insulin requirements result from a diet high in carbohydrates, usually in the form of starchy, high-fiber foods. Conversely, restricting carbohydrate intake in normal individuals produces a temporary metabolic state similar to DM ("starvation diabetes"). A high carbohydrate intake also improves peripheral cellular sensitivity to insulin and promotes glucose utilization.[7] Fiber-rich meals reduce postprandial hyperglycemia and glycosuria in patients with IDDM and may allow insulin doses to be reduced.[7] Thus, current recommendations of the ADA are for carbohydrates to provide 55 to 70% of daily energy requirements and a dietary fiber intake of about 40 g/day.[4–6] This should be provided primarily by increased consumption of whole-grain cereals and bread, starch roots, legumes, and other vegetables and fruits.

Another recent recommendation of the ADA is to liberalize the consumption of table sugar or sucrose and of fruit con-

TABLE 10–3. **Recommended Dietary Goals for Patients with Diabetes**

1. If obese, reduce calories and increase physical activity to gradually attain and maintain ideal weight.
2. Liberalize intake of complex carbohydrates.
3. Reduce intake of total fat, saturated fat, and cholesterol.
4. Minimize intake of simple sugars, except those that naturally occur in fruits and vegetables.
5. Consume nutritionally sound meals using food exchange lists.
6. Individuals on insulin should spread their food intake throughout the waking part of the day and keep the amounts stable.
7. Limit use of salt and alcohol.

taining simple carbohydrates by diabetic individuals.[4-6] This is based on the recent finding that sucrose and starch have a similar postprandial glycemic effect when consumed as part of a meal by patients with either type I or type II DM.[132] However, a high intake of sucrose (17 to 35% of total energy) may impair insulin sensitivity and adversely affect lipid metabolism for at least 6 weeks.[50] In addition, sucrose and other table-top simple sugar sweeteners provide "empty calories" (i.e., they are devoid of other essential nutrients and increase the risk of dental caries). Thus, the current consensus is that sucrose and other simple sugars should not account for more than 10% of total dietary energy and that these should come primarily from fruit and vegetable sources.[4-6] Because the current U.S. diet is believed to contain 16% of energy from sucrose, this recommendation may necessitate a reduction in sucrose intake for most people with DM.

Another important concern regarding the previously traditional low-carbohydrate diabetic diet is that it is high in total fat, saturated fat, and cholesterol. Without doubt, this contributes to elevated blood lipid levels and accelerates the atherosclerotic process, and thereby cardiovascular complications. Enlightened current ADA recommendations are to reduce total fat content of the diabetic diet to 30% or less of daily energy intake, with the proportion of saturated, polyunsatured, and monounsatured fat approximately equal.[4-6] Dietary cholesterol also should be limited to less than 300 mg/day. These recommendations are in line with the American Heart Association's Step 1 diet and the National Research Council's dietary recommendation for the entire U.S. population.[89] For NIDDM patients with hyperlipidemias, the ADA advocates further restriction of dietary fats to 20% of daily energy intake and of dietary cholesterol to 100 to 150 mg/day.[4,6] Protein intake should be similar to that recommended for nondiabetic individuals (0.8 g/kg or about 15 to 20% of energy intake) but a significant amount should come from plant instead of animal sources to reduce

associated saturated fat and cholesterol intake.

OTHER DIETARY CONSIDERATIONS. Sodium intake should be modestly restricted to less than 3 g/day because of its possible contribution to the frequent association of hypertension in DM. Alcohol should be avoided in individuals with poor glycemic control, for those on energy-restricted diets, and in the presence of pregnancy, hypertension, or hyperglyceridemia. In others, it may be used prudently; that is, up to 2 ounces once or twice a week. For those on insulin, it should be consumed only with food to reduce the risk of alcohol-induced hypoglycemia.

A proper selection of foods to cover all essential nutrient needs can be provided using a food exchange system.[66,132,147] This involves selection of a properly prescribed number of food choices from six lists of different food types: 1) milk/dairy, 2) vegetables, 3) fruits, 4) bread/cereals, 5) meats, and 6) fats. The nutritional adequacy of a high-carbohydrate, low-fat diabetic diet has been demonstrated.[51]

For the diabetic patient requiring insulin to attain glycemic control, the basic meal structure usually consists of three main meals daily plus snacks at mid-morning, mid-afternoon, and at bedtime to prevent hypoglycemia.

Controversy exists as to the appropriate dietary content or supplementary administration of omega-3 polyunsaturated fatty acids (n-3 PUFA) for the prevention of atherosclerotic diabetic complications. Fish oils are a rich source of n-3 PUFA (e.g., eicosapentaenoic acid, or EPA, and docosahexaenoic acid, or DA).[48] Other dietary sources of n-3 PUFA are canola oil and soybean oil. Eskimos in Greenland with a high intake of EPA and DA from a diet consisting almost entirely of marine animals have been reported to be at low risk of CHD.[48] Encouraging to those on a Western-style diet was an epidemiologic study from the Netherlands that found that people who consumed an average of 30 g of fish per day also had a reduced risk of CHD mortality.[69] In addition, there is consistent experimental evidence that 5 to 10 g/day of n-3 PUFA can reduce levels of plasma TG and VLDL cholesterol, with no change or at least a transient increase in HDL cholesterol level[37,48]; this includes preliminary observations in patients with NIDDM.[37] However, in patients with hyperlipidemias this may be accompanied by an increase in plasma concentration of atherogenic LDL cholesterol and LDL-apolipoprotein B, which may adversely affect CHD risk. Further, n-3 PUFA may adversely affect glycemic control in patients with NIDDM.[37]

In addition to their effects on blood lipids, n-3 PUFA profoundly reduces blood platelet aggregation to usual stimuli, resulting in a prolonged bleeding time.[48] Although these changes theoretically should counteract increased platelet aggregability commonly found in patients with DM,[3] thereby reducing the possibility of thrombosis in atherosclerotic vessels, this remains to be proven. A tradeoff is increased bleeding tendencies with a high intake of n-3 PUFA. Another potential benefit of n-3 PUFA is the recent demonstration that large doses (6 g/day) of n-3 PUFA in nondiabetic, hypertensive individuals reduce blood pressure levels.[16] Further, a fish oil supplement recently was demonstrated to reduce transcapillary escape of albumin into the urine in IDDM patients, independent of its effect on blood pressure levels.[59] These interesting observations of the potential multiple beneficial effects of n-3 PUFA on reducing risk of diabetic complications warrant additional studies, including safety studies. In the meantime, the routine use of n-3 PUFA supplements for diabetic patients currently is not recommended by the ADA, but fish consumption several times a week is generally encouraged.

Increased Physical Activity and Exercise

METABOLIC EFFECTS OF ACUTE EXERCISE AND THEIR RELATIONSHIP TO DM. The metabolic effects of acute exercise and their therapeutic implications in DM have been extensively reviewed.[114,127,133,134,137,151] During acute prolonged dynamic exercise, major metabolic, hormonal, and cardiovascular adjustments take place in order to increase the supply of fuels and oxygen to the working skeletal muscles, while maintaining adequate levels to vital organs. These exercise-induced changes have therapeutic implications in the management of DM.

Muscle glycogen, blood-borne glucose, and FFA are the principal fuels used during exercise by both the diabetic and the nondiabetic individual. The relative contribution of each to oxidative energy production depends on the intensity and duration of muscular work. An orderly sequence of utilization of these fuels takes place during such prolonged dynamic or endurance exercise as walking, running, cycling, and swimming. During the initial phase of exercise, intramuscular glycogen is the primary source of fuel for contracting muscle. After the first 5 to 10 min, blood glucose and FFA become increasingly important substrates. Glucose utilization during prolonged mild to moderate exercise may increase 20 times over the basal level and account for 25 to 40% of the total oxidative fuel requirements. Despite the marked stimulation of glucose utilization, blood glucose levels usually remain virtually unchanged or decrease only slightly during the first 40 min of exercise by nondiabetic individuals and by individuals with type II and well-controlled type I DM. This is because the blood glucose pool is continuously augmented by a three- to five-fold increase in glucose release from the liver. For at least the first 40 min, most liver glucose production (about 75%) is derived from breakdown of hepatic glycogen (glycogenolysis), the stores of which are limited. During more prolonged exercise, formation of hepatic glycogen and glucose from various precursors (lactate, pyruvate, glycerol, and certain amino acids) through gluconeogenesis becomes increasingly important for maintaining blood glucose levels and may account for 40 to 50% of hepatic glucose output. If exercise is continued long enough, blood glucose levels eventually will fall despite gluconeogenesis. A progressive shift in energy metabolism from carbohydrate to FFA occurs, and the FFA contribution to oxidative metabolism may be twice that of glucose at this point. A direct relationship exists between levels of plasma FFA and muscle utilization, with diabetic individuals being more efficient at using FFA for fuels than nondiabetic individuals.

A number of hormonal changes are involved in the regulation of fuel availability, utilization, and glucose homeostasis during exercise. The essential role of insulin in glucose utilization during exercise is illustrated by classic studies with depancreatized dogs in which exercise did not increase glucose utilization until small doses of replacement insulin were given.[137] However, during acute dynamic exercise, muscle contraction per se appears to stimulate glucose uptake.[137] There is also an immediate and progressive increase in cell insulin sensitivity, causing a fall in circulating insulin levels during prolonged exercise. This improvement in insulin sensitivity in humans appears to be unrelated to insulin-binding affinity to skeletal muscle receptors.[133,134] The reduction in plasma insulin levels along with an exercise-induced increase in counter-regulatory hormones, particularly glucagon and epinephrine, stimulate hepatic glucose production and release by the liver, as well as FFA mobilization from adipose tissues.

Following completion of a prolonged bout of dynamic exercise, the increased insulin sensitivity may persist up to 48 hours, significantly reducing requirements for individuals receiving insulin replacement therapy.[133,134] During the post-exercise period, there is a continued accelerated glucose uptake by tissues, particularly skeletal muscle and the liver. Glycogen depletion and the associated increased activity of glycogen synthetase are believed to contribute to the improved insulin sensitivity and enhanced glucose uptake by muscle and liver cells. However, this is not the entire explanation, because these adaptations persist in the exercise recovery period after glycogen stores have been replenished.

BENEFITS OF EXERCISE CONDITIONING. There are multiple potential benefits of exercise conditioning to the diabetic individual. These include improving glycemic control; prevention of obesity or acting as an adjunct to energy restriction for weight management; helping to correct other atherogenic risk factors, including blood lipid disorders, elevated blood pressure levels, and hypercoagulability of the blood; reducing overall risk of CHD; and improving the quality of life by increasing work capacity and providing psychosocial benefits. Each of these potential benefits of exercise are briefly discussed below.

Improved Diabetic Control. Even prior to the discovery of insulin, dynamic exercise was employed to lower elevated blood glucose levels.[2] It has also been known for over 60 years that acute exercise potentiates the glucose-lowering effect of exogenous insulin administration and reduces insulin requirements.[75] Although exercise is no longer considered essential for glycemic control, it can serve as a useful adjunct to dietary management and drug therapy. As previously indicated, an acute prolonged session of dynamic endurance exercise can increase glucose disposal and improve insulin sensitivity for up to 48 hours in both nondiabetic and diabetic individuals.[107,127,133,134,137] Regular exercise of moderate intensity, if not compensated by an excess intake of food energy, can further potentiate this metabolic adaptation or at least overlap the effects of the previous exercise session. Thus, an endurance exercise program in both type I and type II DM may improve glycemic control and enhance insulin sensitivity and glucose tolerance. These improvements in glucose-insulin dynamics with endurance exercise persist perhaps up to 7 days after cessation of exercise.[127]

Most studies in the literature reporting improved glucose-insulin dynamics with exercise training in nondiabetic or diabetic subjects used moderate-to-high-intensity endurance exercise, 30 to 60 min

167

per session, 3 to 7 days per week. Such training was generally accompanied by a 15% or more increase in $\dot{V}_{O_2max}$. Reduced body weight and fatness was a contributing factor in only a few of the studies. Obese nondiabetic subjects almost invariably significantly improve insulin sensitivity and glucose tolerance with dynamic exercise conditioning, suggesting its potential role in primary prevention of NIDDM. In our laboratory, we observed a 43% reduction from baseline levels in blood insulin-to-glucose ratio and a slight improvement in glucose tolerance during an OGTT challenge in a small group of obese young men after brisk walking on the treadmill, 90 min, 5 times a week for 16 weeks.[81] This was accompanied by a 6-kg weight loss and a significant increase in mean plasma HDL cholesterol.

Despite the high prevalence of NIDDM, there have been few studies examining the effects of exercise training on glucose-insulin dynamics and glycemic control in subjects with NIDDM. Over half of the reported exercise training studies in individuals with NIDDM have observed improvements in glycemic control and/or glucose tolerance and insulin sensitivity with exercise training.[15,52,70,80,89,106,107,109,110,113,128] For example, all five patients exercised by Trovati et al. on a cycle ergometer for 1 hour a day, 7 days a week for 6 weeks at 50 to 60% $\dot{V}_{O_2max}$, achieved significant reductions in levels of fasting plasma glucose and glycosylated hemoglobin, as well as improved glucose tolerance and insulin sensitivity measured 48 hours after the last exercise session.[128] In contrast, in a larger study involving 48 sedentary overweight men aged 33 to 69 years with NIDDM or glucose intolerance, our group failed to improve glucose-insulin dynamics with 12 weeks of a moderate-intensity walking program (30 to 60 min, 2 to 4 times a week) with body weight held constant.[80]

The effect of exercise training on glycemic control has been more thoroughly studied in IDDM than in NIDDM. Most of the exercise training studies with IDDM patients failed to demonstrate any long-term improvement in glycemic control beyond that produced by the overlapping acute effects of exercise.[19,58,133–137,146,151,152] However, an improvement in insulin sensitivity and reduced insulin requirements have generally been observed. Increased carbohydrate intake on exercise days was considered to be a likely cause of failure to improve glycemic control with exercise training, despite the acute glucose-lowering effect with each exercise session.[152] Children and adolescents with IDDM appear more likely than adults to improve diabetic control with regular dynamic exercise. Exercise training also may improve glycemic control in women with gestational DM.

There has been recent interest in the possible role of resistive or strength training exercise on improving glucose-insulin dynamics (including insulin-mediated glucose disposal and glucose tolerance)[133,134] and in the management of associated blood lipid abnormalities and elevated blood pressure levels.[38,39,54] Although preliminary results appear promising, more research is needed to establish the efficacy and safety of strength training in diabetic individuals.

Possible mechanisms identified for the improvement in glucose-insulin dynamics with exercise conditioning beyond the glucose-disposing effect of acute exercise include an increase in the number of cell insulin receptors in proportion to improvement in $\dot{V}_{O_2max}$, an increase in the number of cell insulin receptors, and skeletal muscle adaptations.[65,120] Documented beneficial muscle adaptations to endurance exercise training are improved blood supply, increased glycogen storage, and increased oxidative metabolic capacity due to augmentation in the number of mitochondria and in the activity of their oxidative and respiratory chain enzymes.[133,134,137] Increased skeletal muscle mass probably is the primary mechanism for improved glucose-insulin dynamics with strength or resistive exercise training.

In IDDM, the metabolic response to acute dynamic exercise is markedly affected by adequacy of diabetic control and blood levels of exogenous insulin. When diabetic control is adequate or if only mild hyperglycemia without ketosis is present, exercise can be expected to reduce blood glucose levels and insulin requirements for up to 48 hours. The over-insulinization with hypoglycemia that occurs during exercise or more commonly in the recovery period is a serious concern for the diabetic exerciser receiving insulin therapy. This danger is increased if insulin is administered into arm or leg sites over exercising muscle groups because of enhanced delivery of insulin to the circulation by the massaging effect of muscle contractions.[150] Although this potential problem has received a great deal of attention in the literature, it appears to be of concern only if exercise is performed within an hour of insulin administration into the extremity. If this is the usual situation, insulin should be administered in an abdominal site instead of an active extremity. To further reduce the risk of an insulin reaction, it is best to exercise after eating when plasma glucose levels are at their peak. It is especially important to avoid exercising when exogenously administered insulin levels are at their peak. This is because exogenous insulin suppresses the hepatic glucose production and release required to maintain glucose homeostasis in the presence of accelerated glucose uptake by exercising muscle.

In contrast, prolonged exercise performed in the presence of a marked insulin deficiency and associated poor metabolic control results in an excess release of glucose from the liver, as well as a marked increase in circulating FFA causing excess production of ketone bodies.[133,134] An associated exaggerated rise in counter-regulatory hormones contributes to the worsening of the diabetic state, which may result in increased hyperglycemia and ketoacidosis. Thus, it is important for individuals with IDDM to achieve at least fairly good diabetic control prior to initiating an exercise program.

Prevention or Correction of Obesity. The role of obesity in causing insulin resistance and in the cause of NIDDM was previously discussed. Physical inactivity is a major contributor to obesity in modern society.[77] Regular exercise can reduce the risk of NIDDM through its contribution to weight maintenance. In addition, exercise can improve insulin sensitivity in obese subjects, even without concomitant weight loss or a change in body composition.[106,133,134] Nevertheless, because weight reduction alone usually improves insulin sensitivity and glucose tolerance, the maximal effectiveness of an exercise program is achieved when it is associated with a loss of body fat.

The value of regular prolonged walking exercise in normalizing body weight and mobilizing adipose stores in obese people in the absence of dietary changes has been documented.[42,77,81] The loss of lean body mass (LBM) during weight reduction by restriction of energy intake is less frequently observed when exercise is used in combination with moderate energy restriction for weight reduction. However, individuals with NIDDM are probably unlikely to perform sufficient regular dynamic exercise to contribute substantially to weight reduction. Thus, it would be more practical and likely to be successful to combine a smaller volume of regular dynamic exercise with a moderate reduction in energy intake in order to achieve and maintain a significant loss of excess weight and body fat.

Beneficial Effects of Exercise on Other Atherogenic Risk Factors. Endurance exercise may contribute to the management of other atherogenic risk factors commonly associated with DM, including blood lipid disorders, high blood pressure, and hypercoagulability of the blood. As previously mentioned, these risk factors are additive or synergistic in enhancing the risk of CHD, stroke, and PVD.

Blood lipid abnormalities, particularly elevated plasma levels of TG and its lipoprotein carriers, and a reciprocal reduction in HDL cholesterol levels are commonly associated with DM. Less commonly, plasma total and LDL cholesterol levels are elevated. Because of the important contribution of dyslipidemias to accelerated atherosclerosis, therapeutic strategies for management of DM should give equal emphasis to controlling dyslipidemias and hyperglycemia.[33]

Regular dynamic exercise is considered *adjunctive therapy* for lipid management along with dietary management and reduction of excess weight. Improved glycemic control by hygienic means, insulin, or hypoglycemic drugs may significantly correct or attenuate blood lipid abnormalities.[56,73,84,108] Other therapeutic interventions may include administration of n-3 PUFA or antilipidemic drugs. Gemfibrozil appears to be the antilipidemic drug of choice for most diabetic individuals not responding to diet, weight loss, exercise, and glycemic control, because it markedly reduces plasma TG levels while usually lowering LDL cholesterol and raising HDL cholesterol.[33]

Both acute and chronic endurance exercise can contribute to an improvement in blood lipid abnormalities. An acute, prolonged session of endurance exercise often decreases an elevated plasma TG concentration 50% for up to 24 hours and increases HDL cholesterol levels about 10%.[82] Exercise training has been reported to be effective in reducing elevated (but not normal) plasma TG levels in both the fasting and postprandial state[39,46,84,138,143] and is associated with lower levels of VLDLs and chylomicrons, apparently because of their accelerated catabolism. Increased activity of lipoprotein lipase in skeletal muscles and adipose tissue and increased vascularity of skeletal muscle with exercise training are likely contributing factors. These adaptations make more FFAs from the breakdown of TGs available for fuel. Reduced hepatic synthesis of VLDL and TGs also may be contributing factors.

Increased plasma HDL cholesterol levels have been commonly observed with endurance exercise training in nondiabetic men.[39,46,80,114,121,141–144] In addition, resistive exercise training[38,39,54] has been reported to raise HDL cholesterol levels in some but not all studies.[63] An associated weight loss appeared to be a contributing factor in most studies involving dynamic exercise. It appears that endurance exercise must reach a sufficient intensity and volume to substantially increase $\dot{V}_{O_2max}$ before HDL cholesterol levels are raised. In middle-aged nondiabetic male joggers, 8 to 10 miles a week of running for 9 months or more at a energy cost of about 1400 kcal/week was found to be the threshold for increasing HDL cholesterol levels.[141,142] An exercise-induced increase in lipoprotein lipase activity probably contributes to increased plasma HDL cholesterol levels through conversion of remnants of TG-rich lipoproteins to HDL. It should be noted that individuals with type II DM appear more resistant to blood lipid changes induced by exercise training than nondiabetics.[80] Increases in plasma HDL cholesterol are less likely to occur in women with exercise training.[46,111,112] Because an inverse relationship exists between plasma HDL cholesterol and severity of atherosclerosis, increasing levels of HDL cholesterol through a combination of exercise, weight loss, and improved glycemic control by diet and drugs should theoretically help protect diabetic individuals against macrovascular complications, but this remains to be proven.

High Blood Pressure. The contribution of physical activity to risk of hypertension and the effect of exercise on blood pressure levels in hypertensive and normotensive people recently has been extensively reviewed.[43] Cross-sectional observational data are contradictory, with athletes and people with physically demanding jobs reported to have either lower, higher, or similar blood pressure levels as physically inactive people. Most long-term prospective cohort studies also fail to find an association between physical activity and blood pressure levels, the exceptions being the Tecumseh (Michigan) Heart Study[86] and the College Alumni Study,[36,95] which did find inverse associations. When statistical adjustment was made for body fatness in the Tecumseh Study,[86] the tendency for active men to have lower blood pressure levels was sig-

170

nificantly reduced. In the College Alumni Study, male alumni who exercised 5 hours or more a week during college had up to a 40% lower incidence rate of physician-diagnosed hypertension than did the less-active men at the 20-year follow-up.[95]

Experimentally, prolonged acute endurance exercise generally reduces systolic and diastolic blood pressure levels for 1 to 3 hours post exercise, generally because of vasodilation.[43] Further, over two-thirds of endurance exercise training studies involving hypertensive patients reported significant reduction of about 10 mm Hg in both resting systolic and diastolic blood pressure. Many of these studies, particularly the earlier ones, had serious flaws in experimental design, however. About 30 to 60 min of light to moderate intensity (40 to 60% $\dot{V}_{O_2max}$) dynamic exercise at least every other day appears to be the required exercise stimulus for this blood pressure-lowering effect. In some of the reported studies, a concomitant weight loss appeared to contribute to the blood pressure reduction. Endurance exercise training generally attenuates the blood pressure rise during submaximal workloads, and recent reports suggest that resistive exercise training reduces blood pressure levels in both hypertensive and normotensive nondiabetic individuals.[38,44] Additional research is required to confirm its effectiveness and safety in both diabetic and nondiabetic hypertensive patients.

Reduced sympathetic nervous system activity is postulated to be a contributing mechanism for the blood pressure-lowering effect of exercise training.[43,44,57] This is postulated to attenuate renin-angiotensin activity, reset baroreflexes, produce arterial vasodilitation, and reduce peripheral vascular resistance. Because insulin is involved in renal tubular reabsorption of sodium, improved cell insulin sensitivity and associated reduction in hyperinsulinemia may contribute to blood pressure reduction by increasing the loss of urinary sodium.

Evidence is accumulating that multifactor nonpharmacologic intervention (including regular exercise, weight management, and restriction in salt and alcohol use) can prevent development of fixed hypertension in patients with borderline or labile high blood pressure levels, as well as help control mild hypertension.[122,123] There also is limited evidence that reducing the intake of saturated fatty acids and increasing the ratio of polyunsaturated to saturated fatty acids and increasing intake of n-3 PUFA can contribute to blood pressure reduction.[16,101] However, to the best of my knowledge, the effects of exercise and these other nonpharmacologic measures on blood pressure levels and in the prevention and treatment of hypertension have not been systematically studied in patients with DM.

Another important concern in diabetic patients with hypertension is the proper choice of antihypertensive drugs and special precautions in their use, if nonpharmacologic measures fail to control elevated blood pressure levels. There is growing enthusiasm for making the angiotensin converting enzyme (ACE) inhibitors (such as enalapril) the first-line antihypertensive drug of choice in diabetic patients. ACE inhibitors do not cause or aggravate orthostatic hypotension (a potential problem in the presence of diabetic autonomic neuropathy); have no adverse effects on glycemic control, blood lipid levels, renal blood flow and function, or exercise tolerance; and do not mask hypoglycemia, as do some types of antihypertensive drugs.[96] Further, ACE inhibitors appear to reduce microalbuminuria (a marker of incipient nephropathy) and left ventricular mass, and help correct congestive heart failure.

It is concluded that regular dynamic exercise may be useful along with other nonpharmacologic measures to prevent or manage hypertension commonly associated with diabetes. If antihypertensive therapy is required, an ACE inhibitor is the initial drug of choice.

As previously mentioned, a hypercoagulable state associated with DM may contribute to accelerated atherosclerosis and increased risk of thrombotic occlusion of coronary and cerebral arteries. Both acute and chronic exercise affect blood coagulability and the ability to dissolve clots (fibrinolysis). Although blood coagulability is increased during acute dynamic exertion, this is countered by a concomitant enhancement of fibrinolysis. Endurance exercise conditioning appears to attenuate the hypercoagulable state occurring with physical exertion while further enhancing fibrinolytic activity. Mechanisms include reduced platelet adhesiveness, increased levels of prostacyclin in arterial endothelial cells, reduced levels of thromboxane in platelets,[104] and increased tissue plasminogen activator.[125] More research is needed to confirm these effects of exercise training on blood coagulability and to determine their relevance to the patient with DM.

Independent Reduced Overall Risk of CHD. An inverse relationship between both physical activity and physical fitness levels with incidence of CHD and associated mortality has repeatedly been demonstrated in epidemiologic studies.[13,21,78,79,94,100,118] Optimal protection against major CHD events appears to be afforded by 1500 to 2000 kcal per week of physical activity, with partial protection by as little as 500 kcal per week in the general population. Possible physiologic mechanisms by which exercise reduces CHD risk include the effects on CHD risk factors and possible antithrombotic effects discussed above, decreased myocardial oxygen requirements as a result of decreased systolic blood pressure and heart rate at rest and during submaximal physical exertion, increased myocardial vascularity, and reduced vulnerability to serious cardiac rhythm disturbances.[31,32,67,76] A definitive primary prevention trial proving the protective effects of regular exercise against CHD has not been done in either nondiabetic or diabetic populations and does not appear to be feasible. Nevertheless, the available evidence is sufficient to include exercise as part of a CHD prevention program for both populations.

Increased Work Capacity and Endurance. One of the best-documented benefits of exercise training is improved physical fitness. Of particular health importance is the associated enhancement in cardiorespiratory endurance, as documented by increased $\dot{V}_{O_2max}$ levels, which usually results from improvement in both stroke volume of the heart and increased arteriovenous oxygen difference. The functional value of this training effect is an increase in both maximal work capacity and the ability to perform submaximal work for longer periods with less perceived effort and fatigue.

Psychosocial Benefits. Although difficult to document scientifically, there is general agreement that regular physical activity has a variety of psychosocial benefits that improve quality of life.[53] Activities should be selected that are enjoyable to the individual. The resulting improved feeling of well-being, health consciousness, self-confidence, self-control, and self-esteem are especially important for patients with a chronic disease such as DM. Exercise is also helpful to relieve muscular tension and mental depression and to promote sound sleep.[28]

PRINCIPLES FOR INCREASING PHYSICAL ACTIVITY AND FITNESS. Activities should be selected that the individual enjoys, are appropriate for his/her health and fitness status, and can be maintained for a lifetime. These should involve rhythmic movements of the large muscle groups of the body and generally should be nonexhausting and of mild to moderate intensity. For the purpose of properly adjusting food intake and insulin or oral hypoglycemic medications, it is helpful if the activities can be quantified in terms of energy requirements. Examples of ideal activities that fit these criteria include brisk walking, hiking, slow running (jogging), swimming, bicycling, and cross-country skiing. If performed regularly (at least 3 to 5 days per week) for 30 to 60 min at a time at a moderate level of intensity (60% $\dot{V}_{O_2max}$ or 70% of maximal heart rate or heart rate reserve—i.e., maximal heart rate minus resting heart rate), such activities will significantly improve cardiorespiratory endurance and provide the physiologic and psychologic benefits previously described.

It is important for the diabetic individual to take advantage of opportunities around work or home to expend more energy. This would include walking or cycling instead of driving to work, walking briskly from a distant parking lot, climbing stairs instead of using elevators, walking during coffee and lunch breaks, standing instead of sitting whenever possible, cleaning house, washing and maintaining the car, gardening, walking the dog, dancing, and avoiding such labor-saving devices as extension phones, power lawn mowers, and snow blowers.

EXERCISE PRECAUTIONS AND GUIDE-LINES. The diabetic individual should understand both the benefits and possible adverse effects of exercise (Table 10–4). The need to avoid strenuous exercise until reasonable diabetic control is established was previously discussed. Strenuous dynamic and resistive exercise and contact sports should be avoided in the presence of active proliferative retinopathy. For the diabetic individual receiving insulin therapy, the principal risk during or following exercise is an insulin reaction or hypoglycemia. Oral hypoglycemic drugs are associated with a much smaller risk of hypoglycemia during prolonged exercise. Avoidance of hypoglycemia requires a regular pattern of exercise, food intake, and medication. Exercise is best performed at the same convenient time every day at approximately the same intensity and duration, but should be avoided during the time of peak insulin activity. If this is not possible, the diabetic should have a 10- to 15-g carbohydrate snack about 15 to 30 min before exercising, if blood glu-

TABLE 10–4. **Exercise Dangers and Preventive Measures**

Aggravation of diabetic metabolic derangements:
   Strenuous exercise avoided until diabetes is controlled
   Adequate fluid replacement
   Avoid strenuous and resistive exercise and contact sports in the presence of acute proliferative
      retinopathy

Exercise-induced hypoglycemia (insulin-dependent diabetic patients):
   Frequent monitoring of blood glucose levels
   Avoid insulin administration to active limb within 1 hour of exercise
   Reduce insulin dosage and/or increase food intake with new exercise or use abdominal site
   Avoid exercise during peak insulin activity
   Carbohydrate snacks before, during, and after prolonged exercise
   Reproducible regular exercise is best
   Prompt recognition and response to symptoms

Foot problems:
   Proper footwear
   Foot hygiene

Cardiovascular complications:
   Pre-exercise medical evaluation
   Exercise ECG test
   Individualized exercise prescription
   Modification of other risk factors

Musculoskeletal injuries:
   Appropriate selection of activities
   Slow and gradual progress
   Warm-up and cool-down periods
   Avoid overdoing it

cose is in the ideal range of 100 to 180 mg/dl. More carbohydrate (25 to 50 g) is necessary if blood glucose is < 100 mg/dl, and none is required if it is greater than 180 mg/dl.[29]

Because of the proinsulin effect of exercise, patients with IDDM will have to reduce insulin dose or increase food intake when initiating an exercise program. Careful self-monitoring of blood glucose levels many times throughout the day, particularly after meals, before, during, and after prolonged exercise, and at bed time is the key to balancing diet, exercise, and insulin dosage. Insulin dosage usually has to be reduced 20% or more, but because of great variability in responsiveness, this has to be determined on an individualized basis. The need to avoid administration of insulin to sites on participating limbs just prior to exercise was previously discussed.

During prolonged activities, a 10- to 15-g carbohydrate snack (fruit, fruit juice, or soft drink) is recommended for each 30 min of activity (Table 10–5).[29] Activities should be promptly stopped at initial warning symptoms of hypoglycemia, and blood glucose should be tested, if feasible. An appropriate amount of glucose-containing food or beverage should be consumed based on the blood glucose level

TABLE 10–5. **Food and Beverages Containing 10 to 15 Grams of Carbohydrates per Serving**

Food or Beverage	Quantity
Glucose tablets	2–3
Sugar cubes, large	2
Honey	2 teaspoons
Lifesavers	7
Dried fruit	1/4 cup
Fresh fruit	1 exchange
Bread	1 exchange
Orange juice	1/2 cup
Milk	1 cup
Sports drink (5–10% carbohydrates)	1 cup
Soft drink (not diet)	1/2 cup

and prior experience. The exerciser should then allow time for glucose absorption and for blood glucose level to increase above 100 mg/dl prior to resuming activity. In general, it is a good idea not to exercise alone and for partners, teammates, and coaches to be aware of the possibility of a hypoglycemic reaction and the need for carbohydrates to manage it. Adequate fluid replacement during and after exercise is especially important to avoid dehydration in the individual with DM.

Good footware and careful foot hygiene are extremely important to the diabetic individual to avoid corns, blisters, and other foot injuries that may lead to serious complications because of the frequent association of DM with PVD, peripheral neuropathy, decreasing pain sensation, and tendency for infection.

Before diabetic individuals over age 35 years embark on any exercise program that is more strenuous than brisk walking, a careful medical evaluation is required to rule out exercise contraindications and to prescribe safe levels of exercise. A multistage exercise stress test should be included to rule out manifestations of significant latent CHD and to establish a baseline fitness level. The prescribed exercise should be appropriate to the severity of DM and the fitness status, as well as to the recreational interests of the individual and availability of facilities. To minimize risk of musculoskeletal problems, the initial exercise should be of low intensity and short duration, gradually progressing over a period of weeks or months. A warm-up and cool-down period should be included to further decrease risk of injury. For the middle-aged or older diabetic individual, competitive and static or resistive activities generally should be avoided because of the possibility of excessive cardiovascular stress.

Medications to Control Diabetes

There are two types of medications currently available to control DM, if control cannot be accomplished by a program of weight reduction, diet, and exercise: subcutaneous insulin injections and oral hypoglycemic agents. Highlights in the use of these drugs are discussed in this section to help understand how to regulate their administration to the exercising diabetic individual. More details are available in standard diabetes reference manuals.[5,6,11,66,105]

INSULIN THERAPY. Few developments in medicine have changed the course of a disease so drastically as the development of insulin by Banting and Best in 1921. The indications for insulin are 1) to treat or avoid episodes of ketoacidosis in people with IDDM, and 2) to control symptoms associated with the metabolic derangements accompanying marked hyperglycemia and glycosuria in both type I and type II DM.[150] It is estimated that about one-third of all diabetic patients in this country receive insulin.

Insulin replacement requirements are established by progressively increasing subcutaneous doses, as guided by repeated urine and blood glucose determinations. Optimal control of DM would be sufficient insulin to allow proper utilization of nutrients for energy or storage, relief of acute diabetic symptoms, elimination of glycosuria, maintenance of blood sugar as close to normal as possible (180 mg/dl or lower after meals), yet not so low that increased physical activity causes hypoglycemic reactions.

Most of the available insulin for therapy is obtained by extraction from the pancreas of cattle and pigs. Insulin from almost any animal is effective in humans, but slight variations in arrangements of the amino acids in the insulin molecule may lead to excessive antibody formations and render the insulin less effective. The recent synthesis of human insulin gives hope that the problem of antigenicity can be minimized and effectiveness of insulin therapy improved. Because human insulin is absorbed more quickly than porcine and bovine insulin after subcutaneous administration, it improves glycemic control after meals.[150]

To decrease the required number of daily injections for glycemic control, certain materials have been added to insulin to prolong its duration of action. These modified insulins are generally classified by their peak activity and duration of action as fast, intermediate, or prolonged acting. Table 10–6 summarizes some of the properties of commonly used insulin preparations.

Several recent developments could significantly improve control of DM and make life easier and more normal for people with IDDM. These include various types of insulin pumps that can be implanted in a diabetic patient to supply insulin.[150] Insulin pumps are reservoirs of insulin implanted under the skin and refilled periodically (about once a week) by an injection from the outside. There are two basic types of pumps. One type administers insulin continuously either subcutaneously or by the intravenous or intraperitoneal routes. A more sophisticated system administers insulin "on demand," like the body's own pancreas, and is often referred to as a feedback-controlled or "closed-loop" pump. It has a mechanical glucose-sensing device that "reads" the blood glucose level and responds by injecting appropriate amounts of insulin into the blood stream. Such a device can control blood glucose levels far more effectively than insulin injections and helps avoid hypoglycemic reactions. It currently can be used only at the bedside, but it is hoped that it will be miniaturized.

Pancreatic transplants have been attempted but rejection rates are still high.[47] In addition, several groups of researchers have successfully grown pancreatic β cells in the laboratory in tissue culture media and implanted them in experimental animals. If this approach proves fruitful and the rejection phenomenon is overcome, it may be possible to implant replacement β cells in the diabetic individual's liver. These implanted cells would then provide the host with insulin in response to deviations of blood sugar levels as a normal pancreas does.

ORAL HYPOGLYCEMIC AGENTS. Oral hypoglycemic agents effectively control blood sugar levels in many patients with type II DM who fail to respond or adhere

TABLE 10-6. **Characteristics of Various Insulins**

Action	Preparation	Onset of Action (Minutes)	Peak Effect (Hours)	Duration of Action (Hours)
Fast	Regular (CZI)	15–30	2–4	5–7
	Semilente	30	2.5–5	5–8
Intermediate	NPH	1–4	6–12	18–24
	Lente	1–2	6–12	18–24
Prolonged	Protamine zinc	6–8	14–24	24–16
	Ultra lente	4–6	14–16	20–30

CZI = crystalline zinc insulin; NPH = neutral protamine hagedorn.

to a dietary, weight loss, and exercise program. About 40% of patients with NIDDM receive one of these drugs. The so-called sulfonurea drugs first became available in 1955, and there are currently six available in the United States.[35] As with insulin, they may be classified according to peak activity and duration of action (Table 10–7). Three of these drugs (chloropromide, glipizide, and glyburide) account for about 75% of those prescribed. Although their primary mechanism of action is to stimulate the pancreatic islet cell to release more insulin, they also improve peripheral insulin sensitivity and may inhibit glucagon secretion from the α-islet cells of the pancreas.[35]

Oral hyperglycemic drugs are contraindicated in ketoacidosis-prone patients but have been used widely to treat NIDDM patients whose pancreatic islet cells produce insulin or who require less than 20 units of insulin per day for glycemic control. Patients with mild IDDM requiring less than 20 units also may be candidates for a sulfonurea drug alone or in combination with insulin.

Possible side effects of the sulfonurea drugs include "insulin-like" hypoglycemic reactions resulting from unusual amounts of exercise or other stresses, skin rashes, loss of appetite, gastrointestinal upset, a disulfiram (Antabuse)-like reaction with alcohol, and serious interaction with other drugs and certain nutrients.[35] The use of these agents has been a subject of much controversy that is primarily based on the interpretation of a large multicenter research study, the University Group Diabetes Program (UGDP).[93] In this study, vari-

TABLE 10-7. **Sulfonurea Oral Hypoglycemic Agents**

Type	Usual Daily Dose (mg)	No. of Doses/Day	Peak Action (Hours)	Duration (Hours)
Short-acting			1–3	6–10
Tolbutamide	500–2000	2–3		
Intermediate			8–12	12–24
Acetohexime	250–1500	2		
Tolazamide	100–1000	1–2		
Glipizide	2.5–40	1–2		
Glyburide	1.25–20	1–2		
Long-acting			14–20	24–72
Chloropromide	100–500	1		

176

ous types of therapy were compared in patients with mild ketoacidosis-resistant, NIDDM diabetics. These included treatment with diet in combination with tolbutamide, phenformin (a biguanide-type of oral hypoglycemic agent since removed from the market by the FDA because of toxicity), insulin, or placebo. The study's major conclusions were as follows: 1) the combination of diet and tolbutamide or diet and phenformin was no more effective than diet alone in prolonging life, and 2) cardiovascular mortality was higher in the groups receiving tolbutamide and phenformin groups than in those treated with diet alone or diet plus insulin. Criticism of the study has been focused on criteria for patient selection and various aspects of the study design, and the results are not universally accepted. Furthermore, the results of other studies do not support the conclusion of the UDGP.[35]

The reader is referred to other sources for description of factors involved in the selection of specific sulfonurea drugs and the subtleties of titration and maintenance of proper drug dosage.[5,6,11,35,66]

SUMMARY AND CONCLUSIONS

There is growing evidence that regular exercise can help prevent DM, improve glycemic control, and perhaps help prevent its atherosclerotic complications. Overweight and low levels of physical activity independently contribute to cell insulin resistance and are important risk factors for NIDDM, the most prevalent form of diabetes in Western societies. Exercise has been proposed as therapy for DM since ancient times. Currently, it is widely used as an adjunct to diet therapy and glucose-lowering drugs in diabetic management. Acute, prolonged, rhythmic exercise involving large muscle groups lowers blood glucose levels and improves insulin sensitivity for up to 48 hours. Both endurance and resistive exercise training, if not compensated by excess energy intake, may further contribute to improved glycemic control, glucose tolerance, and insulin sensitivity in patients whose DM is at least under fair control by diet and/or medications. A minimum of 30 to 60 min of dynamic exercise at an intensity of 60% $\dot{V}_{O_2max}$ or more at least 3 or 4 times a week is required to maintain improved glucose-insulin dynamics. The dose-response relationship of resistive exercise training to improved glucose metabolism is less certain.

Mechanisms for improved glycemic control with exercise training include 1) the overlapping effects of the last exercise session on glycemic control, apparently associated with replenishment of muscle glycogen stores, and 2) improvements in skeletal muscle mass, blood supply, metabolic capacity, and peripheral insulin sensitivity. Other potential beneficial effects of an exercise conditioning program to the diabetic individual are 1) a loss of excess fat, which can further substantially improve insulin sensitivity and glucose tolerance, 2) reduced risk of atherosclerotic complications, and 3) improved quality of life.

Proposed mechanisms for reduced severity of atherosclerosis and risk of common cardiovascular complications often contributing to premature mortality in patients with long-term DM include an increase in plasma levels of HDL cholesterol and a decrease in elevated levels of TGs and their principal lipoprotein carriers. An additional improvement in the blood lipid profile results from improved glycemic control by diabetic diet and drugs, loss of excess weight, and smoking cessation. Exercise training may help correct elevated blood pressure levels and hypercoagulability of the blood often associated with DM. Endurance exercise conditioning reduces adrenergic system activity, which then decreases myocardial oxygen requirements by lowering heart rate and systolic blood pressure. Animal studies and limited human studies suggest that vigorous aerobic exercise training increases myocardial blood supply. These favorable effects of exercise conditioning on myocardial oxygen balance would be expected to reduce vulnerability to ventricular fibrillation and sudden death. Quality of life can be significantly enhanced by an exercise program through improved physical fitness and psychological benefits.

There are, however, potential risks accompanying strenuous exercise in diabetic individuals that must be considered when planning an exercise program. These include aggravation of metabolic dysfunctions by exercising in the presence of markedly uncontrolled IDDM. In patients whose diabetes is well controlled by insulin or an oral hypoglycemic agent, hypoglycemia is a common problem during or following prolonged exercise. Frequent self-monitoring of blood glucose levels is crucial for the diabetic athlete or recreational exerciser to properly adjust insulin or oral drugs during hypoglycemic episodes. Consistency in eating, exercise, administration of diabetic medication, and other habits is important. When initiating a vigorous exercise program, diabetic individuals on insulin must either reduce their insulin dose, increase their food intake, or both. Insulin should not be administered in an active extremity for at least an hour prior to exercise because of the associated increased rate of insulin absorption. An alternative is to administer insulin in the abdominal wall. Prolonged exercise should be preceded by a light meal or carbohydrate snack, and supplementary carbohydrates should be administered regularly during and following exercise to prevent hypoglycemia based on self-monitored blood glucose levels.

Vigorous exercise, resistive exercise, and contact sports should be avoided in the presence of uncontrolled proliferative retinopathy because of the danger of retinal hemorrhage or retinal separation. Proper-fitting footwear and hygiene are crucial to the diabetic exerciser to avoid complications leading to lower extremity gangrene and amputation, particularly in those with peripheral neuropathy and peripheral vascular disease. In addition, careful cardiovascular screening including exercise testing is required in all diabetic individuals.

ACKNOWLEDGEMENT

I wish to acknowledge the assistance of Ms. Marilyn Borkon in making this manuscript possible.

REFERENCES

1. Ahern, J.A., Kruger, D.F., Gatcomb, P., et al.: The Diabetes Control and Complication Trial (DCCT): the trial coordinator perspective report by the DCT Research Group. Diabetic Educator, 15:236–241, 1989.
2. Allen, F.M.: Notes concerning exercise in the treatment of severe diabetes. Med. Surg. J., 173:743–744, 1915.
3. Alessandrini, P., McRae, J., Feman, S., and Fitzgerald, G.A.: Thromboxane biosynthesis and platelet function in type I diabetes mellitus. N. Engl. J. Med., 319:208–212, 1988.
4. American Diabetic Association: Nutritional recommendations and principles for individuals with diabetes mellitus: 1986. Diabetes Care, 10:126–132, 1987.
5. American Diabetic Association: Physician's Guide to Non-Insulin-Non-Insulin-Dependent (Type I) Diabetes. Diagnosis and Treatment. Alexandria, VA, ADA, 1988.
6. American Diabetic Association: Physician's Guide to Non-Insulin-Dependent (Type II) Diabetes. Diagnosis and Treatment, 2nd Ed. Alexandria, VA, ADA, 1988.
7. Anderson, J.W., and Chen, W-J.L.: Plant fiber, carbohydrate and lipid metabolism. Am. J. Clin. Nutr., 32:346–363, 1979.
8. Anderson, J.W., and Gustafson, N.J.: A guide for intensive nutrition management of obesity in diabetes mellitus. Intern. Med. Specialist, 7:100–117, 1987.
9. Anderson, S., and Brenner, B.M.: Influence of antihypertensive therapy on development and progression of diabetic glomerulopathy. Diabetes Care, 11:846–849, 1988.
10. Beach, K.W., Bedford, G.R., Berelin, R.O., et al.: Progression of lower extremity arterial occlusive disease in type II diabetes mellitus. Diabetes Care, 11:464–472, 1988.
11. Beigelman, P.M., and Kumar, D. (eds.): Diabetes Mellitus for the House Officer. Baltimore, Williams & Wilkins, 1986.
12. Bennett, P.H.: Epidemiology and diabetes mellitus. In Diabetes Mellitus. Theory and Practice. 4th Ed. Edited by H. Rifkin and D. Porte, Jr., New York, Elsevier, 1990, pp. 357–377.
13. Blair, S.N., Kohl, H.W. III, Paffenbarger, R.S. Jr., et al.: Physical fitness and all-causes mortality. A prospective study of healthy men and women. JAMA, 262:2395–2402, 1989.
14. Boden, G.: Treatment strategies for patients with non-insulin-dependent diabetes mellitus. Am. J. Med., 979(Suppl. 2B):23–26, 1985.
15. Bogardus, C., Ravussin, E., Robbins, D.C., et al.: Effects of physical training and diet therapy on carbohydrate metabolism in patients with glucose intolerance and non-insulin-dependent diabetes mellitus. Diabetes, 33:31–318, 1984.
16. Bonaa, K.H., Bjerve, K.S., Straume, B., et al.: Effect of eicosapentaenoic and decosahexaenoic

acids on blood pressure in hypertension: a population-based intervention trial from the Tromso Study. N. Engl. J. Med., *322*:793–801, 1990.

17. Brunzell, J.D., and Chait, A.: Lipoprotein pathophysiology and treatment. *In* Diabetes Mellitus. Theory and Practice. 4th Ed. Edited by H. Rifkin and D. Porte, Jr., New York, Elsevier, 1990, pp. 756–767.

18. Bunn, H.F., Gabbay, K.H., and Gallop, P.M.: The glycosylation of hemoglobin relevance to diabetes mellitus. Science, *200*:21–27, 1978.

19. Campaigne, B.N., Gilliam, T.B., Spencer, M.L., et al.: Effects of a physical activity program on metabolic control and cardiovascular fitness in children with insulin-dependent diabetes mellitus. Diabetes Care, *7*:57–62, 1984.

20. Cavert, G.D., Mannik, T., Graham, J.J., et al.: Effect of therapy on plasma-high-density lipoprotein concentration in diabetes mellitus. Lancet, *2*:66–68, 1978.

21. Caspersen, C.J., Powell, K.E., and Christenson, G.M.: Physical activity, exercise, and physical fitness. Definitions and distinctions for health related researches. Public Health Reports, *100*:126–131, 1985.

22. Cerami, A., Vlassara, H., and Brounlee, M.: Role of advanced glycosylated products in complications of diabetes. Diabetes Care *11*(Suppl. 1):73–79, 1988.

23. Chen, M.K., and Lowenstein, F.W.: Epidemiology of factors related to self-reported diabetes among adults. Am. J. Prev. Med., *2*:14–19, 1986.

24. Cowie, C.C., Port, F.K., Wolfe, R.A., et al.: Disparities in incidence of diabetic end-stage renal disease according to race and type of diabetes. N. Engl. J. Med., *321*:1074–1079, 1989.

25. Davidson, M.B.: The continuing changing natural history of diabetes. J. Chronic Dis., *34*:5–10, 1981.

26. Despres, J-P., Moorjani, S., Lupien, P.J., et al.: Regional distribution of body fat, plasma lipoproteins, and cardiovascular diseases. Atherosclerosis, *10*:497–511, 1990.

27. Fein, F.S., and Scheuer, J.: Heart disease in diabetics. *In* Diabetes Mellitus. Theory and Practice. 4th Ed. Edited by H. Rifkin and D. Porte, Jr. New York, Elsevier, 1990, pp. 812–823.

28. Folkins, C.H., and Amsterdam, E.A.: Control and modification of stress emotions through chronic exercise. *In* Exercise in Cardiovascular Health and Disease. Edited by E.A. Amsterdam, J.H. Wilmore, and A.N. DeMars. New York, Yorke Medical Books, 1977, pp. 280–294.

29. Frantz, M.J., and Norstrom, J.: Your Game Plan for Diabetes and Exercise. Diabetes Actively Staying Healthy. Minneapolis, DCI Publishing, 1990.

30. Friedman, E.A.: Diabetic renal disease. *In* Diabetes Mellitus—Theory and Practice. 4th Ed. Edited by H. Rifkin and D. Porte, Jr. New York, Elsevier, 1990, pp. 684–709.

31. Froelicher, V.F.: The effect of exercise on myocardial perfusion and function in patients with coronary heart disease. Eur. Heart J., *8*(Suppl. 6):1–9, 1987.

32. Froelicher, V.F.: Exercise, fitness, and coronary heart disease. *In* Exercise, Fitness and Health. A Consensus of Current Knowledge. Edited by C. Bouchard, R.J. Shephard, T. Stephens, et al. Champaign, IL, Human Kinetics, 1990, pp. 429–450.

33. Garg, A., and Grundy, S.M.: Management of dyslipidemia in NIDDM. Diabetes Care, *13*:1153–1169, 1990.

34. Gerich, J.E.: Insulin-dependent diabetes mellitus. Pathophysiology. Mayo Clin. Proc., *6*:787–791, 1986.

35. Gerich, J.E.: Oral hypoglycemic agents. N. Engl. J. Med., *21*:1231–1245, 1989.

36. Gillum, R.F., and Paffenbarger, R.S., Jr.: Chronic diseases in former college students. XVII. Sociocultural mobility as a precursor of coronary heart disease and hypertension. Am. J. Epidemiol., *108*:289–298, 1978.

37. Glauber, H., Wallace, P., Griver, K., and Brechtol, G.: Adverse metabolic effects of omega-3 fatty acids in non-insulin dependent diabetes mellitus. Ann. Intern. Med., *108*:663–668, 1988.

38. Goldberg, J.A.: Aerobic and resistive exercise modify risk factors for coronary heart disease. Med. Sci. Sports Exerc., *21*:669–674, 1989.

39. Goldberg, L., and Elliot, D.L.: The effect of physical activity on lipid and lipoprotein levels. Med. Clin. North Am., *69*:41–59, 1985.

40. Greaves, M., and Preston, F.E.: Haemostatic abnormalities in diabetes. *In* Metabolic Aspects of Cardiovascular Disease. Diabetes and Heart Diseases. Edited by R.J. Jarrett. New York, Elsevier, 1984, pp. 47–80.

41. Greene, D.A., Sima, A.A.F., Albers, J.W., and Pfefer, M.A.: Diabetic neuropathy. *In* Diabetes Mellitus. Theory and Practice. 4th Ed. Edited by H. Rifkin and D. Porte, Jr. New York, Elsevier, 1990, pp. 710–755.

42. Gwinup, G.: Effect of exercise alone on the weight of obese women. Arch. Intern. Med., *135*:676–680, 1975.

43. Hagberg, J.M.: Exercise, fitness and hypertension. *In* Exercise, Fitness and Health. Edited by C. Bouchard, R.J. Shephard, T. Stephens, et al. Champaign, IL, Human Kinetics Books, 1990, pp. 455–66.

44. Hagberg, J.M., Ehrsani, A.A., Goldring, O., et al.: Effects of weight training on blood pressure and hemodynamics in hypertensive adolescents. J. Pediatr., *104*:147–151, 1984.

45. Hales, C.N., and Randle, P.J.: Immunoassay of insulin with insulin antibody precipitate. Biochem. J., *88*:737–746, 1973.

46. Haskell, W.L.: The influence of exercise training on plasma lipids and lipoproteins ion health and disease. Acta Med. Scand. Suppl., *711*:25–38, 1986.

47. Hellerstrom, C., Andersson, A., Carl, C-G. et al.: Experimental pancreatic transplantation in diabetes. Diabetes Care, *11*(Suppl. 1):45–53, 1988.

48. Herold, P.M., and Kinsella, J.E.: Fish consumption and decreased risk of cardiovascular disease: a comparison of findings from animal and human feeding trials. Am. J. Clin. Nutr., *43*:566–598, 1986.

49. Hollander, P.: The diabetes of pregnancy: A screening and management program for gestational diabetes. The Bulletin, *34*:29–36, 1990.

50. Hollenbeck, C.B., Coulson, A.M. and Reaven, G.M.: Effects of sucrose on carbohydrate and lipid metabolism in NIDDM patients. Diabetes Care, *12*(Suppl. 1):62–66, 1989.

51. Hollenbeck, C.B., Leklem, J.E., Riddle, M.C., and Connor, W.E.: The composition and nutritional adequacy of subject-selected high carbohydrate, low fat diets in insulin-dependent diabetes mellitus. Am. J. Clin. Nutr., 38:41–51, 1983.

52. Holloszy, J.O., Schultz, J., Kusnierkiewicz, J., et al.: Effects of exercise on glucose tolerance and insulin resistance. Acta Med. Scand. Suppl., 711:52–65, 1986.

53. Hughes, J.R.: Psychologic effects of habitual aerobic exercise. A critical review. Prev. Med., 13:66–78, 1984.

54. Hurley, B.F., Hagberg, J.M., Goldberg, A.P., et al.: Resistive training can reduce coronary risk factors without altering $\dot{V}_{O_2max}$ or percent body fat. Med. Sci. Sports Exerc., 20:150–154, 1988.

55. L. Jovanovic-Peterson, Durak, E.P., and Peterson, C.M.: Randomized trial of diet versus diet plus cardiovascular conditioning on glucose levels in gestational diabetes. Am. J. Obstet. Gynecol., 16:415–419, 1987.

56. Jarret, R.J. (ed.): Metabolic Aspects of Cardiovascular Disease. Diabetes and Heart Disease. New York, Elsevier, 1984.

57. Jennings, G., Nielson, L., Nestel, P.O., et al.: The effects of changes in physical activity on major cardiovascular risk factors, hemodynamics, sympathetic function, and glucose utilization in man: a controlled study of four levels of activity. Circulation, 75:30–41, 1986.

58. Jensen, M.D., and Miles, J.M.: The roles of diet and exercise in the management of patients with insulin-dependent diabetes mellitus. Mayo Clin. Proc., 61:813–819, 1986.

59. Jensen, T., Sender, S., Goldstein, K., et al.: Partial normalization by dietary cod-liver oil of increased microvascular albumin leakage in patients with insulin-dependent diabetes and albuminuria. N. Engl. J. Med., 321:1522–1527, 1989.

60. Kannel, W.B., and McGee, D.L.: Diabetes and cardiovascular disease. The Framingham Study. JAMA, 241:2035–2038, 1979.

61. Klein, R., Klein, E.K., Moss, S.E., and DeMets, D.L.: Blood pressure and hypertension in diabetes. Am. J. Epidemiol., 122:75–89, 1988.

62. Klein, R., Moss, S.E., Klein, E.K., and DeMets, D.L.: Relation of ocular and systemic factors to survival in diabetes. Arch. Intern. Med., 149:266–272, 1989.

63. Kokkinos, P.F., Hurley, B.F., Vaccaro, P., et al.: Effects of low- and high-repetitious resistive training on lipoprotein-lipid profiles. Med. Sci. Sports Exerc., 20:50–54, 1988.

64. Koivisto, V.A., and DeFranzo, R.A.: Exercise in the treatment of type II diabetes. Acta Endocrinol. Suppl., 262:107–111, 1984.

65. Koivisto, V.A., Soman, V., Conrad, P., et al.: Insulin binding to monocytes in trained athletes. Changes in the resting state and after exercise. Am. Soc. Clin. Invest., 64:1011–1015, 1979.

66. Krall, L.P., and Beaser, R.S.: Joslin Diabetes Manual. 12th Ed. Philadelphia, Lea & Febiger, 1989.

67. Kramsch, D.M., Aspen, A.J., Abramowitz, B.M., et al.: Reduction of coronary atherosclerosis by moderate conditioning exercise in monkeys on atherogenic diets. N. Engl. J. Med., 309:1483–1489, 1981.

68. Kritz-Silverstein, D., Barrett-Connor, E., and Wingard, D.L.: The effect of parity on the later development of non-insulin-dependent diabetes mellitus or impaired glucose tolerance. N. Engl. J. Med., 321:1214–1219, 1989.

69. Kromhout, D., Bosschieter, E., and Coulander, A.: Inverse relationship between fish consumption and 20-year mortality from coronary heart disease. N. Engl. J. Med., 312:1205–1212, 1985.

70. Krotkiewski, M., Lonnroth, P., Mandroukas, K., et al.: The effects of physical training on insulin secretion and effectiveness and on glucose metabolism in obesity and type 2 (non-insulin-dependent) diabetes mellitus. Diabetologia, 28:881–890, 1985.

71. Kuman, D.: Insulin therapy. In Diabetes Mellitus for the House Officer. Edited by P.M. Beigelman and D. Kuman. Williams & Wilkins, Baltimore, 1986, pp. 91–112.

72. Laakso, M., Ronnemaa, T., Pyrola, K., et al.: Atherosclerotic vascular disease and the risk factors in non-insulin dependent diabetic and nondiabetic subjects in Finland. Diabetes Care, 11:449–463, 1988.

73. Laker, M.F.: Plasma lipids and lipoproteins in diabetes mellitus. In The Diabetes Annual/3. Edited by K.G. Alberti and L.P. Krall. New York, Elsevier Science Publishers, 1987, pp. 459–477.

74. Landt, K.W., Campaigne, B.N., James, F.W., and Sperling, M.A.: Effects of exercise training on insulin sensitivity in adolescents with type I diabetes. Diabetes Care, 8:461–465, 1985.

75. Lawrence, R.D.: Effects of exercise on insulin action in diabetes. Br. Med. J., 1:648–650, 1920.

76. Leon, A.S.: Comparative cardiovascular adaptations to exercise in animals and man and their relevance to coronary heart disease. In Comparative Pathophysiology of Circulation Disorders. Edited by C.M. Bloor. New York, Plenum, 1972, pp. 143–174.

77. Leon, A.S.: The role of physical activity in the prevention and management of obesity. In Sports Medicine. 2nd Ed. Edited by A.J. Ryan and F.L. Allman, Jr. San Diego, Academic Press, 1989, pp. 593–617.

78. Leon, A.S., and Blackburn, H.: The relationship of physical activity to coronary heart disease and life expectancy. Ann N.Y. Acad. Sci., 301:561–578, 1977.

79. Leon, A.S., Connett, J., Jacobs, D.R., Jr., and Rauramaa, R.: Leisure-time physical activity levels and risk of heart disease and death. The Multiple Risk Factor Intervention Trial. JAMA, 258:2388–2395, 1987.

80. Leon, A.S., Conrad, J., Casal, D.E., et al.: Exercise in diabetes: effects of conditioning at constant body weight. J. Cardiopulm. Rehabil., 4:278–286, 1984.

81. Leon, A.S., Conrad, J., Hunninghake, D.B., and Serfass, R.: Effects of a vigorous walking program on body composition, and carbohydrate and lipid metabolism of obese young men. Am. J. Clin. Nutr., 32:1776–1787, 1979.

82. Lipman, R.L., Raskin, P., Love, T., et al.: Glucose tolerance during decreased physical activity in man. Diabetes, 21:101–107, 1972.

83. Lipman, R.L., Schnure, J.J., Bradley, E.M., and Lecocq, F.R.: Impairment of peripheral glucose utilization in normal subjects by prolonged bed rest. J. Lab. Clin. Med., 76:221–230, 1970.

84. Lithell, H.O.L.: Lipoprotein metabolism and physical training in normal man and diabetic and cardiac patients. *In* International Series on Sports Sciences. Vol. 16. Biochemistry of Exercise VI. Edited by B. Saltin. Champaign, IL, Human Kinetics, 1986, pp. 280–309.

85. Merimee, T.J.: Diabetic retinopathy. A synthesis of perspectives. N. Engl. J. Med., *322*:978–983, 1990.

86. Montoye, H.J., Meltzer, H.L., Keller, J.B., et al.: Physical activity and blood pressure. Med. Sci. Exerc. Sports, *4*:175–181, 1972.

87. Narins, B.E., and Narins, R.G.: Clinical features and health-care costs of diabetic nephropathy. Diabetes Care, *11*:833–839, 1988.

88. National Diabetes Advisory Board: Diabetes in the 1980s: Challenges for the Future. Washington, D.C., U.S. Department of Health and Human Services, Public Health Service, National Institutes of Health, NIH Publication No. 82-2143, 1982.

89. National Institutes of Health consensus development conference on diet and exercise in non-insulin-diabetes mellitus. Diabetes Care, *10*:639–644, 1987.

90. National Research Council Committee on Diet and Health: Diet and Health. Implication for Reducing Chronic Disease Risk. Washington, D.C., National Academy Press, 1989.

91. Ohlson, L.O., Larsson, B., Svardsudd, K., et al.: The influence of body fat distribution on the incidence of diabetes mellitus: 13.5 years of follow-up of the participants in the study of men born in 1913. Diabetes, *34*:1055–1058, 1985.

92. Ornish, D., Brown, S.E., Scherwitz, L.W., et al.: Can lifestyle changes reverse coronary heart disease? Lancet, *336*:126–132, 1990.

93. Paaikivi, J., and Wahlberg, F.: Preventive tolbutamide treatment and arterial disease in mild hyperglycaemia. Diabetologia, *7*:323–327, 1971.

94. Paffenbarger, R.S., Jr., and Hyde, R.T.: Exercise in the prevention of coronary heart disease. Prev. Med., *13*:3–22, 1984.

95. Paffenbarger, R.S., Thorne, M.C., and Wing, A.L.: Chronic disease in formal college students. VIII. Characteristics in youth predisposing to hypertension in later life. Am. J. Epidemiol., *88*:25–32, 1968.

96. Passa, P., LeBlanc, H., and Marre, M.: Effects of enalapril in insulin-dependent diabetic subjects with mild to moderate uncomplicated hypertension. Diabetes Care, *10*:200–204, 1987.

97. Pederson, O., Beck-Nielsen, H., and Heding, L.: Increased insulin receptors after exercise in patients with insulin-dependent diabetes mellitus. N. Engl. J. Med., *302*:886–892, 1990.

98. Petrides, P., Weiss, L., Loffler, G., and Wieland, O.H.: Diabetes Mellitus: Theory and Management. Baltimore-Munich, Urban and Schwarzenberg, 1978.

99. Porte, D., LaCava, E.C., Halter, J.B., and Halar, E.M.: Diabetic neuropathy. *In* Clinical Guide to Diabetes Mellitus. Edited by K.E. Sussman, B. Drazmin, and W.E. James. New York, Alan R. Liss, 1987, pp. 143–158.

100. Powell, K.E., Thompson, P.D., Caspersen, C.J., and Kendrick, J.S.: Physical activity and the incidence of coronary heart disease. Ann. Rev. Public Health, *8*:253–287, 1987.

101. Puska, P., Nissinen, A., Vartiainen, E., et al.: Controlled randomized trial of the effect of dietary fat on blood pressure. Lancet, *1*:1–10, 1983.

102. Pyorola, K.: Relationship of glucose tolerance and plasma insulin to the incidence of coronary heart disease: results from two population studies in Finland. Diabetes Care, *2*:131–141, 1979.

103. Raskin, P.: Islet-cell abnormalities in non-insulin-dependent diabetes mellitus. Am. J. Med., *76*(Suppl. 2B):2–5, 1985.

104. Rauramaa, R.: Physical activity and prostanoids. Acta Med. Scand. Suppl., *711*:37–42, 1986.

105. Reaven, G.M.: Clinician's Guide to Non-Insulin-Dependent Diabetes Mellitus Pathogenesis and Treatment. New York, Marcel Dekker, 1989.

106. Reitman, J.S., Vasquez, B., Klimes, I., and Nagulespan, M.: Improvement of glucose homeostasis after exercising training in non-insulin-dependent diabetes. Diabetes Care, *7*:334–341, 1984.

107. Rodgers, M.A.: Acute effects of exercise on glucose tolerance in non-insulin-dependent diabetes. Med. Sci. Sports Exerc., *21*:362–368, 1989.

108. Rosenstock, J., Strowig, S., Cercone, S., and Raskin, P.: Reduction in cardiovascular risk factors with intense diabetes treatment in insulin-dependent diabetes mellitus. Diabetes Care, *10*:729–734, 1987.

109. Ruderman, N.B., Ganda, O.P., and Johansen, K.: The effect of physical training on glucose tolerance and plasma lipids in maturity-onset diabetes. Diabetes, *28*(Suppl.):89–92, 1978.

110. Saltin, B., Lingarde, F., Houston, M., et al.: Physical training and glucose tolerance in middle-aged men with chemical diabetes. Diabetes, *28*(Suppl.):30–32, 1979.

111. Santiago, M.C.: Effects of a forty-week walking program of twelve miles per week on physical fitness, body composition, and blood lipids and lipoproteins in sedentary women. Ph.D. thesis. Minneapolis, University of Minnesota, 1990.

112. Santiago, M.C., Alexander, J.F., Stull, G.A., et al.: Physiological responses of sedentary women to a 20-week conditioning program of walking or jogging. Scand. J. Sports Sci., *9*:33–39, 1987.

113. Schneider, S.H., Amorosa, L.F., Khachadurian, A.K., and Ruderman, N.B.: Studies on the mechanism of improved glucose control during regular exercise in type 2 (non-insulin-dependent) diabetes. Diabetologia, *26*:355–360, 1984.

114. Schwartz, S.: The independent effects of dieting, weight loss, and aerobic training on high density lipoprotein and apolipoprotein A-I concentrations in obese men. Metabolism, *36*:165–171, 1987.

115. Service, E.J.: What is "tight control" of diabetes? Goals, limitations and evaluation and therapy. Mayo Clin. Proc., *61*:792–795, 1986.

116. Shulman, G.I., Rothman, D.L., Jue, T., et al.: Quantification of muscle glycogen synthesis in normal patients and subjects with non-insulin-dependent diabetes by C-nuclear magnetic resonance spectroscopy. N. Engl. J. Med., *322*:223–228, 1989.

117. Simonson, D.C.: Etiology and prevalence of hypertension in diabetic patients. Diabetic Care, *11*:821–827, 1988.

181

118. Slattery, M.L., and Jacobs, D.R., Jr.: Physical fitness and cardiovascular mortality. The U.S. Railroad Study. Am. J. Epidemiol., *127*:571–580, 1989.

119. Smith, D.A.: Diabetic cardiomyopathy: pathogenesis, diagnosis, and management. Primary Cardiol., *16*:67–780, 1990.

120. Soman, V.R., Koivisto, V.A., Deibert, D., et al.: Increased insulin sensitivity and insulin binding to monocytes after physical training. N. Engl. J. Med., *301*:1200–1204, 1979.

121. Sopko, G., Leon, A.S., Jacobs, D.R., Jr., et al.: The effects of exercise and weight loss on plasma lipids in young obese men. Metabolism *39*:227–236, 1985.

122. Stamler, J., Farinaro, E., Mojonnier, L.M., et al.: Prevention and control of hypertension by nutritional hygienic means. JAMA, *240*:1819–1823, 1980.

123. Stamler, R., Stamler, J., Grimm, R., et al.: Nonpharmacologic control of hypertension. Prev. Med., *14*:336–345, 1985.

124. Stout, R.W.: The relationship of abnormal circulatory insulin levels to atherosclerosis. Arteriosclerosis, *27*:1–13, 1977.

125. Stratton, J.R., Chandler, W.L., Cerqueira, M.D., et al.: Exercise training increases tissue plasminogen activator. Circulation, *80*(Suppl. II):II–819, 1989.

126. Sullivan, D.R., Sanders, T.A.B., Trayner, I.M., and Thompson, G.R.: Parodoxical elevation of LDL apoprotein B levels in hypertriglyceridaemic patients and normal subjects ingesting fish oil. Atherosclerosis, *62*:129–134, 1986.

127. Sutton, J.R., Farrell, P.A., and Harber, V.J.: Hormonal adaptations to physical activity. *In* Exercise, Fitness and Health. Edited by C. Bouchard, R.J. Shephard, T. Stephens, et al. Champaign, IL, Human Kinetics, 1990, pp. 217–257.

128. Trovati, M., Carta, Q., Cavalot, F., et al.: Influence of physical training on blood glucose control, glucose intolerance, insulin secretion, and insulin activity in non-insulin dependent diabetic patients. Diabetes Care, *17*:416–420, 1984.

129. Truglia, J.A., Livingston, J.N., and Lockwood, D.H.: Insulin resistance: receptor and postbinding defects in human obesity and non–insulin-dependent diabetes mellitus. Am. J. Med., *79*(Suppl. 2B): 13–22, 1985.

130. Turkington, R.W., and Weindling, H.K.: Insulin secretion in the diagnosis of adult-onset diabetes mellitus. JAMA, *240*:833–836, 1979.

131. Unger, R.H.: Diabetic hyperglycemia: Link to impaired glucose transport in pancreatic beta cells. Science, *251*:1200–1205, 1991.

132. Vinik, A., and Wing, R.R.: Nutritional management of the person with diabetes. *In* Diabetes Mellitus. Theory and Practice. 4th Ed. Edited by H. Rifkin and D. Porte, Jr. New York, Elsevier, 1990, pp. 464–496.

133. Vranic, M., and Wasserman, D.: Exercise, Fitness, Diabetes. *In* Exercise, Fitness and Health. A Consensus of Current Knowledge. Edited by C. Bouchard, R.J. Shephard, T. Stephens, et al. Champaign, IL, Human Kinetics, 1990, pp. 467–495.

134. Vranic, M., Wasserman, D., and Bukowieck, I.L.: Metabolic implications of exercise and physical fitness in physiology and diabetes. *In* Diabetes Mellitus. Theory and Practice. 4th Ed. Edited by H. Rifkin and D. Porte, Jr. New York, Elsevier, 1990, pp. 198–219.

135. Wallberg-Henriksson, H., Gunnarson, R., Henriksson, J., et al.: Increased peripheral insulin sensitivity and muscle mitochondrial enzymes but unchanged glucose control in type I diabetics after physical training. Diabetes, *31*:1044–1050, 1982.

136. Wallberg-Henriksson, H., Gunnarson, R., Rossner, S., and Wahren, J.: Long-term physical training in female type I (insulin-dependent) diabetic patients: absence of significant effects on glycemic controls and lipoprotein levels. Diabetologica, *29*:53–57, 1986.

137. Wasserman, D.H., and Vranic, M.: Exercise and diabetes. Diabetes Annual, *3*:527–559, 1987.

138. Weintraub, M.S., Rosen, Y., Otto, R., et al.: Physical exercise conditioning in the absence of weight loss reduces fasting and postprandial triglyceride-rich lipoprotein levels. Circulation, *79*:1007–1014, 1989.

139. West, K.M.: Epidemiology of Diabetes and Its Vascular Lesions. New York, Elsevier, 1978.

140. Wilkins, T.J.: Insulin autoantibodies as markers for type I diabetes. Endocr. Rev., *11*:92–104, 1990.

141. Williams, P.T., Wood, P.D., Haskell, W.L., and Vranizan, K.: The effects of running mileage and duration on plasma lipoprotein levels. JAMA, *247*:2674–2679, 1982.

142. Wood, P.D., Haskell, W.L., Blair, S.N., et al.: Increased exercise level and plasma lipoprotein concentrations: a one-year, randomized, controlled study in sedentary, middle-aged men. Metabolism, *32*:31–39, 1983.

143. Wood, P.D., and Stefanick, M.L.: Exercise, fitness and atherosclerosis. *In* Exercise, Fitness and Health. A Consensus of Current Knowledge. Edited by C. Bouchard, R.J. Shephard, T. Stephens, et al. Champaign, IL, Human Kinetics, 1990, pp. 409–424.

144. Wood, P.D., Stefanick, M.L., Dreone, D.M., et al.: Changes in plasma lipids and lipoproteins in overweight men during weight loss through dieting compared with exercise. N. Engl. J. Med., *319*:1173–1179, 1988.

145. World Health Organization Study Group: Diabetes Mellitus. Report of a WHO Study Group. Geneva, WHO Technical Report Series No. 727, 1985.

146. Yski-Jarvinen, H., DeFronzo, R., and Koivisto, V.A.: Normalization of insulin sensitivity in type I diabetic subjects by physical training during insulin pump therapy. Diabetes Care, *7*:520–527, 1984.

147. Zeyman, F.J., and Ney, D.M.: Application of Clinical Nutrition. Englewood Cliffs, NJ, Prentice-Hall, 1989, pp. 22–256.

148. Zilversmit, D.B.: Atherogenesis: a postprandial observation. Circulation, *60*:473–485, 1979.

149. Zimmerman, B.R., Palumbo, P.J., O'Fallon, W.M., et al.: A prospective study of peripheral occlusive arterial disease in diabetics. Mayo Clin. Proc., *56*:217–253, 1981.

150. Zinman, B.: The physiological replacement of insulin. An elusive goal. N. Engl. J. Med., *3321*:363–370, 1989.
151. Zinman, B., and Vranic, M.: Diabetes and exercise. Med. Clin. North Am., *69*:145–157, 1985.
152. Zinman, B., Zuniga-Guajardo, S., and Kelly, D.: Comparison of the acute and long-term effect of exercise on glucose control in type I diabetes. Diabetes Care, *7*:515–519, 1984.

11
CHAPTER

Obesity

by
Elsworth R. Buskirk

Obesity constitutes a significant health problem, particularly with individuals of advancing years, as susceptibility to chronic disease is enhanced and length of life is decreased.[28,30,117,155] Individuals of all ages are afflicted with obesity, but prevalence rises through middle age and then decreases.[155] There is some evidence that those persons who were obese as infants are most resistant to weight reduction.[149] One also wonders about the early role of physical activity, because infants who were active in utero weighed less at birth for a given body length.[147] Although considerable attention has been focused on child-onset obesity, attendant adipose tissue, hypercellularity, and resistance to body fat loss in later years, optimal treatment is not at all clear, largely because the metabolic causes of this obesity are poorly understood.[87,96] Similarly, no major advance has been made in the prevention, management, or successful therapy of adult-onset obesity. Much more is now known about the adult-onset type, but obesity remains a major health problem complicated by multiple etiologies.[28,30,38,81,149]

The focus of this chapter is on physical activity, with the assumption that regular exercise can influence body weight and composition (particularly fatness) through such regulatory mechanisms as appetite and satiety control and body temperature and heat exchange regulation, as well as metabolic alterations in substrate preference, pathway changes, number and activity of hormonal binding sites, and differential rates of specific tissue metabolism. It should be understood that physical activity usually accounts for only a fraction of daily energy turnover among the obese, and that imposition of a regular exercise regimen is likely to increase this fraction only slightly.

Although the concern for obesity among the biomedical community and the public is longstanding, recent emphasis, highlighted by International Conferences on Obesity, has focused attention on a serious public health problem.[28,30]

A comprehensive report on obesity compiled by James, entitled *Research on Obesity*, was prepared for the Committee on Medical Aspects of Food Policy of the Department of Health and Social Security and for the Medical Research Council, London, England.[95] Attention was paid to the role of exercise in the prevention and management of obesity in all of these deliberations and subsequent publications. Some conclusions of consequence are:

1. There currently exist no entirely satisfactory standards by which obesity may be defined or measured.
2. Obesity is defined as a surplus of fat, and overweight is an excess of body weight relative to height.

Chapter written with the assistance of H.L. Barlett.

3. Obesity probably represents a group of related disorders and account should be taken of child-onset and adult-onset obesity, as well as of different patterns of fat deposition.
4. Exercise is important in the weight control process, and metabolic events are influenced by specific types of exercise and diet.
5. Wide individual differences exist in exercise habits and energy expenditure, with no clear evidence that the obese are significantly more inactive than many of their leaner counterparts.
6. Walking appears to be the most acceptable exercise for the obese.
7. Because obesity is largely a result of lifestyle, control may best be achieved by utilizing behavioral therapies that include regular exercise (see also Bray[29,31]).

The role of regular exercise may be quite different when applied in a weight-reduction regimen or in an obesity prevention program for children or adults. The value of regular exercise among the obese, even in the absence of body weight or fat loss, remains apparent because of other tangible benefits (e.g., increased strength, flexibility, and endurance, and a general feeling of well-being) leading to ostensible improvement in quality of life.

DESCRIPTION OF OBESITY

Even though the "eyeball" test provides a perception of the overly fat, obesity is difficult to define in universally acceptable, quantitative terms. The concepts of relative, ideal, and optimal body weight are useful for epidemiologic purposes because they are based on weight and height indices, but obesity should mean overly fat, i.e., excess lipid stored in adipose tissue. Such a definition means that fatness should be measured. Other than using skinfolds and such anthropometric measurements as lengths and circumferences, direct assessment of fatness is difficult without relatively complicated analytic equipment. Hence, the popularity and practicality of such weight and height indices as the Quetelet or body mass index (BMI = weight in kg $\cdot$ height in m^{-2}) or the Metropolitan Life Insurance weight for height and frame size tables.[8] Garrow regards direct assessment of fatness as unimportant if one is interested only in treating grossly overweight and obese patients.[73] The grossly obese are easy to recognize. Nevertheless, body composition and fatness measurements are needed if it is important to assess changes associated with therapy, including effects of an exercise program.

Garrow recommends maximal limits as a simple classification of obesity, i.e., greater than 110% relative weight.[73] This value corresponds to about 22% fat for men and 28% for women.[105] Garrow[73] recognizes the potential for misclassification of many people (athletes and the elderly), but this is a small price for simplicity. Other researchers argue that the minimum should be greater than 120% relative weight.

Bray published a nomogram (adapted from Thomas et al.[154]) for the BMI (30 is the criterion for obesity), as well as guidelines for acceptable weight.[31] West suggests that the "ideal" BMI for men is 22.1 and that for women is 20.6.[158] Interestingly, a BMI of more than 30 better approximates an upward inflection of the mortality curves prepared by Keys that appear in Figure 11–1.[101]

For experimental work with adults, we have arbitrarily used 25% body fat or more in men and 30% or more in women as the criteria of obesity (i.e., kg stored lipid $\cdot$ 100 kg body weight^{-1}).[39] It could be argued that these percentages are too high with respect to current health attitudes, and that values of 20% for men and 25% for women are more suitable. With the former criteria, about 15% of adults would be regarded as obese; with the latter, the percentage would increase to about 40%. Future research may facilitate development of different criteria for different groups by utilizing the concepts of physiologic strain or pathology, i.e., the stress of carrying excess fat may produce greater physiologic strain in the younger than the older person. Therefore, future obesity criteria should be population specific.

An important problem in defining obesity and in determining its prevalence, therefore, is accurate measurement. Several indirect methods have proven useful (including body density, total body water, and total body potassium), but these and other laboratory procedures (e.g., electrical impedance or conductivity, computed tomography, ultrasonography, neutron activation, and magnetic resonance) are not readily available to the average practicing physician. Thus, height and weight standards including the BMI are more frequently used, although it is recognized that they are somewhat arbitrary and inaccurate. The next most reasonable technique is the measurement of skinfolds with calipers. Reliability of this technique should improve with standardization of calipers, skin site selection, and skinfold handling procedures; better training of technicans; back-up afforded by validation with other measures of body fat of greater specificity; and increased experience with differences associated with age, maturation, gender, body build, and racial or cultural groups.[28,72,150] An alternative form of measurement is that of appropriate body lengths and circumferences and calculation of ratios to establish patterns of adipose tissue distribution.

CLASSIFICATION OF OBESITY

Bray has classified obesity both anatomically and etiologically.[31] The anatomic classification focuses on the pattern of fat storage with either localized or generalized accumulation; the etiologic classification is based on the type of obesity, plus its postulated mechanism and treatment. Recently, Bray[33] added age of onset as a category. The general types of obesity include hypothalamic; endocrinologic; nutritional; pertaining to physical inactivity; genetic; and drug-induced. In any classification scheme, there are several subtypes. Thus, the multiple etiologies of obesity are stressed. This multiplicity means that regular exercise is only one aspect of prevention or treatment, although it probably interacts with several regulatory and metabolic mechanisms, e.g., hyperinsulinemia, ATPase activity, peripheral receptor site activity, and lipogenesis or lipolysis.

The importance of the cellular composition of adipose tissue is not readily apparent. The number and size of the adipocytes varies among individuals and various fat depots, and the mobilization rates from these depots may vary.[16,87,146] For example, a significant association has been found between the amount of subcutaneous fat and HDL cholesterol in serum that is independent of overall obesity.[56] Nevertheless, the differential of classification of hypercellular versus normocellular may prove useful, the child-onset obese individual being frequently hypercellular and the adult-onset being normocellular. It is currently unclear whether these two types of obesity differ in their response to therapy, although Björntorp suggests that they may.[17,115] For such classification to be reasonably accurate, valid and reliable measurements of both cell number and total body fatness are necessary—a difficult task with present methodology.[39]

Another system of classification proposed by Bray and co-workers involves the use of a cybernetic approach with body temperature regulation as a model. The usual components are identified, i.e., set point in the brain; a comparator in the hypothalamus; controllers in neural structures, the gastrointestinal tract, and endocrine glands; a controlled intracellular energy turnover system involving lipolysis or lipogenesis; and feedback pathways involving nerves and circulating humoral mediators. Such models provide a framework for thinking about obesity and the impact regular exercise may have in terms of potential sites for evaluating the effects of such intervention. Evidence exists that body size, fatness, and fat-free mass are influenced by genetics.[23,24] Bray cites data from Bouchard's group that genetic transmission may account for up to 60% of adipose tissue distribution.[33] Several syndromes of obesity have also been associated with autosomal recessive inheritance.

PREVALENCE

In 1966, the U.S. Department of Health, Education, and Welfare suggested that the number of obese individuals was increasing, because of sedentary living, labor-saving devices, and easy access to food, but that the prevalence of obesity could only be surmised.[155] Abraham et al. concluded that the prevalence is high in the United States, and is higher among women.[1] The results of a subsequent survey that pertains to obesity and economic classification are presented in Table 11–1. Black women evidence more obesity than caucasian women. More affluent men tend to be more obese, but this difference was not apparent among women. Table 11–2 clearly indicates that the percentages of overweight compared to obesity are not the same when BMI is used for classification, that is, 25 to 30 $kg \cdot m^{-2}$ overweight and $> 30 \ kg \cdot m^{-2}$ obese.[32] Talbot reported indications that 4.9% of men and 7.2% of women aged 20 to 74 years were severely obese.[150] Severe obesity was defined as the sum of triceps and subscapular skinfold thicknesses greater than the 95th percentile of such measurements for men and non-pregnant women aged 20 to 29 years. Lew and Garfinkel indicated that about 5.6% of men and 10.1% of women were 20% or more above standard weight.[106] Thus, if one assumes that 5% of adult men and 8% of adult women are obese by relatively conservative criteria, the total number of obese adults in the United States is between 5 and 10 million.

MORTALITY

Talbot[150] suggested that the mortality rate in a group of grossly obese men was higher than that for men of more normal fatness. The respective multiples of "nor-

TABLE 11–1. **Obesity in the U.S. Population: Percentage of Obese Adults by Economic Classification***

Economic Status and Age Range	Men		Women	
	Black	Caucasian	Black	Caucasian
Poor 45–64 years	4	5	49	26
More affluent 45–64 years	12	13	40	29
All 20–74 years	14		24	

*Criterion for obesity: more than 120% of "ideal" weight. (Reprinted from *Promoting Health/Preventing Disease*,[156] with permission.)

TABLE 11–2. **Percentage of Overweight and Obese Individuals in the United States and Canada**

Country	Age (years)	Overweight		Obese	
		Males	Females	Males	Females
United States	20–74	31	24	12	12
Canada	20–69	40	28	9	12

(Adapted from Bray.[32])

188

mal" mortality varied with age: more than 11-fold from age 25 to 34 years; more than 5-fold at 35 to 44 years; 3-fold at 45 to 54 years; and about 2.5-fold at 55 to 74 years (see Fig. 11–1).

ASSOCIATED CONDITIONS AND RISK

Gross obesity has been associated with a variety of conditions that affect general health status. These conditions are listed in Table 11–3. Bray[32,33] has attempted to evaluate the health risk of obesity by developing a scheme based on BMI and complicating factors. Bray's appraisal indicates that the risk increases in a curvilinear fashion above a BMI of 25 kg·m^{-2}. He points out that the distribution of body fat provides an ancillary guide to risk. The higher the proportion of truncal or abdominal fat, the greater the risk. The presence of such clinical conditions as diabetes, hypertension, and hyperlipidemia increase risk.

Cardiovascular Function and Disease

An association between the "overweight" state and cardiovascular disease has been suggested for many years.[2,9,46,134,138,152,153] Determination of the overweight state was usually based on weight and height, rather than on calculation of body fatness from more direct measurements. Two studies stand out in this regard. In these 5-year prospective studies, skinfold measurements were utilized to calculate adiposity.[102,131] The conclusion from both studies was that there is an increased risk of developing coronary heart disease (CHD) with increasing fatness in middle-aged men.

Keys discussed the problem of overweight, obesity, CHD, and mortality.[101] He reviewed the literature and calculated quadratic equations relating probability of CHD-caused death to the BMI for men from the Chicago Gas Company study, as

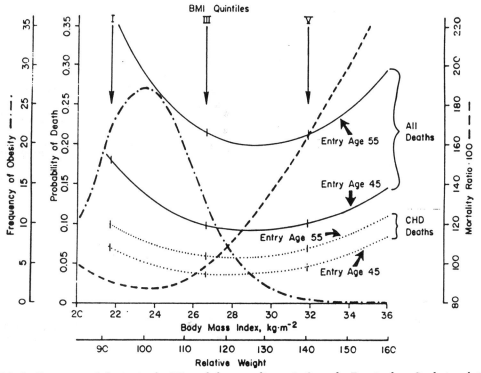

Fig. 11–1. *Frequency of obesity in the U.S. and the mortality ratio from the Framingham Study in relation to relative body weight. (Adapted from Mann.[116]) Probability of death from all causes or from coronary heart disease calculated from multiple logistic solutions with the independent variables of age, systolic blood pressure, and the square of the body mass index (BMI). (Adapted from Keys.[101])*

TABLE 11-3. **Obesity and Associated Conditions***

Hypertension
Atherosclerosis and coronary heart disease
Enlarged heart—congestive heart failure
Reduced myocardial function
Diabetes mellitus
Cirrhosis of the liver
Gout
Renal abnormalities
Menstrual and ovarian abnormalities
Endometrial carcinoma, other cancer, and leukemia
Risks in pregnancy
Gallbladder disease
Appendicitis
Osteoarthritis (in women, of knees)
Reduced pulmonary function
Pneumonia
Peptic ulcer
Poor tolerance of anesthesia
Greater risk at surgery
Accidents
Suicide
Social handicaps

* Adapted from Mann,[116] Garrow,[73] and Stunkard.[149]

well as for deaths from all causes for the United States railroad study and the northern and southern European studies. In each instance, the probability of death was increased at both low and high BMI (Fig. 11-1). The following conclusion was stated: *"The idea has been greatly oversold that the risk of dying prematurely or of having a heart attack is directly related to body weight. For middle-aged men, the best prospect for avoiding death in 10 or 15 years is to be about average, or a bit over in relative weight. The risk rises somewhat with departure in either direction from the happy middle ground, but risk increases substantially only at the extremes of under and overweight."* He further concludes, *". . . there is no acceptable evidence that relative body weight has any relevance to future health for women in the middle 80 percent of the weight distribution."* Keys is careful to point out that the Minnesota data *"indicate that body fatness is more of a risk factor than relative body weight, but even so obesity is still only of minor concern in regard to longev-ity, except at the extreme end of the distribution of fatness."*[101] Relative weight accounted for only 45% of the variance in body fatness, as calculated from body density measurements.

Among the cardiovascular problems associated with obesity, hypertension is perhaps of most consequence, because of the possible long-term effects resulting in arterial wall damage and atherosclerosis, renal vascular disease, and retinopathy. When occurring together after age 20 years, hypertension and obesity increase the risk of the development of cerebrovascular disease, specifically cerebral thrombosis.[86] Cardiac output (Q̇) and myocardial hypertrophy increase directly with body weight.[2, 98] Increased cardiac work and pulmonary hypertension in the grossly obese can result in congestive heart failure.[3] Increased peripheral arteriolar resistance is the prime suspect for the increased blood pressure. Following weight loss in the obese, there usually is a decrease in blood pressure, as well as in the work of the heart.[114]

190

Increased blood volume and $\dot{Q}$ have been found in obesity, with an increase in left ventricular work and heart weight.[2,4,6] Hypertrophy of both ventricles (primarily the left) in proportion to the magnitude of obesity was also noted. In addition, left ventricular failure may result from left ventricular hypertrophy. The left ventricular end-diastolic filling pressure is usually at the upper limit of normal in grossly obese patients.[97] This elevated level was presumably associated with a large central blood volume, for pulmonary blood volume reflects the larger total blood volume.[139] Those individuals with the obesity-hypoventilation syndrome have been shown to have a greater increase in pulmonary blood volume (pulmonary circulatory congestion), perhaps because of the pulmonary arterial vasoconstriction and hypertension induced by hypoxia and hypercapneic acidemia.[110] If these right heart problems are linked with hypertension and CHD, as can easily occur in obesity, functional capacity is severely limited.

Another risk factor for CHD associated with obesity is hyperlipidemia.[71,78,99,119] Serum triglyceride levels increase more than do those of total cholesterol with obesity, and high density lipoprotein cholesterol (HDL-C) concentrations decrease.[78,99] Elevated serum lipid levels have been shown to occur after experimental production of obesity in men by simple overeating, of mostly carbohydrate.[7] An inverse relationship was found between the Quetelet index and plasma HDL-C concentrations.[76] In the Puerto Rico Heart Study involving 25-year incidence of CHD, the overweight state was associated with higher lipid values and less physical activity, but was not related to the development of CHD.[50]

Work with children from the Bogalusa Heart Study showed a tendency for aggregation of multiple risk factors for CHD to increase with age. The risk factors studied were a modified BMI (Wt·Ht$^{-2.77}$) correlated with the triceps skinfold, total serum cholesterol level, and diastolic blood pressure.[15] With increasing obesity in these school age children, the lipoprotein profile

showed an increase in serum triglyceride and very low and low density lipoprotein cholesterol levels, as well as a decrease in the concentration of HDL-C.[70]

Respiratory Abnormalities

Although pulmonary function is relatively normal in many obese individuals,[136] with increasing deposition of fat overlying the thoracic cavity and both in and over the abdominal cavity, progressive changes occur in pulmonary function. Perhaps the most important change involves lung volume diminution at resting end-expiration (functional residual capacity or FRC). Lower FRC is found with moderate and gross obesity, and is brought about by the simple mechanical process of thoracic cavity "squeeze" and a reduction in anatomic dimensions by the mass of overlying adipose tissue.[10,13,52,54,90] The diaphragm is elevated by the distended abdomen. The reduction in FRC occurs primarily in the expiratory reserve volume (ERV), with the residual volume (RV) usually remaining unchanged.[40] If substantial, the reduction in ERV causes abnormalities in ventilation-perfusion distribution, arterial blood gases, lung mechanics, and diffusion of gases.

Another major change with obesity is an increase in mechanical work of breathing and increased oxygen cost of breathing.[22,45,74,100,122] These increases result because the intercostal muscles move an increased mass overlying the thorax and the contracting, descending diaphragm works against the pressure of a distended abdomen. A double jeopardy situation thus develops: inefficient ventilation at a reduced lung volume and a feeling of respiratory distress that may produce an aversion to exercise and, ultimately, reduced capacity for exercise.

Reports of an obesity-hypoventilation syndrome (reduced lung volumes and shallow irregular breathing), dubbed "Pickwickian Syndrome" by Burwell et al., appeared in the mid-1950s, but more satisfactory documentation of pulmonary dysfunction began with the report by

Said.[36,141] Of 20 obese subjects, all had some degree of arterial hypoxemia, but only eight suffered from hypoventilation and hypercapnia. Hypoventilation could not account for each case of hypoxemia, but abnormally elevated venous admixture and physiologic dead space ratios were regularly seen. Said suggested that this disturbed distribution of ventilation and perfusion could account for arterial hypoxemia in the absence of hypoventilation, and further suggested *"that the shallow breathing of the obese at a small lung volume causes small airway closure and regional atelectasis leading to increased venous admixture. It is also possible that shallow and irregular breathing deprives the pulmonary capillary circulation of the important pumping action by which normal respiratory movement promotes uniformity of capillary perfusion. Uneven perfusion of alveoli will, of course, result in a disturbed ventilation/perfusion ratio, with an increase in physiologic dead space and in physiologic shunt."*[141] Further research has extended and confirmed this concept.[11,12,54,59,65,90]

Pulmonary ventilation ($\dot{V}_E$), oxygen consumption ($\dot{V}_{O_2}$), and carbon dioxide production ($\dot{V}_{CO_2}$) are higher than normal in the obese subject during rest and particularly during exercise.[55,161] Increased $\dot{V}_E/\dot{V}_{O_2}$ often results in reduced arterial CO_2 partial pressure ($PaCO_2$). Thus, obese subjects are frequently hypocapneic because they ventilate more and their work of breathing is increased.[110] Sharp et al. found that passive ventilation of grossly obese men required two to four times the mechanical work required for leaner men.[144] The extra work required to move the chest wall is associated with decreased total respiratory compliance because of the decreased chest wall compliance, which results from accumulation of fat in and around the abdomen, diaphragm, and ribs.[110,122] Rochester and Enson described increased demands for diaphragmatic work in obese subjects, with inspiratory pressures only 60 to 70% of normal.[139] This finding led Luce to suggest that there is

skeletal muscle inefficiency involved, particularly during inspiration.[110]

EXPECTATIONS FOR IMPROVEMENT WITH REGULAR EXERCISE AND WEIGHT LOSS

Cardiovascular System

Reduction in body weight and fatness can result in decreased arterial pressure, lower plasma triglyceride and cholesterol concentrations, and a general improvement in cardiovascular function.[5,66,127,137] Hypertension has been shown to be slightly reduced by regular exercise, even with no or only slight weight reduction, in overweight women.[25,47,67] Exercise therapy may well be effective for partial control of hypertension in those obese individuals who are able to engage in regular exercise. High central blood volume, total blood volume, and elevated left ventricular end-diastolic pressure may all return to a normal level when weight is lost.[110]

Plasma triglyceride levels in obese hyperglycemic individuals show marked reductions with regular exercise.[60,109,127] Whether this decrease is because of the effect of regular exercise on metabolism or because of weight loss is not clear. The HDL-C to LDL-C ratio (thought to be an important factor in CHD prevention) increases in obese, as well as in lean individuals with regular exercise.[107]

Some of the well-known, long-term effects of regular exercise on the heart seen in the young have also occurred in middle-aged, formerly sedentary men, some of whom were overweight.[83] After 7 months of regular exercise, these men had resting and exercise bradycardia, reduced resting and submaximal $\dot{Q}$ for a given $\dot{V}_{O_2}$, and reduced cardiac minute work (despite increased stroke volume) at moderate and heavy exercise intensities.

Respiratory System

The effects of regular exercise and training on pulmonary function in the obese subject remains largely unknown; any effects would probably be attributable to weight loss. The ERV and vital capacity of the grossly obese person generally return to near normal levels after significant weight loss.[13,36,62,80] Loss of a substantial amount of body weight results in a return of ERV, ventilation-perfusion ratios, venous admixture, and oxygen partial pressure of arterial blood values to normal.[62,65] There are no known data to indicate at what percent body fat significant improvement might be expected. Farebrother et al. found no improvement in gas exchange until subjects were within 130% of "ideal weight."[65] Although there is a reduced ERV in the slightly or moderately obese population, there is no evidence that they have significant ventilation-perfusion disturbances or altered arterial blood gases. For grossly obese individuals, whose respiratory and cardiovascular function is so severely compromised that they become dyspneic on even slight exertion, weight reduction may have to precede an exercise program.

Metabolism

A significant effect of regular intense and prolonged exercise is the lowering of plasma insulin concentrations, without much effect on glucose tolerance.[19] This effect has been interpreted as an increased insulin sensitivity, and is observed whether or not body fatness is decreased. Thus, regular exercise can be an acceptable adjunct therapeutic measure for obese diabetic patients with signs of insulin insensitivity. Björntorp indicates that controlled studies are scarce, and a study of patients with adult onset diabetes yielded variable results (see Table 11–4).[18] Ruderman et al.[140] studied six sedentary, moderately obese men with maturity onset diabetes who engaged in regular (five times per week) cycle ergometer exercise for 3 to 6 months. Regular exercise did not result in appreciable weight loss, but aerobic power was increased, as was intravenous glucose tolerance. The serum insulin level was not increased, suggesting that some anti-insulin factor was less active or that insulin sensitivity increased. With cessation of regular exercise, reversion to pre-

exercise status occurred within 2 weeks. Interestingly, regular exercise did not change oral glucose tolerance or insulin response to oral glucose. Belfiore et al. suggest that insulin resistance in obesity is due to the failure of insulin to depress the key enzymes of catabolic pathways.[14] Glass has indicated that insulin-induced hypoglycemia normally stimulates an increase in circulating growth hormone, but this phenomenon is decreased in obese patients.[75]

Despite the intraindividual differences that may occur in patterns of caloric turnover related to alternate pathways, substrate availability, enzyme utilization, and the like, energy expenditure still must exceed energy intake if obese individuals are to lose body fat and to reduce weight. Even if evidence of reduced activity of the sodium-pumping mechanism in the obese person is confirmed on a scale broader than that for erythrocytes, the afflicted obese person will still have more difficulty achieving a negative caloric balance.[53] If the sodium pump defect is corrected, normalization of a hypothalamic regulatory mechanism may facilitate significant fat and weight loss. There are many other causes of obesity, e.g., damage to the hypothalamic appetite and satiety centers, such endocrinologic diseases as hypothyroidism and hyperadrenocorticism, and emotional disturbances with binge eating.[28,30,118,149]

Scheen et al. reported the metabolic substrate and hormone concentration changes that occurred when six obese men (mean BMI = 41) walked for 3 hours on a treadmill at 2.5 mph, 0% grade.[142] After fasting overnight, these men walked for 50 minutes and rested for 10 minutes each hour. The mean $\dot{V}_{O_2}$ was about 1.5 L·min^{-1}; heart rate was about 135 b·min^{-1}. A 57% drop in the amount of immunoreactive insulin, a 39% rise in immunoreactive glucagon concentration, and no change or a slight decrease in the plasma glucose level were observed with the long walk. Plasma cortisol concentration rose 59%, and urinary excretion of norepinephrine increased 124%. Plasma lactate and growth hormone concentrations did not change appreciably nor did

TABLE 11-4. **Effects of Physical Conditioning (Regular Exercise) on Some Aspects of Metabolism in the Obese Population***

Lower plasma insulin concentration
Enhanced insulin sensitivity
    Treatment alternative in obese diabetic patients with signs of peripheral insulin insensitivity
Lower plasma triglycerides (TG)
    Lower VLDL level
    Increased HDL level
       A treatment alternative in the obese who have elevated TG (Frederickson Type IV); generally have enlarged fat cells, glucose intolerance, and elevated plasma insulin
Perhaps more efficient utilization of available substrate

* Adapted from Björntorp.[18]

---

urinary excretion of epinephrine. Free fatty acid (FFA) concentration in plasma increased 72%, as reflected by a fall in respiratory quotient from 0.82 to 0.72. Thus, substrate utilization shifted to greater utilization of FFA during the prolonged walk (see Table 11–5).

General Health

Wiley and Camacho reported follow-up results from a survey of non-institutional-

ized residents in California.[144] The goal was to evaluate lifestyle characteristics and health status of Caucasian respondents less than 70 years old in 1965. Both men and women who were 30% or more overweight were at higher risk for poor future health; men were at greater risk. No difference in risk was discernible in the relative weight range of -10 to $+29\%$ for men or women. The mean adjusted health scores for men and women also tended

---

TABLE 11-5. **Change in Plasma Concentrations and Urinary Excretion of Some Metabolic Substrates and Hormones in Obese Men After 3-hour Walk ($\dot{V}_{O_2} \cong 1.5$ L·min^{-1}; HR $\cong$ 135 b·min^{-1})***

Variable	Before Walk	After Walk	Change	Significance (p)
Plasma				
Insulin (μU·ml^{-1})	15.1 ± 2.1	6.4 ± 1.7	− 8.7	<0.001
Glucagon (pg·ml^{-1})	115.0 ± 13.0	160.0 ± 17.0	+ 45.0	<0.05
Growth hormone (ng·ml^{-1})	0.9 ± 0.4	1.9 ± 1.1	+ 1.0	NS
Cortisol (μg·dl^{-1})	11.1 ± 2.4	17.6 ± 4.2	+ 6.5	≅0.05
FFA (μEq·L^{-1})	769.0 + 81.0	1319.0 ± 151.0	+550.0	<0.02
Urine				
NE (ng·mg CR^{-1})	26.1 ± 1.8	58.4 ± 12.1	32.3	≅0.05
E (ng·mg CR^{-1})	10.2 ± 2.8	13.0 ± 2.5	2.8	NS

* Data represent mean plus and minus standard error of the mean. Essentially no change was observed in blood lactate and glucose-levels. FFA = free fatty acids; NE = norepinephrine; E = epinephrine; CR = creatinine; NS = not significant. (Adapted from Scheen et al.[142])

to increase with the amount of physical activity. The difference between those subjects reporting no leisure time activity and those reporting even some activity was especially marked. There was no consistent trend for those persons with moderate or more activity. These conclusions held even when adjustments were made for initial health status, assuming that those with health problems in 1965 would not have been as active in the intervening years. The interaction between the overweight state and physical inactivity was not reported. A summary of the respective health factors is provided in Table 11–6. A summary of some of the possible physiologic and psychologic effects of regular exercise by obese individuals appears in Table 11–7.

Bray has evolved a scheme that classifies treatment with respect to energy intake and expenditure.[33] The treatment sequence for energy intake progressing from low to progressively higher risk is listed as behavior modifications, diets, appetite suppressants, jaw wiring, and gastric surgery. The sequence for energy expenditure proceeds from behavior modification to exercise, thermogenic drugs, inhibited absorption, and jejunal-ileal bypass. In general, procedures that decrease energy intake have a greater potential for producing weight and stored fat loss than those involving energy expenditure.

Body weight fluctuation has frequently been assumed to adversely influence health. A recent examination of data from the Baltimore Longitudinal Study of Aging calculated that weight variability was not predictive of subsequent CHD, cancer, or all-cause mortality, but may have an indirect effect via body fat distribution and glucose tolerance impairment.[108]

APPETITE

It is commonly assumed that appetite and satiety are closely related. Thus, with an increase in physical activity, appetite increases or satiety is less and caloric intake increases. To counter this assumption, results summarized by Mayer from work done on rats and man indicated that caloric intake did not change in proportion to energy expenditure in either the sedentary or the exhaustive range.[117,118]

Holm et al. reported that after early bouts of exercise in a conditioning program, a decrease in appetite was apparent, but they did not determine if it persisted.[91] Staten found that men responded to 5 days of acute exercise (1 hour at 70% $\dot{V}_{O_2max}$) by increasing their intake by about 200 Kcal per day, whereas women did not.[148] Among middle-aged men, Oscai and Williams found that regular exercise increased energy expenditure and that body weight decreased.[128] We have routinely observed similar results in the overweight population exposed to regular exer-

TABLE 11–6. **Prediction of Future Health Status in Alameda County, CA: Significant Health Factors, Regression Coefficients, and Significance***

Factor	Regression Coefficient	Probability
Nonsmoker	−0.54	p < 0.001
1–45 Alcoholic drinks per Month	−0.32	p < 0.01
Physical activity (5–16 units)	−0.60	p < 0.001
Sleep (7–8 hr·d^{-1})	−0.52	p < 0.001
Ideal weight for height (−10 to +29%)	−0.56	p < 0.001

* Comparison of differential factor weighting yielded a non-significant F-ratio. (Adapted from Wiley and Camacho.[159])

TABLE 11-7. **Possible Effects of Regular Exercise Among Obese Individuals***

Physiologic effects
　Increased daily energy expenditure
　Decreased appetite
　Increased or preserved muscle mass
　Reduced body fatness
　Increased functional capacity
　Decreased plasma insulin level
　Increased tissue sensitivity to insulin
　Decreased serum triglyceride level
　Decreased heart rate both at rest and during exercise
　Decreased systolic blood pressure
　Increased stroke volume
　Decreased peripheral vascular resistance
　Decreased cardiac work
　Increased flexibility
　Better motor coordination

Psychologic effects
　Reduced fatigue on-the-job
　Increased self-satisfaction and acceptance
　Improved self-perception
　Improved social interactions
　Improved self-esteem and confidence
　More balanced perspectives

* Adapted from Horton;[93] Mahoney;[115] and Brownell and Stunkard.[35]

cise.[21,37,120] There is some evidence that the scheduling of meals relative to physical activity may be important for caloric intake. There is the common observation that appetite is suppressed after participation in intense exercise. In this connection, Epstein et al. found that food intake was decreased in school children if recess was scheduled before rather than after lunch.[63] It would also be of interest to see whether exercise participation would have been reduced during recess after lunch.

Brownell and Stunkard summarized data from many animal studies on physical activity and concluded that gender, intensity of exercise, and body weight are important factors.[35] Physical activity appears to decrease food intake among male, but not usually among female, animals. Among sedentary animals, increasing activity decreases food intake and facilitates body weight loss. Among more active animals, food intake increases with physical activity and body weight remains stable. In more obese animals, appetite suppression with activity is more prominent than among leaner animals.

In summary, the effect of exercise on food intake in people is complicated and affected by nutritional state (obesity), diet, meal schedules, physical condition or fitness, and intensity and duration of exercise.

DRUGS, HORMONES, AND ENERGY EXPENDITURE

Several drugs have been utilized to increase energy expenditure in the obese individual, including amphetamines (CNS stimulation), caffeine, dinitrophenol (a blocker of oxidative phosphorylation), and salicylates. The metabolic increment is no doubt small with each of these drugs.

196

Among the hormones, most attention has been paid to thyroid-stimulating hormone (TSH), thyroxin (T_4), triiodothyronine (T_3), and reverse T_3; T_3 is the most active metabolically, but reverse T_3 has no known thermogenic effect.[73] Although the exact mechanism of action of the thyroid derivatives on metabolic rate is not well known, they may affect activity of the Na^+/K^+ pump.[61] Growth hormone (dose of 8 mg·day^{-1}) was found to increase $\dot{V}_{O_2}$ by 10%.[27] Similarly, small doses of epinephrine and glucagon may increase $\dot{V}_{O_2}$.[73] Presumably, the small increases in energy expenditure may be significant and superimposed on the metabolic rate at rest and during exercise. Other than for specific deficiency correction, it is unreasonable to assume that any of these compounds should be utilized for long-term elevation of daily energy expenditure to treat obesity. (For a discussion of anorexic drugs, see Bray.[28,30])

RESTING METABOLIC RATE

Among the obese population, resting metabolism accounts for the major fraction of daily energy expenditure, although exercise can add a substantial portion.[42,43,73] With caloric restriction, there is usually a reduction in fat-free body weight or lean body mass (LBM), resulting in a lower resting metabolic rate.[26,42] With successive caloric restrictions, resting metabolic rate falls more rapidly, the return to baseline values taking somewhat longer.[73] With regular exercise, there tends to be better retention of fat-free mass (FFM) even with caloric restriction.[103,107,118,162] With FFM retention, resting metabolic rate tends not to decrease as much as under conditions of caloric restriction and no exercise. Recent work has related FFM and other variables to resting metabolic rate, but these studies have not involved changes in body composition brought about by regular exercise.[82,89]

Resting metabolic rate probably increases with rigorous regular exercise because of the elevated level of resting metabolism that follows exercise.[143] Nevertheless, there can be energy expenditure compensation after exercise, because other activity may be reduced.[37,42] Garrow found that it takes considerable hard physical effort to produce a measurable effect on metabolism a few hours later.[73] Recent studies have indicated that the Harris-Benedict equation, widely used to calculate resting metabolic rate, overestimates it by about 7 to 10%.[48,130] The thought has been expressed that more-modern measurement procedures are more comfortable for the subject being studied.[48]

EXERCISE TESTING

On the assumption that a supervised weight reduction program should include prospects for significant weight loss, investigators should obtain a pertinent medical history, a physical examination, and an exercise tolerance test, and should ensure competent dietary counseling, physical activity leadership, and on-going medical evaluation. In regard to exercise testing of the obese individual, the main concern is to start the test after appropriate warm-up and at a rate that is easily tolerated. This safeguard may mean cycling with no added resistance or walking on the treadmill at 1 mph, 0% grade. For moderately obese women, Franklin et al. used an incremental walking protocol on the treadmill at 2.5 mph, 0% grade for a warm-up, continuing with a grade of 2.5% for 3 minutes, another 2.5% grade increase for 3 minutes, and followed by 3 mph, 5% grade for 3 minutes.[68] Thereafter, speed was kept constant and grade was increased 2.5% every 3 minutes. The test continued to each subject's maximum, in the absence of other contraindications. The average aerobic power ($\dot{V}_{O_2 max}$) for 23 middle-aged women (mean of 38% fat) was less than 8 METs. No untoward events were observed; electrocardiographic monitoring (CM-5 lead) was continuous, and blood pressure was measured at each exercise intensity. Similarly, Imperial et al. have successfully used a similar graded exercise test with elderly subjects and have demonstrated its feasibility, safety, and reproducibility.[94]

In an earlier study, Profant et al. observed that 23 obese women had low aerobic power (about 7 METs) and short treadmill walking times (7 minutes) when following the Bruce treadmill protocol.[135] Only one woman had significant ST segment depression, and none experienced angina. The age-specific prevalence of abnormal responses was similar to that reported elsewhere for CHD surveys. Age was the most important independent variable, not relative body weight. Nevertheless, if apparent CHD risk factors were considered (relative overweight, systolic pressure of 140 mm Hg or more, serum cholesterol concentration of 270 mg·dl^{-1} or more), prevalence of an abnormal ST segment response to exercise was doubled.

DeVore and Nemiro studied 95 obese men and 262 obese women with a mean age of 39 years using a test with a warm-up at 2 mph, 0% grade, followed by an individually adjusted speed of 2.5 to 3.1 mph.[57] Grade was increased 4% every 3 minutes at the constant selected speed. The walk was stopped when the obese patient reached 85% of the age-adjusted and estimated maximal heart rate. Three groups of men and women were studied. The men had a BMI of 25.6, 31.0, and 38.8; the women had a BMI of 25.4, 32.1 and 40.4. The last group of each gender were grossly obese; all groups were obese if the BMI criteria of West are applied, i.e., 22.1 for men and 20.6 for women.[158] If the unisex BMI criterion of 30.0 proposed by Bray is applied, two groups of each gender could be regarded as obese.[30] Exercise capacity was uniformly low, averaging less than 8 METs for all groups. The more obese groups averaged 7 METs or less for the men and 6 METs or less for the women. A total of 13 positive exercise tests were found (based on a 1 mm or more ST segment depression 80 msec from the J-point), in three men and 10 women. Of 20 hypertensive individuals, four men and 16 women had hypertensive responses to exercise. Of 36 normotensive subjects, two men and 34 women had hypertensive responses. The authors regarded the low incidence of positive tests and hypertensive

responses to exercise as evidence that obese patients may safely participate in exercise programs while dieting. Several cases of transient fatigue and leg cramps were observed, and one man with a BMI greater than 30 had severe syncope and significantly elevated systolic pressure.

Sheldahl found that the aerobic power of seven obese women averaged 27.7 ml·kg^{-1}·min^{-1}.[145] The women with the highest value had the least amount of fat (36%), and the woman with the lowest value was the fattest (47%). All of these obese women were physically active to a sufficient degree that the usual protocol for determining $\dot{V}_{O_2 max}$ in middle-aged and older people could be applied, with only a reduction in speed from 3.0 to 2.5 mph. A 5-minute warm-up period, at 2.5 mph, 5% grade was used; the grade increased progressively every 2 minutes until 20%.

On the basis of our experience, either the progressive walking test or a comparable cycle ergometer test can be utilized for obese individuals, with cognizance that their exercise capacities are low and that tests should start at an intensity that is easily tolerated after ample warm-up time. The risks of exercise tests to the obese individual appear to be no greater than that for their leaner counterparts. There are some individuals who are so grossly obese that conventional testing methods are impractical. For these people, a weight loss regimen that does not include exercise should be initiated. Exercise testing can be done once body fat is reduced to about 50% body weight.

Aerobic Power

Moderate obesity in young men does not appear to compromise their cardiovascular function, but it does limit their heat tolerance and ability to transport their body mass over distance.[88] Frequently, $\dot{V}_{O_2 max}$ per kilogram of fat-free tissue (ml·kgFFM^{-1}·min^{-1}) is equal among obese and more normal young men, whereas $\dot{V}_{O_2 max}$ (ml·kg^{-1}·min^{-1}) is not. In a study by Knight (cited in Hodgson and Buskirk[88]), heart rate and systolic blood pressure (SBP) were compared among obese and leaner men aged 40 to 49 and 50 to 59 years at rest and during a progressive exercise test. The age-related effect was small when compared to the effect of fatness and the overweight state. The slope of the regression line for SBP versus exercise intensity in METs was significantly greater for the obese subjects.

The effect of body fatness on aerobic power has been studied by many research groups;[41,84,112,126,161] their findings are summarized by Hodgson and Buskirk.[88] The conclusion was that excess fatness has a greater effect on the ability of young men than of older men to support aerobically the transport of their body weight. The respiratory and cardiovascular systems of the older men, as well as their skeletal musculature, may have become better physically conditioned from exercise performed over the years transporting their excess body fat.

The decline in aerobic power among obese men is shown in Figure 11-2.[88]

Changes in relative exercise intensity (% $\dot{V}_{O_2 max}$) are also shown. It can be seen that performing a task requiring 20 ml·kg^{-1}·min^{-1} falls below 60% $\dot{V}_{O_2 max}$ until age 68 years. Similarly, a task that requires 25 ml falls below 75% $\dot{V}_{O_2 max}$ until age 51 years, and a task that requires 30 ml falls below 85% $\dot{V}_{O_2 max}$ until age 38 years. Thus, not only does aerobic power decrease with age, but tasks requiring fixed energy expenditures require a significantly greater percentage of aerobic power with the advancing age of the obese individual. There is evidence that regular exercise exceeding 60% $\dot{V}_{O_2 max}$ provides measurable training effects.[133]

EXERCISE PROGRAMS

Exercise for purposes of body fat and weight reduction must inevitably involve reasonably high levels of energy expenditure.[129] Movement of the body mass should be emphasized because the greatest expenditures of energy are associated

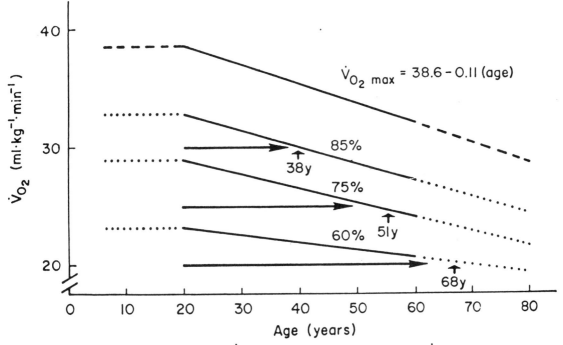

Fig. 11-2. *Decrement in aerobic power ($\dot{V}_{O_2 max}$) and relative oxygen uptake (% $\dot{V}_{O_2 max}$) with age among moderately obese men. The intercepts from $\dot{V}_{O_2}$ of 30, 25, and 20 ml·kg^{-1}·min^{-1} with the 85%, 75%, and 60% regression lines are indicated in terms of age. (Adapted from Hodgson and Buskirk.[88])*

with such activities, e.g., walking, stair climbing, jogging, and cross-country skiing. Such activities as cycling and swimming can be added, although they involve supplemental weight support, i.e., body weight is supported by the seat during cycling and by the buoyancy of the water during swimming.

Brownell and Stunkard prepared a list of activities in which Americans commonly engage, showing the caloric turnover for individuals of different body weight.[35] Table 11–8 is an adapted and abbreviated version. In a recent study involving obese women (30 to 36% body fat), the most rapid sustainable walk-jog speed varied between 5.2 and 5.7 mph (J. Wallace, personal communication).

Perhaps the best way to start an effective program is to encourage the obese individual to walk regularly; this walking should supplement that normally done on the job or at home. Walking a mile requires essentially the same energy as jogging or running a mile. Thus, the concept of distance covered is important for the obese person. In general, obese people are not embarrassed by walking and can usually structure their lives to do more if they are physically able.

Any successful behavior modification should be structured to maximize long-term adherence. Attention needs to be focused on such routine activities as walking, stair climbing, and performing tasks while standing and moving around the job or house. No special equipment is required, lifestyle modification is not painful, and work performance need not be compromised. This simple type of lifestyle change may well be the only type of physical activity that is continued for any length of time. Less reliance on vehicular transportation is also important. Parking a distance from the job, avoiding elevators, using stairs, delivering messages within a building rather than phoning, walking a distance for a modest lunch, etc., are useful and easily

TABLE 11–8. **Calories Expended for 10 Minutes of Physical Activity***

Activity	Body Weight				
	(kg) 56.8 (lbs) 125	68.2 150	79.5 175	90.9 200	113.6 250
Sitting quietly	10	12	14	16	20
Domestic housework	34	41	47	53	68
Walking downstairs	56	67	78	88	111
Walking upstairs	146	175	202	229	288
Walking (2 mph)[†]	29	35	40	46	58
Walking (4 mph)	52	62	72	81	102
Jogging (5.5 mph)	90	108	125	142	178
Running (7 mph)	118	141	164	187	232
Cycling (5.5 mph)	42	50	58	67	83
Cycling (13 mph)	89	107	124	142	178
Mowing grass (power)	34	41	47	53	67
Mowing grass (manual)	38	45	52	58	74
Chopping wood	60	73	84	96	121
Bowling (nonstop)	56	67	78	90	111
Dancing (moderate)	35	42	48	55	69
Dancing (vigorous)	48	57	66	75	94
Golfing (walk)	33	40	48	55	68
Skiing (cross-country)	98	117	138	158	194
Swimming (moderate crawl)	40	48	56	63	80

* Approximate values for activities that can be undertaken by many obese individuals. Values will vary with rate of exercise and efficiency with which the activity is performed. Interpolation and extrapolation can be used for subject's actual weight. (Adapted from Brownell and Stunkard.[35])
† Conversion factor mph to km·hr^{-1}: multiply by 1.6093.

accommodated suggestions for increasing energy expenditure. Brownell and Stunkard cite studies in which spontaneous use of stairs was significantly lower in obese persons.[35] A sign was instrumental in encouraging greater use of the stairs among both the lean and obese groups.

The social environment in which exercise is done can be most important. The primary sources of support are family members, friends, fellow employees, social groups, and club members; in certain instances, the community itself is important when community-wide programs are undertaken. In a collaborative study of exercise in the primary prevention of CHD, Heinzelmann and Bagley found that the attitude of the subjects' wives was important for adherence to the prescribed exercise program.[85] Among those men with wives whose attitude was positive, 80% had excellent or good patterns of adherence. In contrast, with neutral or negative attitudes, only 40% had excellent or good adherence. The wives also influenced other behavior, e.g., diet. Among those men who lost 5 kg or more during the 18-month exercise program, most had modified their diet without any instruction to do so. Brownell and Stunkard reviewed evidence that the training of spouses of overweight persons can dramatically improve the success of dietary programs.[35] Although use of a buddy system was helpful, it was not always useful. Guidelines for structuring social interactions can be found in a book by Brownell.[34]

Our use of exercise for studying weight reduction usually involves group activities.[20,21,68,115,120] Adherence has generally been quite high, i.e., greater than 90% for relatively short periods of 8 to 12 weeks. Other researchers have found good adherence in work-site programs that involve the use of such positive reinforcement techniques as rewards and well-trained leaders.[35] As a modifiable behavior, physical activity should increase in regularity if rewards are forthcoming. Unfortunately, the real rewards of body fat and weight loss, as well as improved health, are available only over the longterm, whereas the

discomfort, boredom, and pain are readily apparent. Thus, intermediate rewards or incentives are essential. Periodic praise from an exercise leader or fellow exerciser is simple but effective. Reinforcement procedures, such as a deposit with refunds contingent on adherence, are also effective.[115]

Brownell and Stunkard contend that the amount of a deposit used as a motivational device is unimportant.[35] They also contend that the important behavioral procedures of monitoring (keeping a diary or log of physical activity) and providing feedback (plotting estimated daily energy expenditure, resting heart rate, or blood pressure) can be utilized effectively. Monitoring provides a record of accomplishment and is useful for reinforcement and feedback. Because of body composition changes during weight reduction, it is interesting that use of a body weight record may be ineffective for feedback. Bray has pointed out that common problems in the successful treatment of obesity remain, such as unwillingness to seek appropriate medical help, unwillingness to maintain prescribed treatment, and termination of treatment, even though side effects might be minimal.[33] The result is a high level of therapeutic failure.

Walking: A Special Case

Obese subjects should do that form of exercise that they can accomplish and enjoy. Walking appears to be a reasonable starting point. Rapid walking may be difficult, as would walking over varied off-sidewalk or off-road terrain. Initially, goals should be set for distance covered, rather than time spent or walking speed. With progress, the distance walked can be increased and alternate or supplementary forms of exercise can be undertaken gradually. Warnold et al. established slow and fast walking regimens for obese patients with about 40% body fat.[157] Slow walking ranged from 25 to 42 m·min^{-1} (0.93 to 1.57 mph) and fast walking ranged from 45 to 75 m·min^{-1} (1.68 to 2.80 mph). Each exercise regimen started with slow walking. It is apparent that these rates are much slower than comparable walking rates for leaner people. Advantages of a walking program are listed in Table 11–9. There are many other simple activities that can be undertaken by the obese individual (Table 11–10).

Exercise in Water

Several investigations have been performed on subjects exercising in water; most were conducted on subjects who were swimming.[92,111,123] Swimming is an excellent form of exercise, and obese subjects with swimming skill could swim fast enough and far enough to expend considerable energy. Swimming-type movements and their effect upon respiratory and other responses have also been studied.[49]

Most obese people cannot swim well enough to use swimming as an effective means of regular exercise. For these individuals, alternative water exercise is appropriate, e.g., using a kickboard with or without rubber foot fins, kicking while hanging on to the side of the pool, walking or jogging in waist-deep water for a prescribed period of time or distance, playing simple games in waist-deep water, cycling on an immersed ergometer, or simulating jogging in deeper water while buoyed up with a special vest.[44,64,145] Exercise in water reduces strain on joints induced by weight bearing because the water buoyancy partially supports the body.

Other investigators have used cycling in water to study body temperature regulation and heat exchange.[51] Morlock and Dressendorfer modified a standard Monark cycle ergometer for underwater use, and found that energy expenditure was directly related to pedaling rate.[121] Obese women easily tolerated 90 $min \cdot day^{-1}$ of cycling in water, five times per week, at an intensity of 30 to 40% $\dot{V}_{O_2max}$. They were immersed to the neck in a tank and a 6.8-kg (15-lb) weighted seat belt was affixed to the waist. Pedalling rates varied among the seven subjects, but did not exceed 45 rpm. No injuries or heat stress problems arose during the 8-week study, and no learning was necessary because no special skills were required. Although the exercise intensity was relatively low, about 430 kcal were expended per 90 minutes of cycling. It is anticipated that exercise intensities that were easily tolerated could go as high as 75 to 80% $\dot{V}_{O_2max}$ for other moderately obese women, and that caloric turnover in 90 minutes could reach 700 to 900 kcal. The $\dot{V}_{O_2max}$ of the seven women was 27.7 $ml \cdot kg^{-1} \cdot min^{-1}$, ranging from 20.3 to 40.0 $ml \cdot kg^{-1} \cdot min^{-1}$. Although body weight or fat loss was not significant, reductions in fat have been shown, particularly when exercise energy expenditure exceeded 500 $kcal \cdot day^{-1}$.[120] Similar body weight and fat losses may be found with much more intense exercise in water.

Exercise in the Cold

An interesting approach to body fat and weight reduction was undertaken by O'Hara et al., who had six obese men exercise vigorously for 10 days with about 3.5

TABLE 11–9. Advantages of Walking

Avoids musculoskeletal problems associated with running
Avoids traffic hazards of cycling
Avoids inconvenience of trying to find a swimming pool
Requires no extraordinary skill
Can be done most anywhere and any time
Can produce a training effect

TABLE 11–10. Recommended Simple Physical Activities

Walking
Stair climbing
Walk-jog
Selected strength and flexibility exercises
Dancing, with or without partner
  Aerobic
  Simple steps to music
Distance swimming
Walking purposefully in waist-deep water
Cycling, perhaps on tricycle
Cycling in water

hr·day^{-1} of cycling an ergometer, walking on the treadmill, or marching and backpacking while residing in a cold chamber maintained at -34°C. The mean daily energy expenditure for these activities was 1242 kcal. There was an early water loss of about 1 kg (associated with cold-induced diuresis or mobilization of glycogen stores) and a subsequent fat loss. Fat determinations based on both skinfolds and underwater weighing indicated that body fat loss was well sustained 2 months after completion of the exercise program. The authors cite additional evidence that substantial fat loss can occur when soldiers work hard in an Arctic environment.[125] In attempting to confirm such results with a different type of cold exposure, Sheldahl had seven obese women exercise at about 40% $\dot{V}_{O_2max}$ five times per week for 8 weeks in cool water (17 to 22°C or 62.6 to 68°F) for about 90 min·day^{-1}.[145] Although some women lost a small amount of body weight and fat, these losses were non-significant. The women experienced considerable heat debt as a result of the cool water exposure, but subsequent appetite and satiety were apparently not altered. If such exercise in the cold is to be an effective mode of body weight and fat reduction, either the exercise must be more intense or more than 1.5 hr·day^{-1} must be spent in the cold.

ADHERENCE TO EXERCISE PROGRAMS

A serious problem exists in that obese individuals are not likely to become voluntarily involved in an exercise program. Their regular participation, should they start, tends to decrease appreciably after a few months.[58] Adherence can be well maintained for a few weeks to 6 months if attentive leadership and supervision are provided, making the program enjoyable and worthwhile. The problem is at least threefold: starting; maintaining adherence; and developing sufficient motivation to continue regular exercise once the supervised program has stopped.

Most studies of "drop-outs" indicate a curvilinear relationship, with a rapid early phase and then a slower phase. At 6 months, the percentage of drop-outs may vary from 20 to 50% of the original exercisers; by 12 months, the percentage has increased from 35 to 60%. In studies lasting as long as 18 months, the percentage of drop-outs was found to be 40% or more.[18,151] In referring to some of their earlier work, McMinn and Katahn found that only 15% of their subjects remained consistently active at 27 months of follow-up.[113] Studies of post-myocardial infarction patients tend to show lower rates, but the problem is serious, even with groups in which motivation to continue exercise is thought to be high.[18]

In a separate consideration of obese patients, Björntorp reported a 15% drop-out rate at 3 months and a 29% drop-out rate within 6 months among those with hyperplastic obesity, and a 24% rate at 6 months among patients with other types of obesity.[18] He also cites an unpublished study by Bjuro, who presumably recruited subjects at random from the urban area of Göteborg, Sweden. Those persons who were least active at their job or during leisure time were invited to participate. The greatest number of drop-outs occurred prior to and following the first examination (85% remained) and explanation of the exercise and research program (40% remained). Several subjects were also excluded because of medical contraindications for exercise. About 30% of those individuals originally invited subsequently participated in the exercise program and tended to remain with it. Motivating people to start was the major problem.

Our experience with an exercise program for middle-aged men indicated that the percentage of exercise sessions attended was approximately 50% at 6 months and remained about 40% at 12 months.[151] Kukkonen et al. reported comparable results, i.e., after 16.5 months of exercise, adherence was 42% among men and 44% among women.[104] Gwinup found that only 32% of obese women completed a 1-year program of modest walking.[79]

Franklin et al. conducted a program for 36 middle-aged women, of whom 23 were obese.[69] They participated in a regular exercise program for 12 weeks. Nineteen women (15 of whom were obese) were queried about their exercise during the 18 months after the supervised program, and it was clear that they were minimally active. The obese women reported an average of only 10 min·wk^{-1} of jogging, and the leaner women no more than 40 min·wk^{-1}. Fewer obese women (33%) jogged during the 18-month period, compared to 67% of the leaner women. Obese women sustained neither the regular exercise habit nor the modest weight losses resulting from the original program.

Thus, there is a need to develop methods for motivating obese subjects to start and continue an exercise program, as well as to devise combinations of diet and exercise that provide the "carrot" of reasonable fat and weight loss. Exercise is generally unpopular among the obese, and extraordinary behavior therapy may need to be applied to get them to start and particularly to continue regular exercise. An estimated retention percentage based on our experience with obese individuals is presented in Figure 11–3. The fatter the individual, the less likely the individual will adhere rigorously to the program.

Reasons for poor adherence to an exercise program are given in Table 11–11, and important considerations that could improve adherence are listed in Table 11–12.

INJURIES AND HAZARDS

Goodman and Kenrick noted that the obese population has a higher incidence of injury in walk-jog programs.[77] Pollock et al. found that percent body fat was signifi-

TABLE 11–11. **Some Reasons for Poor Adherence to an Exercise Program**

Illness
Dissatisfaction (e.g., small weight loss)
Embarrassment
Boredom
Discomfort or pain
Disability or accident
Inability to schedule activity regularly
Vacation
Work pressures
Changed jobs
Moved away
Family conflict

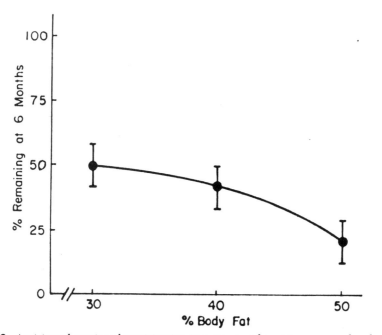

Fig. 11–3. *Anticipated continued participation in a structured exercise program by obese subjects.*

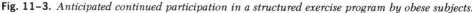

TABLE 11–12. Factors that Could Help to Improve Adherence to an Exercise Program

Select appropriate exercise
  Emphasize movement of body mass
  Emphasize all opportunities for walking
  Emphasize that all daily activities are exercise

Provide realistic expectations, no miracles
  Amount of exercise, intensity, and duration
  Time commitment and frequency
  Physiologic and psychologic changes

Provide for a slow start

Select convenient hours

Select pleasant surroundings

Provide for individual attention

Encourage group activity

Have highly motivated group leader

Record results—self-monitoring

Provide positive feedback about changes in:
  weight, fatness, work capacity, heart rate,
  blood pressure, serum lipids, glucose, insulin,
  and uric acid

Utilize deposit and refund—rewards

Emphasize re-education
  Self, family members—a commitment
  Understanding of energy turnover with diet
  and exercise

cantly related to the incidence of injuries in men undergoing a conditioning program of moderate intensity.[132] Franklin et al. found that of 36 middle-aged women, 11 sustained leg and foot injuries that were severe enough to cause a reduction in exercise intensity or discontinuation (7 of 23 obese and 4 of 13 leaner women, or about 30% for each group).[68] Nine of the 11 injuries occurred in the first 6 weeks; all were sustained within 8 weeks. Three women had a prior history of injury; two had shinsplints, three had joint sprains, and five had muscle strains, with one Achilles tendon problem. Only obese women suffered patellar dysfunction. The original program was planned to achieve an intensity of 75% $\dot{V}_{O_2max}$ for at least 15 minutes of the exercise period. After in-

jury, two women continued to exercise on a cycle ergometer after missing 1 to 1.5 weeks of exercise. The anticipated relative immobility of the obese women was compensated for by the gradual initiation of the exercise program. Virtually all obese women started with brisk walking. It was concluded that moderately obese women with no apparent musculoskeletal limitations can participate in a supervised walk-jog program with no more disorders than their leaner counterparts. The program must be based on intensities comparable with their capacities. Extra caution is needed during the first few weeks, with adequate warm-up and stretching; progressive increases in intensity, frequency, and duration; selection of appropriate apparel; and selection of appropriate environments. It is also necessary to pay special attention to the feet and footwear of the obese exerciser. The provision of orthotic devices that provide heel support or compensatory foot pronation may make exercise safer and more comfortable. Gait instruction may also be necessary. Several potential hazards associated with exercise for the obese person are listed in Table 11–13.

WEIGHT CONTROL

A major challenge in treating obesity is not the initial weight reduction, but the

TABLE 11–13. Potential Hazards of Exercise for the Obese Individual*

Precipitation of angina pectoris or myocardial infarction
Excessive rise in blood pressure
Aggravation of degenerative arthritis and other joint problems
Ligamentous injuries
Injury from falling
Excessive sweating
Skin disorders, chafing
Hypohydration and reduced circulating blood volume
Heat stroke and/or heat exhaustion

* Adapted from Horton[93] and Stunkard.[149]

205

continuing task of maintaining desired body weight and fatness. Regression to obesity is all too common. Thus, emphasis is currently placed on the achievement of a relatively permanent lifestyle change via multiple behavioral modification techniques that include dietary regulation and regular exercise.[150] Hopefully, multiple intervention approaches will prove more successful than dietary or exercise counseling that is undertaken independently. Some of the characteristics of the obese individual most likely to benefit from an exercise program are listed in Table 11–14.

If it is assumed that a variety of strategies can be employed to maintain a near-desirable weight after considerable weight has been lost, what strategies for maintaining the weight loss have proven successful? Wing and Jeffery queried 64 formerly obese individuals (42 men and 22 women) who originally averaged 43% overweight, had lost 10 kg or more, and had maintained the reduced weight for 1 year.[160] Their results appear in Table 11–15. The most common reason for losing weight was concern about appearance, but increased exercise was also important.

Gross obesity can be a disabling condition that reduces both function and performance. Clearly, establishment of the role that increased caloric turnover via regular exercise may play in the prevention of obesity, in the weight reduction

TABLE 11-15. Most Popular Strategies for Maintaining Weight Loss Among Formerly Obese Individuals *

Strategy	Percent Using Strategy
Frequent weighing	75
Reduced snacking	60
Reduced meal portions	60
Better food selection	57
Increased exercise	55

* Adapted from Wing and Jeffery.[160]

process, or in the reduced weight management process awaits additional research. If neuromotor, cardiovascular, or respiratory complications develop, such disability enhances sedentary existence through decreased muscle mass and exercise tolerance. On the basis of present knowledge, there is ample evidence that the moderately obese individual can profit in a variety of ways from participation in regular exercise. Thus, regular exercise should be encouraged and made part of any multiple intervention scheme associated with sound principles of behavioral modification.

ACKNOWLEDGMENTS. I gratefully acknowledge the assistance of Vincent Rabatin in securing many of the references and preparing the illustrations cited; Becky Nilson for typing the original manuscript and assisting with the revision; and Pat MacKeen for proofreading and helpful suggestions.

TABLE 11-14. Characteristics of the Obese Individual Most Likely to Benefit from an Exercise Program *

Slightly or moderately obese
Became obese as an adult
Had not previously tried to lose weight
Sincerely desires weight reduction
Psychologically adjusted to pursuit of weight reduction goal
Can intelligently follow directions
Has no complicating disease or disability

* Adapted from Buskirk.[39]

REFERENCES

1. Abraham, S., Lowenstein, F.W., and O'Connell, D.E.: Preliminary Findings of the First Health and Nutrition Examination Survey. United States, 1971–1972: Anthropometric and Clinical Data. DHEW Publication No. (HRA) 75-1229. Rockville, MD, USDHEW Health Resources Administration, National Center for Health Statistics, 1975.
2. Alexander, J.K.: Obesity and the circulation. Mod. Concepts Cardiovasc. Dis., 32:799, 1963.
3. Alexander, J.K., Amad, K.H., and Cole, V.W.: Observations on some clinical features of extreme obesity with particular reference to cardiorespiratory effects. Am. J. Med., 32:512, 1962.
4. Alexander, J.K., Dennis, E.W., and Smith, W.E.: Blood volume, cardiac output and distribution

of systemic blood flow in extreme obesity. Cardiovas. Res. Cent. Bull., *1*:39, 1963.

5. Alexander, J.K., and Peterson, K.L.: Cardiovascular effects of weight reduction. Circulation, *45*:310, 1972.

6. Amad, K.H., Brennan, J.C., and Alexander, J.K.: The cardiac pathology of chronic exogenous obesity. Circulation, *32*:740, 1965.

7. Anderson, J.T., Lawler, A., and Keys, A.: Weight gain from simple overeating. II. Serum lipids and blood volume. J. Clin. Invest., *36*:81, 1957.

8. Angel, A.: Pathophysiology of obesity. Can. Med. Assoc. J., *110*:540, 1978.

9. Ashley, F.W., and Kannel, W.B.: Relation of weight change to changes in atherogenic traits: the Framingham Study. J. Chronic Dis., *27*:103, 1974.

10. Aslett, E.A., Hart, P.D., and McMichael, J. The lung volume and its subdivisions in normal males. Proc. R. Soc. Lond. [Biol.], *126*:502, 1939.

11. Barrera, F., et al.: The distribution of ventilation, diffusion and blood flow in obese patients with normal and abnormal blood gases. Am. Rev. Respir. Dis., *108*:819, 1973.

12. Barrera, F., et al.: Ventilation-perfusion relationships in the obese patient. J. Appl. Physiol., *26*:420, 1969.

13. Bedell, G.N., Wilson, W.R., and Seebohm, P.M.: Pulmonary function in obese persons. J. Clin. Invest., *37*:1049, 1958.

14. Belfiore, F., Iannello, S., and Rabuazzo, A.M.: Insulin resistance in obesity: a critical analysis at enzyme level. A review. Intl. J. Obes., *3*:301, 1979.

15. Berenson, G.S., et al.: Occurrence of multiple risk-factor variables for cardiovascular disease in children. *In* Cardiovascular Risk Factors in Children. New York, Oxford University Press, 1980, pp. 311–320.

16. Björntorp, P.: Effects of age, sex and clinical conditions on adipose tissue cellularity in man. Metabolism, *23*:1091, 1974.

17. Björntorp, P.: The fat cell: a clinical view. *In* Recent Advances in Obesity Research II. Edited by G.A. Bray. London, Newman, 1978.

18. Björntorp, P.: Physical training in the treatment of obesity. *In* Comparative Methods of Weight Control. Edited by G.A. Bray. Westport, CT, Technomic Publishing, 1980, pp. 51–58.

19. Björntorp, P., et al.: The effect of physical training on insulin production in obesity. Metabolism, *19*:631, 1970.

20. Blair, D.A.: The energy expenditure and activity levels of lean, adult-onset and child-onset obese women. Ph.D. dissertation. Ithaca, NY, Cornell University, 1980.

21. Boileau, R.A., et al.: Body composition changes in obese and lean men during physical conditioning. Med. Sci. Sports, *3*:183, 1971.

22. Bosman, A.R., and Goldman, H.J.: The oxygen cost and work of breathing in normal and obese subjects. S. Afr. J. Lab. Clin. Med., *7*:62, 1961.

23. Bouchard, C., Savard, R., Després, J.P., et al.: Body composition in adopted and biological sibblings. Human Biol., *57*:61–75, 1985.

24. Bouchard, C., Tremblay, A., Després, J.P., et al.: The response to long-term overfeeding in identical twins. N. Engl. J. Med., *322*:1477–1482, 1990.

25. Boyer, J.L., and Kasch, F.W.: Exercise therapy in hypertensive men. JAMA, *211*:1668, 1970.

26. Bray, G.: Effect of caloric restriction on energy expenditure in obese subjects. Lancet, *2*:397, 1969a.

27. Bray, G.: Calorigenic effect of human growth hormone in obesity. J. Clin. Endocrinol. Metab., *29*:119, 1969b.

28. Bray, G.A. (ed.): Obesity in Perspective. Fogarty International Center Conference, Oct. 1973, Vol. 2, Part 1 and Vol. 2, Part 2, DHEW Publication No. (NIH) 75-708. Washington, D.C., U.S. Government Printing Office, 1975.

29. Bray, G.A.: The Obese Patient. Philadelphia, W.B. Saunders, 1976.

30. Bray, G.A. (ed.): Obesity in America. Washington, D.C., U.S. DHEW, NIH Publ. No. 79–359, 1979, 275 pp.

31. Bray, G.A. (ed.): Comparative Methods of Weight Control. Westport, CT, Technomic Publishing, 1980, 192 pp.

32. Bray, G.A.: Overweight is risking fate. Definition, classification, prevalence and risks. Ann. N.Y. Acad. Sci., *249*:14–28, 1987.

33. Bray, G.A.: Obesity. Present Knowledge in Nutrition. Edited by M.L. Brown. Washington, D.C., International Life Sciences Institute-Nutrition Foundation, 1990, pp. 23–38.

34. Brownell, K.D.: The Partnership Diet Program. New York, Rawson, Wade, 1980.

35. Brownell, K.D., and Stunkard, A.J.: Physical activity in the development and control of obesity. *In* Obesity. Edited by A.J. Stunkard. Philadelphia, W.B. Saunders, 1980, pp. 300–324.

36. Burwell, C.S., et al.: Extreme obesity associated with alveolar hypoventilation—a Pickwickian syndrome. Am. J. Med., *21*:811, 1956.

37. Buskirk, E.R.: Increasing energy expenditure: the role of exercise. *In* Obesity. Edited by N.L. Wilson. Philadelphia, Davis, 1969, pp. 163–176.

38. Buskirk, E.R.: Obesity. *In* The Physiologic Basis of Rehabilitation. Edited by J.A. Downey, and R.C. Darling. Philadelphia, W.B. Saunders, 1971, pp. 229–242.

39. Buskirk, E.R.: Obesity: a brief overview with emphasis on exercise. Fed. Proc., *33*:1948, 1974.

40. Buskirk, E.R., and Barlett, H.L.: Pulmonary function and obesity. *In* Advances in Modern Human Nutrition. Vol. 1. Edited by R.B. Tobin, and M.A. Mehlman. Park Forest South, IL, Pathotox, 1980, pp. 211–224.

41. Buskirk, E.R., and Taylor, H.L.: Maximal oxygen intake and its relation to body composition, with special reference to chronic physical activity and obesity. J. Appl. Physiol., *11*:72, 1957.

42. Buskirk, E.R., et al.: Energy balance of obese patients during weight reduction: influence of diet restriction and exercise. Ann. N.Y. Acad. Sci., *110*:918, 1963.

43. Buskirk, E.R., et al.: Human energy expenditure studies in the National Institute of Arthritis and Metabolic Diseases metabolic chamber—1. Interaction of cold environment and specific, 2. Sleep. Am. J. Clin. Nutr., *8*:602, 1960.

44. Castronis, M.: Jog in the pool—no pain. J. Phys. Ed., *74*:8, 18, 1976.

45. Cherniak, R.M., and Guenter, C.A.: The efficiency of the respiratory muscles in obesity. Can. J. Biochem., *39*:1215, 1961.
46. Chiang, B.N., Perlman, L.V., and Epstein, F.H.: Overweight and hypertension, a review. Circulation, *29*:403, 1969.
47. Choquette, G., and Ferguson, R.J.: Blood pressure production in "borderline" hypertensives following physical training. Can. Med. Assoc. J., *108*:699, 1973.
48. Clark, H.D., and Hoffer, L.J.: Reappraisal of the resting metabolic rate of normal young men. Am. J. Clin. Nutr., *53*:21–26, 1991.
49. Cooper, K.E., Martin, S., and Riben, P. Respiratory and other responses in subjects immersed in cold water. J. Appl. Physiol., *40*:903, 1976.
50. Costas, R., Jr., et al.: Relation of lipids, weight and physical activity to incidence of coronary heart disease: the Puerto Rico heart study. Am. J. Cardiol., *42*:653, 1978.
51. Craig, A.B., and Dvorak, M.: Comparison of exercise in air and in water of different temperatures. Med. Sci. Sports, *1*:124, 1969.
52. Cullen, J.H., and Formel, P.F.: The respiratory defects in extreme obesity. Am. J. Med., *32*:525, 1962.
53. DeLuise, M., Blackburn, G.L., and Flier, J.S.: Reduced activity of the red-cell sodium-potassium pump in human obesity. N. Engl. J. Med., *303*:1017, 1980.
54. Dempsey, J.A., et al.: Alveolar-arterial gas exchange during muscular work in obesity. J. Appl. Physiol., *21*:1807, 1966.
55. Dempsey, J.A., et al.: Work capacity determinants and physiologic cost of weight-supported work in obesity. J. Appl. Physiol., *21*:1815, 1966.
56. Després, J.P., Tremblay, A., Pérusse, L., et al.: Abdominal adipose tissue and serum HDL-cholesterol association independent from obesity and serum triglyceride concentration. Int. J. Obesity, *12*:1–13, 1988.
57. DeVore, P.A., and Nemiro, D.D.: Exercise testing of obese subjects. Physician Sportsmed., *8*:47, 1980.
58. Dishman, R.K.: Compliance/adherence in health related exercise. Health Psych., *1*:237–267, 1982.
59. Douglas, F.G., and Chong, P.Y.: Influence of obesity on peripheral airways patency. J. Appl. Physiol., *33*:559, 1972.
60. Dudleston, A.K., and Bennion, M.: Effect of diet and/or exercise on obese college women. J. Am. Diet. Assoc., *56*:126, 1970.
61. Edelman, I.S., and Ismail-Beigi, F.: Thyroid thermogenesis and active sodium transport. Recent Prog. Horm. Res., *30*:235, 1974.
62. Emirgil, C., and Sobol, B.J.: The effects of weight reduction on pulmonary function and the sensitivity of the respiratory center in obesity. Am. Rev. Respir. Dis., *108*:831, 1973.
63. Epstein, L.H., Masek, B., and Marshall, W.: Pre-lunch exercise and lunch-time caloric intake. Behav. Therapist, *1*:15, 1978.
64. Evans, B.W., Cureton, K.J., and Purvis, J.W.: Metabolic and circulatory responses to walking and jogging in water. Res. Q., *49*:442, 1978.
65. Farebrother, M.J.B., McHardy, G.J.R., and Munro, J.F.: Relation between pulmonary gas exchange and closing volume before and after substantial weight loss in obese subjects. Br. Med. J., *3*:391, 1974.
66. Fletcher, A.P.: The effect of weight reduction upon the blood pressure of obese hypertensive women. Q. J. Med., *23*:331, 1954.
67. Franklin, B.A.: Effects of a 12-week physical conditioning program on cardiorespiratory function, body composition, and serum lipids of normal and obese middle-aged women. Ph.D. dissertation. University Park, PA, The Pennsylvania State University, 1976.
68. Franklin, B., et al.: Effects of physical conditioning on cardiorespiratory function, body composition and serum lipids in relatively normal-weight and obese middle-aged women. Int. J. Obes., *3*:97, 1979.
69. Franklin, B.A., MacKeen, P.C., and Buskirk, E.R.: Body composition effects of a 12-week physical conditioning program for normal and obese middle-aged women, and status at 18-month follow-up. Int. J. Obes., *2*:394, 1978.
70. Frerichs, R.R., et al.: Relation of serum lipids and lipoproteins to obesity and sexual maturity in white and black children. Am. J. Epidemiol., *108*:486, 1978.
71. Garn, S.M., Bailey, S.M., and Block, W.D.: Relationships between fatness and lipid level in adults. Am. J. Clin. Nutr., *32*:733, 1979.
72. Garn, S.M., and Clark, D.C.: Trends in fatness and the origins of obesity. Pediatrics, *57*:443, 1976.
73. Garrow, J.S.: Energy Balance and Obesity in Man. 2nd Ed. New York, Elsevier, 1978, 243 pp.
74. Gilbert, R., Sipple, J.H., and Auchincloss, J.H., Jr.: Respiratory control and work of breathing in obese subjects. J. Appl. Physiol., *16*:21, 1961.
75. Glass, A.R.: Endocrine aspects of obesity. Med. Clin. North Am., *73*:139–160, 1989.
76. Glueck, C.J., et al.: Plasma high-density lipoprotein cholesterol: association with measurements of body mass. Circulation, *62*(Suppl. IV):IV62, 1980.
77. Goodman, C.E., and Kenrick, M.M.: Physical fitness in relation to obesity. Obes. Bar. Med., *4*:12, 1975.
78. Gordon, T., et al.: Diabetes, blood lipids, and the role of obesity in coronary heart disease risk for women. The Framingham Study. Ann. Intern. Med., *87*:393, 1977.
79. Gwinup, G.: Effect of exercise alone on the weight of obese women. Arch. Intern. Med., *135*:676, 1975.
80. Hackney, J.D., et al.: Syndrome of extreme obesity and hypoventilation: studies of etiology. Ann. Intern. Med., *51*:541, 1959.
81. Hafen, B.Q.: Nutrition, Food and Weight Control. Boston, Allyn and Bacon, 1981, pp. 201–226, 227–250.
82. Halliday, D., et al.: Resting metabolic rate, weight, surface area and body composition in obese women. Intl. J. Obes., *3*:1, 1979.
83. Hanson, J.S., et al.: Long-term physical training and cardiovascular dynamics in middle-aged men. Circulation, *38*:783, 1968.
84. Haymes, E.M., McCormick, R.J., and Buskirk, E.R.: Heat tolerance of exercising lean and obese prepubertal boys. J. Appl. Physiol., *39*:457, 1975.

85. Heinzelmann, F., and Bagley, R.W.: Response to physical activity programs and their effects on health behavior. Public Health Rep., 85:905, 1970.
86. Heyden, S., et al.: Weight and weight history in relation to cerebrovascular and ischemic heart disease. Arch. Intern. Med., 128:956, 1971.
87. Hirsch, J., and Batchelor, B.: Adipose tissue cellularity and human obesity. Clin. Endocrinol. Metab., 5:299, 1976.
88. Hodgson, J.L., and Buskirk, E.R.: Physical fitness and age, with emphasis on cardiovascular function in the elderly. J. Am. Geriat. Soc., 25:385, 1977.
89. Hoffmans, M., et al.: Resting metabolic rate in obese and normal weight women. Intl. J. Obes., 3:111, 1979.
90. Holley, H.S., et al.: Regional distribution of pulmonary ventilation and perfusion in obesity. J. Clin. Invest., 46:475, 1967.
91. Holm, G., Björntorp, P., and Jagenburg, R.: Carbohydrate, lipid, and amino and metabolism following physical exercise in man. J. Appl. Physiol., 45:128, 1978.
92. Holmér, I., and Bergh, V.: Metabolic and thermal response to swimming in water at various temperatures. J. Appl. Physiol., 37:702, 1974.
93. Horton, E.S.: The role of exercise in the prevention and treatment of obesity. In G.A. Bray (ed.): Obesity in Perspective. Vol. 2, Part 1. DHEW Publication No. (NIH) 75-708. Washington, D.C., U.S. Government Printing Office, 1975, pp. 62–66.
94. Imperial, E.S., Gass, G., Mitchell, R., et al.: Graded exercise testing protocol for the elderly. J. Cardiopulm. Rehabil., 10:465–470, 1990.
95. James, W.P.T.: Research on Obesity: A Report to the DHSS/MRC Group. London, Her Majesty's Stationery Office, 1976, p. 94.
96. Jung, R.T., et al.: Does adipocyte hypercellularity in obesity exist? Br. Med. J., 2:319, 1978.
97. Kaltman, A.J., and Goldring, R.M.: Role of circulatory congestion in the cardiorespiratory failure of obesity. Am. J. Med., 60:645, 1976.
98. Kannel, W.B., and Gordon, T.: Obesity and cardiovascular disease: the Framingham Study. In Obesity. Edited by W. Burland, P.D. Samuel, and J. Yudkin. London, Churchill Livingstone, 1974.
99. Kannel, W.B., Gordon, T., and Castelli, W.P.: Obesity, lipids, and glucose intolerance. The Framingham Study. Am. J. Clin. Nutr., 32:1238, 1979.
100. Kaufman, B.J., Ferguson, M.H., and Cherniak, R.M.: Hypoventilation in obesity. J. Clin. Invest., 38:500, 1959.
101. Keys, A.: Overweight, obesity, coronary heart disease and mortality. Nutr. Rev., 38:297, 1980.
102. Keys, A., et al.: Coronary heart disease: overweight and obesity as risk factors. Ann. Intern. Med., 77:15, 1972.
103. Keys, A., and Brozek, J.: Body fat in adult man. Physiol. Rev., 33:245, 1953.
104. Kukkonen, K., et al.: Individually programmed training for use in health care centers: effects on middle-age obese subjects. In Biochemistry of Exercise IV-A. Edited by J. Poortmans, and G. Niset. Baltimore, University Park Press, 1981, pp. 289–290.
105. Lesser, G.T., Deutsch, S., and Markofsky, J.: Use of independent measurement of body fat to evaluate overweight and underweight. Metabolism, 20:792, 1971.
106. Lew, E.A., and Garfinkel, L.: Variations in mortality by weight among 750,000 men and women. J. Chronic Dis., 32:563, 1979.
107. Lewis, S., et al.: Effects of physical activity on weight reduction in obese middle-aged women. Am. J. Clin. Nutr., 29:151, 1976.
108. Lissner, L., Andres, R., Muller, D.C., and Shimokata, H.: Body weight variability in men: metabolic rate, health and longevity. Int. J. Obesity, 14:373–383, 1990.
109. Lopez-S., A., et al.: Effect of exercise and physical fitness on serum lipids and lipoproteins. Atherosclerosis, 20:1, 1974.
110. Luce, J.M.: Respiratory complications of obesity. Chest, 78:626, 1980.
111. McArdle, W.D., et al.: Metabolic and cardiovascular adjustment to work in air and water at 18, 25 and 33°C. J. Appl. Physiol., 40:85, 1976.
112. McCormick, R.J., and Buskirk, E.R.: Heat tolerance of exercising lean and obese middle-aged men. Fed. Proc., 33:441, 1974 (Abstract).
113. McMinn, M.R., and Katahn, M.: Energy expenditure in obesity—Part II. J. Obesity Wt. Reg., 5:146–165, 1986.
114. MacMahon, S.W., Wilcken, D.E.L., and MacDonald, G.J.: The effect of weight reduction on left ventricular mass: a randomized controlled trial in young overweight hypertensive patients. N. Engl. J. Med., 314:334–379, 1986.
115. Mahoney, K.B.: Adipose cellularity as a predictor of responsiveness to treatment of obesity. Ph.D. dissertation. University Park, PA, The Pennsylvania State University, 1977.
116. Mann, G.V.: Obesity, the nutritional spook. Am. J. Public Health, 61:1491, 1971.
117. Mayer, J., Roy, P., and Mitra, K.P.: Relation between caloric intake, body weight and physical work: studies in an industrial male population in West Bengal. Am. J. Clin. Nutr., 4:169, 1956.
118. Mayer, J.: Overweight: Causes, Cost, and Control. Englewood Cliffs, NJ, Prentice-Hall; 1968, 213 pp.
119. Miettinen, T.A.: Cholesterol production in obesity. Circulation, 44:842, 1971.
120. Moody, D., Kollias, J., and Buskirk, E.R.: The effect of a moderate exercise program on body weight and skinfold thickness in overweight college women. Med. Sci. Sports, 1:75, 1969.
121. Morlock, J.F., and Dressendorfer, R.H.: Modification of a standard bicycle ergometer for underwater use. Undersea Biomed. Res., 1:335, 1974.
122. Naimark, A., and Cherniak, R.M.: Compliance of the respiratory system and its components in health and obesity. J. Appl. Physiol., 15:377, 1960.
123. Nielsen, B., and Davies, C.T.M.: Temperature regulation during exercise in water and air. Acta. Physiol. Scand., 98:500, 1976.
124. O'Hara, W.J., Allen, C., and Shephard, R.J.: Treatment of obesity by exercise in the cold. Can. Med. Assoc. J., 8:773, 1977a.

125. O'Hara, W.J., Allen, C., and Shephard, R.J.: Loss of body weight and fat during exercise in a cold chamber. Eur. J. Appl. Physiol., *37*:205, 1977b.

126. Oja, P.: Intensity and frequency of physical conditioning as determinants of the cardiovascular responses of middle-aged men at rest and during exercise. Ph.D. dissertation. University Park, PA, The Pennsylvania State University, 1973.

127. Olefsky, J., Reaven G.M., and Farquhar, J.W.: Effects of weight reduction on obesity. Studies of lipid and carbohydrates metabolism in normal and hyperlipoproteinemic subjects. J. Clin. Invest., *53*:64, 1974.

128. Oscai, L.B., and Williams, B.T.: Effect of exercise on overweight middle-aged males. J. Am. Geriat. Soc., *16*:794, 1968.

129. Oscai, L.B.: The role of exercise in weight control. *In* Exercise and Sports Sciences Review. Vol. 1. Edited by J. Wilmore. New York, Academic Press, 1973, pp. 103–123.

130. Owen, O.E., Holup, J.L., D'Alessio, D.A., et al.: A reappraisal of the caloric requirements of men. Am. J. Clin. Nutr., *46*:875–885, 1987.

131. Paul, O.: A longitudinal study of coronary heart disease. Circulation, *28*:20, 1963.

132. Pollock, M.L., et al.: Effects of frequency and duration of training on attrition and incidence of injury. Med. Sci. Sports, *9*:31, 1977.

133. Pollock, M.L., et al.: Effects of walking on body composition and cardiovascular function of middle-aged men. J. Appl. Physiol., *30*:126, 1971.

134. Prodger, S.H., and Dennig, H.: A study of the circulation in obesity. J. Clin. Invest., 11:789, 1932.

135. Profant, G.R., et al.: Responses to maximal exercise in healthy middle-aged women. J. Appl. Physiol., *33*:595, 1972.

136. Ray, C.S., Sue, D.Y., Bray, G.A., et al.: Effects of obesity on respiratory function. Am. Rev. Respir. Dis., *128*:501–506, 1983.

137. Reisin, E., et al.: Effect of weight loss without salt restriction on the reduction of blood pressure in overweight hypertensive patients. N. Engl. J. Med., *298*:1, 1978.

138. Robinson, S.C., and Brucer, M.: Hypertension, body build and obesity. Am. J. Med. Sci., *199*:819, 1940.

139. Rochester, D.F., and Enson, Y.: Current concepts in the pathogenesis of the obesity-hypoventilation syndrome. Am. J. Med., *57*:402, 1974.

140. Ruderman, N.B., Ganda, O.P., and Johansen, K.: The effect of physical training on glucose tolerance and plasma lipids in maturity-onset diabetes. Diabetes, *28*(Suppl. 1):89, 1979.

141. Said, S.I.: Abnormalities of pulmonary gas exchange in obesity. Ann. Intern. Med., *53*:1121, 1960.

142. Scheen, A., et al.: Fuel-hormone response during prolonged exercise in obese subjects. *In* Biochemistry of Exercise IV-A. Edited by J. Poortmans and G. Niset. Baltimore, University Park Press, 1981, pp. 292–293.

143. Scheuer, J., and Tipton, C.M.: Cardiovascular adaptations to physical training. Annu. Rev. Physiol., *39*:221, 1977.

144. Sharp, J.T., Henry, J.P., and Sweany, S.K.: The total work of breathing in normal and obese men. J. Clin. Invest., *43*:728, 1964.

145. Sheldahl, L.M.: Effects of exercise in cool water on body weight loss and thermoregulation of women. Ph.D. dissertation. University Park, PA, Pennsylvania State University, 1978, 140 pp.

146. Sjöstrom, L., et al.: Cellularity in different regions of adipose tissue in young men and women. Metabolism, *21*:1143, 1972.

147. Sontag, L.: Implication of fetal behavior and environment for adult personalities. Ann. N.Y. Acad. Sci., *134*:782, 1965.

148. Staten, M.A.: The effect of exercise on food intake in men and women. Am. J. Clin. Nutr., *53*:27–31, 1991.

149. Stunkard, A.J. (ed.): Obesity. Philadelphia, W.B. Saunders, 1980, 470 pp.

150. Talbot, J.M.: Research Needs in Management of Obesity by Severe Caloric Restriction. Bethesda, MD, Life Sciences Research Office, Federation of American Societies for Experimental Biology, 1979.

151. Taylor, H.L., Buskirk, E.R., and Remington, R.D.: Exercise in controlled trials for the prevention of coronary heart disease. Fed. Proc., *32*:1623, 1973.

152. Terry, A.H.: Obesity and hypertension. JAMA, *81*:1283, 1923.

153. Thomas, C.B., and Hirschhorn, B.: The familial occurrence of hypertension and coronary artery disease with observations concerning obesity and diabetes. Ann. Intern. Med., *42*:90, 1955.

154. Thomas, A.E., McKay, D.A., and Cutlip, M.B.: A nomogram method for assessing body weight. Am. J. Clin. Nutr., *29*:302, 1976.

155. U.S. Department of Health, Education and Welfare: Obesity and Health. Washington, D.C., U.S. DHEW, PHS Publication No. 1485, 1966, 77 pp.

156. U.S. Department of Health and Human Services: Promoting Health/Preventing Disease: Objectives for the Nation. Washington, D.C., Public Health Service, 1980, 102 pp.

157. Warnold, I., et al.: Energy intake and expenditure in selected groups of hospital patients. Am. J. Clin. Nutr., *31*:742, 1978.

158. West, K.M.: Obesity in America (editorial). Ann. Intern. Med., *92*:854, 1980.

159. Wiley, J.A., and Camacho, T.C.: Life-style and future health: evidence from the Alameda County Study. Prev. Med., *9*:1, 1980.

160. Wing, R.R., and Jeffrey, R.W.: Successful losers: a descriptive analysis of the process of weight reduction. Obes. Bar. Med., *7*:190, 1978.

161. Wolfe, L.A., et al.: Pulmonary function at rest and during exercise in uncomplicated obesity. Res. Q., *47*:829, 1976

162. Young, C.M., and DiGiacomo, M.M.: Protein utilization and changes in body composition during weight reduction. Metabolism, *14*:1084, 1965.

12
CHAPTER

Asthma

by
Alan R. Morton and Kenneth D. Fitch

The relationship of asthma to exercise can be described as paradoxical. Most asthmatics will experience bronchoconstriction during, but mostly after exertion, a fact known for nearly nineteen centuries.[1] Conversely, current opinion considers exercise to be an integral component in the total management of asthma. Indeed, the first documented exercise prescription was given to the Archbishop of Edinburgh by Professor Cardan of Pavia in 1551. The 40-year-old cleric, severely incapacitated by asthma, was recommended to take a daily horseback ride and in conjunction with other appropriate measures was greatly improved.[41] Another notable asthmatic who benefited from exercise was Theodore Roosevelt, later President of the United States. Advised by his physician to undertake a strenuous exercise program during adolescence, Roosevelt did so with enthusiasm and became a fine athlete at Harvard, only mildly inconvenienced by asthma.[64]

This chapter will review the relationship of exercise to asthma, exercise testing, and exercise prescription, including anticipated benefits for asthmatics and drugs to reduce, prevent, and relieve exercise-induced asthma (EIA).

DEFINITION AND INCIDENCE

Asthma may be defined as a condition "characterized by an increased responsiveness of the airways to various stimuli and manifested by a diffuse narrowing of the airways that changes in severity either spontaneously or as a result of treatment."[5] Asthma occurs among members of all races, with the first episode occurring at any age.

Asthma is one of the most common respiratory disorders; its incidence is greatest in the first decade of life. It is more common in boys than girls (3:2 ratio) but more common in older women than older men. At any one time, the occurrence of asthmatic symptoms is considered to be between 4 and 16% of the population, depending on the country. In the United States, it is the leading cause of disease in those under 17 years of age, with an estimated 1.5 million asthmatics in this age group, and asthma is responsible for 23% of all days off school.[63] Currently, asthma is believed to be an inflammatory condition and the consequence of the release of potent mediators.[10] Airflow limitation is principally caused by contraction of airway smooth muscle compounded by mucosal edema and impaired mucociliary function.

EIA may be defined as "15% or greater postexercise reduction of either the forced expiratory volume in the first second (FEV_1) or the peak expiratory flow rate (PEFR) on pre-exercise values after standard submaximal exercise stress."[50] It is customary to use an exercise challenge of 6 to 8 min at 65 to 75% of predicted maximal oxygen uptake ($\dot{V}_{O_2max}$), which is approximately 75 to 85% of predicted maximal heart rate (HR_{max}). Following such an exercise challenge, 80 to 90% of asthmatics can be expected to develop EIA. The resultant postexercise bronchoconstriction can be classified as follows:

MILD   15–29% fall in FEV_1 or PEFR

MODERATE   30–44% fall in FEV_1 or PEFR

SEVERE   45% or greater fall in FEV_1 or PEFR

CAUSES OF EIA

Despite the early recognition of the association between exercise and asthma and extensive research into EIA during the last 30 years, no mechanism that satisfactorily explains its occurrence has been proposed and received general acceptance. A number of initiating stimuli have been postulated but the best hypothesis is that EIA is caused by the release of some bronchoconstrictor substance, probably in response to the changes in osmolarity of the periciliary fluid. This change is thought to occur as a result of the loss of fluid from the airways during the conditioning of the inspired air.[31]

Conditioning the air refers to the warming, humidifying, and filtering of the inspired air and is important in preventing damage to the delicate alveolar tissue, damage that can occur when it is exposed to cold dry air. Most of the conditioning occurs in the nose, the pharynx, and the first seven generations of the bronchi. The asthmatic should inhale through the nose during rest and light exercise to maximize this warming and humidification process. Even when dry air at 0° iC is inspired through the nose, it is modified so that it has been warmed to 37° iC by the time it reaches the alveolar membrane. This saturation of alveolar air occurs by absorbing water from the airways during its passage from the nose to alveolar regions. This "dries" the airways, thereby concentrating the ions in the periciliary fluid. Asthmatics appear to be unusually sensitive to these changes in osmolarity.

The released broncho-active mediators may include histamine, leukotrienes, or prostaglandins released from the mast cells and epithelial cells. They may act directly on smooth muscle, stimulate lung irritant receptors (which in turn causes bronchoconstriction via vagal influences), and/or produce the inflammation reaction via such constituents as neutrophil chemotactic factor. Cooling of the airways may enhance the response to water loss.[20]

RELATIONSHIP OF EXERCISE TO ASTHMA

Although breathlessness is normal during high-intensity exercise, it is abnormal if it occurs during or after light exercise. Unfortunately, many asthmatics do not realize this fact and are unaware that they develop EIA. They assume that their dyspnea is just lack of fitness, fail to seek medical advice, and perform at a disadvantage because of a lack of appropriate medication.

At least 80% of asthmatics develop EIA after standardized exercise tests,[7] and almost all asthmatics occasionally develop airway narrowing with physical exertion. Exercise, therefore, may be used as a challenge test to confirm the diagnosis of asthma. It is also used to determine the category of EIA severity into which a given asthmatic is classified. In addition, exercise is widely used in asthma research to determine 1) the efficacy of various medications in preventing and/or reversing asthma and 2) the effects of agents that reduce and aggravate EIA, such as face masks and certain environmental conditions.

Between episodes of asthma, the cardiorespiratory system is normal in many asthmatics and does not interfere with physical performance. This is indicated by the vast number of asthmatics who are classified as elite athletes. An asthmatic's exercise performance and the ability to endure will certainly be impaired, however, if he or she participates while airways are constricted. Narrowed airways will limit ventilation and thus oxygen uptake. When hyperinflation occurs, usually as a result of early airway closure, it is an attempt to use the assistance of increased elastic recoil to maintain adequate air flow. However, ventilation at high lung volumes requires the respiratory muscles to operate at a me-

212

chanical disadvantage, utilizing the more inefficient part of the length-tension range. This can lead to respiratory muscle fatigue.

Provocation of Asthma by Exercise

When exercise provokes a bout of asthma, there is a characteristic response. First, there is bronchodilation, which may last the duration of the activity or may persist for just a few minutes. This bronchodilation is followed by narrowing of the airways, an event that accelerates as soon as exercise is ceased. The narrowed airway increases the resistance of air flow, reaching a peak 2 to 10 min after cessation of exercise.

Airway narrowing is probably a result of not only contraction of the smooth muscle surrounding the airway but also of airway inflammation. When the airway wall is thickened because of inflammation, there will be an exaggerated reduction in the size of the airway lumen as a result of a given degree of muscle shortening.[34]

Bronchoconstriction usually reverses spontaneously, and the resistance to airflow gradually returns to pre-exercise levels in 45 to 60 min.[35] Whenever spontaneous recovery does not occur, medication may need to be administered to reverse the EIA.

The pattern of change in airway resistance with exercise is usually evaluated by measuring the change in FEV_1 (PEFR) (Fig. 12–1). The relative instability of the airways, that is, the susceptibility for change in airway diameter is indicated by the lability index, which is computed by summing the exercise-induced percentage increase in FEV_1 or (PEFR) during bronchodilation and the postexercise maximal percentage decrease in FEV_1 (or PEFR) during bronchoconstriction (see Fig. 12–1). A lability index greater than 20 is usually considered abnormally high.[11]

The above indicates that some asthmatics do not exhibit EIA until after exercise has ceased, whereas others will develop it during the active period; this latter group will be at a greater disadvantage during sport. The longer the event, the more se-

vere the EIA in these asthmatics and the greater the limitation placed on the delivery of oxygen to the active tissue. The symptoms that may develop during an episode of EIA include wheezing, shortness of breath, chest tightness, cough, increased production of mucus, and the inability to continue exercise.

Another exercise response that some asthmatics, particularly children, display is termed the late or second reaction. This may not develop for 3 to 4 hours after cessation of exercise, and may take 3 to 9 hours to reach its peak. This late response is probably due to an inflammatory reaction due to such mediators as neutrophil chemotactic factor.[40]

About 50% of asthmatics exhibit a refractory period after exercise. During this period, a second bout of exercise will provoke an airway response that is less than 50% of the initial response.[56] This refractory period may last an hour or longer but refractoriness is usually lost within 2 to 4 hours.

Exercise in the Management of Asthma

Regular exercise is an important component in the management of the disease because of its beneficial effects on respiratory and circulatory function and on the psychological development of asthmatics, which is reflected in its effect on their social life. These training benefits are manifested in the improved working capacity due to an increased $\dot{V}_{O_2max}$, as well as improved skill and efficiency during motor tasks. This means that the same daily tasks can be performed with less ventilation and thus less drying of the airways. In general, asthmatics should be able to participate in regular exercise and sports with a minimum of restriction.

Modification of the Asthmatic Response to Exercise

Selection of Exercise

The asthmatic's response to exercise is extremely variable from person to person and even in the same person at different times. There is evidence showing that the

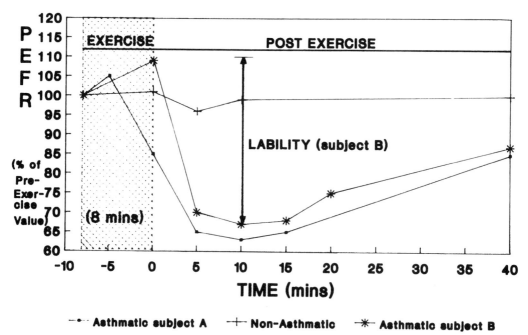

Fig. 12–1. *Typical changes in peak expiratory flow rate (PEFR) following exercise in asthmatic and nonasthmatic subjects.*

type,[26,27,35,36,59,61] duration,[35,36,47,58] and intensity[58] of exercise, as well as the type of exercise loading,[46] the environmental conditions,[12,31,62] and pharmacologic intervention, can all modify the responses to a bout of exercise.

Briefly, the evidence indicates that if modes of exercise are ranked by asthmogenicity, swimming and walking would be the least asthmogenic activities, progressing through cycling and kayaking to running, which provokes the most severe asthma. There is evidence that exercise of short duration induces less EIA than prolonged activity, but that this increasing airway response with increasing duration plateaus at about 6 to 8 min. There is also an increase in airway resistance with a higher exercise intensity up to about 65 to 75% of one's $\dot{V}_{O_2max}$ or about 75 to 85% of predicted HR_{max}.

At least for changes in type, duration, and intensity, these differences in response can be partially explained by the difference in ventilatory requirements. For instance, the more intense and the longer the duration of activity, the larger the minute ventilation required and thus the greater the loss of fluid from the airways, resulting in a larger degree of airway drying and a greater increase in osmolarity of the periciliary fluid. Studies that have used the various exercise modes but standardized the effort to ensure equal ventilation and air humidity have found the asthmogenicity of running, walking, cycling, and arm cranking to be similar.[11] Swimming allows one to inhale moist air from just above the surface of the water and may explain some of its lower asthmogenicity when compared to other modes of activity.

Although the amount of water loss can account for much of the variability in response, it does not appear to be the only factor involved. For instance, Inbar et al. showed that when the water content of inspirate was kept constant (using dry air) and a similar ventilation was induced, swimming still produced smaller reduction in lung function than running.[33] They also found that if asthmatics breathing dry air and breathing moist air were compared while swimming, there was no significant difference. Bar-Yishay et al. showed a small but significant difference in the asthmogenicity of swimming and running, even under conditions of the same metabolic stress and respiratory heat loss.[13] The fact that the effects of changes in exercise duration plateau at 6 to 8 min and intensity peaks at 75 to 85% HR_{max} is also difficult to explain if accepting the osmolarity theory alone. That is, one would expect that the longer one exercises and the higher the intensity, the greater the total ventilation and total water loss. One explanation might be that there is a maximal amount of airway narrowing possible for a given individual; once this has been accomplished, further stimuli produce no further change.

A comparison of the efficacy of salbutamol, ipratropium bromide, and cromolyn sodium in the prevention of bronchospasm induced by exercise and hyperosmolar challenges also suggest that hyperosmolarity, though playing a role in EIA, may not be the sole factor involved.[18]

Use of Aids to Warm and Humidify Inspired Air

Under resting conditions, breathing through the nose warms and humidifies the air to ensure that when the inspired air reaches the delicate alveolar membrane, it is warmed to 37° iC[69] and completely saturated with water vapor ($pH_2O = 47$ mm Hg). As the metabolic rate is raised with increasing exercise intensity, there is a change in ventilation from about 6 L · min^{-1} at rest to levels above 200 L · min^{-1} in some elite athletes performing maximal exercise. The protection from EIA that could be expected by breathing through the nose is limited to light exercise, as the size of the nostrils allow a maximum of about 40 to 60 L · min^{-1} of nasal ventilation. Nasal resistance to air flow increases with exercise and eventually reaches a critical ventilation value (usually about 40 L · min^{-1}), at which time respiration is switched from the nose to the mouth. To facilitate the benefits of nasal breathing, Bar-Or has recommended that a nasal va-

soconstrictor be prescribed for those with allergic rhinitis.[11]

There have been a number of aids suggested to maintain a warmer and more moist inspirate during exercise in an attempt to minimize the asthmatic response. For instance, surgical face masks and similar devices have been used with benefit during training sessions, especially during cold weather. Another mask that can be successfully adapted for use with asthmatics exercising in cold weather has been used with angina patients wishing to exercise during the Canadian winter (Fig. 12–2).[37] This mask is a simple plastic disposable oxygen mask to which a piece of flexible plastic tubing approximately 30 cm long has been attached. The mask fits over the mouth and nose and is held in place by an elastic headband. The tubing is placed beneath the asthmatic's T-shirt.

There are also a number of commercially produced products such as BLO.GO which consists of a mouthpiece attached to a small tube containing material that traps heat and moisture from the exhaled

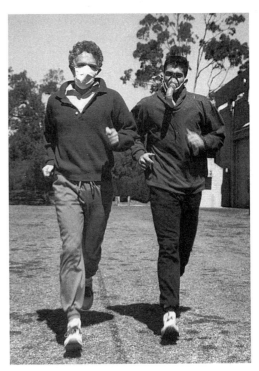

Fig. 12–2. *Cold weather exercising masks.*

215

air and so ensures a warmer and moister inspirate. That is, it is a heat exchanger that conserves the heat and moisture of the exhaled breath within the exchanger, instead of allowing them to be wasted to the atmosphere.

It is obvious that although these aids can be useful during training sessions, they are usually impractical to use during competition itself.

When and Where to Exercise

Asthma may be provoked by many factors other than exercise. It is wise to avoid as many of these other provoking agents as possible during exercise, because the effects may be cumulative. For instance, because breathing cold dry air is a potent stimulus for EIA, one should either avoid exercise during the coldest part of the day (early morning or evening) or exercise indoors. Because air pollution can provoke an episode of asthma, exercise should be avoided during those daily periods when pollution is highest. Exercising near busy roadways and factories is also contraindicated. At times when air pollution levels are high, asthmatics should perform their exercise training programs indoors.

Those asthmatics who are allergic to certain grasses and pollens should avoid outdoor exercise when pollen counts are high. For those who are allergic to dust, the opposite might be true, especially if indoor programs require the use of the older, dusty, stuffing-filled gymnastic mats or dusty rooms. Jumping rope in dusty rooms or in dusty outdoor playgrounds can also stir up dust particles and trigger an episode of bronchospasm. Asthmatics must avoid smoke-filled rooms when exercising. Smoking should not be permitted in any indoor sporting arena because of the effects of passive smoking.

If an asthmatic chooses swimming as the mode of exercise and is susceptible to the effects of cold water, a heated pool should be used. Experience has shown that there appears to be little likelihood of EIA being provoked by chlorinated water.

Warm-Up

A thorough warm-up has a threefold benefit for the asthmatic participant. Firstly, the usual benefits attributed to warm-up prior to vigorous exercise apply to the asthmatic. Secondly, a warm-up, which may or may not provoke EIA, can reduce the severity and duration of EIA triggered by a second exercise session. For asthmatics who experience a refractory period following an initial bout of EIA,[56] a warm-up can be scheduled so that the asthmatic has time to recover from the EIA that it triggers, and then be in the refractory state during the competitive event. Reiff et al. demonstrated that a prolonged warm-up period of low-intensity exercise can induce refractoriness to EIA without itself inducing marked bronchoconstriction.[54] Anderson suggests that those who demonstrate a refractory period and who are required to perform vigorous exercise at regular intervals throughout the day or those who exercise for long periods may have an advantage.[6] She claims that these asthmatics can prevent a second attack of EIA with a reduction or even elimination of further medication. Thirdly, there is some evidence that a thorough warm-up included as part of an exercise session can reduce the EIA that occurs as a result of that session.[55]

Medications

The asthmatic's response to exercise can be modified most by the judicious use of medication. This requires that asthmatics and their physicians determine the best medication program for control of their chronic asthma and then determine which pre-exercise medication(s) and dose(s) provide the best protection from EIA. A discussion of the various medications follows.

DRUGS FOR EIA

During the last 25 years, several pharmacologically different groups of drugs have been developed to assist the asthmatic by minimizing EIA. They appear to act via several different sites and mechanisms, including smooth muscle relaxation, inhibition of release of bronchoconstrictor mediators, reduction of mucosal edema and permeability, and alteration of vagal tone. The beta-2 agonists, khellin derivatives, methyl xanthines, glucocorticosteroids, and belladonna alkaloids will be discussed.

Beta-2 Agonists

These sympathomimetic amines are the most effective drugs to prevent and reverse EIA.[8] Beta-2 adrenoceptor stimulants have replaced their predecessors (e.g., ephedrine, which is also an alpha receptor stimulant, and isoproterenol), which stimulate both beta-1 and beta-2 receptor stimulants. The latter two drugs can no longer be justifiably termed acceptable therapeutic agents in the management of EIA.

Metaproterenol, albuterol (salbutamol), terbutaline, fenoterol, rimiterol, and biltolterol are about equally effective when administered by the aerosol route.[25] About 90% of asthmatics obtain clinical protection from pre-exercise beta-2 agonists. Because of the much lower dosage, greater rapidity of action, and fewer side effects, the aerosol route is always preferred to oral administration, except in very young children who cannot manipulate hand-held aerosols. It is essential that the correct inhaler technique be used, because many asthmatics use faulty techniques, reducing the effectiveness of the medication. A recent innovation, a "spacer" (which is a plastic inhalational chamber used in conjunction with hand-held nebulizers), greatly facilitates the amount of the drug reaching the lungs in those who have trouble coordinating inhalation and activation of the metered dose inhaler. The required number of activations are released into the chamber, and the patient slowly and deeply inhales the aerosol cloud through a one-way valve. This obviates the need to synchronize the rapid release of drug particles with a rapid, deep inhalation.

The usual dosage is one to two activations shortly prior to exercise. Because these beta-2 agonists are potent bronchodilators, a similar dose may be administered if EIA supervenes and is promptly effective in most asthmatics. Principal side effects (e.g., tremor, nervousness, tachycardia, and palpitations) are more frequent following oral administration.

Khellin Derivatives

Cromolyn sodium, now in clinical use for 25 years, remains the principal example, and is totally or partially effective in about 70% of asthmatics.[39] Intrinsic asthmatics are generally less responsive. However, a recently released khellin derivative, nedocromil sodium, appears to be equipotent with cromolyn, but perhaps more effective in intrinsic asthma.[48]

Initially, cromolyn was administered by inhalation of the dry powder via a spinhaler. However, the preferred method is now via a metered-dose inhaler, which is a more effective delivery system.[57] Children appear more responsive to cromolyn than adults are, as do asthmatics who do not experience airway obstruction prior to exercise. Cromolyn administration should be preceded by a beta agonist in persons with airway obstruction.

The infrequent late response, that is, postexercise bronchoconstriction occurring some hours after exercise, is blocked by cromolyn but not by beta agonists.[6] Cromolyn is free of side effects, except for its bitter taste.

Methyl Xanthines

Theophylline and, to a lesser degree, aminophylline (theophylline ethylene diamine) are usually prescribed for regular oral administration to attain and maintain serum concentrations of 10 to 20 $\mu g/ml$ to control asthma and EIA.[23] With such therapy, the protection achieved against EIA approximates that of cromolyn. Although pre-exercise theophylline (as a single dose) can be administered and will result in some measure of protection, it cannot be recommended because of the long interval required (90 min), even for a rapidly absorbed preparation and because of a significant risk of gastric side effects. However, because of more effective aerosol agents with rapid action and fewer side effects, theophylline is not considered to

217

have a major role in the pharmacologic amelioration of EIA.[25]

Glucocorticosteroids

Recent theories that asthma is an inflammatory disease[10] fit comfortably with the excellent therapeutic effect of glucocorticosteroids in the treatment of both chronic and life-threatening asthma. In such circumstances, oral and intravenous administration are used. Topical anti-inflammatory preparations became available 20 years ago with the introduction of the chlorinated analogue of butomethasone (butomethasone diproprionate), an aerosol preparation.[43]

Early studies demonstrated the efficacy of aerosol butomethasone and such related preparations as triamcinolone acetonide in the management of asthma, but these agents were disappointing in their protective effect against EIA when administered before exercise. However, recent studies with a new nonhalogenated corticosteroid with topical anti-inflammatory properties (budesonide) confirmed enhanced protection against EIA.[32] Nevertheless, the principal value of aerosol glucocorticosteroids is to control asthma by regular administration, supplemented by inhaled beta agonists before exercise.

Belladonna Alkaloids

The development of ipratropium bromide, a quarternary ammonium derivative of atropine with potent anticholinergic properties but minor atropine-like side effects, has provided an agent that is beneficial in both asthma and EIA in certain patients.[21] In both circumstances, responders are commonly those who do not achieve full protection from beta agonists, cromolyn, and/or glucocorticosteroids. Indeed, the principal indication to add ipratroprium bromide is the case of an asthmatic with severe and incompletely blocked EIA despite pre-exercise cromolyn and a beta agonist.[65]

In summary, aerosol beta agonists provide effective protection against EIA in a majority of asthmatics. To those who do not achieve relief, the addition of cromolyn or theophylline or glucocorticoids will assist many. Ipratropium bromide may benefit a few of those still unresponsive.[44]

For those asthmatics who may be subjected to sports drug testing, almost all these agents are permitted without restriction. Those that are banned include fenoterol, injected and oral beta-2 agonists, and oral and parenteral glucocorticosteroids. Of course, all drugs that are alpha or beta-1 receptor stimulants (e.g., ephedrine and isoproterenol) are banned.[25]

EXERCISE TESTING

Regardless of the reason for conducting tests on asthmatics, a pretest medical history should be obtained. This history should emphasize the cardiorespiratory system (particularly relating to EIA), the current list of medications, habitual activity level, and any sporting involvement.

For those males older than 40 years and females older than 50 years or those who fall into the high-risk category for coronary artery disease, the testing and exercise precautions set out in the guidelines of the American College of Sports Medicine must be observed.[4] Those procedures are in addition to the ones outlined below.

Exercise Testing to Disprove or Confirm EIA

Briefly, the test involves examination of airway resistance, as reflected by changes in FEV_1 or PEFR before and after a bout of exercise. Tests to determine whether one is susceptible to EIA should include the following procedures to optimize the response.

1. The test should be a single-stage, continuous test lasting at least 6 to 8 min.
2. The intensity should be such that one works at 65 to 75% $\dot{V}_{O_2max}$, which is approximately 75 to 85% HR_{max}.
3. Ensure that all inhaled air enters via the mouth and is not subject to the warming and humidifying processes of the nose. To ensure this, the subject should wear a nose clip.

218

4. To determine the severity and duration of EIA, pre-exercise lung function measurement of FEV_1 or PEFR (at least) is made. The same lung function measurements are repeated immediately after and at frequent intervals (e.g., every 5 min) for 40 min following the cessation of exercise. All exercise and postexercise values should be expressed as a percentage of the pre-exercise value.

5. Nonasthmatics will show only a slight change in these measures. The criteria for EIA vary, because some use a maximal drop of 10% in FEV_1 or PEFR as indicative of an episode of EIA,[6,29] whereas others use a 15% drop.[11,26,52] Other EIA diagnostic tests such as specific conductance (SGaw), the rate of flow at 50% of vital capacity (FEF_{50}), or the average flow rate between 25% and 75% of vital capacity (FEF_{25-75}) are also in common use. These tests require a 35% postexercise reduction for EIA to be diagnosed.[11] The FEF_{50} or FEF_{25-75} reductions are indicative of small airway involvement, whereas FEV_1 and PEFR are indications of large airway involvement.

6. If possible, the test should be conducted under environmental conditions conducive to the triggering of EIA, i.e., a cold, dry environment.

7. Although EIA can be provoked by all modes of exercise, running is the mode of choice during testing because it is the most asthmogenic.

8. Subjects should abstain from medication prior to testing. Cromolyn sodium methyl xanthines and antihistamines should be withheld for a minimum of 24 hours, aerosol corticosteroid and anticholinergics for 8 hours, and beta-2 agonists for a minimum of 4 and 12 hours for short- and long-acting products, respectively.

9. Vigorous exercise should be avoided for at least 12 hours prior to testing to ensure that the subject is not in a refractory state or likely to have test results influenced by a late or second response to the initial bout of exercise.

10. Food (particularly chocolate and such caffeinated drinks as coffee, tea, and cola) should be avoided for at least 3 hours before testing, because caffeine is a methyl xanthine and has some bronchodilatory effect.[15,28] Ingestion of water is not restricted.

Where the fitness level of the subject is unknown, the starting work load should be low. The work load is then increased gradually over the next 2 to 3 min until the target HR is achieved. The last 5 min of the test should be completed at this workload.

If testing is conducted on a serial basis (for example, to determine the protective value of a given medication), certain conditions should be controlled to ensure reliability. To standardize environmental conditions, tests should be conducted in a climate chamber at 19 to 20° iC and 40% RH, at the same time of day and with a minimum of 1 and a maximum of 7 days between tests. The ingestion of products containing methyl xanthine (e.g., coffee, tea, cola, chocolate) should also be similar. The subjects' best lung function, that is, their unobstructed lung function values, should be determined by testing FEV_1, PEFR, etc. 15 min after the inhalation of an aerosol bronchodilator. Because it is known that the degree of airway wall thickness can change the amount of lumen narrowing for a given degree of smooth muscle contraction,[34] EIA tests should not be conducted on days when the pre-exercise FEV_1 or PEFR is less than 75% of the best (unobstructed) value.

The workload should be maintained at the same level for a given subject during all tests, because this will ensure a similar $\dot{V}_{O_2}$, ventilation, and HR during each test. To minimize the problems of test-retest variability, successive tests should be performed with a minimum of 24 hours and maximum of 1 week between them. To control for the psychological component in the triggering of EIA, it is essential that exercise tests are undertaken not only after administration of a placebo and the drug under examination in a randomized, double-blind manner, but also after no treatment.

If testing is part of a long-term research project to examine the changes following the use of a certain medication or a regular training program, there are other items that should also be examined. These items are usually best evaluated by having the asthmatics or their parents complete a daily diary. This diary will allocate daily scores for such items as wheezing at night, wheezing during the day, cough, sputum, medication taken, and days absent from work or school due to asthma, together with a record of physical activity if it is a training study. This type of project might also include the monitoring of the arterial oxygen saturation level using an ear oximeter as an estimate of venous admixture and the degree of hypoxemia at different work loads. The ratio of dead space volume to tidal volume can also be monitored. These tests are often performed during the assessment of the subject's $\dot{V}_{O_2max}$, which is determined so that appropriate and comparative workloads can be set at the correct percentage of $\dot{V}_{O_2max}$ during EIA challenge tests. The $\dot{V}_{O_2max}$ value is also used to indicate work capacities of the asthmatic individuals. Research concerning the asthmogenicity of various modes of exercise should control the severity of activity to ensure that the ventilation is the same during each activity.

Fitness Assessment in Asthmatics

When selecting tests to assess the fitness of an asthmatic, one needs to know whether the asthmatic requires fitness evaluation for participation in some competitive event or sport, or whether it is general fitness to maintain an optimal normal healthy lifestyle. In each case, the test items selected should be the same as those for the nonasthmatic. In both situations, however, emphasis must be placed on the determination of pulmonary function and

aerobic power of asthmatic subjects. Asthmatics should also have an assessment of the severity of their EIA.

Some vocations require a minimal level of fitness for one to be able to perform the essential functions of the job safely and adequately. In some cities, the fitness test requirement for such vocations as the police force, the armed services, or firefighting place unreasonable restrictions on asthmatic applicants. In some cases, the mere history of asthma is enough to eliminate an applicant; this same criterion would make about 10% of Olympic athletes ineligible. In our opinion, the asthmatic applicant should qualify providing:

1. The chronic asthma is under control.
2. The EIA can be prevented with pre-exercise medication.
3. He/she can perform the physical tasks and tests within the required time limits. All physical tasks should be tested following normal preventive medication.

The pulmonary function test should include as a minimal requirement, FEV_1, FVC (forced vital capacity), $FEV_1\%$ ($FEV_1/FVC \times 100$), and PEFR. If possible, flow volume loops should be obtained, together with data usually determined during these tests including flow rates at different lung volumes, especially FEF_{25-75} and FEF_{50}. Other recommended pulmonary function tests include the test of maximal voluntary ventilation (maximal breathing capacity) and determination of the resting lung subdivisions, that is, tidal volume (TV), inspiratory reserve volume (IRV), expiratory reserve volume (ERV), inspiratory capacity (IC), expiratory capacity (EC), vital capacity (VC), residual volume (RV), and functional residual capacity (FRC). There are many portable electronic devices that provide most of these pulmonary function scores on a visual display, and in a printed and graphic report. The rating of perceived exertion (RPE) using the Borg scale[16] and rating of breathlessness (a rating of dyspnea during exercise[17]) should be assessed at given workloads.

Fitness tests for asthmatics should be conducted when they demonstrate unobstructed lung volumes. To ensure this, all tests, except severity of EIA, should be performed 5 min after inhalation of two doses of an aerosol beta-2 agonist.

Testing is of greatest benefit if repeated on a regular basis to determine not merely status, but change in status due to change in activities.

EXERCISE PRESCRIPTION

Training for Competition

When an asthmatic is competing in some sporting event, the training program will need to be similar to that used by nonasthmatics in the same sport. The asthmatic should ensure adequate preventive medication prior to each training session and competitive event. World championship level performances have been recorded by asthmatics in almost all sporting events. These athletes train as hard as nonasthmatics, using the same procedures. They may occasionally have to curtail a training session or even a game or competitive event should a severe bout of asthma be experienced.

Training for General Fitness

Regular fitness training programs appear to be effective in improving work capacity, increasing efficiency, and lessening dyspnea without affecting the disease process. The general fitness program for improved daily living (the wellness program) should emphasize general aerobic fitness and follow the guidelines described by the American College of Sports Medicine concerning exercise prescription for asymptomatic adults.[4] That is, the prescription includes an adequate warm-up, which includes low-intensity (below 75% maximal HR), large-muscle rhythmical activities such as walking and jogging. This is followed by a segment of flexibility exercises. The aim of a 5- to 10-min warm-up is to gradually increase HR and increase body temperature until mild sweating occurs. A period of strengthening exercises should also be included. During strength training, activities that involve the Valsalva maneuver should be avoided because of the increased intrathoracic pressure that it produces, which can eventually result in a reduction in the oxygen saturation level of the arterial blood.

The aerobic segment, which is the major component of the exercise program, begins at low intensity and gradually increases in severity as the fitness level improves. Again, the activities should utilize large muscle groups in a rhythmic fashion and include such activities as walking, jogging, running, cycling, swimming, dancing, aerobics, circuit training, kayaking, canoeing, skiing, and various endurance game activities. The intensity should be equivalent to 50 to 85% of one's $\dot{V}_{O_2max}$ or 65 to 90% of HR_{max}. The more disabled the asthmatic, the more emphasis on interval-training activities.

The session concludes with a 5- to 10-min cool-down period. The intensity of activity in this segment should be gradually reduced until HR returns to within 20 bpm of the pre-exercise level. The cool-down segments should conclude with a repetition of the flexibility regimen performed during the warm-up segment. At this stage, activities to produce neuromuscular relaxation and exercises for breathing control are often valuable. The breathing exercises involve diaphragmatic (abdominal) breathing and activities that require breathing against resistance to increase the strength and endurance of the respiratory muscles. Abdominal breathing can be demonstrated by having the subject place a hand on the abdomen. The abdomen (and the hand) should rise with each inspiration and descend with each exhalation, while keeping the upper thorax relatively still. The abdomen appears to swell because of the downward movement of the diaphram, which increases intra-abdominal pressure. Deep slow breathing while exhaling against pursed lips helps to keep the small airways open, because these airways tend to collapse (close) when intrapleural pressure exceeds the pressure within the airway.

When selecting the exercise loading, consideration must be given to the current fitness level of the asthmatic. If he/she is very unfit, the program should consist of continuous walking, because this exercise has a low asthmogenicity and prepares the muscles for higher intensity exercise in future weeks. As fitness improves, especially that of the musculoskeletal system, one can increase the intensity by progressing to low-level interval training consisting of walking and jogging. The next progression is to high-intensity interval training using work intervals of 10 to 30 sec followed by 30- to 90-sec rest periods; this is prescribed because intermittent exercise is less asthmogenic.[46] The overload principle of training is also important in planning an exercise program for the asthmatic. It is important, however, to avoid overloading to the extent that severe breathlessness occurs because the subject's reaction to this discomfort may be to drop out of the program. A regular physical activity program provides frequent opportunities for the asthmatic to experience moderate breathlessness and to practice breathing control to gain relief. The skills that are learned can be useful in relieving anxiety during severe asthma attacks.

If the asthmatic prefers to train using such other methods as fartlek or cross-country running, this can usually be performed successfully, providing adequate pre-exercise medication has been administered. Many team sports are ideal because they require the less asthmogenic, intermittent pattern of energy expenditure.

The mode of exercise selected is also important. The success of any training program relies on regular and frequent participation. One of the major stimulants to exercise regularity is an adequate level of enjoyment. Therefore, despite the asthmogenicity of various activities, those of major interest to the individual should be prescribed. The exercise leader should attempt to influence the asthmatic to select activities that are aerobic in nature and spend some period of their childhood involved in swimming training. Swimming is less asthmogenic than other activities

and helps to increase heart and lung volumes.[24] The one physical activity that most physicians advise against is scuba diving. Though a great many asthmatics dive without incident, the threat of barotrauma while surfacing following the advent of air trapping due to small airway closure is a real danger. The present medical regulations in some countries prohibit anyone with a history of asthma from this activity, but this rule appears excessively stringent. There is a need to find a suitable method to screen those whose asthma is not under control and therefore at risk, without excluding all who wish to participate. In those who experience EIA sporadically, there often appears to be little indication when bronchoconstriction is likely to occur. It is suggested, therefore, that preventive medication be administered before each training session or competition.

Asthmatics who are unwilling to use, or who do not obtain full protection from pre-exercise medication, should be encouraged to select those physical activities with low asthmogenicity such as swimming and walking and to perform activities using an intermittent work/rest regimen.

The asthmatic should utilize exercise sessions lasting 15 to 60 min. The very unfit may need to limit sessions to 15 min initially, but should aim to increase the duration to a minimum of 30 min. If the subject is using low-intensity activity, the duration should be increased.

The frequency of training should be at least 3 to 5 times per week. Many asthmatics find that training each day, providing they alternate a hard day with an easy day, gives maximal benefit as far as controlling their chronic asthma is concerned.

When suffering from an acute respiratory infection, the asthmatic has a greater susceptibility to EIA; this susceptibility may last for as long as 6 weeks after the acute infection. Whenever possible, therefore, the exercising asthmatic should avoid others with such respiratory infections as influenza and the common cold. They should also be sure to have a warm shower and dress in warm clothing as soon as possible after an exercise session, because many asthmatics are susceptible to sudden changes in temperature.

Regular assessment of fitness is a valuable means of motivating the asthmatic and thus maintaining training regularity. It also provides an indication of the effectiveness of the training program and helps to redirect the program when changes are needed.

When the exercise program is performed in a formal fitness class situation, such as a health club or during school physical education, the exercise leader (teacher) should be aware of those participants who are asthmatic. The leader should construct a register of asthmatics together with an indication of their best PEFR reading, 80% and 50% of their best PEFR, their usual medication, and their doctors' names and phone numbers. The leader should have one of the inexpensive peak flow meters available to allow assessment of the severity of any bronchoconstriction that occurs. These results allow decisions to be made concerning the advisability of continued participation in a given session and the need for medical assistance.

Many schools require children on medication to keep their medication in a central administrative office or nurse's station. This is considered unwise in the case of the asthmatic, who should have free and easy access to their metered dose inhaler.[3]

When to Avoid or Cease Exertion

If the asthmatic has taken the prescribed pre-exercise medication and is still exhibiting bronchoconstriction, it is probably unwise to attempt vigorous exercise. Some asthmatics under these conditions find that exercise opens the airways and may alleviate the situation, but the majority get worse. School children reporting to physical education class or a sports event with airway constriction should be excused for that session. Some can run through mild attacks of EIA, whereas others cannot. As a general rule, the asthmatic should cease participating in a game or vigorous exercise session if EIA develops during that activity. If inhalation of a beta-2 agonist reverses the bronchoconstriction, the asthmatic can resume the exercise or sporting event. If it is not successful, he/she should refrain from further participation.

Performing vigorous activity with moderate or severe bronchoconstriction can lead to a severe drop in the oxygen saturation level of arterial blood, carbon dioxide accumulation, and hyperinflation of the lungs with an increased residual volume. This results in severe dyspnea and general discomfort, possible worsening of the resistance to air flow, and fatigue of the respiratory muscles. If the asthmatic regularly measures the PEFR and is thus aware of his/her normal unobstructed level, a peak flow measure made at the time of concern can be a good guide to the advisability of either commencing or continuing activity. It should be at least 80% of his/her "best" value. The availability of inexpensive peak flow meters means that school physical education departments and individual asthmatics can afford their own instruments and have them available for such use.

BENEFITS OF REGULAR EXERCISE

Physical and Physiologic Benefits

Regular and frequent aerobic exercise at moderate to high intensity does not cure asthma, although it provides the same physiologic benefits for the asthmatic as for the nonasthmatic. For instance, one study[28] showed that asthmatics had significantly improved posture, physical work capacity, and swimming ability, as well as a reduced amount of body fat, after 5 months of intensive swimming training. However, their susceptibility to EIA when challenged with a standard treadmill running test was unchanged. This confirms that bronchial hyper-responsiveness is not relieved by enhanced aerobic fitness through training. A similar finding was reported in a study of 9- to 14-year-old boys participating in twice-weekly training sessions that lasted 90 min each.[38] The training sessions in this study consisted of a short warm-up period, stretching exercises, calisthenics, strengthening exercises, breathing exercises, interval training, and such team games as soccer. Swim training was also included.

Both of these studies also found a reduction in the amount of medication required to control the chronic asthma of the subjects and a reduction in the number of episodes of asthma. These results suggest that regular aerobic training will improve clinical asthma, but like pubertal remissions, the underlying defect remains. These findings are confirmed by some investigators[19,59] but not others.[49,51]

Training outcomes of particular importance to the asthmatic are the increased physical exercise capacity, as determined by the $\dot{V}_{O_2max}$ and the $\dot{V}_{O_2}$ at which one can exercise before lactate begins to accumulate in the blood. This event appears to coincide with the respiratory compensation threshold, at which time there is a sudden and disproportionate increase in ventilation.

The residual volume is usually reduced with training because of a reduction in the amount of air trapped in the lungs.[42] Other respiratory system benefits include a more efficient pattern of respiration involving a slower and deeper breathing,[68] maximizing alveolar ventilation and minimizing the proportion of total ventilation accounted for by the dead space volume (improving VD/VT). The proportion of abdominal breathing may also increase.[14]

Training increases the maximal attainable rate of ventilation, while the inspired volume required to perform a given level of submaximal work is reduced. This decreased respiration means less air has to be "conditioned" and, as a result, there is a smaller change in the osmolarity of the periciliary fluid and less EIA.

All of the above training-induced changes result in asthmatics being able to perform a given task with a smaller disturbance of their internal environment. This means that the aerobically trained asthmatic can cope better than the untrained asthmatic with the same degree of mild or moderate airway obstruction. Research has also indicated that an increase in aerobic fitness increases the tolerance and threshold levels of asthmatics, so that a higher level of provocation is required to produce symptoms.[2,28,60] It has been shown to decrease absenteeism as a result of the disease and to decrease the medication requirement.[20,28]

Social and Psychological Benefits

Another important benefit of regular exercise is that the parents of the asthmatic develop a better insight into their child's disease and their capabilities and become less protective. The children cite increased freedom and permission to participate in physical and social activities as evidence of parental thinking.[28]

It is possible that psychological and sociological benefits of increased aerobic fitness, along with the resulting improvement in self-image and the greater recognition and acceptance by both peer groups and parents, help to remove the "cripple" stigma from which many asthmatics suffer. It is of great importance, therefore, that asthmatics practice and improve their skills in sports to gain greater status and recognition by others. It is important for the young asthmatic to realize that with dedication and application, most asthmatics can compete quite well with nonasthmatic peers, providing adequate training and pre-event medication programs are followed.

Medical records kept on Australian Olympic participants over the past 20 years have indicated that between 7% and 10% of the members of the team for each Olympiad were asthmatic (Table 12–1). These asthmatics participated in a variety

TABLE 12–1. **Asthmatic Athletes in Recent Australian Olympic Teams**

Year	Asthmatic Athletes	Total Athletes	%
1976	18	185	9.7
1980	9	106	8.5
1984	16	225	7.2
1988	21	255	8.2

TABLE 12-2. **Asthmatics on the 1988 Australian Olympic Team**

Number:	21 (11 males, 10 females)		

Medals Won: Two (2 gold)
Three (3 silver)

Participation in 11 of the 24 sports in which Australia entered:

Swimming	6	Boxing	1
Basketball	2	Weightlifting	1
Athletics	2	Table tennis	1
Cycling	2	Canoeing	1
Soccer	2	Hockey	1
Diving	2		

of the Olympic sporting events (Table 12–2). Voy reported that of 597 U.S. athletes participating in the 1984 summer Olympics, 67 (11.2%) suffered EIA and won 41 medals (15 gold, 20 silver, and 6 bronze).[66]

CONCLUSION

Exercise can induce an episode of asthma, and yet regular physical activity is an important component in the management of the disease. The severity of EIA can be easily assessed, and the regular measurement of FEV_1 or PEFR to indicate the state of the airways is recommended. There are a number of effective medications for both the prevention and reversal of EIA. The use of pre-exercise medication allows most asthmatics to perform in exercise and sporting events with little disadvantage.

REFERENCES

1. Adams, F.: The Extant Works of Areteus, The Cappadocium. Edited and translated by Francis Adams. London, Sydenham Society, 1856.
2. Afzelius-Frisk, I., Grimby, G., and Lindholm, N.: Physical training in patients with asthma. Poumon Coeur, 33:33, 1977.
3. Altenburger, K.M.: More concerning asthma and exercise. Pediatrics, 85:385, 1990.
4. American college of Sports Medicine: Guidelines for Exercise Testing and Exercise Prescription. 4th Ed. Philadelphia, Lea & Febiger, 1990.
5. American Thoracic Society: Definitions and classification of chronic bronchitis, asthma and pulmonary edema. Am. Rev. Respir. Dis., 85:763, 1962.
6. Anderson, S.D.: Exercise-induced asthma. In Allergy: Principles and Practice. Edited by E. Middleton, C. Reed, E. Ellis, et al. St. Louis, C.V. Mosby, 1988.
7. Anderson, S.D., Silverman, M., Konig, P., and Godfrey, S.: Exercise-induced asthma: a review. Br. J. Dis. Chest, 69:1, 1975.
8. Anderson, S.D., et al.: An evaluation of pharmacotherapy for exercise-induced asthma. J. Allergy Clin. Immunol., 64:612, 1979.
9. Anderson, S.D.: EIA: new thinking and current management. J. Resp. Dis., 7:48, 1986.
10. Barnes, P.J.: A new approach to the treatment of asthma. N. Engl. J. Med., 321:517, 1989.
11. Bar-Or, O.: Pediatric Sports Medicine. New York, Springer-Verlag, 1983.
12. Bar-Or, O., Neuman, I., and Dotan, R.: Effects of dry and humid climates on exercise-induced asthma in children and pre-adolescents. J. Allergy Clin. Immunol., 60:163, 1977.
13. Bar-Yishay, E., et al.: Difference between swimming and running as stimuli for exercise-induced asthma. Eur. J. Appl. Physiol., 48:387, 1982.
14. Bass, H., Whitcomb, J.F., and Forman, R.: Exercise training therapy for patients with chronic obstructive pulmonary disease. Chest, 57:116, 1970.
15. Becker, A.B., Simons, K.J., Gillespie, R.N., and Simons, P.E.R.: The bronchodilator effects and pharmokinetics of caffeine in asthma. N. Engl. J. Med. 310:743, 1984.
16. Borg, G.A.V.: Psychophysical bases of perceived exertion. Med. Sci. Sports Exerc., 14:377, 1982.
17. Borg, G., and Ottoson, D. (eds.): The Perception of Exertion in Physical Work. New York, Macmillan, 1986.
18. Boulet, L.P., Turotter, H., and Tennina, S.: Comparative efficacy of salbutamol, ipratropium and cromoglycate in the prevention of bronchospasm induced by exercise and hyperosmolar challenges. J. Allergy Clin. Immunol., 83:882, 1989.
19. Bundgaard, A., Ingemann-Hansen, T., Schmidt, A., and Halkjaer-Kristensen, J.: Exercise-induced asthma after walking, running, cycling. Scand. J. Clin. Lab. Invest., 42:15, 1982.
20. Bundgaard, A. et al.: Short term physical training is bronchial asthma. Br. J. Dis. Chest, 77:147, 1983.
21. Chan-Yeung, H.: The effect of Sch 1000 and disodium cromoglycate on exercise-induced asthma. Chest, 71:320, 1977.
22. Chatham, M. et al.: A comparison of histamine, methacholine and exercise airway reactivity in normal and asthmatic subjects. Am. Rev. Respir. Dis., 117:911, 1978.
23. Ellis, E.F.: Inhibition of exercise-induced asthma by theophylline. J. Allergy Clin. Immunol., 73(Suppl.):722, 1984.
24. Eriksson, B.O. et al.: A physical analysis of former girl swimmers. Acta Paediatr. Scand., 60(Suppl. 217):68, 1971.
25. Fitch, K.D.: The use of anti-asthmatic drugs: do they affect sports performance? Sports Med., 3:136, 1986.
26. Fitch, K.D., and Morton, A.R.: Specificity of exercise in exercise-induced asthma. Br. Med. J., 4:577, 1971.

27. Fitch, K.D., and Godfrey, S.: Asthma and athletic performance. JAMA, *236*:152, 1976.
28. Fitch, K.D., Morton, A.R., and Blanksby, B.A.: Effects of swimming training on children with asthma. Arch. Dis. Child., *51*:190, 1976.
29. Godfrey, S.: Exercise-induced asthma (Review article). Allergy, *33*:229, 1978.
30. Godfrey, S.: Introduction: symposium on special problems and management of allergic athletes. J. Allergy Clin. Immunol., *73*(Suppl.):693, 1984.
31. Hahn, A. et al.: A re-interpretation of the effect of temperature and water content of the inspired air in exercise-induced asthma. Am. Rev. Respir. Dis, *130*:575, 1984.
32. Henriksen, J.M., and Dahl, R.: Effects of inhaled budesonide alone and in combination with low dose terbutaline in children with exercise-induced asthma, Am. Rev. Respir. Dis., *128*:993, 1983.
33. Inbar, O. et al.: Breathing dry or humid air and exercise-induced asthma during swimming. Eur. J. Appl. Physiol. *44*:43, 1980.
34. James, A.R., Pare, P.D., and Hogg, J.C.: The mechanics of airway narrowing in asthma. Am Rev. Respir. Dis., *139*:242, 1989.
35. Jones, R.S., Buston, M.H., and Wharton, M.J.: The effect of exercise on ventilatory function in the child with asthma. Br. J. Dis. Chest, *56*:78, 1962.
36. Jones, R.S., Wharton, M.J., and Buston, M.H.: The place of physical exercise and bronchodilator drugs in the assessment of the asthmatic child. Arch. Dis. Child., *38*:539, 1963.
37. Kavanagh, T.: The Healthy Heart Program. Toronto, Key Porter Books, 1985.
38. King, M.J., Noakes, T.D., and Weinberg, E.G.: Physiological effects of a physical training program in children with exercise-induced asthma. Pediatr. Exerc. Sci. *1*:137, 1989.
39. Koenig, P.: The use of cromolyn in the management of hyperactive airways and exercise. J. Allergy Clin. Immunol., *73*(Suppl.):686, 1984.
40. Lee, T.H. et al.: Exercise-induced late asthmatic reactions with neutrophil chemotactic activity. N. Engl. J. Med., *308*:1502, 1983.
41. Major, R.H.: A note on the history of asthma. *In* Science, Medicine and History, Vol. 2. Edited by E.A. Underwood. London, Oxford University Press, 1953.
42. Mertens, D.J., Shephard, R.J., and Kavanagh, T.: Long-term exercise therapy for chronic obstructive lung disease. Respiration, *35*:96, 1978.
43. Morrow-Brown, H. et al.: Butomethasone dipropionate: a new steroid aerosol for the treatment of allergic asthma. Br. Med. J., *1*:585, 1972.
44. Morton, A.R., and Fitch, K.D.: Exercise-induced bronchial obstruction. In Current Therapy in Sports Medicine–2. Edited by J.S. Torg, R.P. Welsh, and R.J. Shephard. Toronto, B.C. Decker, 1990.
45. Morton, A.R., Fitch, K.D., and Hahn, A.G.: Physical activity and the asthmatic. Phys. Sportsmed., *9*:50, 1981.
46. Morton, A.R., Hahn, A.G., and Fitch, K.D.: Continuous and intermittent running in the provocation of asthma. Ann. Allergy, *48*:132, 1982.
47. Morton, A.R., Lawrence, S.R., Fitch, K.D., and Hahn, A.G.: Duration of exercise in the provocation of exercise-induced asthma. Ann. Allergy, *51*:530, 1983.
48. Morton, A.R., Ogle, S.L., and Fitch, K.D.: Effects of nedocromil sodium, cromolyn sodium and a placebo in exercise-induced asthma. Ann. Allergy, *68*:143, 1992.
49. Nickerson, B.G., et al.: Distance running improves fitness in asthmatic children without pulmonary complications or changes in exercise-induced bronchospasm. Pediatrics, *71*:147, 1983.
50. Nicklaus, T.M., Burgin, W.W., and Taylor, J.R.: Spirometric tests to diagnose asthma. Am. Rev. Respir. Dis., *100*:153, 1969.
51. Orenstein, D.M., Reed, M.E., Grogan, F.T., and Crawford, L.V.: Exercise conditioning in children with asthma. J. Pediatr., *106*:556, 1985.
52. Oseid, S.: Exercise-induced asthma: a review. *In* International Series on Sports Science. Vol. 10: Children and Exercise IX. Edited by K. Berg and B.O. Eriksson. Champaign, IL, Human Kinetics.
53. Proctor, D.F.: The upper airways, I. Nasal Physiology and defense of the lungs. Am. Rev. Respir. Dis., *115*:97, 1977.
54. Reiff, D.B., Nozhat, B., Choudry Pride, N.B., and Ind, P.W.: The effect of prolonged submaximal warm-up exercise on exercise-induced asthma. Am. Rev. Respir. Dis., *139*:379, 1989.
55. Schnall, R.P., and Landau, L.I.: Protective effects of repeated short sprints in exercise-induced asthma. Thorax, *35*:828, 1980.
56. Schoeffel, R.E., Anderson, S.D., Gillam, I., and Lindsay, D.A.: Multiple exercise and histamine challenge in asthmatic patients. Thorax, *35*:164, 1980.
57. Schoeffel, R.E., Anderson, S.D., and Lindsay, D.A.: Sodium cromoglycate as a pressurised aerosol (Vicrom) in exercise-induced asthma. Austr. N. Z. J. Med., *13*:157, 1983.
58. Silverman, M., and Anderson, S.D.: Standardization of exercise tests in asthmatic children. Arch. Dis. Child., *47*:882, 1972.
59. Sly, R.M.: Exercise related changes in airway obstruction: frequency and clinical correlates in asthmatic children. Ann. Allergy, *28*:1, 1970.
60. Sly, R.M., Harper, R.T., and Rosselot, I.: The effect of physical conditioning upon asthmatic children. Ann. Allergy, *30*:86, 1972.
61. Sly, R.M.: Exercise-induced asthma. *In* Bronchial Asthma: Mechanisms and Therapeutics. Edited by R.B. Weiss and M.S. Segal. Boston, Little Brown, 1976.
62. Strauss, R.H., McFadden, E.R., Jr, Ingram, R.H., Jr, and Jaeger, J.J.: Enhancement of exercise-induced asthma by cold air. N. Engl. J. Med., *297*:743, 1977.
63. Swinburn, P.: Asthma definition. *In* Proceedings of meetings held in Auckland Wellington, Dunedin and Christchurch, New Zealand, 1976.
64. Szanton, V.L.: Theodore Roosevelt, the asthmatic. Ann. Allergy, *27*:485, 1969.
65. Thomson, N.C., Patel, K.R., and Kerr, J.W.: Sodium cromoglycate and ipratroprium bromide in exercise induced asthma. Thorax, *33*:694, 1978.
66. Voy, R.: The U.S. Olympic Committee experience with exercise-induced bronchospasm 1984. Med. Sci Sports Exerc., *18*:328, 1986.
67. Weiler, J.M. et al.: Prevalence of bronchial hyperresponsiveness in highly trained athletes. Chest, *90*:23, 1986.

68. Wolf, C.R., and Suero, J.T.: Alterations in lung mechanics and gas exchange following training in chronic obstructive lung disease. Dis. Chest, 55:37, 1969.

69. Zeballos, R.J., et al.: Benefits of nose breathing in prevention of EIA. Am. Rev. Respir. Dis., 118:877, 1978.

13
CHAPTER

Chronic Obstructive Respiratory Disorders

by
Norman L. Jones, Leslie B. Berman,
Peter D. Bartkiewicz and Neil B. Oldridge

The use of exercise rehabilitation programs in the management of patients with airway obstruction (asthma, bronchitis, and emphysema) has been controversial, and there is continued debate regarding the selection of patients, the most successful types of programs, and the expected outcome.[21,35] The problems posed by respiratory "cripples" are different in many respects from those of their cardiovascular counterparts, but the epidemiologic magnitude is at least as great in terms of morbidity and mortality. The mortality rate from chronic respiratory ailments in the United States has been estimated at over 40,000 persons per year. In terms of days lost from work or dollars lost to the economy ($2 billion per year), the size of the problem cannot be dismissed lightly. If exercise could be shown to help the respiratory patient to continue or to return to a productive life, there is little doubt it would become more widely used. Although more research is needed to establish the value of exercise programs, most studies reveal that many patients show improvement in their symptoms. The mechanisms underlying these improvements are still debated.[7]

This chapter is a review of some factors that bear on clinical exercise programs in patients with chronic airway obstruction in terms of the pathophysiology and natural history of these disorders, the assessment of patients entering the program, program design, and evaluation.

DEFINITIONS

In spite of several conferences devoted to the nomenclature of chronic airflow obstruction from which several pathologic and clinical conditions have been identified, the custom in North America has been to "lump" all patients into one term, "chronic obstructive pulmonary disease" (COPD). One unfortunate implication of this term is that there is one "disease" and thus, that all patients may be managed similarly. We do not believe this fact to be true, particularly when considering disability and the role of exercise. For this reason, we provide definitions for a number of terms.[18]

CHRONIC AIRFLOW OBSTRUCTION. This condition may be defined functionally by spirometric measurements, of which the most useful and simplest are the forced expired volume in 1 second (FEV_1) and the vital capacity (VC). Airflow obstruction is established by values for FEV_1 and for FEV_1 as a percentage of the VC (FEV_1 : VC) that are two standard deviations below the mean for the population defined by gender, age, and height.[8]

ASTHMA. Asthma is defined in terms of diffuse narrowing of airways that varies significantly over time (either spontaneously or as the result of treatment). This diagnosis implies a variable degree of airway obstruction, which may be demonstrated by spirometry. The airflow obstruction is due to bronchial inflammation with associated smooth muscle contrac-

229

tion. A number of factors have been shown to underly the episodic bronchoconstriction.[9] First, there is often a family history of asthma and atopy (predisposition to hay fever, hives, eczema, and migraine). Second, specific allergic reactions may be identified (pollens, animal dander, and many other naturally occurring or man-made agents). Third, an increase in non-specific airway reactivity may be demonstrated by histamine or methacholine provocation tests, which are related to the provocation of asthma by such non-allergic agents as cold air, exercise, and smoke.[12]

CHRONIC BRONCHITIS. This condition is defined as the chronic production of sputum for at least 3 years. The process may be subdivided into simple bronchitis, in which sputum production is constant and there is no airflow obstruction; infective bronchitis, in which episodes of respiratory infection occur on the background of simple bronchitis; and chronic obstructive bronchitis, in which there is evidence of airflow obstruction, as defined previously.[11] The airflow obstruction is due principally to thickened bronchial walls and secretions. By far, the most common cause of chronic bronchitis is cigarette smoking, but childhood respiratory infections and industrial pollution may also be contributory.

EMPHYSEMA. Emphysema is defined in terms of alveolar distention and destruction. Two types are recognized: panlobular, in which the alveoli of the pulmonary lobule are diffusely affected; and centrilobular, in which the distention is mainly at the site of the respiratory bronchiole at the center of the pulmonary lobule. Although the functional effects of these two processes differ slightly, the distinction is difficult to establish in life. The airflow obstruction is due to a loss of pulmonary elastic recoil, which leads to dynamic airway narrowing. The occasional familial incidence in emphysema is explained by a genetically determined deficiency of anti-proteolytic enzymes that predispose the lung to damage by proteases released by inflammatory cells.[18]

Smoking and air pollution may also be important pathogenic factors.

From these definitions, it may be appreciated that these processes are not mutually exclusive; a patient may meet the criteria for chronic obstructive bronchitis, may show clinical or functional features of emphysema, and finally may show some variation in airway obstruction, meeting the criteria for asthma. These diagnostic distinctions should be made wherever possible, however, because the approach to management may differ.

PATHOPHYSIOLOGY

AIRFLOW OBSTRUCTION. The main cause of symptoms in most patients is airflow obstruction, which may be due to three main pathologic mechanisms that exist alone or, more commonly, in combination: 1) bronchial muscle contraction and airway inflammation (asthma); 2) thickened bronchial walls (bronchitis); and 3) loss of pulmonary elastic recoil (emphysema). If asthma is excluded, airflow obstruction is usually slowly progressive and symptoms develop insidiously over many years. Usually by the time the patient is experiencing symptoms, FEV_1 is below 60% of the predicted value. Once FEV_1 is below 30%, disability may be severe. There is great variability in symptoms, however, due to the presence of other factors that may be adaptive and beneficial or that may contribute to disability by adding further functional abnormalities through disordered pulmonary gas exchange or impaired cardiac function. In general, patients with emphysema are more dyspneic than patients with chronic bronchitis who have similar degrees of airway obstruction; this difference is due to a greater pulmonary gas exchange abnormality and a high thoracic volume, which impairs the function of the inspiratory muscles.[13]

DISORDERED PULMONARY GAS EXCHANGE. This condition is due to poor matching of alveolar ventilation ($\dot{V}_A$) to pulmonary capillary blood flow ($\dot{Q}_c$) and by poor diffusion characteristics secondary to loss of alveolar surface area. Alveolar ventilation is poorly distributed due to variations in airway caliber and in pulmonary compliance throughout the lung. The normal even distribution of pulmonary capillary blood flow is disturbed due to loss of capillaries in emphysema and to variations in blood vessel caliber. The combination of these abnormalities causes 1) some areas of the lung to be poorly ventilated and overperfused (low $\dot{V}_A:\dot{Q}_c$), so that the blood flowing from them is poorly oxygenated and has high levels of CO_2 (high venous admixture or "wasted blood"); and 2) other areas to be relatively overventilated in relation to their blood flow (high $\dot{V}_A:\dot{Q}_c$), leading to reduced gas exchange with inspired air (high dead space:tidal volume, i.e., V_D to V_T ratio or "wasted air"). In patients with chronic bronchitis and minimal emphysema ("type B") in whom pulmonary gas exchange is impaired mainly by poor distribution of $\dot{V}_A$, improvement may occur during exercise due to the increased tidal volume, leading to an increase in arterial oxygen saturation.[13] When a gas exchange disturbance is due to a fixed abnormality caused by the alveolar wall destruction and loss of pulmonary capillaries that occur in emphysema ("type A"), however, gas exchange is worse during exercise and arterial oxygen saturation decreases.[13]

VENTILATORY FAILURE. This term is defined as an inability of resting ventilation to maintain a normal arterial PCO_2 (below 45 torr).[18] Although ventilatory failure is also associated with a low arterial PO_2 value (below 70 torr), a low arterial PO_2 value may be found in many patients without a significant increase in PCO_2.

PULMONARY HEART DISEASE. This condition is usually the result of chronic ventilatory failure with an increased level of PCO_2 and a low PO_2 value in arterial blood. The hypercapnia and hypoxemia lead to an increase in pulmonary vascular resistance, an increase in pulmonary artery pressure, and a resulting deterioration in right ventricular function. These changes are usually accompanied by clinical signs of fluid retention and polycythemia, i.e., an increase in the mass of red blood cells and an increase in blood hemoglobin to over 16 g·dl^{-1}.

EXERCISE PERFORMANCE. Exercise performance may be impaired for a number of reasons. Patients with asthma may have a normal exercise capacity, but exercise may be followed by bronchoconstriction, particularly if exercise is done in cold air.[23] In patients with chronic airflow obstruction, exercise performance may be reduced through the restrictions imposed by the abnormal mechanical characteristics of the lungs, often combined with weakness of the respiratory muscles, that produce a limited ability to increase tidal volume and respiratory frequency.[19] Abnormal pulmonary gas exchange associated with a high V_D to V_T ratio may lead to high values of ventilation at a given power output; the patient will then reach his ventilatory capacity at a lower power output. Respiratory control mechanisms may not lead to an increase in ventilation that is appropriate to the demand, leading to an increase in arterial PCO_2 and a fall in the level of PO_2. Impaired pulmonary gas exchange will also cause a reduction in arterial PO_2, impairing oxygen delivery to exercising tissues; oxygen supplementation may improve exercise in these patients. Adaptation to pulmonary malfunction may include an increase in $\dot{Q}$ during exercise and also an increased oxygen extraction by exercising muscles.

Weakness of the leg muscles frequently contributes to poor exercise capacity; this is usually the result of the inactivity that accompanies chronic respiratory disease, but electrolyte disturbances and steroid myopathy should also be considered in this context.

In addition to these physiologic factors, exercise may be limited through psychologic mechanisms. In some patients, anxiety and hysteria may lead to hyperventilation, and anxiety and depression may lead to a disproportionate fatigue.[4] The psychologic factors sometimes may be difficult to separate from the physiologic factors during exercise tests. Nevertheless, improvement in the attitude of patients toward their illness may produce a marked improvement in their ability to exercise.

NATURAL HISTORY

The course of chronic bronchitis and emphysema is generally one of slow progression with increasing disability (Fig. 13–1). Results of a number of long-term studies show that pulmonary function decreases at a steady rate. Once FEV_1 has fallen to below 30% of predicted values and the arterial PCO_2 has risen to above normal values, the 5-year outlook is poor, with a mortality rate of at least 25%.[5]

PSYCHOSOCIAL EFFECTS

There is often an early denial of symptoms, which are attributed to a smoker's cough and the effects of increasing age. At this stage, patients find that they are less able to meet their job demands, leading to reliance on fellow workers and a loss of self-confidence. Reduced exercise capacity produces inactivity and frequent absences from work due to depression and an inability to provide for the family. These effects are joined by an avoidance of any activity outside the home, resulting in a gradual narrowing of their social sphere. Secondary effects are seen through the impact of the patient's illness on the family, with associated tensions, sleep disturbances, panic, and anxiety. A complex interaction between physical and psychosocial factors contributes to the total picture of disability and handicap.

MEDICAL MANAGEMENT OF AIRFLOW OBSTRUCTION

The management of patients with asthma, chronic bronchitis, and emphysema is based on the appropriate use of a

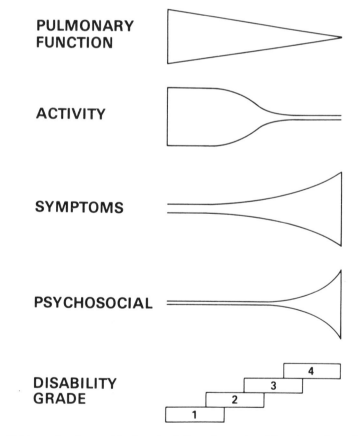

Fig. 13–1. *Natural history of patients with chronic airflow obstruction. There is a relatively steady decline in pulmonary function; early maintenance of activity with few symptoms, followed by relatively rapid decline in activity and increase in symptoms; and few psychosocial effects until activity is seriously curtailed. Disability grades are also shown, but vary widely depending on factors acting in a given patient.*

variety of agents in optimal dosage, and weighs the benefits against the potential dangers.[10] Treatment is based on the identification of the important factors in a given patient (e.g., allergy, bronchoconstriction, and infection) and on careful documentation of efficacy via pulmonary function assessment and other techniques.

Bronchoconstriction is managed mainly by the use of such bronchodilator aerosols as salbutamol, orciprenaline, and fenoterol. Oral steroid use (usually prednisone) is reserved for patients with severe asthma, because of the many serious side-effects (e.g., osteoporosis, myopathy, and adrenal suppression). These systemic side-effects may be avoided by the use of inhaled steroid preparations (beclomethasone), which are now considered first-line treatments of bronchial inflammation. Specific desensitization for allergens is performed occasionally, and the use of antihistamines and cromoglycate is often recommended. Bronchodilators are often helpful in the treatment for chronic bronchitis and emphysema, but steroids are less effective than they are in the treatment for asthma. Short courses of antibiotics are used for episodes of bronchial infection. Therapy for fluid retention and cardiac dysfunction may be required. It is of great importance that each patient be optimally treated before entering an exercise program.

THE EXERCISE REHABILITATION PROGRAM

It must be stated at the outset that exercise rehabilitation programs are just one part of the total approach to patient care, which includes 1) optimal medical care, with appropriate therapy for airway obstruction and other supportive measures; 2) increased physical and social activity; and 3) adaptation to disability on a personal, physical, and psychologic level, and also at the level of the family.[22] Because of the great variation in symptoms and disability, and in view of the different factors that may influence disability, the exercise program must be flexible with regard to the spectrum of patients who may take

part and also to the program that is offered.

Assessment of Patients for Admission

Careful assessment of the patient is required to decide on the type of program of most potential benefit and also so that progress during the program may be evaluated. Ideally, assessment is made by a team consisting of a physician, an exercise program director, a physiotherapist, an occupational therapist, and a social worker.

REFERRAL. The patient is normally referred through a personal physician. The use of a standard referral form is best, on which all the relevant information regarding the medical management of the patient is recorded. The referral is important in that the patient requires the firm support of the physician and a close liaison must be maintained between the physician and the professionals running the program.

INITIAL HISTORY AND PHYSICAL EXAMINATION. These steps need not be medically complex and will have been carried out by the referring physician. However, elements of the history that are important in designing the rehabilitation program include an assessment of symptoms and disability, a survey of lifestyle (together with a daily and weekly diary to obtain a picture of the patient's activities and cigarette and alcohol consumption), the patient's description of his difficulties, and his aspirations for the future. An interview with the spouse or other close family member can yield a second perspective on the disability and activities in everyday life, together with an appraisal of the patient's personality and the family dynamics. It may be helpful to obtain an assessment of the patient's work environment by an occupational health professional.

PULMONARY FUNCTION TESTS. These tests are essential to quantify impairment of airflow and gas exchange characteristics and to judge the extent to which the pathophysiologic findings contribute to the disability.[18] Where disability is greater than expected for the impairment in pulmonary function, investigation and treatment of other aspects of the patient's medical condition may be needed.

Measurement of FEV_1 and VC with the use of spirometry yields important indices of airflow obstruction and is usually all that is required. If these measurements reveal a serious abnormality (below 50% of predicted values), however, further tests may be necessary to quantify pathophysiology and to identify ventilatory failure.[8]

The pulmonary residual volume, functional residual capacity, and total lung capacity may be measured by helium dilution or body plethysmography. Characteristically, all these lung volumes are increased in chronic airflow obstruction, with very large increases evident in patients with emphysema.[6]

Pulmonary mechanical characteristics include measurement of airway resistance, pulmonary compliance, and flow-volume curves. Pulmonary compliance is usually increased in patients with emphysema and gross reductions in expiratory flow may also occur in persons with chronic bronchitis and asthma. Inspiratory flow is often surprisingly well maintained.

The degree of carbon monoxide uptake can help to assess the gas exchange function of the lungs, and is characteristically reduced in emphysema patients.[6] Arterial blood gas levels are often used to assess gas exchange and acid-base status.[15] Arterial PCO_2 values (measured directly or estimated non-invasively by rebreathing) help to assess alveolar ventilation. With expired gas collection, the measurement is used to calculate the V_D to V_T ratio. The level of arterial PO_2 is used to estimate venous admixture and to document the degree of hypoxemia during exercise.[15] Arterial O_2 saturation may be measured directly from arterial blood samples and indirectly by ear oximetry.[34]

RESPIRATORY MUSCLE POWER. This determination is made by recording the maximal pressure the patient can generate against an occluded airway during inspiration (MIP) and expiration (MEP). This measurement should be made in any patient who complains of exercise-related dyspnea, especially if this is disproportionate to the degree of airway obstruction.[20]

EXERCISE TESTING. Exercise tests are used to obtain information regarding the integrated pulmonary responses to increased metabolic demands (O_2 intake and CO_2 output).[16] In the context of a rehabilitation exercise program, exercise tests are used to obtain: an objective measurement of exercise tolerance; an explanation and rating for exercise-related symptoms; identification of the factors limiting exercise (e.g., limited ventilatory capacity, disordered pulmonary gas exchange and hypoxemia, abnormal cardiac function, and muscle weakness); and prescription of exercise levels. There are numerous exercise test protocols that may be used to obtain this information, but they are not detailed in this chapter.[17]

For subjects not severely disabled, an incremental progressive test on a cycle ergometer or treadmill may be used. Measurements are made at several increasing work rates of heart rate (HR) and blood pressure, of ventilation and breathing frequency, and of magnitude scaling of dyspnea; such exercise-related symptoms as muscle fatigue and chest pain are also assessed by using the Borg rating scale.[17] Arterial O_2 saturation may be monitored with an ear oximeter and end-tidal PCO_2 levels may be evaluated with a rapid analyzer. Electrocardiographic monitoring is also performed because coronary artery disease frequently co-exists with chronic airflow obstruction.

For more disabled subjects, a 6- or 12-minute walk test may be used to obtain an indication of functional ability, and is easily repeated.[24] This test may be carried out in an indoor corridor that is at least 30 m in length. Observations are made of distance covered in 6 or 12 minutes, stride length, breathing pattern, HR, and if available, ear oximetry.

Because patients requiring O_2 therapy are usually very disabled, the most convenient protocol involves a constant exercise level that produces limiting symptoms in 4 to 6 minutes during air breathing.[40] For example, tests can be performed on a cycle ergometer (200 to 600 kpm·min^{-1}) or a treadmill (1 to 3 mph, 0% grade). Oxygen (24 or 28%) and air are administered identically without the patient's knowledge (i.e., "single blind"). An increase in endurance time of at least 100% indicates a useful effect of oxygen. Although not essential, measurements of arterial O_2 saturation and end-tidal or arterial PCO_2 are helpful during the tests to show that oxygen desaturation is reversed and that PCO_2 does not increase too much. In patients who identify muscle fatigue as the main factor limiting performance in an exercise test, muscle testing with an isokinetic dynamometer may reveal significant muscle weakness.

OVERALL DISABILITY ASSESSMENT. This assessment is made on the basis of the interviews, clinical information, and the pulmonary function and exercise results. A grading of disability (Table 13–1) may be used to prescribe the optimal type of program, but it may also be important to obtain the patient's subjective ratings of symptoms and performance, particularly if disability is severe. Because improvement in severely disabled patients is often subjective and is difficult to relate to the commonly recorded objective measurements, the measurement of symptomatic changes in a semi-objective manner through the use of rating scales is worth attempting. Although the Borg scale for rating perceived exertion may be used for this purpose, we also suggest the use of visual analogue scaling of symptoms experienced in such everyday physical tasks as dressing, bed making, bathing, or climbing stairs from one floor in the house to another.[17] As long as the activity is precisely defined, the scalings may be used to follow progress. The patient is asked to indicate the rating of a symptom (e.g., shortness of breath) that occurs during or immediately after the given activity. This information is then compared to ratings from someone their own age who does not have a breathing problem. Ratings may also be obtained of the "pace" or "speed" at which a task is performed and the time taken to complete the activity, again compared to values for healthy subjects. Changes in the ratings may be used to identify the reasons for symptomatic change. For example, an improvement in shortness of breath that accompanies a reduction in the speed of a task may be associated with improved techniques of pacing and energy conservation, rather than with improved fitness or pulmonary function.

Prescription of Activity

For those patients with Grade 1 disability who are not limited by impaired pulmonary function, prescription is carried out in the usual way on the basis of submaximal exercise power outputs and HR responses, as in patients with cardiovascular disease.[29] Monitoring of training intensity is carried out by using an appropriate percentage of the HR response observed in the patient's exercise test. The exercise

TABLE 13–1. **Guide to Grading Disability (Based on 40-Year-Old Man)**

Grade	Cause of Dyspnea	FEV$_1$ (%Pred)	Max $\dot{V}_{O_2}$ (ml·min^{-1}·kg^{-1})	Exercise Max $\dot{V}_E$ (L·min^{-1})	Blood Gases
1	Fast walking and stair climbing	> 60	> 25	Not limiting	Normal PCO_2, SaO_2
2	Walking at normal pace	< 60	< 25	> 50	Normal $PaCO_2$; SaO_2 above 90% at rest and with exercise
3	Slow walking	< 40	< 15	< 50	Normal $PaCO_2$; SaO_2 below 90% with exercise
4	Walking limited to less than one block	< 40	< 7	< 30	Elevated $PaCO_2$; SaO_2 below 90% at rest and with exercise

session should be 30 to 60 minutes in duration and should be performed daily, with a minimal frequency of every other day.

Because of the different factors that may limit activity in patients with more severe chronic respiratory problems, prescription for patients with disabilities of Grades 2 to 4 is carried out by using guidelines that differ in some important respects from those for cardiovascular disease.

In patients with Grade 2 disability in whom moderate impairment exists, maximal exercise may be limited by a reduced ventilatory capacity. A training intensity is chosen that will not lead to more than 60 to 80% of the ventilatory capacity (estimated from $FEV_1 \times 35$) and that was shown in the exercise test to lead to a breathing frequency of less than 30 breaths$\cdot$min^{-1}. An equivalent HR is chosen by reference to the exercise test results and may be used for monitoring purposes. Initially, exercise duration may be severely restricted. Exercise frequency may then be such that the patient exercises more than once a day every day for short periods of time before breathlessness restricts further activity.

Patients with Grade 3 disability are often the most difficult to give a prescription. Although the guidelines listed for Grade 2 disability generally apply, the exercise intensity may be so small that it is unlikely to produce a training effect. In these patients, consideration is given to oxygen supplementation, "interval" training methods, and training of muscle groups (e.g., separate exercises for each leg), particularly if muscle weakness is present. Breathing training may be effective and re-education regarding the pattern of breathing may be helpful in those patients who show a high frequency and small tidal volume or who have a low respiratory muscle power, as demonstrated by measurement of MIP and MEP.

Patients with Grade 4 disability may be in chronic respiratory and cardiac failure. The emphasis for these individuals is on adaptation to the disability. The activity prescribed is thus directed toward efficiency and energy conservation in every-day tasks and toward education and encouragement to avoid a negative lifestyle. The benefits and risks of exercise and oxygen administration must be carefully considered in view of the fact that long-term benefit from oxygen during training sessions has not been established.[24] Patients who are in chronic hypoxic ventilatory failure may require treatment with continuous (24 hours per day) low-flow oxygen.[32]

In practice, prescription of activity for very disabled patients considers such exercise-related symptoms as dyspnea, fatigue, anxiety, and headaches that may lead to modification of the usual prescription. Although most patients limited by impaired pulmonary function at low exercise levels show a limited HR response, the HR remains a useful indicator of training level. Once patients understand the optimal relative stress for training through the use of such symptom-rating scales as the Borg scale, they can pace themselves. An increase in HR during activity sessions may indicate the need for a clinical review.

Types of Programs

As may be appreciated from the preceding discussion of the varying limiting factors and the many objectives that may apply to different patients, the program must have sufficient flexibility to accommodate patients of wide-ranging disabilities and demands (Table 13–2). As it may not be easy for a single program to handle patients with widely differing problems, three main types of programs may be identified.

IN-HOSPITAL PROGRAMS. This type may be required for very disabled (Grades 3 and 4) patients who require medical supervision, supplemental oxygen, and highly skilled physiotherapy. Patients in this category often exhibit complications from severe chronic airway obstruction (respiratory and cardiac failure, and hypoxemia) and present with multiple psychosocial problems (depression, anxiety, introversion, hypochondriasis, and poor family dynamics). These patients, how-

TABLE 13-2. **Objectives of Rehabilitation Exercise Programs**

Education of patients and relatives
   Disease process and management
   Improved compliance with therapy
   Practical advice regarding living with disability
Improvement in fitness and exercise performance
   Increased endurance
   Reduced respiratory muscle fatigue
   Increased strength
   Improved coordination and efficiency in everyday activities
Improved voluntary control of breathing pattern
   Increased tidal volume in exercise
   Reduced dyspnea in exercise and stressful situations
Increased flexibility
Improved confidence in physical abilities
Increased self responsibilities
Improved quality of life
   Increased physical and social activity
   Improved family relationships
   Increased sense of achievement through realistic goal setting and less reliance on others in work and at home

ever, are usually able to attend a program run during working hours, given no transport problems.

DAYTIME OUTPATIENT CLINICS. The outpatient clinic or community-based program is particularly suited to reasonably mobile patients (Grades 1 and 2) who have access to transport and receive adequate family support. It may also be useful for patients who have progressed well within the hospital-based clinic. It is an advantage if some personnel attend both programs to provide continuity.

EVENING EXERCISE PROGRAMS. This program is essential for patients who are employed and cannot afford time away from work. Ideally, this type of program is based within a community, supported by the local lung association, and run by an executive committee that includes patient representatives.

HOME EXERCISE PROGRAMS. This type of program may be suitable for some patients and can be effective.[25]

Suitable Activities

For the least disabled patients, the usual aerobic training activities (jogging, cycling, and treadmill running) are appropriate. Extremes of temperature and other environmental changes (e.g., air pollution) should be avoided. The more disabled the patient, the greater will be the emphasis on interval training techniques, due to the limited endurance capacity of these patients.

A balanced program of exercise (including activities to improve cardiorespiratory endurance, muscular strength and endurance, flexibility, and relaxation) is designed for the individual patient. If possible, the primary type of training should be aerobic in nature and task specific, i.e., aerobic to improve the oxygen transport system and to simulate everyday activities, and task specific to ensure maximal application to functional activity in daily life.

The exercises should suit the interests and capabilities of the individual, with prescribed endurance activities that vary little in oxygen cost. A relatively constant intensity avoids repeated episodes of uncomfortable dyspnea and long recovery periods. Examples of low variability exercises are walking and stationary cycling, in contrast to such high variability activities as traditional calisthenics, some types of dancing, and recreational games. Regardless of the type of exercise, each session should be preceded by warm-up exercises of increasing intensity that permit breathing to accommodate gradually to the training load. Each session should be completed with exercises of decreasing intensity. Both the warm-up and cooldown periods are excellent opportunities to implement flexibility, relaxation, and breathing control exercises.

Muscular endurance activities (defined as low-tension, high-repetition contractions of small muscle groups) do not require a major increase in the total circulation or respiration and may initially be a large component of the exercise program for patients who are bedridden or are recuperating from cardiac or respiratory failure. At this stage, a program of active, dynamic bed exercises and prophylactic breathing exercises is suitable until the patient's overall medical and physical condition improves.[33] The decision to progress to endurance activities is a mutual one made by the physician, patient, and exercise leader, and depends on the physical, psychologic, and medical status of the patient. At some time during the training period, strengthening exercises should gradually be introduced, employing high tension, low repetition muscular contractions of either a dynamic or static nature. Activities accompanied by breathholding or the Valsalva maneuver should be avoided, because they are associated with high intrathoracic pressures, changes in systemic and pulmonary vascular pressures, and decreases in arterial O_2 saturation.

The role of breathing exercises in the treatment of chronic airway obstruction is still controversial and is beyond the scope of this chapter.[14,21] Many patients tend to hyperventilate when anxious or performing activities to which they are not accustomed. They are encouraged to slow and deepen their breathing and to employ pursed-lip expiration (which helps to lessen airway collapse on expiration) if they find it helpful. Although patients are instructed in the technique of abdominal breathing, not all obtain benefit and the optimal breathing pattern is determined by trial and error.[39] Specific resistive-breathing exercises to enhance the strength and endurance of the respiratory muscles may offer some benefit, particularly to patients who have symptoms or signs of diaphragm fatigue after exercise.[1,3,31] Patients with large amounts of sputum (more than 30 ml daily) may find postural drainage to be of benefit immediately before training to improve airflow. Similarly, inhaled bronchodilating agents are helpful at this time.

Success in activity programs for disabled subjects largely depends on the personality and expertise of the exercise leader. An effective, safe, and comfortable level of training is set by the patient and activity leader working closely together. Changes in airflow obstruction, fatigue, anxiety level, and other health-related problems may require day-to-day modifications in therapy and exercise prescription. The leader also makes changes in exercise prescription as a training effect occurs. Although participants are able to increase their MET load progressively to approach or reach their target HR or their highest tolerable level of ventilation, intensities that induce severe breathlessness are avoided. Extreme discomfort reduces enjoyment, compliance, and motivation. Repeated exposure to a breathless state may be unavoidable and even useful in helping patients to control breathing and reduce anxiety, but it must be carried out in a systematic fashion with a defined end point.

The leader should be familiar with typical warning signals of cardiorespiratory problems, including worsening dyspnea, change in sputum color, swollen ankles, sudden weight gain, and high resting HR. Easy communication with referring physicians and other team members is important, and simple measures of airflow obstruction by peak flow meter or dry spirometer need to be readily available.

Evaluation of Progress

Regular review of progress is important to provide encouragement and to improve compliance. Repeat exercise studies and the use of symptom scales are particularly valuable to measure progress and to decide on possible changes in exercise prescription and program design.

Results of Programs

A review of published studies suggests that regular exercise training may be effective in improving work performance and lessening dyspnea, without influencing the disease process. Investigators agree that improvement in pulmonary function is not to be expected. Although it is not possible to identify all the mechanisms that are influenced by training, an increase in activity may be achieved in a number of ways:

1. Improved efficiency of walking (with better posture, improved stride, and less accessory movements) leading to a reduction in oxygen uptake at a given level of activity, thus lessening the metabolic load on breathing.[30]
2. A reduction in the carbon dioxide load accompanying a reduction in lactic acid production; this result stems from improved central cardiac response and distribution of blood flow and enhancement of muscle enzyme activity. In most patients, however, these factors are not limiting and it is often difficult for these patients to train at a power output that is sufficient to improve these processes.[37]
3. Ventilation at a given submaximal power output is decreased and the level of PCO_2 is higher after training; this is particularly true when oxygen supplementation is used in training sessions and may contribute to a lessening of dyspnea.[27,38]
4. An increase in tidal volume may improve gas exchange through reductions in the dead space to tidal volume ratio and venous admixture.[13]
5. Increases in red cell mass may occur, but not if oxygen supplements are given during training sessions.[37,38]
6. Respiratory muscle training is capable of increasing ventilation capacity and endurance.[3] Although the changes are often small, only small changes are required to allow patients to get around with less distress. Small changes in ventilatory capacity may also have a major effect on work tolerance and the sensation of dyspnea.[28]

There is little doubt that we need to know more about the mechanisms that may be improved in patients with chronic lung problems, e.g., breathing patterns, gas exchange efficiency, diaphragm function, oxygen cost of breathing and of day-to-day activities, and muscle performance. We also need to know how to choose the most effective program for an individual, as well as to judge the benefits of such ancillary measures as oxygen supplementation. These questions are difficult to investigate rigorously, however, because of the extreme variability in the clinical features and the natural history of these conditions. In addition, improvements in activity, confidence, and quality of life are difficult to measure. Enough evidence has been accumulated to inspire confidence in the beneficial effects of exercise rehabilitation programs that are established on the basis of a common-sense approach to the improvement of function and are individualized for each patient.[2,7,25,26,28,36,37,40]

REFERENCES

1. Anderson, J.B., and Dragsted, L.: Resistive breathing. Scand. J. Respir. Dis., 60:151, 1979.
2. Bass, H., Whitcomb, J.F., and Forman, R.: Exercise training: therapy for patients with chronic obstructive lung disease. Chest, 57:116, 1970.
3. Belman, M.J., and Mittman, C.: Ventilatory muscle training improves exercise capacity in chronic obstructive pulmonary disease patients. Am. Rev. Respir. Dis., 121:273, 1980.
4. Burns, B.H., and Howell, J.B.L.: Disproportionately severe breathlessness in chronic bronchitis. Q. J. Med., 38:277, 1969.
5. Burrows, B., and Earle, R.H.: Course and prognosis of chronic obstructive lung disease: a prospective study of 200 patients. N. Engl. J. Med., 280:397, 1969.
6. Burrows, B., Niden, A.H., Fletcher, C.M., and Jones, N.L.: Clinical types of chronic obstructive lung disease in London and Chicago: a study of 100 patients. Am. Rev. Respir. Dis., 90:14, 1964.
7. Chester, E.H., et al.: Multidisciplinary treatment of chronic pulmonary insufficiency. 3. The effect of physical training on cardiopulmonary

performance in patients with chronic obstructive pulmonary disease. Chest, *72*:695, 1977.

8. Cotes, J.F.: Lung Function. Assessment and Application in Medicine. 3rd Ed. Oxford, Blackwell Scientific, 1976.

9. Dolovich, J., and Hargreave, F.E.: The asthma syndrome: inciters, inducers and host characteristics. Thorax, *36*:641, 1981.

10. Dolovich, J., et al.: Control of asthma. Can. Med. Assoc. J., *126*:613, 1982.

11. Fletcher, C., Peto, R., Tinker, C., and Speizer, F.E.: The natural history of chronic bronchitis and emphysema. New York, Oxford University Press, 1976.

12. Hargreave, F.E., et al.: Bronchial responsiveness to histamine or metacholine in asthma: measurement and clinical significance. J. Allergy Clin. Immunol., *68*:347, 1981.

13. Jones, N.L.: Pulmonary gas exchange during exercise in patients with chronic airway obstruction. Clin. Sci., *31*:39, 1966.

14. Jones, N.L.: Physical therapy—present state of the art. Am. Rev. Respir. Dis., *110*:132, 1974.

15. Jones, N.L.: Blood gases and acid-base physiology. New York, Thieme-Stratton, 1979.

16. Jones, N.L.: Exercise testing. Med. Clin. North Am. *21*:2089, 1982.

17. Jones, N.L., and Campbell, E.J.M.: Clinical Exercise Testing. 2nd Ed. Philadelphia, W.B. Saunders, 1981.

18. Jones, N.L., and Campbell, E.J.M.: Chronic airway obstruction due to asthma, bronchitis, and emphysema. *In* Principles of Internal Medicine. 7th ed. Edited by M.M. Wintrobe, et al. New York, McGraw-Hill, 1974.

19. Jones, N.L., Jones, G., and Edwards, R.H.T.: Exercise tolerance in chronic airway obstruction. Am. Rev. Respir. Dis., *103*:477, 1971.

20. Killian, K.J., and Jones, N.L.: The uses of exercise testing and other methods in the investigation of dyspnea. *In* Exercise-Physiology and Clinical Application. Clin. Chest Med., 5:99, 1984.

21. Lefcoe, N.M., and Paterson, N.A.M.: Adjunct therapy in chronic obstructive pulmonary disease. Am. J. Med., *54*:343, 1973.

22. Lertzman, M.M., and Cherniack, R.M.: Rehabilitation of patients with chronic obstructive pulmonary disease. Am. Rev. Respir. Dis., *114*:1145, 1976.

23. McFadden, E.R., Jr., and Ingram, R.H., Jr.: Exercise-induced asthma. N. Engl. J. Med., *301*:763, 1979.

24. McGavin, C.G.R., Gupta, S.P., and McHardy, G.J.R.: Twelve-minute walking test for assessing disability in chronic bronchitis. Br. Med. J., *1*:822, 1976.

25. McGavin, C.R., Gupta, S.P., Lloyd, E.L., and McHardy, G.J.R.: Physical rehabilitation for the chronic bronchitic: results of a controlled trial of exercises in the home. Thorax, *32*:307, 1977.

26. Mertens, D.J., Shephard, R.J., and Kavanagh, T.: Long-term exercise therapy for chronic obstructive lung disease. Respiration, *35*:96, 1978.

27. Neff, T.A., and Petty, T.L.: Long-term continuous oxygen therapy in chronic airway obstruction. Ann. Intern. Med., *72*:621, 1970.

28. Nicholas, J.J., Gilbert, R., Gabe, R., and Auchincloss, J.H., Jr.: Evaluation of an exercise therapy program for patients with chronic obstructive pulmonary disease. Am. Rev. Respir. Dis., *102*:1, 1970.

29. Oldridge, N.B., Wicks, J.R., and McIntosh, J.: Exercise in coronary rehabilitation: prescription and program design. Physiotherapy, *30*:64, 1978.

30. Paez, P.N., Phillipson, E.A., Masangkay, M., and Sproule, B.J.: The physiologic basis of training patients with chronic airway obstruction. I. Effects of exercise training. Am. Rev. Respir. Dis., *95*:944, 1967.

31. Pardy, R.L., Reid, W.D., and Beeman, M.J.: Respiratory muscle training. Clin. Chest Med., 9:287–296, 1988.

32. Pierce, A.K.: Exercise training with the aid of portable oxygen supply in patients with emphysema. Am. Rev. Respir. Dis., *91*:654, 1965.

33. Rochester, F.D., and Goldberg, S.K.: Techniques of respiratory physical therapy. Am. Rev. Respir. Dis., *122*:133, 1980.

34. Saunders, N.A., Powles, A.C.P., and Rebuck, A.S.: Ear oximetry: accuracy and practicability in the assessment of arterial oxygenation. Am. Rev. Respir. Dis., *113*:745, 1976.

35. Shephard, R.J.: On the design and effectiveness of training regimens in chronic obstructive lung disease. Bull. Eur. Physiopathol. Respir., *13*:457, 1977.

36. Sinclair, D.J.M., and Sinclair, C.G.: Controlled trial of supervised exercise training in chronic bronchitis. Br. Med. J., *1*:519, 1980.

37. Vyas, M.N., Banister, E.W., Morton, J.W., and Grzybowski, S.: Response to exercise in patients with chronic airway obstruction. I. Effects of exercise training. Am. Rev. Respir. Dis., *103*:390, 1971.

38. Vyas, M.N., Banister, E.W., Morton, J.W., and Grzybowski, S.: Response to exercise in patients with chronic airway obstruction. Am. Rev. Respir. Dis., *103*:401, 1971.

39. Watts, N.: Improvement of breathing patterns. Am. Phys. Ther. J., *48*:563, 1968.

40. Woolf, C.R.: A rehabilitation program for improving exercise tolerance of patients with chronic lung disease. Can. Med. Assoc. J., *106*:1289, 1972.

14
CHAPTER

Cystic Fibrosis

by
Frank Cerny and David Orenstein

Cystic fibrosis (CF) is the most common fatal inherited disease of whites and is transmitted as an autosomal recessive trait. The gene causing the disease has been described recently[44] and appears to be responsible for the production of a protein labeled as the CF transmembrane regulator (CFTR) protein. This protein participates in controlling the flux of chloride into and out of the cells lining the airways and the other exocrine glands. The alteration in the CFTR results in abnormal ion flux, abnormally high negative transmembrane electrical charges, and relative dehydration of intraluminal fluids in affected organs. The primary organs affected are the lungs, pancreas, intestines, and sweat glands.[42,50] The decreased water in the airways leads to abnormally thick secretions, which impede breathing and prevent the normal secretion of digestive enzymes through the pancreatic ducts into the intestines. In the 1950s, the mean survival age was under 5 years, and even today, the patient may not survive infancy in severe cases. With aggressive therapy, however, most affected individuals survive into adulthood, with the present median age of survival being 28 years.[16]

Symptoms of CF vary among patients.[18,51] Pulmonary symptoms include recurrent or persistent cough, wheezing, and dyspnea. Because these symptoms are similar to those of patients with asthma, the correct diagnosis may be overlooked for months or years. Frequent lower-airway infection, particularly with *Staphylo-coccus aureus, Hemophilis influenzae,* or mucoid *Pseudomonas aeruginosa,* is typical in CF. Gastrointestinal (GI) involvement may present at birth with intestinal obstruction (meconium ileus) or, somewhat later, with failure to thrive. Obstruction of the pancreatic ducts leads to trypsin, amylase, and lipase deficiencies in 90% of patients, resulting in frequent, bulky, and foul-smelling stools with a high lipid content.

The diagnosis of CF is made definitively by analysis of sweat sodium and chloride.[16] The defect results in abnormally high concentrations of these ions in the sweat, with a clear separation between affected (> 60 mEq/L) and unaffected (< 40 mEq/L) individuals during childhood; there is a low incidence of false-positive results into adulthood.[19] Sweat testing must be performed in a laboratory experienced in the techniques of pilocarpine iontophoresis with quantitative analysis of sodium and/or chloride. These laboratories are most often associated with CF Centers certified by the Cystic Fibrosis Foundation. The rate of false-positive and false-negative tests is very high in inexperienced hands, which can lead to tragic results. Although DNA testing is now possible in several medical centers, it is not yet capable of identifying all affected patients and is currently slower and more expensive than sweat testing.

The pulmonary complications of the disease are related to the plugging of the airways by the excessive, thick mucous secretions. Repeated airway infections, a hallmark of the disease, also result in inflammation and bronchiectasis, associated with further increases in secretions. Other pulmonary complications may include hemoptysis, atelectasis, allergic aspergillosis, pneumothorax, pulmonary hypertension, cor pulmonale, and respiratory failure.[27] The extent of involvement is assessed by radiographs and most sensitively by pulmonary function testing.

Treatment of the digestive complications of CF includes supplemental pancreatic enzymes with meals and supplementation with fat-soluble vitamins.

The bronchial plugging eventually results in elevated airway resistance and considerable trapping of air in the lungs such that they become hyperinflated. Over time, there is a mismatching of ventilation and perfusion and a deterioration in arterial blood gases. The progressive, chronic hypoxemia results in cor pulmonale. The continuing airway obstruction and hyperinflation increase the flow-resistive and the elastic work of breathing, respectively. In most patients, the progressive deterioration in lung function is not reflected in an altered exercise blood gas response until pulmonary reserves are decreased below a critical threshold. Once this threshold of lung dysfunction is reached, exercise-induced decreases in arterial oxygen and increases in arterial carbon dioxide are noted.[6,15,26] The lung hyperinflation alters lung mechanics such that the respiratory pattern during exercise becomes abnormal.[8,13] The increased work of breathing results in chronic increases in resting oxygen consumption.[28,30]

The greatest impact on patient morbidity and mortality is from pulmonary complications.[27] Treatment of these complications includes control of pulmonary infections with antibiotics and pulmonary hygiene to remove mucus. The underlying pulmonary infection and inflammation will worsen periodically. These pulmonary exacerbations may require hospitalization with intravenous antibiotics and chest physical therapy. In cases of mild exacer-

bations, treatment may be accomplished at home with oral, aerosolized, or even intravenous antibiotics.

The removal of secretions by chest physical therapy has been a standard part of the treatment of CF patients for many years.[36] Chest physical therapy consists of postural drainage, chest percussion, forced expirations and, more recently, exercise.[20] These techniques appear to be effective in inducing sputum expectoration only if cough is induced.[9,38,45] After decades of use, these chest physical therapy techniques have only recently been shown to be effective in preventing or attenuating deterioration of pulmonary function.[21,43]

Airway reactivity is frequently associated with CF and may require treatment with bronchodilators or other drugs that may influence airway function. Corticosteroids and other nonsteroidal anti-inflammatory agents have been suggested as possible treatment for the airway inflammation of CF[4,32] but have not yet been evaluated in large controlled studies to permit a clear understanding of their roles.

With the identification of the specific defect in CF, new treatments are being developed and are currently undergoing clinical trials. Finally, there is speculation that therapies eventually will be developed that can replace the defective CFTR protein or that can alter the defective gene, or even replace it with a normal gene, a procedure that would cure the airway cells of CF.

The following section presents 1) the rationale for exercise testing in patients with CF, 2) protocols for the exercise test, 3) the expected pulmonary response to exercise in a healthy and a CF population, 4) a basis for the interpretation of the test and for prescribing exercise, and 5) various strategies for incorporating exercise into the therapeutic regimen of patients.

WHY AN EXERCISE TEST?

It has been estimated that even at maximal exercise in a healthy population, the lungs are required to use only about 80%

of their total capacity for gas exchange; the remaining 20% has been called the pulmonary reserve. As disease compromises lung function, this reserve is decreased and eventually disappears.[6,15] A progressive, incremental exercise test, by encroaching into these reserves, can be useful to estimate the chronic and acute effects of the lung disease on the appropriateness of the response to exercise. If a program of exercise is being considered or if advice regarding participation in activities is being sought, the exercise test can be useful to identify the level of activity that can be safely accomplished. Tables of energy expenditure for a variety of activities can be used to obtain a qualitative determination of effort for various activities.[35] By matching these estimates with the heart rate (HR) response to the exercise test, one can estimate the patient's response to activities of daily living. The exercise threshold above which acute respiratory insufficiency may be observed can be identified through the exercise test. Finally, the effects of disease progression, treatment, or exercise therapy can be evaluated with the exercise test.

THE EXERCISE TEST

Patients Younger Than 7 Years

Most patients younger than 7 years will not be able to cooperate sufficiently for a formal laboratory test with careful monitoring of cardiopulmonary adaptation. Exercise-induced respiratory compromise in infants and children 1 to 3 years old may be detectable by careful observation during feeding, periods of crying, or normal activity. For objective documentation of suspected compromise, an ear oximeter can be attached to the scapha of the ear to detect changes in arterial hemoglobin oxygen saturation (SaO_2%). Most children will tolerate the earprobe well and do not mind the slight restriction of activity due to the 6- to 8-foot cable connection.

In children from 3 to 6 years of age, a more quantitative estimate of exercise tolerance can be made by using a motor-driven treadmill.[46] With support, even children this age can walk on the treadmill while SaO_2% and ECG are monitored. It is difficult to standardize the test in this age group, and the attainment of high work levels is difficult. Young patients rarely exceed an HR rate of 160 beats per minute for this test. Because most children this age do not carry out sustained activity at HRs higher than 50 to 60% of maximum,[17] the information obtained is still useful to describe whether the pulmonary response to exercise is normal and to determine safe levels of activity.

Patients Older Than 7 Years

Before the exercise test, each patient should undergo a clinical evaluation and pulmonary function tests if these have not been done recently. We have found that FEV_1 correlates best with exercise tolerance, and that a scoring system using six resting pulmonary function tests also correlates well.[15] It should be noted that there is a large individual variation, and although the resting lung function may identify a group of patients at increased risk for exercise-induced desaturation, the exercise test itself is the only tool that can determine with certainty what will happen to oxygen saturation during exercise or what exercise level will be tolerated.

Patients should be dressed appropriately for testing. A loose-fitting T-shirt, shorts, and sneakers are best. Long pants with wide cuffs can become tangled in the cycle pedals or cause the patient to trip on the treadmill. The sites for the chest ECG electrodes should be cleaned and lightly abraded to ensure good contact. All procedures should be carefully explained to make the test less frightening and to optimize cooperation.

Several testing protocols can be selected depending on the reason for the exercise evaluation.

INCREMENTAL TESTS. If the primary purpose of the test is to determine peak exercise capacity, a progressive incremental test using 1-min work periods should be used. If one is interested in the adaptive response to exercise, in addition to a determination of the patient's functional work capacity, 2-min stages are recommended. The 2-min stage allows observation of various parameters during a quasi steady-state in the last 30 sec of each stage. If 3-min stages are chosen, the test may become unnecessarily long. For those who have a treadmill available or prefer its use, increments in elevation of 2 to 2.5% grade every 2 min are comfortable for most patients and result in an increase in HR of approximately 10 beats per work stage. The speed of the treadmill should be selected so that a moderately fast walk must be assumed and should allow most patients, including those with severe dysfunction, to exercise at two to three levels. For smaller children, this speed ranges from 2 to 3 km/hr, in adolescents from 4 to 5 km/hr, and in adults 6 to 7 km/hr.

Most published studies of exercise in CF patients have used the cycle ergometer. It is quieter, less intimidating than the treadmill, safer (patients may fall on the treadmill), and more easily mastered. The patient moves less, making collection of expired gases and measurement of blood pressure and $SaO_2\%$ by oximetry considerably easier. Power output also depends less on body weight when using the cycle ergometer. In choosing an ergometer for the laboratory, one should take into account the need for fitting small children and the need for relatively small increments in power output. Electronically braked ergometers are more expensive than mechanically braked units, but have the advantage that power output is relatively independent of pedaling rate. Lower peak oxygen consumption will be obtained on the cycle than would be measured using the treadmill because fewer muscles are involved.

On the cycle ergometer, several different protocols can be used. We prefer either of the following:

1. Power output increments of 0.3 watts/kg yield results similar to those with the treadmill protocol discussed above. The initial power output should be 0.3 watts/kg for small or severely compromised patients and 0.6 watts/kg for others.

2. Godfrey's protocol is based on height, starting with as low a power output as possible on the cycle and 1-min increments of 10, 15, and 20 watts for children shorter than 125 cm, between 125 and 150 cm, and those taller than 150 cm, respectively.[25] Power output relationships to oxygen consumption and predicted values for maximal exercise are shown in Tables 14–1 and 14–2, respectively.

OTHER TESTS. When it is not necessary to record a peak or maximal exercise value, the above protocols may be modified. When one is interested in the cardiopulmonary adaptation to exercise, measurements should be taken during a steady state. In most circumstances, steady state can be assumed to have been reached between 4 and 5 min after the start of exercise or after a change in exercise level. This time may be prolonged to some degree in patients with severe lung disease.[22,37] These tests are generally done to allow special measurements during exercise, such as lung diffusing capacity and cardiac output, or when information is needed at a particular work level (e.g., to simulate job requirements). The one- or two-level test is also useful to evaluate the effects of supplemental oxygen on exercise response.

When periodic check-ups are needed or when the effects of therapy must be determined at frequent intervals, a full incremental test may not be required. In these cases, a shorter test with fewer power outputs can be used. For example, if the exercise prescription asks that the patient exercise below an HR of 150 beats/min and arterial oxygen desaturation was observed at this point during the initial evaluation, follow-up evaluations need take the patient only to an HR of 150. The effects of exercise therapy can be documented by frequent 2- to 3-stage submaximal tests.

MONITORING DURING THE TEST. To establish a safe exercise prescription, it is

TABLE 14–1. **Power Output/Oxygen Uptake Relationships on Cycle Ergometer***

Power Output (watts/kg)	Oxygen Uptake $(ml \cdot kg^{-1} \cdot min^{-1})$ $(\bar{X} \pm SE)$	Minute Ventilation $(ml \cdot kg^{-1} \cdot min^{-1})$
0.3	10.2 ± 0.45	0.30 ± 0.01
0.6	13.8 ± 0.28	0.43 ± 0.01
0.9	17.2 ± 0.34	0.54 ± 0.02
1.2	20.0 ± 0.23	0.66 ± 0.02
1.5	22.9 ± 0.037	0.79 ± 0.02
1.8	26.7 ± 0.048	0.94 ± 0.03
2.1	31.2 ± 0.56	1.10 ± 0.03
2.4	35.2 ± 1.02	1.20 ± 0.04
2.7	39.9 ± 1.16	1.31 ± 0.05

* Unpublished results, Cerny, F.J. Children's Lung Center, Children's Hospital of Buffalo.

TABLE 14–2. **Predicted Values at Peak Power Output Using Godfrey's Progressive Cycle Ergometer Protocol***

	Power Output (watts)	Oxygen Uptake $(L \cdot min^{-1})$	Minute Ventilation $(L \cdot min^{-1})$
Male:	3.54 × ht − 377	0.045 × ht − 4.64	1.82 × ht − 192
Female:	2.17 × ht − 197	0.031 × ht − 2.28	1.03 × ht − 88

ht = height in cm
* Unpublished results, Orenstein, D.M., Henke, K.G., Reed, M.E., and Wachnowsky, D.

important to monitor SaO_2 or arterial oxygen pressure (PaO_2) during exercise; this is virtually mandatory in patients with an FEV_1 <50% of the predicted normal value. We recommend the ear oximetric measurement of SaO_2 because of its convenience and noninvasive nature. Regarding the interpretation of SaO_2 measurements, it should be noted that for patients high on the O_2 dissociation curve (>80 mm Hg PaO_2), relatively large and potentially clinically significant drops in PaO_2 may be reflected in a decrease of only 1 to 2% SaO_2.

In healthy individuals, end-tidal PCO_2 reflects $PaCO_2$ and can be a useful parameter to monitor during exercise. Healthy individuals have a negligible alveolar to arterial (A-a) gradient, making alveolar or end-tidal CO_2 a good estimate of arterial CO_2. However, the gradient is increased in patients with lung disease, making it likely that end-tidal CO_2 underestimates arterial CO_2. The measurement of end-tidal CO_2 can still be valuable as a reflection of changes in arterial CO_2.

A description of the pulmonary response to exercise requires the measurement of minute ventilation ($\dot{V}_E$) either directly by collecting exhaled air in a gasometer or indirectly by integrating expiratory flow measured with a pneumotach. Quantification of the energy expenditure (oxygen consumption, $\dot{V}_{O_2}$) during exercise can be made by measuring the mixed expired fractions (F) of O_2 and CO_2. $\dot{V}_{O_2} = \dot{V}_I(FIO_2) - \dot{V}_E(FEO_2)$ and $\dot{V}_I = \dot{V}_E([1 - (FEO_2 + FECO_2)]/FIN_2)$.

To access the cardiovascular responses to exercise, ECG, HR, and blood pressure should be monitored throughout the test. Measurement of HR also allows prescription of activity using HR to monitor the intensity of the exercise.

Termination of the test is based on one or a combination of the criteria discussed by Bar-Or in Chapter 4. In addition, particular attention should be paid to decreases in SaO_2 below 80% and clinical observations of pallor, extreme dyspnea, or other signs of respiratory decompensation.

SAFETY PRECAUTIONS. Equipment in the laboratory should be properly maintained and calibrated. Oxygen and resuscitation supplies (e.g., drugs, intravenous sets) and equipment (e.g., defibrillator and bag respirator) should be readily available. Emergency codes and procedures, including drug availability and dosages, should be posted. Personnel should be trained and, if possible, certified in cardiopulmonary resuscitation.[14]

RESPONSE TO EXERCISE IN PATIENTS WITH CF

Exercise capacity in CF patients has been shown to be related to severity of lung disease[6,10,11,24,40] and can be affected by nutritional status.[10] There is no evidence that cardiac dysfunction contributes to the disease-related changes in exercise tolerance.[12,34] In addition, the slope of the HR response to exercise in patients is similar to that of healthy subjects,[6] changing only in intercept with clinical status.[7] The reduced exercise tolerance is due to pulmonary limitations, as evidenced by the strong relationship between pulmonary dysfunction and exercise capacity.[6,15,24,26,33] The strength of this general relationship also is shown by parallel changes in lung function and exercise tolerance in patients hospitalized for an acute exacerbation of their lung disease.[7] Exercise capacity or response to exercise, however, cannot be predicted simply from lung function because of the variability in the response[26] and because the relationship is not linear, showing nearly normal exercise capacity until lung dysfunction is severe.[6,15]

The increase in $\dot{V}_E$ by CF patients during exercise is exaggerated, especially with increasing severity of pulmonary dysfunction.[6] The progressive deterioration of blood-gas matching, as measured by the ratio of alveolar ventilation ($\dot{V}_A$) to cardiac output ($\dot{Q}$), with CF requires an increased $\dot{V}_E$ to maintain $\dot{V}_A$. In a few, very severely obstructed patients, dyspnea may force an end to exercise before $\dot{V}_E$ has risen significantly above normal.

In spite of the higher $\dot{V}_E$, some patients with severe dysfunction are unable to maintain arterial O_2 and CO_2 levels.[6,15,26] The higher $\dot{V}_E$ in these patients is accomplished by an increased breathing frequency and a small tidal volume. The hyperinflation already seen at rest in CF patients likely minimizes the probability of further increases during exercise. The combination of gas exchange abnormalities and mechanical inefficiency results in exercise limitations that depend on disease severity.

INTERPRETATION OF THE EXERCISE TEST AND EXERCISE PRESCRIPTION

Maximal $\dot{V}_{O_2}$ changes little in healthy people from the age of 7 to adulthood when corrected for weight or body surface area. Values for peak work capacity or peak $\dot{V}_{O_2}$ measured in a clinical setting generally are lower than those measured in a school or research setting. Average values for peak $\dot{V}_{O_2}$ in a clinical setting range from 38 to 44 ml·kg^{-1}·min^{-1} for boys and 34 to 38 ml·kg^{-1}·min^{-1} for girls on the cycle ergometer. These $\dot{V}_{O_2}$ levels correspond to power outputs of approximately 2.7 to 3.0 watts/kg and 2.1 to 2.4 watts/kg for males and females, respectively. Values for peak $\dot{V}_{O_2}$ from a treadmill test are approximately 10% higher. The coefficient of variation for these values is about 10%.

The linear relationship between HR and $\dot{V}_{O_2}$ can be used to prescribe and monitor exercise therapy. Unfortunately, there is considerable variation between individuals in this relationship, so the exercise test should be used to establish the specific relationship for each patient. By knowing the unique individual relationship between $\dot{V}_{O_2}$ and HR, one can require that the patient exercise at an established HR to accomplish the therapeutic goals based on energy expenditure. The relationship will change as conditioning progresses, so that a higher $\dot{V}_{O_2}$ will be achieved at the same HR—that is, any given submaximal work rate is done at a lower HR.

The Exercise Program

Any conditioning program must consider the usual elements of endurance, flexibility, and strength. It is not yet known if any exercise program can prevent or slow the deterioration of lung function in patients with CF, but it is known that aerobic exercise programs can increase cardiopulmonary fitness,[31,41] and it is thought that certain types of exercise may facilitate sputum expectoration. The primary concerns for the patient with CF, therefore, are the improvement of cardiovascular reserves and the promotion of sputum expectoration. Cough and sputum expectoration should be encouraged in all patients, but particularly in those in whom the cough is productive.

The prescription of endurance (aerobic) exercise must be individualized. In choosing the type of activities for the exercise prescription, the types of activities the patient enjoys must be ascertained and used as a base. Compliance with a program will be poor if the patient feels that the exercise is boring.[29] A second important factor to ensure compliance is to promote the use of exercise partners, whether this be other members of the family or friends. Special outing clubs or sporting groups may be helpful in promoting regular activity. Patients should not engage in highly competitive sports in which there may be pressure to exercise beyond what may be safe. Competitive activities should allow some means of self-regulation whereby the patient can slow down without feeling a lot of pressure. Diving, whether underwater or in the sky, should be engaged in only after careful consideration of the potential for negative consequences (e.g., alveolar rupture).

The exercise prescription in young children can be filled simply by encouraging participation in normal activity. The family can be a partner in this by assuming an active lifestyle. This type of partnership also helps ensure that exercise will become part of the patient's lifestyle. As the pa-

tient enters the teen years, the exercise prescription can concentrate on more specific activities.

Some strength training can be prescribed in patients with CF. The effects of strenuous body building in patients with CF are unknown, but one study showed that a regular program of weight lifting resulted in improvements in strength and marginal improvements in selected pulmonary function tests.[49] We recommend that the more strenuous types of lifting be avoided, particularly in children through adolescence.

In summary, it is important to choose activities that the patient enjoys, that will specifically improve cardiovascular endurance and strength, and that will allow the use of family or friend support.

Exercise Intensity

There is a level of exercise intensity below which no training effect will be achieved. There is also a level above which the extra effort required will result in little additional benefit. The exercise prescription should be chosen to ensure that the middle intensities of effort will be reached. For cardiovascular benefit, this level is usually between 50 and 70% of the individual's maximal capacity. Guidelines for the calculation of appropriate target HRs are available.[1] However, because CF patients may be limited by ventilatory factors before their HR has reached its maximum, one cannot prescribe exercise intensity based on age-predicted maximal HR, but must use each patient's own measured maximum. The target HR should be below the point at which desaturation was observed during the exercise test. In cases in which desaturation has been noted as soon as exercise begins, or at HRs < 120 beats per min, supplemental oxygen should be considered to keep the SaO_2 above 90% and to allow exercise at HRs of 120 to 130 beats per min.

Strength exercises should be prescribed so that the weight or resistance chosen will allow the patient to do a minimum of 10 repetitions at a time. If this cannot be done, the resistance is too high. Three sets of each exercise should be done at each session. A reasonable session would include 5 to 10 different exercises. Two series of 5 to 10 exercises should be available so that the patient can alternate between these series on different days (e.g., one series would be done on Monday and Friday and a different series on Wednesday and Sunday).

Exercise Duration

Accepted guidelines for cardiovascular exercise prescription suggest that continuous activity be done for about 30 min a day; the minimal recommended duration is 10 to 15 min. There should also be some warm-up time before and cool-down after the main exercise period. In many patients with moderate to severe lung dysfunction who may be less fit or who have a severely limited work capacity, light exercise may be tolerated for only 5 min at the start. The exercise time should increase to 10 or 15 min over a period of 1 to 2 weeks. In many cases, the exercise may have to be completed in two sessions.

Exercise Frequency

These exercises should be done a minimum of 3 days a week. Ideally, these activities should be done 5 to 6 days/week in patients with little or only mild dysfunction. In patients with more severe dysfunction, rest days must be inserted.

IN-PATIENT THERAPY

All patients admitted to the hospital with an acute exacerbation of their disease and those admitted for elective intensive therapy should be considered for exercise therapy. For those patients restricted to their beds, the exercise can be simple resistive exercises using the body's own weight. These exercises include leg lifts, arm lifts, and modified sit-ups. For ambulatory patients, whether on or off supplemental oxygen, a preliminary exercise assessment should be done to determine the degree of monitoring needed during the therapy sessions. Patients who desaturate during their exercise test, regardless of their peak exercise capacity, should be monitored by ear oximetry during exercise. Patients who do not desaturate during the initial evaluation can exercise in the physical therapy department where less-careful monitoring is necessary. All patients who are able should be encouraged to move around the ward. Leg, heart, and ventilatory muscle function should not be allowed to deteriorate while lung function is improving!

Expected Benefits of Regular Exercise in CF Patients

Except in circumstances in which heavy exercise is done several times a day,[52,53] there is no convincing evidence that exercise training will improve lung function, as measured by standard pulmonary function tests. Specific respiratory muscle training will improve respiratory muscle function,[3] but how these improvements affect lung dysfunction or exercise capacity is not known. Engaging in regular cardiovascular endurance activities will improve respiratory muscle endurance and exercise capacity[31,41] and may slow the progressive deterioration of lung function in CF patients. Studies on the potential benefits of long-term regular exercise have not been able to show positive effects on lung function or even always on exercise capacity because of problems of compliance and high individual variability.[2,5,23,29,39,41,47,48] When they are available, however, a close examination of individual data indicates that individual patients can benefit greatly by regular exercise. All patients with CF can safely perform some form of exercise, and exercise should be encouraged as part of the regular routine for these patients.

REFERENCES

1. American College of Sports Medicine: Guidelines for graded exercise testing and exercise prescription. 4th Ed. Philadelphia, Lea & Febiger, 1990.
2. Andreasson, B., et al.: Long-term effects of physical exercise on working capacity and pulmonary function in cystic fibrosis. Acta Paediatr. Scand., 76:70, 1987.
3. Asher, M., Pardy, R., Coates, A., et al.: The effects of inspiratory muscle training in patients with cystic fibrosis. Am. Rev. Respir. Dis., 126:855, 1982.

4. Auerbach, H.S., Kirkpatrick, J.A., Williams, M., and Colten, H.R.: Alternate-day prednisone reduces morbidity and improves pulmonary function in cystic fibrosis. Lancet, 28:686, 1985.
5. Blomquist, M., Freyschuss, U., Wiman, L-G., and Strandvik, B.: Physical activity and self treatment in cystic fibrosis. Arch. Dis. Child., 61:362, 1986.
6. Cerny, F.J., Pullano, T.P., and Cropp, G.J.A.: Cardiorespiratory adaptations to exercise in cystic fibrosis. Am. Rev. Respir. Dis., 126:217, 1982.
7. Cerny, F.J., Cropp, G.J.A., and Bye, M.R.: Hospital therapy improves exercise tolerance and lung function in cystic fibrosis. Am. Rev. Respir. Dis., 138:261, 1984.
8. Cerny, F.J.: Ventilatory control during exercise in children with cystic fibrosis (CF). Am. Rev. Respir. Dis., 123:195, 1981.
9. Cerny, F.J.: Relative effects of chest physiotherapy and exercise for in-hospital care of cystic fibrosis. Phys. Ther., 69:633–639. 1989.
10. Coates, A., Boyce, P., Muller, D., et al.: The role of nutritional status, airway obstruction, hypoxia and abnormalities in serum lipid composition in limiting exercise tolerance in children with cystic fibrosis. Acta Paediatr. Scand., 69:353, 1980.
11. Coates, A., Boyce, P., Shaw, D., et al.: Relationship between the chest radiograph, regional lung function studies, exercise tolerance, and clinical condition in cystic fibrosis. Arch. Dis. Child., 56:106, 1981.
12. Coates, A.L., Desmond, K., Asher, M.I., et al.: The effect of digoxin on exercise capacity and exercise cardiac function in cystic fibrosis. Chest, 82:543, 1982.
13. Coates, A.L., et al.: The effects of chronic airflow limitation, increased dead space, and the pattern of ventilation on gas exchange during maximal exercise in advanced cystic fibrosis. Am. Rev. Respir. Dis., 139:1524, 1988.
14. Cropp, G.J.A.: The exercise bronchoprovocation test: standardization of procedures and evaluation of response. J. Allergy Clin. Immunol., 64:627, 1979.
15. Cropp, G.J.A., Pullano, T.P., Cerny, F.J., and Nathanson, I.: Exercise tolerance and cardiorespiratory adjustments at peak work capacity in cystic fibrosis. Am. Rev. Respir. Dis., 126:211, 1982.
16. Cystic Fibrosis Foundation: Guide to Diagnosis and Management of Cystic Fibrosis. Bethesda, MD, 1984.
17. Danner, F., et al.: Description of the physical activity of young children using movement sensor and observation methods. Pediatr. Exerc. Sci., 3:11, 1991.
18. Davis, P., and SantAgnese, P.: Diagnosis and treatment of cystic fibrosis: an update. Chest, 85:802, 1984.
19. Davis, P., Del Rio, S., Muntz, J., and Dieckman, L.: Sweat chloride concentration in adults with pulmonary diseases. Am. Rev. Respir. Dis., 93:62–72, 1966.
20. DeCesare, J.A., and Graybill, C.A.: Physical therapy for the child with respiratory dysfunction. In Cardiopulmonary Physical Therapy. 2nd Ed. Edited by S. Irwin and J. Tecklin. St. Louis, C.V. Mosby, 1990.

21. Desmond, K.J., et al.: Immediate and long-term effects of chest physiotherapy in patients with cystic fibrosis. J. Pediatr., 103:538, 1983.
22. Dolan, P., and Cerny, F.: Oxygen uptake kinetics at onset of exercise in cystic fibrosis. Med. Sci. Sports Exerc., 15:138, 1983.
23. Edlund, L.D., et al.: Effects of a swimming program on children with cystic fibrosis. Am. J. Dis. Child., 140:80, 1986.
24. Godfrey, S., and Mearns, M.: Pulmonary function and response to exercise in cystic fibrosis. Arch. Dis. Child., 46:144, 1971.
25. Godfrey, S.: Exercise Testing in Children. Applications in Health and Disease. Philadelphia, W.B. Saunders, 1974.
26. Henke, K., and Orenstein, D.: Oxygen saturation during exercise in cystic fibrosis. Am. Rev. Respir. Dis., 129:708, 1984.
27. Hillman, B.: Respiratory complications: the chief danger in CF. J. Resp. Dis., 2:75, 1981.
28. Hirsch, J., Zhang, S., Rudnick, M., et al.: Resting oxygen consumption and ventilation in cystic fibrosis. Pediatr. Pulmonol., 6:19–26, 1989.
29. Holzer, F.J., Schnall, R., and Landau, L.I.: The effect of a home exercise programme in children with cystic fibrosis and asthma. Aust. Paediatr. J., 20:297, 1984.
30. Katsardis, C.V., Desmond, K.J., and Coates, A.L.: Measuring the oxygen cost of breathing in normal adults and patients with cystic fibrosis. Respir. Physiol. 65:257, 1986.
31. Keens, T., et al.: Ventilatory muscle endurance training in normal subjects and patients with cystic fibrosis. Am. Rev. Respir. Dis., 116:853, 1977.
32. Konstan, M.W., Vargo, K.M., and Davis, P.B.: Ibuprofen attenuates the inflammatory response to Pseudomonas aeruginosa in a rat model of chronic pulmonary infection. Implications for antiinflammatory therapy in cystic fibrosis. Am. Rev. Respir. Dis., 141:186, 1990.
33. Lebeque, P., Lapierre, J-G., Lamarre, A., and Coates, A.L.: Diffusion capacity and oxygen desaturation effects on exercise in patients with cystic fibrosis. Chest, 91:693, 1987.
34. Marcotte, J.E., Grisdale, R.K., Levinson, H., et al.: Multiple factors limit exercise capacity in cystic fibrosis. Pediatr. Pulmonol., 2:274, 1986.
35. McArdle, W., Katch, F., and Katch, V.: Exercise Physiology. 3rd Ed. Philadelphia, Lea & Febiger, 1991.
36. Mellins, R.B.: Pulmonary physiotherapy in the pediatric age group. Am. Rev. Respir. Dis., 110:137–142, 1974.
37. Nery, L.E., et al.: Ventilatory and gas exchange kinetics during exercise in chronic airways obstruction. J. Appl. Physiol., 53:1594, 1982.
38. Oldenberg, F.A., Dolovich, M.B., Montgomery, J.M., and Newhouse, M.T.: Effects of postural drainage, exercise and cough on mucus clearance in chronic bronchitis. Am. Rev. Respir. Dis., 120:739–745, 1979.
39. O'Neill, P.A., et al.: Regular exercise and reduction of breathlessness in patients with cystic fibrosis. Br. J. Dis. Chest, 81:62, 1987.
40. Orenstein, D.M., Henke, K.G., and Cerny, F.C.: Exercise and cystic fibrosis. Phys. Sportsmed., 11:57, 1983.

41. Orenstein, D., et al.: Exercise conditioning and cardiopulmonary fitness in cystic fibrosis. Chest, *80*:392, 1981.
42. Quinton, P.: Cystic fibrosis: a disease in electrolyte transport. FASEB J., *4*:2709, 1990.
43. Reisman, J.J., et al.: Role of conventional physiotherapy in cystic fibrosis. J. Pediatr., *113*:632, 1988.
44. Riordan, et al.: Identification of the cystic fibrosis gene: cloning and characterization of complementary DNA. Science, *245*:1066, 1989.
45. Rossman, C.M., Waldes, R., Sampson, D., and Newhouse, M.T.: Effect of physical therapy on the removal of mucus in patients with cystic fibrosis. Am. Rev. Respir. Dis., *126*:131, 1982.
46. Shuleva, K.M., Hunter, G.R., Hester, D.J., and Dunaway, D.L.: Exercise oxygen uptake in 3- through 6-year-old-children. Pediatr. Exerc. Sci., *2*:130, 1990.
47. Stanghelle, J.K., Hjeltnes, N., Bangstad, H.J., and Michalsen, H.: Effect of daily short bouts of trampoline exercise during 8 weeks on the pulmonary function and the maximal oxygen uptake of children with cystic fibrosis. Int. J. Sports Med., *9*(Suppl.):32, 1988.
48. Stanghelle, J.K., and Skyberg, D.: Cystic fibrosis patients running a marathon race. Int. J. Sports Med., *9*(Suppl.):37, 1988.
49. Strauss, G.D., et al.: Variable weight training in cystic fibrosis. Chest, *92*:273, 1987.
50. Welsh, M.: Abnormal regulation of ion channels in cystic fibrosis epithelia. FASEB J., *4*:2718, 1990.
51. Wood, R., Boat, T., and Doershuk, C.: Cystic fibrosis. Am. Rev. Respir. Dis., *113*:833, 1976.
52. Zach, M.S., Oberwaldner, B., and Hausler, F.: Cystic fibrosis: physical exercise versus chest physiotherapy. Arch. Dis. Child., *57*:587, 1982.
53. Zach, M.S., Purrer, B., and Oberwaldner, B.: Effect of swimming on forced expiration and sputum clearance in cystic fibrosis. Lancet, *2*:1201, 1981.

15
CHAPTER

Coronary Heart Disease

by
William L. Haskell and J. Larry Durstine

Coronary heart disease (CHD) is primarily the result of advanced coronary atherosclerosis, the cause of which has not been definitively established. During the past three decades, however, significant advances have been made in the earlier detection, prevention, and treatment of CHD. Contributing to these advances has been the use of exercise testing for the functional assessment, diagnosis, prognosis, and clinical management of patients with CHD, and the use of exercise training for prevention and in cardiac rehabilitation. This chapter presents a brief review of the current trends in CHD mortality, prevention, and therapy; cardiovascular adjustments to exercise in CHD patients; the potential benefits of training for these individuals; and some special considerations for the exercise testing and training of patients with CHD.

The recommendations provided in this chapter are general principles related to the design and conduct of training programs for CHD patients. The characteristics of the exercise plan for a specific patient should be determined by the cardiac rehabilitation team. The cardiac rehabilitation plan is comprehensive in scope and may include input from the medical director, the program director, the nurse, an exercise specialist, a dietician, a psychologist, or a vocational counselor. The interaction of various circumstances that influence exercise program details requires that each plan be individualized and that it be revamped as patient status changes.

The guidelines presented for exercise testing and training of patients or for program design should be used as a general guide and will not be applicable to every patient. As with all other cardiovascular therapies, no absolute assurance regarding benefit or safety can be ascribed to exercise training for all patients.

CAUSES, PREVENTION, AND THERAPY

Coronary heart disease continues to be the most frequent cause of death in economically developed Western countries. Currently in the United States, approximately one third of all deaths in adults aged 35 to 75 years is attributed to the two major fatal manifestations of CHD— cardiac arrest and myocardial infarction. Fatality rates for CHD remain low under the age of 35 years, but these figures increase exponentially until age 75 years, with men generally experiencing mortality at approximately twice the rate of women until age 65. Total CHD mortality in women after age 65 now exceeds that of men.[11]

During the past two decades, the mortality from CHD in the United States has decreased at the rate of approximately 2% per year.[11] Decreases of a smaller magnitude also have been experienced in such countries as Australia, Canada, and Norway; such Western countries as Italy, Scotland, England, and Wales have maintained a relatively constant rate. In some countries (Poland, North Ireland, and Bulgaria), however, CHD mortality rate has actually increased during this same period.[52] The percentage decline in this rate among Americans during the 1970s and 1980s has been reasonably constant across all ages of adults.

Why the number of deaths related to CHD has significantly decreased in some countries but not in others remains a controversial issue. At least in the United States, there are some indications that changes in health-related habits, especially in cigarette smoking, eating habits, and possibly physical activity, may have contributed to the decline, as well as certain advances in medical therapy. There is no evidence that obesity has declined during this time or that psychologic stress among the general population is any less. Recognized improvements in therapy include more widespread control of hypertension via case finding and medications, increased availability of emergency cardiac care (cardiopulmonary resuscitation and coronary care units), the use of more effective anti-anginal and anti-arrhythmic medications, and recently, judicious use of coronary artery bypass graft surgery. That this steady decrease in the CHD mortality rate has occurred among men and women of all ages and many races makes the attribution of this decline to any single health habit change or therapy highly speculative.

The variability in CHD risk among the North American population appears to be due more to health-related habits and environment than to heredity. This contention is supported by several different sources of information: 1) animal studies showing that changes in diet, especially saturated fat and cholesterol feeding, or cigarette smoke exposure influences rate of atherosclerosis; 2) human twin studies showing a strong influence of environment on differential rates of CHD; 3) cross-sectional studies of humans within a culture associating atherosclerosis in coronary arteries and clinical manifestations of CHD with various environmental factors and living traits; 4) cross-cultural studies showing differences in disease prevalence or incidence associated with living habits; 5) migration studies demonstrating a rapid and significant increase in CHD events when people with primitive living habits acculturate to more affluent lifestyles; 6) intervention studies demonstrating that changes in lifestyle or risk status result in decreased CHD mortality rates; and 7) clinical trials using lipoprotein medications or changes in lifestyle, producing a reduction in the rate of progression of coronary atherosclerosis in humans using quantitative angiography.[10,23,34,40] For selected individuals, genetic predisposition (especially abnormalities in lipoprotein metabolism) can play a very important role in their risk of developing atherosclerosis, but for most people it is to what they expose their coronary arteries that will be the major determinant.

Atherosclerosis and Ischemia

The precise biologic mechanism at the cellular level of how atherosclerosis of the coronary arteries occurs, why it develops at a specific site in one artery and not in another exposed to seemingly the same conditions, or why atherosclerosis progresses at widely differing rates in the same artery or different arteries in the same person still requires further investigation. The most popular and plausible of the current theories is that *arterial wall damage* permits the *infiltration* of macromolecules (especially cholesterol in the low density fraction) from blood through the damaged endothelium to the underlying smooth muscle cells causing their *proliferation* and enlargement. This process is followed by the *necrosis* of these smooth muscle cells and further accumulation of intracellular and extracellular lipid and fibrous material. The *intrusion* of the smooth muscle cells and accompanying debris into the arterial lumen decreases blood flow. When the cross-sectional area of the artery is reduced by 70% or more, myocardial ischemia and tissue damage begin to occur. The initial damage to the endothelial tissue may be caused by either physical or chemical trauma, and probably needs to be a chronic condition for clinically significant atherosclerosis to result.[42]

The clinical manifestations of CHD (including angina pectoris, left ventricular dysfunction, cardiac arrest, myocardial infarction, and, in some cases, cardiac dysrhythmias) result primarily from myocardial ischemia; technically, this is a reduction in blood flow at the tissue level resulting from constriction of a blood vessel. From a clinical perspective, this reduction in blood flow is equated with a decrease in myocardial oxygen delivery, and ischemia is said to exist if myocardial oxygen demand exceeds myocardial oxygen supply. By this definition, ischemia can result from conditions other than atherosclerosis, including coronary artery spasm and compression of coronary arteries due to increased intramyocardial tension. Ischemic-type responses also occur when tissue hypoxia results from a reduction in cardiac output ($\dot{Q}$) (and thus, coronary blood flow) or decreased arterial oxygen saturation. It is important to remember that manifestations of ischemia indicate a *functional imbalance* between oxygen delivery and tissue oxygen requirements, and are not determined solely by a fixed atherosclerotic obstruction in a coronary artery.

Prevention and Therapy

Most preventive and therapeutic measures for CHD focus on maintaining or re-establishing a balance between myocardial oxygen supply and demand so that oxygen supply throughout the myocardium exceeds both immediate and long-term demands under a variety of living situations. Because this balance between supply and demand can be upset by either decreasing supply or increasing demand, maintenance or restoration of this balance may be achieved by increasing supply or decreasing demand. Myocardial oxygen supply can be influenced by decreasing the rate with which coronary atherosclerosis develops or its possible regression, formation of collateral coronary arteries, enlargement of the diameter of major coronary vessels, redistribution of coronary blood flow, and improved functioning of the clotting or fibrinolytic system. Decreases in myocardial oxygen demand can be achieved by reductions in heart rate (HR), intramyocardial tension (indirectly indicated by systolic blood pressure or SBP), myocardial contractility, and possibly ventricular volume.

The preventive measures most likely to ameliorate myocardial oxygen supply include cessation of cigarette smoking; treatment of hypertension by medication; reduction of dietary saturated fat, cholesterol, and salt; maintenance of optimal body weight (calorie restriction and exercise); and exercise to modify lipoprotein and carbohydrate metabolism. Exercise training, hypertension control, weight loss, smoking cessation, and stress management all can contribute to a reduction in myocardial oxygen demand. Because most of these risk factors seem to have a synergistic effect in causing or accelerating the development of atherosclerosis, a multiple risk-factor reduction approach is strongly advocated, especially when designing programs for individuals at high risk or individuals known to have CHD.[42]

Medical treatment for CHD is primarily focused on reducing myocardial oxygen demand by decreasing HR, blood pressure, or myocardial contractility (use of nitroglycerin, beta blockers, or calcium antagonists). None of these drugs have much, if any, effect on increasing myocardial oxygen delivery by decreasing coronary vascular resistance. Anti-arrhythmic therapy frequently is used for treating CHD patients, but evidence of its benefit in reducing new events has been difficult to obtain, except in patients who also have clinically significant left ventricular dysfunction. Coronary artery bypass graft surgery and percutaneous transluminal coronary angioplasty (PTCA) now are the primary means of therapy for increasing myocardial blood flow and hence oxygen supply. Improved functional capacity, clinical status, and longevity have been reported for subsets of patients with multivessel coronary disease or its equivalent who have undergone coronary artery bypass graft surgery.[8,32,35] Although PTCA relieves symptoms and increases functional capacity, adequate studies of its effects on mortality have not been performed.[7] Also, the long-term effect of this procedure on arterial wall integrity is not known, but short-term clinical results have been favorable.[38]

CARDIOVASCULAR ADJUSTMENT TO EXERCISE

The capacity of the oxygen transport system is generally considered to be the limiting factor in large muscle dynamic (aerobic) exercise—that used for most exercise tolerance testing of patients with CHD or in training for CHD prevention and rehabilitation. During this type of exercise, performed by healthy persons from 6 to 60 minutes, neither pulmonary function (ventilation or diffusion) nor skeletal muscle oxidative capacity is limiting. Usually the limitation is the rate at which oxygen can be transported from the pulmonary circulation and delivered to the contracting skeletal muscles. Thus, if the capacity of one or more of the components of the oxygen transport system becomes limited due to disease, exercise tolerance declines.

Oxygen transport can be described by a rearranged Fick equation: oxygen uptake $= \dot{Q}$ (HR $\times$ stroke volume, SV) $\times$ total arteriovenous oxygen difference or AVD-O_2, as determined by distribution of $\dot{Q}$ and local tissue factors influencing oxygen extraction. In healthy adults of similar age and gender, most of the variation in maximal oxygen uptake ($\dot{V}_{O_2max}$) or aerobic exercise capacity can be accounted for by differences in SV at maximal exercise. At a given age, maximal HR is relatively similar (usual standard deviation is 9 to 11 beats per minutes, or 4 to 6% of the mean), as is maximal AVD-O_2. The inability for SV to continue to increase further with exercise is not due to limitations in coronary blood flow, but more likely is the result of either or both reduced left ventricular filling time at a high HR and inability to increase ventricular emptying further due to increased "after load" with rising systemic arterial pressure.

Response to Dynamic Exercise

Patients with documented CHD may respond quite normally to dynamic exercise, or they might exhibit marked abnormalities due to myocardial ischemia, non-reversible myocardial necrosis, or damage to the conduction system. The magnitude of the impairment in the cardiovascular adjustment to exercise will depend on the severity of the disease. While some patients are non-distinguishable from healthy subjects, the majority are likely to display a diminished $\dot{Q}$, $\dot{V}_{O_2max}$, and work tolerance. The reduced work tolerance associated with CHD is due to diminished peak SV or HR, whereas AVD-O_2 is usually within normal limits. The arterial blood pressure response at submaximal and maximal exercise can be elevated, normal, or diminished, the latter being especially critical in patients with myocardial ischemia. The impaired left ventricular response to exercise can be due either to permanent myocardial lesions (scarring and fibrosis), which can increase compliance and produce akinetic or dyskinetic contraction patterns, or to reversible ischemia. This transient ischemia is produced by increased myocardial oxygen requirements associated with increased HR, ventricular wall tension, and contractility.

Patients with normal hemodynamic function at rest can demonstrate an abnormal hemodynamic status during exercise, with evidence of diminished work tolerance without transient ischemia. Such responses are due to poor left ventricular compliance or abnormal contraction patterns, and may become apparent only with increases in left ventricular work. More frequently, however, major decrements in work capacity in patients with normal hemodynamics at rest are due to effort-induced ischemia. In patients with normal resting hemodynamics, $\dot{Q}$ for any given level of submaximal work (and $\dot{V}_{O_2}$) is usually within the normal range, as is AVD-O_2. On the other hand, this $\dot{Q}$ value may be achieved by a lower SV and higher HR. As left ventricular impairment becomes greater (due either to fixed or transient abnormalities), increased HR does not fully compensate for the further decrease in SV, so that $\dot{Q}$ for a given $\dot{V}_{O_2}$ is decreased and a widening of the AVD-O_2 provides the needed delivery of oxygen.

Because coronary reserve is not markedly impaired until atherosclerosis reduces the cross-sectional area of the coronary artery lumen by at least 70%, most patients with less than this degree of narrowing do not demonstrate exercise-induced cardiac abnormalities. In fact, some patients with greater than 70% narrowing of one or more arteries have normal responses. There is an inverse association between the extent of arterial disease and work capacity or peak $\dot{V}_{O_2}$, but it is not great. Average work capacity declines progressively with the degree of narrowing and number of major vessels involved, but the magnitude of physical impairment cannot be used to predict with accuracy the extent of anatomic involvement in the individual patient.[21] If the pathophysiologic aspects are kept in mind, then this relative lack of correlation between coronary anatomy and exercise performance or hemodynamic responses is not surprising. In a patient with a critical lesion of a single coronary artery, work tolerance may be very low, with angina pectoris precipitated by mild effort, whereas another patient with double or triple-vessel disease but with well-developed collateral vessels may be free of angina, arrhythmias, or left ventricular dysfunction at relatively high workloads. Even though average or representative values are usually lower than those of age-matched counterparts, substantial variation exists and the tolerance of any one patient cannot be estimated accurately from clinical data. The New York Heart Association's functional classification of patients with heart disease can be related to exercise tolerance (expressed as peak $\dot{V}_{O_2}$) obtained by exercise testing. Class I patients with no symptoms have a peak $\dot{V}_{O_2}$ greater than 6 METs. Class II patients with symptoms during ordinary physical activity have a peak $\dot{V}_{O_2}$ of 4 to 6 METs. Class III patients (symptoms with less than ordinary physical activity) have a 2- to 4-MET capacity. Class IV patients with symptoms at rest have a peak $\dot{V}_{O_2}$ of less than 2 METs.[36]

In addition to a decrease in exercise tolerance, CHD also appears to reduce the speed with which the patient can make circulatory adjustments to exercise. In patients with either poor left ventricular function or cardiac acceleration, the time required for $\dot{V}_{O_2}$ and its components to meet the demands for a given exercise intensity is increased.[5] The magnitude of this delayed response is probably related to the magnitude of left ventricular involvement, and should be considered in exercise test protocol selection and the design of the warm-up component of training.

EXERCISE-INDUCED ISCHEMIA. The patient with increasing ischemia usually terminates exercise because of the inability to transport sufficient oxygen to the working myocardium as well as to the working muscles; the latter is often limiting in healthy persons. Increasing ischemia usually results in a diminished SV response (an increase instead of a decrease in end-systolic volume and a decrease in left ventricular ejection fraction); a more rapid increase in HR (but lower peak HR); an earlier widening of the AVD-O_2; and a subnormal rise in SBP, with the possibility of no increase or even a precipitous decline. Such abnormal responses can occur without such objective indicators of ischemia as angina pectoris or ST-segment displacement on the ECG. Decreases in ventricular function may even occur without evidence of myocardial perfusion abnormalities, as assessed by Thallium[201] imaging.

The onset of detectable ischemia (angina or ST-segment depression) occurs at a relatively constant threshold of myocardial work for an individual patient. This threshold can be best defined noninvasively by the HR $\times$ SBP product (rate-pressure product, RPP). In a patient who is clinically stable, it has been demonstrated that angina or ST depression occurs at a similar RPP during repeated bouts of exercise days or even months apart.[46] Even when the RPP at a specific exercise intensity is altered by the addition of static arm exercise, cigarette smoking, reduced environmental temperature, or food ingestion, the threshold for ischemia remains relatively constant.[4,28] This close relationship between the onset of angina and RPP indicates that such determinants of myocardial oxygen demand as ventricular volume and contractility vary in proportion to the RPP, both in healthy subjects and in CHD patients. In situations in which left ventricular volume differs from that occurring during upright dynamic leg exercise, however, the RPP threshold for ischemia may change. During supine exercise, left ventricular end-diastolic volume is increased due to an elevated central blood volume, and the onset of ischemia occurs at a lower RPP.[48] The lower threshold might also result from a decrease in myocardial flow due to the effect of increased myocardial tension on the blood flow to small intramural vessels. The opposite reaction occurs with dynamic arm exercise, in which SV and left ventricular end-diastolic volumes (and possibly left ventricular end-diastolic pressure) are lower at the same RPP, and the anginal threshold therefore tends to be somewhat higher.[14]

EXERCISE SOON AFTER INFARCTION AND BYPASS SURGERY. The exercise capacity of patients relatively soon after myocardial infarction and bypass surgery is determined by the same parameters as in healthy individuals or in other cardiac patients: genetic endowment, gender, age, physical training status, and the amount of myocardial dysfunction (either permanent or transient) that occurs with exercise. As well, their circulatory control mechanisms during exercise are similar to those of other patients with CHD. The magnitude of their functional impairment due to CHD depends on the amount and location of myocardial damage due to infarction, as well as the nature of the blood supply to the remaining viable myocardium. The other consideration is the time since infarction, because exercise toler-ance is decreased until significant myocardial healing has been accomplished. Definitive data are lacking on this issue, but in patients less than 70 years of age with medically uncomplicated infarction, it appears that any limitation of exercise tolerance due to healing is no longer observed 8 to 12 weeks after infarction.[43] Peak HR 3 weeks after infarction usually does not exceed 135 beats·min^{-1}, and for any given level of submaximal $\dot{V}_{O_2}$, $\dot{Q}$ is decreased in patients 6 weeks after infarction.[57]

Responses to Static Exercise

Static or isometric exercise primarily produces a pressure load on the myocardium, in contrast to the predominantly volume load elicited by large muscle dynamic exercise. A vigorous (> 25% of maximal) static contraction of even a relatively small muscle mass in normal subjects produces a significant rise in HR, $\dot{Q}$, and systemic arterial pressures (systolic, diastolic, and mean), with minimal or no change in SV or total peripheral resistance. With the rise in arterial pressure, there normally is only a small rise in left ventricular end-diastolic pressure and a significant rise in left stroke work index. In patients with abnormal ventricular function at rest or with poor tolerance during dynamic exercise (NYHA Classes II and III), sustained static exercise produces a significant rise in left ventricular end-diastolic pressure, no increase or even a decrease in SV, and only a small increase in left ventricular stroke work.[31] Thus, in patients with poor dynamic exercise tolerance, the left ventricle has scant physiologic capacity to increase its output during static exercise, and a sustained contraction may produce myocardial ischemia, left ventricular failure, or complex ventricular arrhythmias. In these patients, systemic arterial pressure rises normally with static exercise due to an increase in peripheral arterial tone produced by a powerful activation of the adrenergic nervous system.

Patients with relatively good dynamic exercise capacity (> 6 METs) tolerate static exercise quite well. Because the increase in HR with static exercise is only about 50% (25 to 35 beats·min^{-1}) of that noted during symptom-limited cycle ergometer or treadmill testing (50 to 80 beats·min^{-1}), and the systolic pressure increase is similar with the two types of exercise, the increase in myocardial oxygen demand is less for isometric exercise. Also, there is some evidence that the rise in diastolic pressure with static exercise increases diastolic filling of the coronary arteries; this occurrence actually results in a higher RPP threshold for ischemia.[30]

In addition, recent information suggests that the incorporation of static activity during dynamic exercise favorably modifies the myocardial oxygen supply/demand relationship in CHD patients. Ischemic electrocardiogram responses attained during dynamic exercises were attenuated when dynamic and isometric exercises were combined and performed at the same RPP values that elicited significant ST segment depression during dynamic exercise.[9] These results have changed the previous cautious attitude held toward the inclusion of strength training in cardiac rehabilitation programming.[1,2,22]

BENEFITS OF EXERCISE TRAINING

Participation in a program of endurance-type training generally improves the clinical status and exercise capacity of patients with CHD. For persons with exertional ischemia, the intensity needed to precipitate chest pain or ST-segment depression becomes greater, and less antianginal medication may be required. These improvements are due more to a reduction in myocardial work and oxygen demand at rest and submaximal exercise than to any substantial increase in myocardial oxygen supply. Reductions in myocardial oxygen demand result primarily from decreases in HR, with possibly some drop in systemic arterial blood pressure. The decrease in RPP is greatest during submaximal exercise with trained limbs, suggesting that the site of this important training effect is mainly the muscles used

during training.[49] Alterations in the metabolic capacity of skeletal muscle probably make a major contribution to the quite rapid decrease in HR and increase in AVD-O$_2$ that occurs during submaximal exercise soon after the beginning of training. A slight reduction in $\dot{Q}$ during submaximal exercise after training is associated with a decrease in blood flow to working muscles and a small increase in flow to non-exercising tissue.[13]

In contrast to the substantial data demonstrating a reduction in myocardial oxygen demand with training, there is a minimal amount of evidence that any significant increase in myocardial perfusion or oxygen supply routinely occurs. So far, in humans it has not been possible to demonstrate systematically that training increases oxygen delivery to myocardial tissue by delaying the rate of atherosclerotic progression, by increasing lumen diameter of major atherosclerotic coronary arteries, or by the stimulation of coronary collateral vascularization.[15,20,45] Myocardial perfusion at rest and exercise has been studied by using Thallium[201] imaging before and after training in patients with established CHD. Even though a few patients show some improvement in perfusion with training, most test results have been negative.[55]

Training favorably alters both lipoprotein and carbohydrate metabolism, and thus would seem to have the potential to modify the course of coronary atherosclerosis.[6,33] Human studies directly addressing this issue are limited to the use of repeat coronary arteriography, which until recently has lacked accuracy, interreader agreement, test-retest reproducibility, and subject acceptance, although the results of one very preliminary study are encouraging.[44] New procedures for image enhancement with computerized edge detection and volume calculations now make the study of progression or regression more feasible.[24] The previous finding by researchers conducting animal studies that training might enhance coronary artery collateral development has not been seen in humans. In four studies in which training periods ranged in length from 15 weeks to 1 year, no evidence of any collateral development was observed. By direct measurement of coronary sinus blood flow during rest and exercise, there is no evidence that maximal coronary blood flow or coronary blood flow at the onset of angina significantly increases as a result of training.[20] In some cases, angina-limited exercise tolerance was increased by more than 35%, with no evidence of any improvement in coronary blood flow. Increases in angina threshold associated with short-term or low-intensity training probably are due to an increase in pain tolerance or patient confidence after training or repeat testing.[17]

As training increases in intensity, duration or both, more general or central circulatory effects begin to occur, e.g., reductions in HR and sometimes blood pressure at rest, and reductions in HR during exercise with use of nontrained limbs. At this point, there frequently is an increase in SV at rest and during submaximal exercise.[41] Some evidence now available indicates that with longer, more vigorous training, the RPP at which ischemia (ST-segment depression) develops can be increased.[18] These changes are probably associated with alterations in central nervous system control of the myocardium or with enhanced intrinsic myocardial function. It is unlikely that increases in blood volume or red blood cell mass contribute much to these changes.

The rate and magnitude of hemodynamic and metabolic improvement in patients with CHD due to training appear to be a function of the viability of the myocardium as well as of the characteristics of the exercise regimen. Ambulatory patients with severely compromised ventricular function prior to training may have already utilized much of their adaptive capacity (e.g., widening of the $AVD\text{-}O_2$ and shunting of blood to working tissues), and therefore have minimal potential for improvement. Some of these patients, however, do surprisingly well with training and show improvement in exercise capacity with no change in ventricular function.[26,47] The occurrence of angina pectoris does not necessarily diminish a patient's potential for improvement in clinical status, because many angina patients achieve remarkable increases in exercise tolerance and symptom relief with appropriate activity programs. Even with long-term training (more than 26 weeks), however, the exercise capacity of patients is lower than that of age-matched normal individuals.

The cardiac function of some patients with CHD will not improve with training. Myocardial damage (necrosis, dyskinesis, and ischemia) may minimize the potential for improvement or the progression of coronary atherosclerosis (despite concerned medical treatment) may negate or override any achievable training benefit. When the clinical status and exercise tolerance level of a patient continue to deteriorate despite adherence to an appropriate training program, alternate forms of medical or surgical therapy should be considered.

Aside from improvement in functional capacity and clinical status, training has been promoted for patients with CHD to accelerate their return to work after myocardial infarction or surgery, to improve their psychologic status, and to reduce the occurrence of reinfarction and death. The improved functional status of many patients as a result of exercise probably increases their job potential and productivity, but it has not been possible to prove the specific benefits attributable to training because of the numerous social and economic factors influencing the individual's return to work. A more-rapid return to work has been reported for patients who participate in work evaluation soon after hospitalization for myocardial infarction.[16] Increased self-confidence of many patients participating in cardiac exercise programs has been frequently observed but is difficult to document scientifically; however, improved self-confidence can make a major contribution to an increase in self-care or work potential.

Although comprehensive cardiac rehabilitation apparently reduces the mortality rate due to reinfarction, the role that exercise alone plays in improving prognosis is not well established.[37,39] Studies in which the morbidity and mortality rate of CHD rehabilitation program participants was compared to that of non-participants considered to be clinically similar resulted in a CHD mortality rate for the participants that was one half to one third that of non-participants. Part of this difference in the number of CHD events is probably due to the fact that lower-risk patients entered the rehabilitation program, multiple risk-factor reduction occurred as part of the program, and there was improved medical care of the program participants, as well as any direct benefit of exercise. An evaluation of 10 clinical trials in which patients after hospitalization for myocardial infarction were randomized to exercise-based cardiac rehabilitation or usual care was performed using a meta analysis.[39] Participation in these rehabilitation programs resulted in approximately 25% lower CHD or all-cause death rates, but no difference in nonfatal myocardial infarction. A similar analysis by O'Connor and colleagues, but using the results from 22 studies of cardiac rehabilitation, demonstrated similar results.[37] The power of the individual studies to demonstrate a training benefit has been curtailed by a high degree of non-adherence to the exercise regimen, a substantially lower than expected mortality rate in the usual-care patients, an inadequate sample size, and a relatively short period of follow-up.[37,39]

SPECIAL EXERCISE TESTING CONSIDERATIONS

Exercise testing of patients known to have CHD is performed to determine exercise tolerance and what exercise intensity, if any, elicits such abnormal responses in cardiac function as myocardial ischemia, left ventricular dysfunction, cardiac dysrhythmias, and conduction disturbances. The results of such testing can be used to quantify objectively the functional or clinical significance of disease; aid in determining appropriate therapy; contribute to the prognosis of new clinical events; help to evaluate the effectiveness of various treatment regimens including surgery, medication, and exercise; and establish the appropriateness of performing specific job-related, leisure time, or physical conditioning activities. Exercise testing, with one or more of these objectives as the primary indication, is routinely performed on chronic, stable, asymptomatic patients; those with exercise-induced ischemia manifested as angina, ST depression, or both; patients with known or suspected left ventricular dysfunction at rest or with exercise; and patients in the process of recovering from acute myocardial infarction, bypass surgery, or PTCA. The discussion in this section is limited to those special considerations required in the exercise testing of patients with CHD for the primary purpose of developing the intensity component of a conditioning program. Most of the requirements and procedures used when conducting a test for this purpose, however, may also be applied when the purpose is one of those mentioned previously.

The special considerations required for the safe and effective exercise testing of patients with CHD primarily consist of emphasis on 1) excluding patients for medical reasons that might put them at undue risk; 2) selecting an appropriate test protocol consistent with the likelihood of a restricted capacity; and 3) monitoring of the patient to detect those abnormalities that provide information on the functional significance of the disease or, even more importantly, are contraindications to further exercise. Attention is given to the requirements for exercise testing in the clinical setting with medical supervision and not from special procedures used primarily for research purposes. In many cases, no one single procedure has been demonstrated to be better (safer, elicit more precise or valid information, more cost effective, more acceptable to the patient), there being various trade-offs in the use of one procedure as opposed to another.

Patient Evaluation and Contraindications to Testing

Immediately before testing, every patient with CHD should have a cardiovascular assessment, including medical history, physical examination by a qualified physician, and a resting 12-lead electrocardiogram. The medical history should include questions concerning recent changes in clinical status, especially any indications of a change in chest discomfort or pain, shortness of breath, or unusual fatigue; current medication use; recent changes in weight or diet; general physical health (pulmonary, orthopedic, metabolic, and neuromuscular); and psychologic status. An attempt should be made to detect any condition that would contraindicate the completion of the test for safety reasons, aid in the test interpretation, or influence when the test should be stopped. The physical examination should include palpation and auscultation of the precordium, paying particular attention to any gallop rhythm or murmur; observation and palpation of the extremities for edema or vascular insufficiency and the neck for venous distention; listening to the lungs; and measurement of HR and blood pressure. The resting 12-lead ECG should be reviewed carefully by the physician and, if abnormal against previous ECGs, should be rechecked to determine if recent changes have occurred. Conditions generally considered to be contraindications to testing are included in Table 15–1. In special cases, these conditions may not be absolute contraindications, but special attention should at least be paid. For example, in testing the efficacy of a new antiarrhythmic drug, patients with more frequent ventricular arrhythmias might be tested under close medical monitoring and safety considerations. Written informed consent should be obtained before all testing is begun, but especially when the clinical status of the patient significantly increases the risk of exertion-induced complications.

Protocol Selection

The general principles and guidelines for testing patients with CHD to assess the integrity of their oxygen transport system are similar to those described for healthy adults in Chapter 1. Special considerations concern the initial exercise intensity and the rate at which intensity is increased during the test; the need for closer and more frequent monitoring of the ECG, blood pressure, and symptoms during exercise and recovery; the value of multiple-lead ECG recordings; and a longer post-exercise recovery period before the patient is discharged from the facility. The value of including such measures of cardiac function during exercise as Thallium[201] for evaluating myocardial perfusion and Technetium[99] for determining ventricular function also should be considered.

The use of motor-driven treadmills or cycle ergometers is preferred because exercises involving these devices maximally stress the cardiovascular system (instead of being limited by local muscle factors), require little special skill, can be calibrated, and the interindividual variation in biomechanical efficiency is relatively small. For patients with poor leg strength (especially those who have restricted their exercise for some time, older patients, and those with low total body weight), the treadmill is preferred. Because $\dot{V}_{O_2}$ is usually not measured but is estimated from the intensity of exercise performed, it is extremely important that the exercise device be accurately calibrated. Accurate calibration of treadmills can be achieved easily; calibration of most cycle ergometers with electric brakes is difficult, because dynamometers needed for their calibration are not generally available.

Before testing, many patients will be known to have a limited exercise capacity and, even more importantly for some patients, their exercise capacity will be totally unpredictable.[25] Thus, a test protocol should be selected in which the initial exercise intensity is low and the increase in intensity is gradual, e.g., beginning at 2 to

TABLE 15-1. **Contraindications to Exercise Testing.**

Absolute Contraindications
1. A recent significant change in the resting ECG suggesting infarction or other acute cardiac events
2. Recent complicated myocardial infarction
3. Unstable angina
4. Uncontrolled ventricular dysrhythmia
5. Uncontrolled atrial dysrhythmia that compromises cardiac function
6. Third-degree A-V block
7. Acute congestive heart failure
8. Severe aortic stenosis
9. Suspected or known dissecting aneurysm
10. Active or suspected myocarditis or pericarditis
11. Thrombophlebitis or intracardiac thrombi
12. Recent systemic or pulmonary embolus
13. Acute infection
14. Significant emotional distress (psychosis)

Relative Contraindications
1. Resting diastolic blood pressure > 120 mm Hg or resting systolic blood pressure > 200 mm Hg
2. Moderate valvular heart disease
3. Known electrolyte abnormalities (hypokalemia, hypomagnesemia)
4. Fixed-rate pacemaker (rarely used)
5. Frequent or complex ventricular ectopy
6. Ventricular aneurysm
7. Cardiomyopathy, including hypertrophic cardiomyopathy
8. Uncontrolled metabolic disease (e.g., diabetes, thyrotoxicosis, or myxedema)
9. Chronic infectious disease (e.g., mononucleosis, hepatitis, AIDS)
10. Neuromuscular, musculoskeletal, or rheumatoid disorders that are exacerbated by exercise
11. Advanced or complicated pregnancy

From American College of Sports Medicine.[2]

4 METs, with the increase in intensity not to exceed 1 MET per minute. For patients with poor exercise tolerance, intensity should be increased by 1 MET every 2 or 3 minutes. Starting the patient at too high an intensity may increase the risk of precipitating a cardiovascular complication, and it is uncomfortable. Gradual increases in intensity are recommended due to the slower rate of cardiovascular adjustment in patients with CHD as compared to healthy adults. If intensity is increased by more than 2 to 3 METs every 3 minutes for patients with poor left ventricular function, the measured $\dot{V}_{O_2}$ drops below that value estimated from previously reported data.[18] This reduced rate of cardiovascular adjustment can result in an overestimation of exercise tolerance.

Substantial data have been published demonstrating that exercise testing can be performed safely and can provide useful clinical information when only one electrocardiographic lead is recorded. For the screening of asymptomatic subjects, single-lead monitoring may be optimal when considering cost and the frequency of false-positive results. As CHD severity increases, however, the use of more leads provides more information about the status of the myocardium. Additional leads may pick up ischemia otherwise not detected and aid in the detection and interpretation of cardiac dysrhythmias or altered electrical conduction. The use of from three to six leads provides most of the information contained in as many as 12 to 14 leads.[12] Three or twelve-lead recordings appear to be most prevalent, due primarily to the recording configuration of the strip chart recorders and oscilloscopes available. The capability for the continuous monitoring of the ECG on an oscilloscope should be considered a required testing procedure, because it is possible to identify a sudden change in ECG rhythm, HR, and ischemia (ST-segment displacement). The ECG should be recorded prior to increasing workload, at times of major ECG abnormalities, at peak exercise, at the end of recovery, and possibly at the end of each minute of exercise. The major concern is not to miss data that may have clinical relevance.

The inability of a patient with CHD to increase or maintain SBP during increasing exercise is a good indication of left ventricular dysfunction or failure; close, accurate monitoring of blood pressure is therefore important. Blood pressure should be recorded in the last 20 to 30 seconds of each workload; if 3-minute work stages are used, it is recommended that blood pressure also be recorded in the last 20 to 30 seconds of the first minute at each workload. Measurements should be made by using a high quality stethoscope and mercury manometer. Most automatic or semi-automatic blood pressure machines have poor accuracy or reliability or are too expensive for routine clinical use. Accurate blood pressure recording during exercise, especially on the treadmill, requires careful execution and experience.

Test Termination Considerations

Except for such special circumstances as very soon after acute myocardial infarction, a general consensus now exists that symptom-limited or clinical maximal exercise testing is preferred to submaximal testing for assessing the cardiovascular response of patients with CHD. Symptom-limited testing is of particular value when determination of exercise capacity is the primary reason for the test. With healthy individuals, responses to submaximal exercise can be used to predict exercise capacity (usually expressed as $\dot{V}_{O_2max}$) with a fair degree of accuracy. For these predictions, it is assumed that the subject has a maximal HR somewhat close to the average for his age. For patients with CHD, this is not the case because their

maximal or peak HR cannot be accurately estimated from age, clinical information, or submaximal exercise data. When a patient is tested, it is not possible to predict when an abnormality will develop that will contraindicate further exercise. The maximal or peak HR achieved by patients during testing usually is lower than that of their age-matched, healthy counterparts. Just as important, the variation in peak HR for patients at a given age is large. The usual standard deviation for peak HR in healthy adults at a given age is 9 to 11 beats$\cdot$min^{-1}, whereas that for patients with CHD is more than double that amount.

The "clinical maximal" concept of exercise test termination seems the most appropriate for patients with CHD. This concept is based on the premise that patients should continue to exercise until they need to stop due to fatigue or until signs or symptoms develop that, given the reasons for testing and the testing environment, indicate that further exercise is not warranted. The specific signs or symptoms that make up the clinical indication for stopping vary with the clinical status of the patient, the primary reason for conducting the test, and the general test environment. For example, more conservative criteria are used early after infarction, when the myocardium is still healing; in patients with known left ventricular dysfunction who may develop congestive failure with exercise; or in patients with known ventricular irritability but for whom some objective measure of exercise tolerance is desired. If the primary reason for conducting a test is to clear a patient for high level exercise or for the return to a demanding occupation (especially if a sudden cardiovascular complication would put other people in danger), then a more aggressive attitude regarding criteria for terminating the test should be employed. Unless absolute contraindications to exercise occur first, patients should be pushed to levels of myocardial work above that they would be expected to reach in the activity for which they are being cleared. The more experienced the testing personnel and the more comprehensive the capability for immediate emergency medical care, the more liberal should be the criteria for test termination. Testing conducted in a major medical center may use criteria considered inappropriate for use in a private physician's office or in a community exercise facility.

The same basic principle used to terminate maximal testing of healthy adults applies to symptom-limited testing of patients with CHD. The patient should be stopped when significant fatigue occurs or if signs or symptoms develop that indicate the patient's exercise tolerance level has been reached or exceeded. At this point, to continue exercise would not only not provide additional useful information but, more importantly, might rapidly lead to significant medical complications. Various individuals and organizations have proposed quite similar criteria for stopping exercise tests performed by patients with CHD. Reasons for terminating a test specific to CHD manifestations include indications of increasing left ventricular failure, myocardial ischemia, myocardial irritability, or intraventricular conduction abnormalities. Specific signs or symptoms that should be considered special considerations or indications for stopping the test are listed in Table 15–2. This list includes most of the common reasons for stopping symptom-limited tests in patients with CHD.

Total Patient Monitoring

The concept of "total patient monitoring" should be emphasized when testing patients with CHD. There is a tendency to focus on the ST-segment or angina pectoris and to ignore other important signs or symptoms that indicate impending problems or aid in understanding the nature of the patients' limitations. For example, in patients with known or highly suspect left ventricular dysfunction, close monitoring for the development of undue fatigue, dyspnea, or systolic hypotension may give the first major clue that their exercise tolerance level has been reached. During testing, the patient's appearance needs to be observed (gait, skin color, and breathing rate), verbal communication should be maintained (pain, fatigue, and dyspnea), and the ECG and blood pressure should be monitored. Failure to incorporate this comprehensive approach to patient monitoring into the testing protocol reduces the clinical value of the results and increases the risk of an exercise-related complication. The importance of this approach increases with the severity of the illness in the patient being tested. The excellent safety record during the testing of patients with CHD in many medical facilities over the past three decades can be attributed, in part, to implementation of comprehensive patient monitoring.

TEST INTERPRETATION. Because we are concerned here with tests of patients with known CHD, results are not to be used to aid in the diagnosis of CHD but primarily for determining the functional significance of the disease. Test interpretation will focus on how much exercise the patient can perform (Watts, treadmill speed and grade, and METs), what limited the patient's capacity to perform the test (reasons for termination), and the occurrence of symptoms (pain and dyspnea) or signs (ECG and SBP) indicating an abnormal response. Significant CHD can decrease exercise capacity, cause undue fatigue or shortness of breath, reduce peak HR and SBP, produce myocardial ischemia (ST displacement or angina), and precipitate or aggravate cardiac arrhythmias and intraventricular conduction abnormalities. Other ECG changes may occur (e.g., alterations in R wave amplitude or T wave inversion), but they generally are not of great use when evaluating the functional significance of CHD or establishing the prognosis of future cardiac events. These responses must be considered when making decisions regarding the patient's therapy, plans for return to work, use of leisure time, and training programs.

Strong indicators of severe CHD include very poor exercise tolerance (≤ 4 METs), significant myocardial ischemia (Grade $3+$ angina or ST-segment depression ≥ 0.2 mV) at low workloads or low

TABLE 15-2. **Indications for Stopping an Exercise Test**

Symptoms
  New-onset anginal chest pain
  Increasing angina to Grade 3 as estimated by patient, with or without ECG changes
  Fainting or lightheadedness
  Severe dyspnea
  Severe fatigue or muscle pain
  Nausea or vomiting

Clinical signs
  Pallor, cyanosis, cold moist skin
  Staggering gait, ataxia
  Confusion in response to enquiries or blank stare

Electrocardiographic signs
  ST displacement (elevation or depression) of horizontal or descending type greater than 0.3 mV
    above or below that of the resting tracing
  Conduction disturbance other than first-degree atrioventricular block (prolonged P-R interval)
  Ventricular arrhythmias
    Ventricular tachycardia
    Ventricular fibrillation
    Ventricular premature beats with a frequency of 35% of beats lasting more than 30 seconds
  Supraventricular arrhythmias
    Atrial fibrillation occurring with exercise
    Supraventricular tachycardia occurring with exercise

Blood pressure abnormalities
  Fall in SBP with increase in workload of 10 mm Hg or more below any previously recorded blood
    pressure, with other symptoms or signs, especially at low HR
  Rise in SBP above 250 mm Hg or diastolic pressure above 120 mm Hg

Patient indicates desire to stop

Failure of ECG or blood pressure monitoring system

(Adapted from American Heart Association.[3])

HR, and an inadequate SBP response (failure to rise or a decrease, especially below the pre-exercise level, with increasing workloads). The clinical significance of exercise-induced ventricular arrhythmias is not well established, but they are prognostic of new cardiac events in patients with poor left ventricular function. Until additional data are collected and revised guidelines are developed, complex ventricular arrhythmias need to be considered potentially hazardous events and patients should be informed as to how to avoid them (e.g., medication, controlled exercise intensity if related to HR, and reduced use of nicotine or caffeine). The severity of myocardial damage (both necrosis and transient ischemia) resulting from CHD is related inversely to exercise capacity, workload, or HR at the onset of ischemia or to a hypotensive pressure response. Combinations of these abnormalities increase the likelihood that multivessel disease exists and that substantial myocardium is necrotic or becomes dyskinetic during exercise.

Drug Effects on Response to Exercise

Several categories of drugs influence exercise test results because they produce abnormal ST responses that are not due to myocardial ischemia. Among the drugs that may affect the ECG response are digitalis preparations, sympathetic nervous system blocking agents (beta blockers, guanethidine, and methyldopa), diuretics, and nitroglycerin compounds. Other drugs known to alter the HR or ECG response are quinidine, procainamide, atropine sulfate, phenothiazine derivatives, and lithium. Diuretics may reduce serum potassium levels and cause abnormal ST-T changes or ventricular dysrhythmias during exercise.

The two classes of drugs causing the most difficulty in exercise test interpretation are digitalis preparations and beta-adrenergic blocking agents. If a patient has ST changes while receiving digitalis, the ECG cannot be interpreted. If documentation of ischemia is important, the test should be repeated after withdrawing the drug for at least 3 weeks. If a patient receiving digitalis has a normal ST response during the test, it can be considered negative.

Beta-adrenergic blocking agents cause a reduction in resting and exercise HR. However, peak HR during testing can still be used to establish guidelines for training intensity. Information on the intensity or HR at the onset of symptoms or signs of myocardial ischemia or ventricular dysfunction is of clinical value. Significant attenuation of the HR response may be seen in patients taking other drugs affecting the sympathetic nervous system (such as methyldopa and guanethidine).

If one of the major reasons for conducting an exercise test is to establish the appropriate intensity for training, the patient should then continue the regimen of medication that will be followed during training. Withholding medications during the day of testing can significantly change a patient's symptom-free exercise tolerance, as well as the relationship between HR and total body or myocardial oxygen demand. These differences in exercise response can negate the usefulness of test data for establishing the correct training regimen. For example, if a patient is tested while all medications are withheld and then returns to the use of a beta blocker, it is likely that the training HR will be too high and will place the patient at undue risk.

For more detailed information on the effects of various drugs on the exercise response during exercise testing and training in patients with CHD, refer to *Exercise Guidelines for Exercise Testing and Training* by the American College of Sports Medicine.[2]

SPECIAL CONSIDERATIONS FOR PRESCRIBING EXERCISE

All ambulatory patients with CHD should have an activity plan that includes both the proscription and prescription of exercise. Ideally, this plan would have all patients undergo a clinical evaluation to include a symptom-limited exercise test to determine the severity of their disease and to establish risk stratification for future cardiac events (Table 15–3). This evaluation should include the determination of the amount of ischemic myocardium, the impairment of ventricular function, and the frequency and severity of various signs or symptoms, including silent and symptomatic ischemia, dysrhythmias, abnormal blood pressure, and heart responses to exercise and fatigue. The special considerations advised for the formulation and execution of physical conditioning programs for patients with CHD (beyond those recommended for healthy middle-aged and older adults) are needed because of the increased risk that exercise may precipitate cardiovascular complications. More than 85% of all non-traumatic sudden deaths during vigorous exercise in individuals over age 35 years occur in those people with severe CHD.[56] On the basis of information collected primarily in medically supervised exercise programs for cardiac patients, it has been determined that cardiac arrest is the most frequent major cardiovascular complication during exercise, whereas acute myocardial infarction is relatively rare.[50,53,54] This increased risk of exercise-induced cardiovascular complications apparently results from a decrease in coronary reserve and/or electric stability of the myocardium as a result of hemodynamically significant CHD or myocardial necrosis.

Exercise Selection

Most of the health and performance benefits for patients produced by training

TABLE 15-3. **Low-, Intermediate-, and High-Risk Classification**

Low-risk patients
  Following uncomplicated myocardial infarction or bypass surgery
  Functional capacity ≥ 8 METs* on 3-week exercise test
  Asymptomatic at rest with exercise capacity adequate for most vocational and recreational activities
  No ischemia, left ventricular dysfunction, or dysrhythmias

Intermediate-risk patients
  Functional capacity < 8 METs on 3-week exercise test
  Shock or CHF during recent myocardial infarction (< 6 months)
  Inability to self-monitor heart rate
  Failure to comply with exercise prescription
  Exercise-induced ischemia or < 0.2 mV

High-risk patients
  Severely depressed left ventricular function (ejection fraction $< 30\%$)
  Resting complex ventricular dysrhythmias (Lown grade IV and V)
  PVCs appearing or increasing with exercise
  Exertional hypotension (decrease in sytolic pressure of ≥ 15 mm Hg)
  Recent myocardial infarction (< 6 months) complicated by serious ventricular dysrhythmias
  Exercised-induced ischemia of > 0.2 mV
  Survivors of cardiac arrest

Health and Public Policy Committee, American College of Physicians: Cardiac rehabilitation services. Ann. Intern. Med., *15*:671–673, 1988.
*One MET is considered the equivalent of a $\dot{V}_{O_2}$ of 3.5 ml·kg^{-1}·min^{-1}.

result from the performance of large muscle, dynamic activities frequently referred to as aerobic or endurance-type exercises. Activities such as walking, hiking, jogging, running, cycling, swimming, selected calisthenics, and active sports all can produce endurance training effects. Decisions as to the most appropriate activities should be based on the patient's clinical status, exercise tolerance, interests, skills, location of facilities, and the availability of supervised exercise programs. During the early convalescent period after infarction or surgery, such stationary equipment as cycle ergometers or exercisers, treadmills, and rowing machines are useful.

For patients who perform heavy resistance exercise with the arms during employment or leisure time, a special program of arm endurance and strength training may be considered. Because the stress placed on the myocardium by this type of exercise is primarily determined by the percentage of maximal strength at which a muscle must perform, an increase in muscle strength will reduce myocardial work for any given amount of exercise. Thus, the best way to reduce the workload

on the heart during arm exercise is to perform arm training. Information indicates that patients (including those with angina pectoris) can safely increase arm endurance capacity during supervised arm training programs or standard programs that contain an arm component.[22] Program guidelines have been established for the use of resistance training by low-risk patients (Table 15–3) whose program objectives include a significant increase in muscle strength.[1–3,22]

Establishing Exercise Intensity

A major goal of the exercise prescription is to establish an appropriate intensity for each patient. The basic premise is that exercise should be of sufficient intensity to produce improvements in performance and health status but not so vigorous as to precipitate cardiovascular complications. The necessary stimulus for producing changes in hemodynamic and metabolic function by endurance training appears to be an increase in energy expenditure above some threshold (best expressed as a percentage of functional capacity) and done for an extended period of time. The nature and magnitude of the training effects depend on the total amount of energy expended above this threshold, with variations produced by different combinations of intensity, frequency, and duration.

Because HR increases proportionately with increases in total body energy expenditure and with increases in myocardial work during large muscle dynamic exercise, HR is the single best guide of intensity for cardiac patients. If the target HR range concept is used properly, then the lower HR (usually given as 70% of peak exercise test HR or the HR at 60% of exercise capacity) represents the "stimulus threshold," and the upper HR (usually given as 85% of peak exercise test HR or at 80% of exercise capacity) represents the "safety threshold" (Fig. 15–1). The more medically complicated the patient, the greater the emphasis on establishing a proper safety threshold.

The basic assumption in using exercise test results to determine training intensity for cardiac patients is that the peak myocardial work during training should always be lower than that achieved during the exercise test when contraindications to unmonitored exercise occurred. For the patient who performs a symptom-limited exercise test free of abnormalities, percentage of peak HR is an appropriate value to use, similar to the approach used with healthy adults. When abnormalities that occur during testing are associated with a significant risk of cardiovascular complications, the intensity at the onset of these abnormalities should then be used. For example, if a patient reports chest pain at a HR of 135 beats·min^{-1} but the test is not stopped due to Grade 3+ angina pectoris until a HR of 144 beats·min^{-1} is achieved, a HR of 135 and the accompanying exercise are used to establish the training intensity. In this case, 70 to 85% of 135 (95 to 115 beats·min^{-1}) could be used as the training HR range. Another approach would be to subtract about 15 beats from the HR of 135 beats·min^{-1}, then using the difference as the high target HR. The lower target HR would be reduced to 18 to 24 beats, giving a training

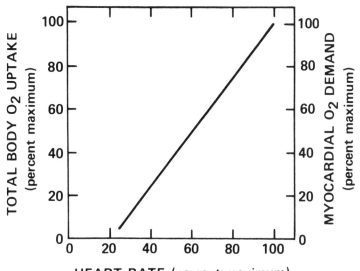

Fig. 15–1. *Use of heart rate for exercise prescription.*
Near-linear relationship of heart rate to total body oxygen uptake and myocardial oxygen demand during large muscle dynamic exercise (all variables expressed as a percentage of their maximal value for specific individual). An increase in total body oxygen uptake is the necessary stimulus for cardiovascular conditioning; myocardial oxygen demand is the major limiting factor for exercise in patients with significant coronary heart disease. (Reprinted from Haskell, W.: Design of a cardiac conditioning program. In Exercise and the Heart. Edited by N.K. Wenger, Philadelphia, F.A. Davis Company, 1978. p. 98).

HR range of about 102 to 120 beats·min^{-1}. Similar approaches can be used when other contraindications to unmonitored exercise occur during testing (e.g., ST changes, ventricular arrhythmias, or an inadequate blood pressure response).

Another way to establish exercise intensity is to use the rating of perceived exertion (RPE). Briefly, this method employs a 15-point numerical scale ranging from 6 to 20 with a verbal description given at every odd number. Because RPE responses to graded exercise correlate highly with such cardiorespiratory and metabolic variables as $\dot{V}_{O_2}$, HR, and ventilation, this scale provides a valid and reliable indicator for the level of physical exertion during steady-state exercise. Thus, RPE can be used to determine exercise intensity for endurance training programs. When the RPE scale is used, the fairly light (numerical value of 11) and somewhat hard (numerical value of 15) portion of the scale encompasses the range that most cardiac patients use during their exercise training session.[2]

Because the degree of likelihood of the development of cardiovascular and orthopedic complications during exercise increases with intensity, it is advisable for high-risk patients to reduce intensity and increase duration or frequency of training to attain an adequate volume of exercise. Patients with poor exercise capacity may be encouraged to exercise at lower intensities (50 to 70%, instead of 60 to 85% for healthy adults) but for longer periods (walking for 1 hour) or more frequently (once or twice daily). After hospitalization for myocardial infarction, such low level exercises as walking significantly improves functional capacity, with greater increases seen in patients without angina.[16] As with healthy adults, patients should try to increase their exercise capacity so that they can train at an energy expenditure of as much as 300 kcal per session. Many patients will not be able to reach this level and will need individualized goals based on their own exercise tolerance.

In addition to the physical demands exercise makes on the myocardium, the added stress potentially produced by the patient's psychologic response to exercise should be considered. Substantial increases in myocardial work at rest and submaximal exercise probably can occur during highly competitive situations, and patients may ignore the usual warning signals of overexertion under such conditions. Fear or excitement may produce similar responses and may actually reduce the symptomatic patient's exercise tolerance due to enhanced sympathetic drive. In many competitive activities, exercise intensity is quite variable, depending on the capacity and skill of opponents, and is difficult for the patient to control.

Caution regarding environmental conditions during exercise should be provided, especially to those individuals who are symptomatic at a low exercise intensity. High temperatures, especially when accompanied by high humidity, can increase cardiovascular demands for temperature regulation and decrease exercise tolerance; dehydration can aggravate this situation. On the other hand, cold temperatures increase myocardial work. Increases in blood pressure as a result of vasoconstriction in the skin reduces the exercise tolerance of symptom-limited patients, and exposure to cold air on the skin or the breathing of cold air may limit the exercise tolerance of some patients.[19] Any decline in arterial oxygen saturation due to acute exposure to altitude (more than 2,000 m) reduces the exercise capacity of patients and may be especially troublesome to symptomatic patients and those with chronic pulmonary disorders. For all cases in which environmental stress may be added to the myocardial demands of exercise, the use of an appropriate target HR will greatly aid the patient in maintaining the proper exercise intensity.

Medical Supervision

A major consideration of substantial clinical and economic significance in the training of patients with CHD is the degree of medical monitoring or supervision provided. Some general recommendations can be provided, but additional objective information is needed on the benefits, risks, and costs of various approaches before mandatory requirements or criteria are established. For those situations in which patients are at intermediate and high risk for fatal cardiovascular complications precipitated by exercise (Table 15–3), close medical supervision is indicated and continuous ECG monitoring may be needed. Such intensive supervision is suggested for patients with poor functional capacity (< 8 METs); indications of left ventricular dysfunction (inadequate SBP response and decrease in ejection fraction); myocardial ischemia (angina or ST depression greater than 0.2 mV); or complex ventricular dysrhythmias during exercise testing, who plan to exercise above 50 to 60% of their symptom-or sign-free exercise tolerance. Exercise performed at lower intensities, even within several weeks after myocardial infarction, may be at an acceptably low risk level, so that medical supervision is not required (even though desirable). Such exercise, if performed regularly, may provide significant beneficial effects.

Patients at low risk (Table 15–3) and who have a symptom-free exercise capacity (> 7 METs) should require substantially less medical supervision during their exercise training, even when exercising at 60 or 75% of their tolerance (as defined by the recent performance of a symptom-limited exercise test). After instruction and practice with regard to following an exercise prescription properly, high capacity and low risk patients may be encouraged to train without medical supervision in a community-based adult fitness program or on their own using individually prescribed programs.[10]

Detailed guidelines for the supervision of cardiac exercise programs have been published by the American Heart Association, the American College of Sports Medicine and the American Association of Cardiovascular and Pulmonary Rehabilitation.[1-3] These guidelines generally recommend the attendance of a physician or cardiovascular nurse at all exercise sessions conducted for cardiac patients during the first 12 weeks of rehabilitation or as long as they exhibit cardiac abnormalities associated with an increased risk. This supervision should include emergency cardiopulmonary resuscitation equipment and a comprehensive emergency plan. The effectiveness of well-trained medical personnel in resuscitating patients after cardiac arrest during supervised exercise has been established and is the most persuasive argument for recommending medical supervision.[50] Use of lower intensity types of exercise may significantly reduce the risk of major cardiovascular complications in patients with good function so that expensive medical monitoring can be restricted to those patients at risk.

Exercise During Convalescence

Patients frequently enter into medically supervised training programs during their hospitalization for acute myocardial infarction or immediately after discharge from the hospital. These are low level programs in which passive and active calisthenics are performed while sitting and standing, along with walking, slow stair climbing, and stationary cycling. Low level treadmill exercise testing is performed at or soon after discharge from the hospital to determine the appropriateness of a low level exercise program. Exercise testing is performed up to a HR of 110 to 130 beats$\cdot$min^{-1}, an increase in HR of 20 beats$\cdot$min^{-1} or a workload of 5 METs. The general principles of exercise prescription and training apply to these patients, with special emphasis placed on low-intensity dynamic exercise, intermittent work bouts, and conservative criteria for exercise termination.

When a medically supervised exercise program is not available or feasible, it is recommended that patients with uncomplicated histories be given a plan of unsupervised, low-level physical-activity during early post-hospitalization. Individualized to each patient's clinical status, this plan should focus on walking or low-intensity stationary cycling, easy calisthenics, light household chores or recreational activities, and low-level, job-related tasks when feasible in those patients who have returned to work.[29] High-intensity exercise of any type, heavy resistance activities, and competitive situations are to be avoided.

Each exercise plan should include 1) information on selected characteristics of the exercise to be performed; 2) specific instructions on how to perform these exercises; and 3) how to monitor responses. All too frequently, such instructions are given verbally and are not sufficiently specific for the patient to be confident of what to do and what to avoid. For unsupervised exercise, the patient should be provided a written prescription that contains specific information on how to carry out an exercise plan.

If the patient has performed an exercise test recently, an exercise prescription with use of the target HR concept can be provided. If contraindications to exercise do not exist, patients are given a target HR range that is approximately 15 to 30 beats below the peak HR achieved during the test. For the patient who does not perform an exercise test during the early convalescent period, exercise recommendations will be made on the basis of clinical judgment, taking into consideration current clinical status, duration of convalescence, previous exercise habits, and age. All such patients should be given a conservative exercise plan in which the intensity is kept low and the duration and frequency are increased. It is generally recommended that patients participate in activities requiring an increase in HR of no more than 30 or 40 beats$\cdot$min^{-1} above resting or not above 110 to 120 beats$\cdot$min^{-1} (lower if the patient is receiving such medications as propanolol, which suppress HR with exertion) or have an energy requirement of not more than 4 to 6 METs. Activities of the proper type but that are too intense for patients during early convalescence include jogging, running, hiking in hills or mountains, and most active sports or games (e.g., basketball, handball, squash, and singles tennis). Activities of the wrong type include any heavy resistance or isometric exercise (e.g., heavy lifting or water

skiing). Because their intensity can be easily controlled, walking, stationary cycling, and low-level bench stepping are useful conditioning activities. A combined program of walking and stationary cycling can be used for all ambulatory patients. Walking can be performed when weather, daylight, and terrain permit, and bike riding or bench stepping can be done when it is necessary or advisable to exercise indoors.

Exercise After Convalescence

Once the patient has completed early convalescence (i.e., 12 to 20 weeks after infarction or surgery) and has been performing a low-level exercise program on a reasonably regular basis, he or she may be ready and interested in additional physical activities, especially some that are of higher intensity. If at all possible, it is recommended that the patient perform a multistage exercise test to evaluate individual exercise capacity. The results of this test, along with data from the medical history and physical examination, should form the basis for an updated exercise plan. If the decision is made to increase intensity to the level of jogging or running, attempts should be made to enter a medically supervised program.

The exercise plan for patients not in a supervised program should keep intensity at 60 to 75% of the peak HR determined during the most recent exercise test, and should emphasize a longer exercise session duration (30 to 60 minutes) and increased frequency (possibly four or five times per week, instead of three or four times). They should have a prolonged warm-up period (10 minutes) at the beginning of each exercise session and a cool-down period (5 to 10 minutes) at the end. To control exercise intensity accurately, brisk walking, intermittent walking and jogging, continuous jogging, stationary cycling, or regular bicycle riding should be the primary activities. For many patients, slow to moderate-speed stair climbing, bench stepping, or walking over hilly terrain are activities within their capacity that might be added. Such vigorous or competitive sports or games as handball or singles tennis should be delayed until the patient increases his or her exercise capacity and is cleared by the performance of a maximal, multistage exercise test.

The same approach and considerations for prescribing unsupervised exercise during the early convalescence phase still apply. As the patient's cardiovascular capacity increases, there is a need for the individual to learn to recognize early signs of overexertion, chronic fatigue, and orthopedic problems. The patient needs to know when not to exercise, when to slow down, and when to stop. As exercise capacity increases with training, a decision is needed regarding the level of exercise capacity that should serve as a goal. No specific answer to this question is applicable to all individuals, because the potential of each patient depends on the magnitude of the disease, age, gender, previous exercise habits, and heredity. The best general guide to achieve and maintain the maximal health benefits from an exercise program is to exercise regularly (three to five times per week) for approximately 30 minutes at 60 to 80% of the maximal symptom-free HR. Exercise capacity can be maintained by regular participation at the lower limits of this recommendation.

As the experience of having a heart attack or heart surgery becomes more distant, chances increase that patients will revert to their former lifestyle. If the individual was sedentary prior to the attack, frequent encouragement and guidance may be needed for the patient to remain sufficiently motivated to exercise. Such encouragement and guidance can be provided by the physician, particularly when the patient is re-evaluated and found to be progressing well. Whereas a great deal of support is needed to keep some patients exercising regularly, other individuals may need guidance to keep from overexercising. Competitive individuals need to understand the dangers of overexertion and why they need to exercise well within their exercise tolerance.

Exercise After Coronary Artery Bypass Graft Surgery

Although coronary artery bypass graft surgery effectively increases the functional potential of many patients, all too many persons remain unnecessarily incapacitated after surgery due to restrictive medical management. Limited activity before and after surgery results in substantial deconditioning, along with increased risk of pulmonary and thromboembolic complications. Overly conservative medical management compounds these problems and increases the depression and loss of self-confidence frequently experienced by these patients. Patients often confuse postoperative chest wall pain with angina and are hesitant to exercise because of fear they will injure their legs at the site of saphenous vein removal. If angina or other cardiac disease symptoms are not relieved by surgery, patients can become extremely anxious and depressed regarding their prognosis and may be extremely difficult to motivate regarding exercise.

The potential benefits of training for the post-surgery patient are similar to those for other patients with CHD—improvement in functional capacity, clinical status, and possibly prognosis.[27] The general principles of exercise prescription and training are also similar, but some specific consideration must be given to exercise of the chest wall and legs. In addition to slow walking, calisthenics designed to increase the strength and flexibility of the pectoral and leg muscles should be performed. Special exercises to improve chest wall function include deep breathing, shoulder shrugs and adduction, arm circles and lifts, trunk twisters, and wall push-ups. During this time, elastic stockings are worn to prevent fluid accumulation at the site of the leg incisions. These activities should begin within 5 days after surgery, continuing in hospital, and then on an out-of-hospital basis in a manner similar to that recommended for post-myocardial infarction patients.

REFERENCES

1. American Association of Cardiovascular and Pulmonary Rehabilitation: Guidelines for Cardiac Rehabilitation Programs. Champaign, Illinois, Human Kinetics Publishers, 1991.
2. American College of Sports Medicine: Guidelines for Graded Exercise Testing and Exercise Prescription. 4th Ed. Philadelphia, Lea & Febiger, 1991.
3. American Heart Association: Exercise standards: a statement for health professionals. Circulation, 82:2286, 1991.
4. Aronow, W., et al.: Effect of smoking cigarettes on cardiovascular hemodynamics. Arch. Environ. Health, 28:330, 1974.
5. Auchincloss, J.H., et al.: One- and three-minute exercise response in coronary artery disease. J. Appl. Physiol., 46:1132, 1979.
6. Ballantyne, F., Clark, R., Simpson, H., and Ballantyne, D.: The effect of moderate physical exercise on the plasma lipoprotein subfractions of male survivors of myocardial infarction. Circulation, 65:913, 1982.
7. Ben-Ari. E., and Rothbaum, D.: Clinical and exercise considerations for the percutaneous transluminal coronary angioplasty patient. J. Cardiopulm. Rehabil., 11:145, 1991.
8. Ben-Ari, E., et al.: Benefits of long-term physical training in patients after coronary artery bypass grafting—a 58 month follow-up and comparison with a non-trained group. J. Cardiopulm. Rehabil., 6:165, 1986.
9. Bertagnoli, K., et al.: Attenuation of exercise-induced ST depression during combined isometric and dynamic exercise in coronary artery disease. Am. J. Cardiol., 65:314, 1990.
10. Blankenhorn, D.H., et al.: Beneficial effects of combined colestipol-niacin therapy on coronary atherosclerosis and coronary venous bypass grafts. JAMA, 257:3233, 1987.
11. Centers for Disease Control. Chronic disease reports: deaths from coronary heart disease—United States, 1986. MMWR, 38:285, 1989.
12. Chaitman, B.R., et al.: The importance of clinical subsets in interpreting maximal treadmill exercise test results: the role of multiple lead ECG systems. Circulation, 59:560, 1979.
13. Clausen, J.P., and Trap-Jensen, J.: Effects of training on the distribution of cardiac output in patients with coronary heart disease. Circulation, 42:611, 1970.
14. Clausen, J.P., and Trap-Jensen, J.: Heart rate and arterial blood pressure during exercise in patients with angina pectoris. Circulation, 44:1120, 1971.
15. Conner, J.F., et al.: Effects of exercise on coronary collateralization-angiographic studies of six patients in a supervised exercise program. Med. Sci. Sports, 8:145, 1976.
16. DeBusk, R.F., et al.: Exercise training soon after myocardial infarction. Am. J. Cardiol., 44:1223, 1979.
17. Detry, J.M., and Bruce, R.A.: Effects of physical training on exertional ST-segment depression in coronary heart disease. Circulation, 44:390, 1971.
18. Ehsani, A., et al.: Effects of 12 months of intense exercise training on ischemic ST-segment depression in patients with coronary artery disease. Circulation, 64:1116, 1981.
19. Epstein, S.E., et al.: Effects of a reduction in environmental temperature on the circulatory response to exercise in man. N. Engl. J. Med., 280:7, 1969.
20. Ferguson, R.J., et al.: Effect of exercise capacity collateral circulation and progression of coronary disease. Am. J. Cardiol., 34:764, 1974.
21. Fisher, L., et al.: Diagnostic quantification of CASS (coronary artery surgery study): clinical and exercise test results of coronary artery disease. A multivariate approach. Circulation, 63:987, 1981.
22. Franklin, B.A., et al.: Resistance training in cardiac rehabilitation. J. Cardiopulm. Rehabil., 11:99, 1991.
23. Hamalainen, H. et al.: Long-term reduction in sudden deaths after a multifactorial intervention programme in patients with myocardial infarction: 10-year results of a controlled investigation. Eur. Heart J., 10:55, 1989.
24. Haskell, W.L., Fair, J., Sanders, W., and Alderman, E.L.: New methodologies for studying the prevention of atherosclerosis. Ann. Clin. Research, 20:39–45, 1988.
25. Haskell, W.L., Savin, W., Oldridge, N., and DeBusk, R.: Factors influencing estimated oxygen uptake during exercise testing soon after myocardial infarction. Am. J. Cardiol., 50:299, 1982.
26. Hedback, B., and Perk, J.: Can high-risk patients after myocardial infarction participate in comprehensive cardiac rehabilitation? Scand. J. Rehabil. Med., 22:15, 1990.
27. Hedback, B., et al.: Cardiac rehabilitation after coronary artery bypass grafting: Effects on exercise performance and risk factors. Arch. Phys. Med. Rehabil., 71:1069, 1990.
28. Hung, J., et al.: Comparison of cardiovascular response to combined static-dynamic effort, postprandial dynamic effort and dynamic effort alone in patients with chronic ischemic heart disease. Circulation, 65:1411, 1982.
29. Juneau, M., et al.: Effectiveness of self-monitored, home-based moderate-intensity exercise training in middle-aged men and women. Am. J. Cardiol., 60:66, 1987.
30. Kerber, R.E., Miller, R., and Najjar, S.: Myocardial ischemia effects of isometric, dynamic and combined exercise in coronary artery disease. Chest, 67:4, 1975.
31. Kivowitz, C., et al.: Effects of isometric exercise on cardiac performance: the grip test. Circulation, 44:994, 1971.
32. Lawrie, G.M., et al.: The results of coronary bypass more than five years after operation in 434 patients: clinical, exercise treadmill and angiographic correlations. Am. J. Cardiol., 40:665, 1977.
33. Laws, A., and Reaven, G.M.: Effect of physical activity on age-related glucose intolerance. Clin. Geriatr. Med., 6:849, 1990.
34. Lipid Research Clinics Program. The lipid research clinics coronary primary prevention trial results: I. Reduction in incidence of coronary heart disease. JAMA, 251:351, 1984.
35. Nalai, Y., et al.: The benefits of exercise training after coronary artery bypass grafting. Compr. Ther., 24:45, 1988.

36. Naughton, J., and Haider, R.: Methods of exercise testing. *In* Exercise Testing and Exercise Training in Coronary Heart Disease. Edited by J. Naughton, H.K. Hellerstein, and I.C. Mohler. New York, Academic Press, 1973, p. 79.

37. O'Connor, G.T., et al.: An overview of randomized trials of rehabilitation with exercise after myocardial infarction. Circulation, *80*:234, 1989.

38. O'Keefe, J.H., Jr., et al.: Multivessel coronary angioplasty from 1980 to 1989: procedural results and long-term outcome. J. Am. Coll. Cardiol., *16*:1097, 1990.

39. Oldridge, N.B., et al.: Cardiac rehabilitation after myocardial infarction: combined experience of randomized clinical trials. JAMA, *260*:945, 1988.

40. Ornish, D., et al.: Can lifestyle changes reverse coronary heart disease? Lancet, *336*:129, 1990.

41. Paterson, D.H., et al.: Effects of physical training on cardiovascular function following myocardial infarction. J. Appl. Physiol., *47*:482, 1979.

42. Ross, R.: The pathogenesis of atherosclerosis—an update. N. Engl. J. Med., *314*:488, 1986.

43. Savin, W., Haskell, W., Houston-Miller, N., and DeBusk, R.: Improvement in aerobic capacity soon after myocardial infarction. J. Cardiac Rehabil., *1*:337, 1981.

44. Selvester, R., Camp, J., and Sanmarco, M.: Effects of exercise training on progression of documented coronary atherosclerosis. *In* The Marathon: Physiological, Medical, Epidemiological, and Psychological Studies. Edited by P. Milvy. New York, New York Academy of Sciences, 1977, p. 495.

45. Sim, D.N., and Neill, W.A.: Investigation of the physiological basis for increased exercise threshold for angina pectoris after physical conditioning. J. Clin. Invest., *54*:763, 1974.

46. Smokler, P.E., MacAlpin, R., Alvaro, A., and Kattus, A.: Reproducibility of a multi-stage near maximal treadmill test for exercise tolerance in angina pectoris. Circulation, *49*:346, 1973.

47. Sullivan, M.J., et al.: Exercise training in patients with severe left ventricular dysfunction: hemodynamic and metabolic effects. Circulation, *78*:525, 1981.

48. Thadani, V., West, R.O., Mathew, T.M., and Parker, J.O.: Hemodynamics at rest and during supine and sitting bicycle exercise in patients with coronary artery disease. Am. J. Cardiol., *39*:776, 1977.

49. Thompson, P., Cullinane, E., Lazarus, B., and Carleton, R.: Effect of exercise training on the untrained limb exercise performance of men with angina pectoris. Am. J. Cardiol., *48*:844, 1981.

50. Thompson, P.D.: The benefits and risks of exercise training in patients with chronic coronary artery disease. JAMA, *259*:1537, 1988.

51. Thompson, P.D.: The cardiovascular risks for cardiac rehabilitation. J. Cardiopulm. Rehabil., *5*:321, 1985.

52. Uemura, K.: Excess mortality ratio with reference to the lowest sex-age specific death rates among countries. World Health Stat. Q., *42*:26, 1989.

53. Van Camp, S.P., and Peterson, R.A.: Cardiovascular complications of outpatient cardiac rehabilitation programs. JAMA, *256*:1160, 1988.

54. Van Camp, S.P.: The safety of cardiac rehabilitation. J. Cardiopulm. Rehabil., *11*:64, 1991.

55. Verani, M., et al.: Effects of exercise training on left ventricular performance and myocardial perfusion in patients with coronary artery disease. Am. J. Cardiol., *47*:797, 1981.

56. Vuori, I., Makarainen, M., and Jaaselainen, A.: Sudden death and physical activity. Cardiology, *63*:287, 1979.

57. Wohl, A.J., et al.: Cardiovascular function during early recovery from acute myocardial infarction. Circulation, *56*:931, 1977.

273

Hypertension

by
Rune Sannerstedt

DEFINITION

According to a WHO Expert Committee, arterial hypertension in adults is arbitrarily defined as a chronically elevated systolic blood pressure (SBP) $\geq$ 160 mm Hg and/or a fifth-phase diastolic blood pressure (DBP) $\geq$ 95 mm Hg.[48] Blood pressure (BP), however, is a highly unstable function, showing considerable differences between daytime and night-time determinations; variation also occurs with numerous mental and physical stimuli.[14,46]

The interplay between physical rest and various degrees of exertion has immediate and marked effects on SBP, which rises linearly with increasing oxygen consumption ($\dot{V}_{O_2}$). Thus, in healthy middle-aged men, the mean regression line for SBP crosses the threshold between normotension and hypertension (as defined above) at a $\dot{V}_{O_2}$ between 1.0 and 1.6 L$\cdot$min^{-1}.[2,35,50] Obviously, therefore, the diagnosis of "arterial hypertension" must be based on BP determined while the patient is at reasonable physical and mental rest; this is usually described as a "casual" BP reading.

The influence of age, gender, and race must also be taken into account when BP figures are considered. For example, it is well known that SBP rises with age and that this rise is more marked in women.

Any evaluation of BP determinations must also consider the recording technique being used. This factor is important, especially if BP is measured during exercise, when a faulty technique may give erroneous figures.[28,56]

PRIMARY AND SECONDARY HYPERTENSION

In the true meaning of the term, arterial hypertension is not a disease, but a symptom. It may appear in a great variety of conditions that have an elevated systemic BP as their common denominator but are otherwise quite different regarding such aspects as etiologic background and general course. In only a minor part of a hypertensive population (5 to 10%) is it possible to demonstrate an identifiable cause of hypertension; this state is then denoted as secondary hypertension.[7] Accordingly, the majority of hypertensive patients (90 to 95%) have primary or essential hypertension, defined as high BP without evident organic cause and affected by the interaction of many genetic and environmental influences. Considering its dominant role, the following discussion applies only to primary or essential hypertension.

COURSE OF THE DISEASE

When untreated, primary or essential hypertension is a long-term, chronic disorder, leading progressively to involvement of target organs and eventually to irreparable organ damage. The rate of progression varies markedly among individuals, depending on such factors as genetic traits, dietary habits, degree of social stress, and concomitant diseases.

The World Health Organization (WHO) Expert Committee suggests classifying arterial hypertension into three stages, according to the extent of organ involvement and damage.[48]

WHO STAGE 1. No objective signs of organic change are evident.

WHO STAGE 2. At least one of the following signs of organ involvement is present: left ventricular hypertrophy on physical examination, chest radiography, electrocardiography, or echocardiography; generalized and focal narrowing of retinal arteries; proteinuria and/or slight elevation of plasma creatinine concentration.

WHO STAGE 3. Appearance of symptoms and signs due to damage to various organs from hypertensive disease, including three features that are pathognomonic of the malignant or accelerated phase:

Heart: left ventricular failure
Brain: cerebral, cerebellar, or brain stem hemorrhage and hypertensive encephalopathy
Optic fundi: retinal hemorrhages and exudates with or without papilledema

Other conditions that are frequently apparent in Stage 3 but are less clearly a direct consequence of hypertension include the following:

Heart: angina pectoris and myocardial infarction
Brain: intracranial arterial thrombosis
Blood vessels: dissecting aneurysm and arterial occlusive disease
Kidney: renal failure

HEMODYNAMICS AT REST

Although the main hemodynamic change in hypertensive cardiovascular disease is an increased systemic vascular resistance (SVR), patients in various stages of the disorder may be characterized by different hemodynamic patterns.[2,9,35,50] Using the WHO classification for subgrouping hypertensive patients, the following group patterns may be distinguished (Fig. 16–1).

WHO STAGE 1. Clinically described as mild, latent, or borderline arterial hypertension, this group of patients is characterized by a hyperdynamic circulation at rest, with an increased cardiac output ($\dot{Q}$); this increase is mainly due to an elevated heart rate (HR) with or without an enlarged stroke volume (SV). The calculated SVR is within the normal range, whereas plasma volume may be lower than normal. Corresponding to the elevated $\dot{Q}$, $\dot{V}_{O_2}$ is raised, leaving normal values for arteriovenous oxygen difference (AVD-O_2). Over the years, the hemodynamic picture may change in young subjects, with a gradual fall in $\dot{Q}$ and a continuous increase in SVR.[37]

WHO STAGE 2. Clinically termed as having manifest, fixed, or established arterial hypertension, patients in this group have a normodynamic circulation at rest (with normal $\dot{Q}$) and usually normal figures for HR and SV, but the SVR is elevated. Plasma volume, $\dot{V}_{O_2}$, and AVD-O_2 are within normal ranges.

WHO STAGE 3. Clinically denoted as having severe or advanced arterial hypertension, patients at this stage characteristically have a hypodynamic circulation at rest, with subnormal $\dot{Q}$ due to a lowered SV. SVR is grossly elevated and the intravascular fluid volume tends to expand. AVD-O_2 widens to compensate for the lower blood flow.

These hemodynamic patterns are summarized in Figure 16–1. It should be noted that these hemodynamic changes are group patterns, and that there may be a marked scatter of values within the group. Accordingly, there are great overlaps among the various groups. This variance must be kept in mind when considering a particular hypertensive patient.

MEDICAL TREATMENT

Viewed hemodynamically and according to the law of Poiseuille (BP = $\dot{Q}$/SVR), there are three ways to decrease the BP: lower $\dot{Q}$, decrease SVR, or combine these two means. Considering the differences in hemodynamic patterns among hypertensive patients at different stages of the disorder, it immediately emerges that the various ways of lowering BP preferably should be used differently for the three WHO stages. Clinically, it should be possible to take advantage of the varying

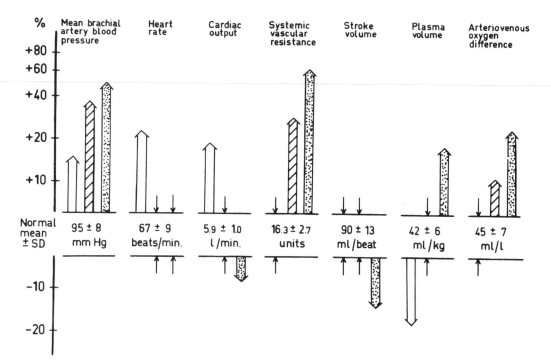

Fig. 16–1. *Hemodynamic patterns at rest in men with untreated essential arterial of various stages.*[32] *Mean differences in percent are compared to a control group of age-matched normotensive men by using a logarithmic scale. ( ) = WHO Stage 1; ( ) = WHO Stage 2; ( ) = WHO Stage 3.*

hemodynamic properties of today's anti-hypertensive drugs, prescribing them in a spirit of what has been depicted as "enlightened empiricism."[10,25,60] A schematic outline of drug treatment emphasizing hemodynamic principles is presented in Table 16–1.

WHO STAGE 1. The logical approach to treating these patients is to aim at normalizing the circulation through the lowering of $\dot{Q}$, which may be achieved by beta-adrenoceptor blockers. In patients with mild, borderline hypertension, monotherapy with a beta-adrenoceptor

TABLE 16–1. **Drug Treatment of Arterial Hypertension, with Emphasis on Hemodynamic Principles**

Treatment	WHO Stage 1	WHO Stage 2	WHO Stage 3
Objective	Normalization of circulation; reduction of HR and $\dot{Q}$	Normalization of circulation; reduction of systemic vascular resistance	Prevention of cardiac failure and combatting symptoms of CHD; protection of vital vascular areas against pressure damage
Main approach	Beta-adrenoceptor blockers	Peripheral vasodilators such as calcium channel blockers and angiotensin converting enzyme (ACE) inhibitors	Peripheral vasodilators such as calcium channel blockers and angiotensin converting enzyme (ACE) inhibitors and diuretic agents
Supplement		Beta-adrenoceptor blockers Diuretic agents	Beta-adrenoceptor blockers

blocker is therefore the preferred approach, especially in patients with an exaggerated adrenergic drive that manifests itself as an increased HR.

Physical conditioning and meditation therapy are tentative nonpharmacologic measures to lower the adrenergic influence and to enhance parasympathetic tone.

WHO STAGE 2. In these hypertensive patients, the main therapeutic attack should be directed against the increased SVR, the aim being to reduce it to as normal a level as possible. From the pathophysiologic standpoint, such peripheral vasodilators as calcium-channel blockers and angiotensin-converting enzyme (ACE) inhibitors would be the drugs of choice.

By way of the baroreceptors, peripheral vasodilators may produce a compensatory increase in HR and $\dot{Q}$ to counteract the lower BP level caused by the drug. This reflex can be effectively inhibited by a beta-adrenoceptor blocker, without jeopardizing the antihypertensive action of the peripheral vasodilator.

Thus, a combined therapeutic approach with the use of an effective peripheral vasodilator and a beta-adrenoceptor blocker may be preferable for patients with manifest, established hypertension.

WHO STAGE 3. In patients with severe, advanced hypertension, an ideal treatment should aim to reverse all circulatory changes in an attempt to repair any possible organic damage. In most cases, however, such a reversal is no longer possible, and the main objective should therefore be to lower BP to reduce the burden on the heart and to protect vital organs from further damage.

To accomplish this objective, such peripheral vasodilators as calcium-channel blockers and ACE inhibitors may be regarded as the drugs of first choice. The addition of a diuretic agent enhances the antihypertensive effect.

A beta-adrenoceptor blocker may well be added to the combination of a calcium-channel blocker or an ACE inhibitor and a diuretic agent. Thus, triple therapy may turn out to be needed and appropriate for many patients with severe, advanced arterial hypertension.

EXERCISE ABILITY

The maximal physical working capacity of individuals with mild, borderline hypertension (WHO Stage 1) is not different from that seen in normotensive subjects of the same gender and age.[13,41,59] Once WHO Stage 2 has been reached, however, hypertensive patients tend to develop a decreasing ability to exercise.[6,61] The degree of impairment is proportional to the extent of myocardial involvement, and is naturally most obvious in those patients in overt cardiac failure.

HEMODYNAMIC EFFECTS OF EXERCISE

Dynamic Exercise

In spite of the fact that hypertensive patients start with higher resting BPs, the elevated SBP is consistently maintained with increasing $\dot{V}_{O_2}$ (Fig. 16–2). Actually, the deviation from values found in normotensive subjects even increases in some patients, especially in patients with more advanced arterial hypertension (WHO Stages 2 and 3). Thus, the average SBP responses of these patients are significantly steeper than those found in normotensive persons. For individual patients, exceedingly high SBP levels may be recorded, with values well above 300 mm Hg.

Occasionally, considerable increases in SBP from around 150 mm Hg at rest to around 250 mm Hg during exercise may also occur in patients with mild, borderline arterial hypertension (WHO Stage 1). Considered as a group, however, these patients do not have SBP responses to exercise that are different from those seen in normotensive subjects of the same gender and age.

Similar to the responses of normotensive subjects, hypertensive patients of all stages have a slight to moderate rise in DBP with increasing $\dot{V}_{O_2}$ during dynamic exercise (Fig. 16–3). As a result, the initial

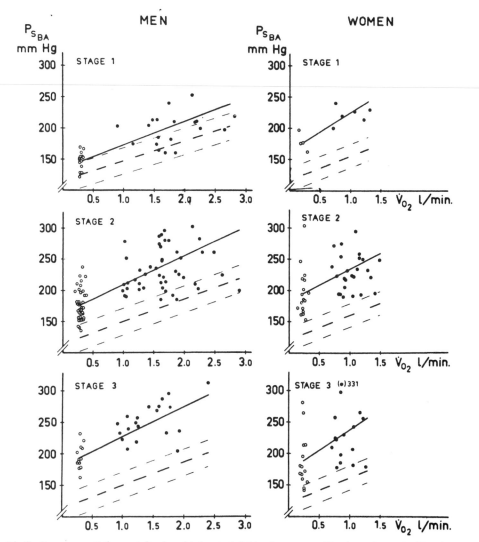

Fig. 16–2. *Response of the systolic brachial arterial blood pressure ($P_{S_{BA}}$) to dynamic bicycle ergometer exercise in relation to oxygen consumption ($\dot{V}_{O_2}$) in patients with arterial hypertension (WHO Stages 1–3) and in age-matched normotensive controls.[28] (○) = rest; (●) = exercise; (———) = regressions for the hypertensive patients; (- - -) = regressions (with ± 2 SD) for normotensive controls.*

deviation at rest from the normal range is unchanged. Patients with marked DBP elevations at rest may therefore develop very high DBP levels of 150 to 170 mm Hg during dynamic exercise.

WHO STAGE 1. In patients with mild, borderline hypertension, the hyperkinetic circulation at rest with increased HR and elevated $\dot{Q}$ is cancelled during physical exercise, when $\dot{Q}$ apparently adjusts to the metabolic needs. This means that the increase in $\dot{Q}$ is relatively smaller in these patients than in normotensive controls

(Fig. 16–4), indicating that their circulation is somewhat normalized during the performance of exercise. However, their BP may increase markedly, the percentage increase being the same as in normotensives, which means that the BP difference at rest is kept during exercise.

Thus, although there is a considerable fall in SVR, the average relative and absolute decrease is less than that found in normotensives. Not even during strenuous exercise does the resistance reach the same low level as in persons with normotension;

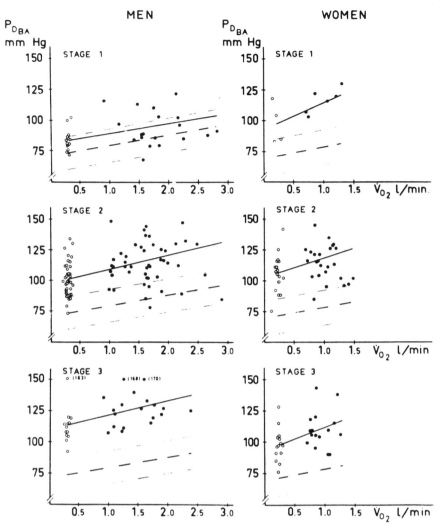

Fig. 16–3. *Responses of the diastolic brachial arterial blood pressure ($P_{D_{BA}}$) to dynamic bicycle ergometer exercise in relation to oxygen consumption ($\dot{V}_{O_2}$) in patients with arterial hypertension (WHO Stages 1–3) and in age-matched normotensive subjects.[28] See Figure 16–2 for symbols and details.*

this fact indicates that restrictive changes in the peripheral vascular bed are already present at this very early stage.[27]

WHO STAGE 2.   In comparison to normotensive individuals, patients with manifest, established arterial hypertension may react to dynamic exercise with a more marked increase in HR and less of a rise in SV. The net result is a relative and absolute rise in $\dot{Q}$ similar to that observed in persons with normal BP values (Fig. 16–4). Although the relative fall in SVR is similar at comparable levels of exercise, the absolute values for SVR stay elevated at all levels of exercise, just as in WHO Stage 1 hypertensive patients.

WHO STAGE 3.   In patients with severe, advanced hypertension, characteristics of impending cardiac failure during exercise are added to the hemodynamic pattern described for patients in WHO Stage 2. Thus, in absolute figures, a subnormal rise in $\dot{Q}$ and abnormal widening in AVD-O_2 may be seen, together with marked increases in HR and pulmonary artery blood pressure beginning at low exercise levels.

Static Exercise

Basically, patients with uncomplicated arterial hypertension (WHO Stages 1 and 2) show reactions to static, isometric exercise similar to those in normotensive con-

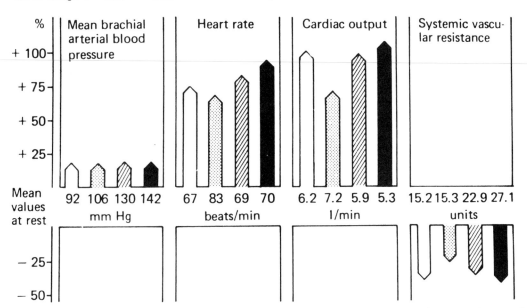

WHO Stage 1 = ▨ 2 = ▨ 3 = ■. Healthy controls = ☐

%	Mean brachial arterial blood pressure	Heart rate	Cardiac output	Systemic vascular resistance
Mean values at rest	92 106 130 142 mm Hg	67 83 69 70 beats/min	6.2 7.2 5.9 5.3 l/min	15.2 15.3 22.9 27.1 units

Fig. 16–4. *Patterns of hemodynamic responses to bicycle ergometer exercise in men with untreated essential arterial hypertension (WHO Stage 1, 2, or 3).*[33]

trols.[11,22,53] Thus, although starting from elevated BP levels already at rest, there are further marked elevations during static exercise in both SBP and SDP, the absolute increase being about the same as in normotensive individuals (Fig. 16–5).

A wide scatter of BP changes is seen among both normotensive and hypertensive individuals in Figure 16–5. However, although no normotensive subject exceeded an SBP of 170 mm Hg during hand squeezing, hypertensive patients regularly surpassed this level when using 30% of their maximal hand-squeezing capacity for 4 min.

As seen in normotensive controls, HR and Q̇ increase moderately and the calculated SVR is mainly unchanged.

Hemodynamically, static isometric exercise may therefore mean a considerably heavier strain on the vascular system than dynamic exercise. It has to be pointed out, however, that this strain is normally only of short duration. Thus, after stopping the static exercise, BP will immediately drop, reaching the initial resting level within 15 to 30 seconds.

EFFECTS OF ANTIHYPERTENSIVE DRUGS ON EXERCISE RESPONSES

Ideally, an antihypertensive drug regimen should normalize any hemodynamic abnormalities not only at rest but also during the strain of mental and/or physical stress of various kinds.[25,54] Today, this can be achieved using drug combinations tailored to the need of the individual hypertensive patient. Still, there is no single antihypertensive drug available that will normalize the circulation in all categories of hypertensive patients (e.g., young and old patients; mild, borderline hypertension versus manifest, established hypertension; degree of myocardial derangement present).

Dynamic Exercise

Basically, four types of modified BP responses to dynamic exercise may be distinguished:

1. The BP is lowered to the same extent both at rest and during dynamic exercise. Although the absolute increase with exercise is the same as before

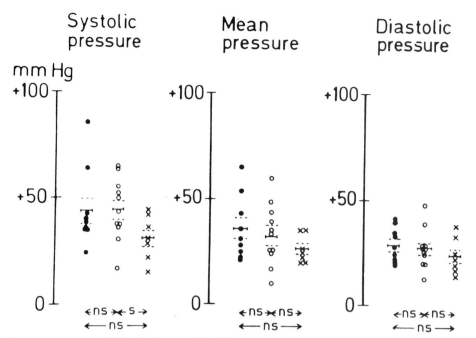

Fig. 16–5. *Responses of the brachial arterial blood pressure to static hand exercise in men with WHO Stage 1 arterial hypertension (●) or WHO Stage 2 (○) and in normotensive men (X). Mean changes ± SEM are shown with significance levels for paired differences. s = p < 0.05; ns = non-significant.*

treatment, the relative pressure rise is higher during treatment. This type of response is probably the most common and is generally seen during monotherapy with diuretics, calcium-channel blockers, and ACE inhibitors.[18,19,43,44,58,62,63]

2. The BP-lowering effect becomes more marked during dynamic exercise than at rest. The absolute increase with exercise is less than before treatment, whereas the relative pressure rise is equal to or lower than the one seen before treatment. Such findings have been described after monotherapy with both alpha- and beta-adrenoceptor blockers.[23,29,58,62] In cases of manifest, established hypertension with high resting BP levels, this type of response may be needed to achieve complete or nearly complete normalization of the exercising BP. A combination therapy (e.g., a peripheral vasodilator plus a beta-adrenoceptor blocker) may yield better results than either drug alone.[16]

3. Any BP increase during dynamic exercise is abolished, and a decreasing BP may be seen. This has been a typical feature of treatment with such presently abandoned potent sympatholytic drugs as guanethidine and bethanidine, which sometimes led to syncopal attacks during strenuous dynamic exercise. It may also occur in elderly patients treated with excessive dosages of diuretics and in patients with advanced myocardial damage.

4. Any BP-lowering effect of treatment becomes evident only during exposure to strain. BP is then unchanged at rest but shows lower values during dynamic exercise than before treatment.[49] Occasionally, this may be seen during monotherapy with beta-adrenoceptor blockers,[38] especially in young patients who present with near-normal BP figures at rest but who react to the strain of dynamic exercise with excessive BP increases in the untreated state.

Apart from these four basic patterns of BP response to physical exercise in hypertensive patients undergoing antihypertensive drug treatment, the question also arises as to what extent antihypertensive drugs may modify or normalize other hemodynamic abnormalities.

Regarding myocardial function, a reduction of left ventricular hypertrophy has been described after sustained treatment with various antihypertensive drugs.[21] The combination of calcium-channel blockers and ACE inhibitors seems to be particularly effective.[1,39,40] However, a study showed that the reduction in left ventricular mass index during treatment with combinations of either an ACE inhibitor plus a diuretic or a calcium-channel blocker plus a beta-adrenoceptor blocker was not accompanied by any change in left ventricular performance during the stress of isometric handgrip exercise.[1]

The fall in BP during chronic treatment with alpha-adrenoceptor blockers, ACE inhibitors, and calcium-channel blockers has been found to be entirely due to a reduction in SVR, both at rest and during dynamic exercise, with a maintained $\dot{Q}$.[36,37] This must be interpreted with caution, however, and it is still an open question as to whether such conclusions can be broadened to cover a general population of treated hypertensive patients and result in reduced cardiovascular complications and mortality.

Static Exercise

In general, such antihypertensive drugs as beta-adrenoceptor blockers, ACE inhibitors, and calcium-channel blockers will not attenuate the BP response to static, isometric exercise.[18,19,22,42,53]

EFFECT OF ANTIHYPERTENSIVE DRUGS ON EXERCISE ABILITY

Few studies deal specifically with the effect of antihypertensive drugs on physical working capacity. Some researchers report unchanged exercise ability and even improved left ventricular function.[12,33] It seems clear, however, that beta-adrenoceptor blockers may negatively affect exercise tolerance, reducing maximal working and endurance capacity and

increasing the degree of perceived exertion,[15,20,45] whereas clonidine and alpha-adrenoceptor blockers do not.[17,23] When choosing antihypertensive therapy for patients who are interested and engaged in endurance sport activities, such facts have to be kept in mind.[36]

EXERCISE TESTING

Standardized dynamic exercise tests in hypertensive patients may be useful in the clinical routine:

—to disclose a hypertensive pattern of BP regulation in subjects who are normotensive at rest;

—to disclose an insufficient BP response to the challenge of physical strain in patients with impaired myocardial function;

—to support the indication for active antihypertensive treatment in subjects with mild, borderline hypertension (WHO Stage 1);

—to evaluate the efficacy of antihypertensive drug therapy in normalizing BP responses to an exercise challenge;

—to verify inadequate or absent BP increases during antihypertensive drug therapy that produces subjective complaints of weakness and dizziness during exercise; and

—to ensure that the patient's physical working capacity is not impaired by the antihypertensive medication in relation to requirements of his/her occupational duties and life enjoyment.

BLOOD PRESSURE RECORDING TECHNIQUES

The systemic BP can be recorded directly in an artery during exercise by using indwelling needles or catheters. This method yields exact values for both SBP and DBP, and the mean BP can be immediately derived via electrical integration. This invasive technique, however, is inconvenient for the patient and may cause complications. Its clinical usefulness is therefore limited to strict indications.

Indirect BP measurements during exertion using a cuff and auscultatory readings of the Korotkoff sounds are simple and safe, but are less precise and prone to technical shortcomings.[28,56] Thus, auscultatory readings of DBP obtained during exercise are generally unreliable and may be disregarded. Indirect measures of SBP during exercise may also occasionally diverge markedly from the true value, as mentioned previously. In addition, the mean BP value cannot be immediately obtained and must be estimated as the DBP plus one-third of the pulse pressure (i.e., SBP minus DBP). Systematic studies have generally shown, however, that there may be a good correlation between direct and indirect measures of SBP, both at rest and during exercise.

PERFORMANCE OF THE EXERCISE TEST

During an exercise test of progressively increasing intensity, SBP normally rises with increasing $\dot{V}_{O_2}$. Should the SBP fail to rise or even drop with an increase in power output, the myocardium may be going into failure and the test should be stopped. Similarly, a marked rise in DBP should also be considered a contraindication to continuing the exercise test.

After stopping dynamic exercise, BP will immediately start to fall, usually reaching its initial resting level within 2 to 3 min. Therefore, to obtain true information about the exercising BP level in hypertensive patients, the recordings must be made during exercise, because anything else may yield erroneous values. Blood pressures should also be recorded repeatedly after exercise to disclose any tendency toward an exaggerated fall, with the patient being observed for such symptoms as giddiness.

It should be noted that the systemic BP responses to dynamic exercises are generally greater for arm work than for leg work.[55] On the other hand, BP responses are not systematically different for dynamic exercise performed in the recumbent, sitting, or upright positions.[8]

POSSIBLE RISKS

A rather self-evident question is whether exercise and physical training have any deleterious effects on patients with arterial hypertension. Very little is known about such risks, but in light of the fact that various procedures encompassing dynamic and/or static exercise may lead to marked BP increases in hypertensive patients, with peaks well above 300 mm Hg, the risk of acute cerebrocardiovascular disasters should not be ignored. Naturally, this warning is especially valid for patients who have high BP levels at rest and who have signs of cardiovascular complications.

It should be mentioned, however, that in a survey of about 50,000 exercise tests performed in Sweden, the general frequency of complications was only 18.4 per 10,000 tests.[4] Pre-existing CHD accounted for most of the complications, whereas hypertension was relatively rare among those persons who developed symptoms associated with the exercise test. It was concluded that under controlled circumstances, exercise tests may be regarded as a method of examining even seriously ill patients, with little risk of subsequent complications. In Sweden, however, some laboratory staff do not accept patients for exercise tests if their resting SBP is above a certain level, the range of exclusion being 220 to 270 mm Hg.[3] In addition, exercise tests are often stopped if SBP exceeds a certain level, the range being 240 to 300 mm Hg.

PHYSICAL CONDITIONING

Over the last few years, there has been an increasing interest in physical conditioning as a tool to reduce BP in hypertensive patients. The numerous studies now available have also led to an official recommendation from an expert group that all patients with mild hypertension should take appropriate exercise as part of their nonpharmacologic treatment.[57]

The hemodynamic effects of physical training in cardiovascularly healthy people are well outlined and consist mainly of an increase in maximal $\dot{V}_{O_2}$, a lowered HR and a lower $\dot{Q}$ both at rest and during exercise at equivalent $\dot{V}_{O_2}$ levels, and a somewhat lower BP level both at rest and during exercise. The values for the calculated SVR remain basically unchanged.

Similar findings may also be obtained in hypertensive patients, and many studies have shown that sustained regular exercise training, especially when combined with other nonpharmacologic measures, produces a significant BP reduction and a lesser need of pharmacologic intervention.[24,26,47,51] The lower BP level may be paralleled by only small changes in $\dot{Q}$, thus yielding lower figures for an initially increased value for the derived SVR, the mainstay of hemodynamic changes in arterial hypertension. It might be anticipated that exercise training could increase left ventricular mass, thereby counteracting the beneficial effects of the decrease in BP. Recent data show, however, that this is not the case.[34] On the contrary, left ventricular mass index tends to decrease.[5]

There are some indications that subjects with mild, borderline arterial hypertension (WHO Stage 1), especially those with a hyperkinetic circulation at rest with elevated HR and $\dot{Q}$, will benefit more from physical conditioning than patients with manifest, established arterial hypertension (WHO Stage 2) (Fig. 16–6).[31,51] Both male and female patients have been followed, and there are no indications that the results of physical conditioning are any different between the sexes.

To date, no data are available on the effects of physical training in patients with severe, advanced arterial hypertension (WHO Stage 3). However, it can be anticipated that exercise training in such patients will not have a positive effect on their hemodynamic profile, including their BP level.

It may therefore be summarized that sustained exercise training will primarily benefit patients with mild, borderline arterial hypertension corresponding to WHO Stage 1 (Fig. 16–7). Improved physical fitness may also be of therapeutic value in patients with manifest, established arterial hypertension (WHO Stage 2).[30] Under all circumstances, these patients should be recommended to maintain their physical condition; this also may be true for patients with severe, advanced arterial hypertension (WHO Stage 3).

The type of physical conditioning best suited to the hypertensive patient probably includes dynamic exercise, although it has been proposed that a well-balanced combination of dynamic and static exercises may give the best conditioning effect. Generally speaking, weight-lifting and other heavy static exercise, as well as exhausting long-distance running and similar activities, are not recommended for hypertensive patients, especially not to patients with arterial hypertension at WHO Stages 2 and 3.[32]

To retain any BP reduction obtained through physical conditioning, it is necessary to maintain an improved level of physical fitness. In practice, this may be difficult for many patients to accomplish, especially if they find the exercise activities boring and a time-consuming burden. It is therefore important to find out at an early stage which kind of physical activity will fit the individual over time. In some parts in Sweden, we can now recommend that our sedentary patients join "Friskis & Svettis" (Healthy & Sweaty), which has developed into some kind of people's movement over the past 10 years (Fig. 16–8).

The basis for Friskis & Svettis is simple gymnastics in step with rhythmic, exciting, and loud music under the leadership of specially educated and enthusiastic leaders. There are various programs available, from easy ones for previous lazybones to advanced ones requiring a high level of physical fitness, and from exercise groups for pregnant women to elderly, retired people.

Finally, it should be emphasized that any recommendations to hypertensive patients about physical activity have to be accompanied by advice on general measures against overweight, excess salt intake, overconsumption of alcohol, etc. In

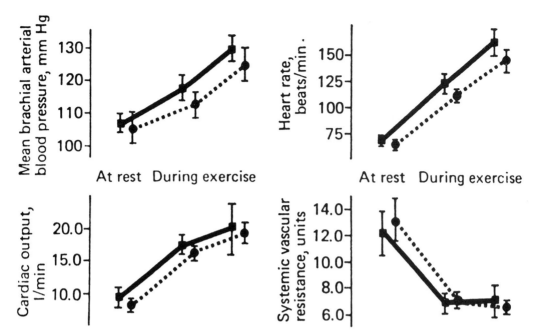

Fig. 16–6. *Hemodynamic findings at rest and during dynamic exercise before (——) and after (- - -) physical training in five men with WHO Stage 1 arterial hypertension.*[33] *Mean values ± SEM are shown.*

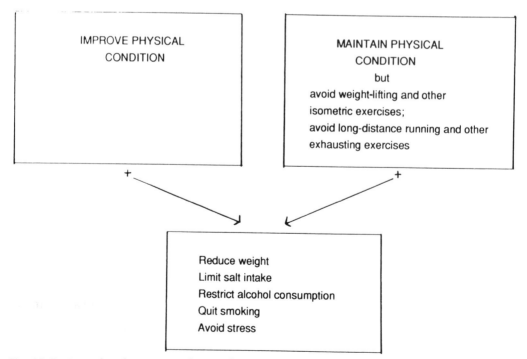

LATENT, BORDERLINE ARTERIAL HYPERTENSION
WHO Stage 1

ESTABLISHED ARTERIAL HYPERTENSION
WHO Stage 2

IMPROVE PHYSICAL
CONDITION

MAINTAIN PHYSICAL
CONDITION
but
avoid weight-lifting and other
isometric exercises;
avoid long-distance running and other
exhausting exercises

Reduce weight
Limit salt intake
Restrict alcohol consumption
Quit smoking
Avoid stress

Fig. 16–7. *General outline for nonpharmacologic measures in patients with arterial hypertension WHO Stages 1 and 2.*

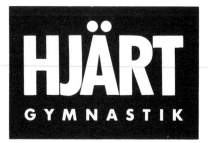

GÖTEBORG

Fig. 16–8. *Logotype of the "Friskis & Svettis" movement in Sweden, which in translation means something like the "Healthy & Sweaty" movement.*

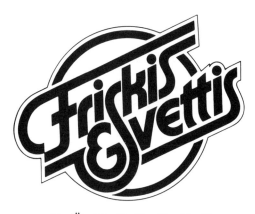

doing so, it might be expected that a substantial number of hypertensive individuals, especially those with mild, borderline arterial hypertension (WHO Stage 1), will be able to normalize their BP, thereby avoiding any annoying, costly, and lifelong pharmacotherapy and the potential risk of side effects inherent with drugs.

REFERENCES

1. Agabiti-Rosei, E., et al.: Long-term antihypertensive treatment may induce normalization of left ventricular mass before complete regression of vascular structural changes: consequences for cardiac function at rest and during stress. J. Hypertension. 6(Suppl. 4):S94, 1988.
2. Amery, A., Julius, S., Whitlock, L.S., and Conway, J.: Influence of hypertension on the hemodynamic response to exercise. Circulation, 36:231, 1967.
3. Atterhög, J.-H., Jonsson, B., and Samuelsson, R.: Exercise testing in Sweden: a survey of procedures. Scand. J. Clin. Lab. Invest., 39:87, 1979.
4. Atterhög, J.-H., Jonsson, B., and Samuelsson, R.: Komplikationer vid klinisk arbetsprövning i Sverige (Complications in clinical work tests in Sweden). Läkartidningen, 77:2689, 1980.
5. Baglivo, H.P., et al.: Effect of moderate physical training on left ventricular mass in mild hypertensive persons. Hypertension, 15(Suppl. I):I153, 1990.
6. Bahler, R.C., and Gatzoylis, K.: Exercise performance in patients with hypertension. J. Electrocardiol., 23:41, 1990.
7. Berglund, G., Andersson, O., and Wilhelmsen, L.: Prevalence of primary and secondary hypertension: studies in a random population sample. Br. Med. J., 2:554, 1976.
8. Bevegård, S., and Danielson, M.: Effect of body position on circulatory adaption to exercise in patients with essential hypertension. Scand. J. Clin. Lab. Invest., 37:63, 1977.
9. Birkenhäger, W.H., and Schalekamp, M.A.D.H.: Control Mechanisms in Essential Hypertension. Amsterdam, Elsevier, 1976.
10. Bravo, E.L.: Rational drug therapy based on understanding the pathophysiology of hypertension. Cleve. Clin. J. Med., 56:362, 1989.
11. Brorson, L., Wasir, H., and Sannerstedt, R.: Haemodynamic effects of static and dynamic exercise in males with arterial hypertension of varying severity. Cardiovasc, Res., 12:269, 1978.
12. Bruce, R.A., Eleady-Cole, R., Bennett, L.J., and Kusumi, F.: Divergent effects of antihypertensive therapy on cardiovascular responses and left ventricular function during upright exercise. Am. J. Cardiol., 30:768, 1972.
13. Bruce, R.A., Fischer, L.D., Cooper, M.N., and Gey, G.O.: Separation of effects of cardiovascular disease and age on ventricular function with maximal exercise. Am. J. Cardiol., 34:757, 1974.
14. Clement, D.L. (ed.): Blood Pressure Variability. Lancaster, MTP Press Ltd., 1979.
15. Conradson, T.-B., Stenberg, J., and Sannerstedt, R.: Influence of β-adrenergic blocking agents on submaximal and maximal physical working capacity in healthy subjects. Eur. J. Clin. Invest., 4:370, 1974 (Abstract).
16. Daniels, A.R., and Opie, L.H.: Atenolol plus nifedipine for mild to moderate systemic hypertension after fixed doses of either agent alone. Am. J. Cardiol., 57:965, 1986.
17. Davies, S.F., et al.: Comparative effects of transdermal clonidine and oral atenolol on acute exercise performance and response to aerobic conditioning in subjects with hypertension. Arch. Intern. Med., 149:1551, 1989.
18. Fariello, R., et al.: Effect of enalapril at rest and during isometric and dynamic exercise in essential hypertensive patients. J. Int. Med. Res., 17:76, 1989.
19. Fariello, R., et al.: Calcium entry blockade, autonomic activity and exercise performance in essential hypertensive patients. Clin. Exp. Hypertension. [A], 11(Suppl. 1):427, 1989.
20. Franciosa, J.A., Johnson, S.M., and Tobian, L.J.: Exercise performance in mildly hypertensive patients. Impairment by propranolol but not oxprenolol. Chest, 78:291, 1980.
21. Franz, I.-W., Tönnesmann, U., Behr, U., and Ketelhut, R.: Regression der Linksherzhypertrophie

Hochdruckkranker durch antihypertensive Therapie. Z. Kardiol., *78*(Suppl. 5):43, 1989.

22. Garavaglia, G.E., Messerli, F.H., Schmieder, R.E., and Nunez, B.D.: Antihypertensive therapy and cardiovascular reactivity during isometric stress. J. Hum. Hypertension, *2*:247, 1988.

23. Gillin, A.G., et al.: Comparison of doxazosin and atenolol in mild hypertension, and effects on exercise capacity, hemodynamics and left ventricular function. Am. J. Cardiol., *63*:950, 1989.

24. Gleichmann, U.M., et al.: Group exercise improves patient compliance in mild to moderate hypertension. J. Hypertension, *7*(Suppl. 3):S77, 1989.

25. Houston, M.C.: New insights and new approaches for the treatment of essential hypertension: selection of therapy based on coronary heart disease risk factor analysis, hemodynamic profiles, quality of life, and subsets of hypertension. Am. Heart J., *117*:911, 1989.

26. Jennings, G.L., et al.: Exercise, cardiovascular disease and blood pressure. Clin. Exp. Hypertens. [A], *11*:1035, 1989.

27. Julius, S., et al.: Borderline hypertension. Acta Med. Scand., *208*:481, 1980.

28. Karlefors, T., Nilsén, R., and Westling, H.: On the accuracy of indirect auscultatory blood pressure measurements during exercise. Acta Med. Scand., *180*(Suppl. 449):81, 1966.

29. Kästner, C., Zott, H.-J., and Wallrabe, D.: Einwirkungen von Propranolol auf die zentrale Hämodynamik bei Hypertonikern. Z. Gesamte Inn. Med., *44*:442, 1989.

30. Keul, J., Lehmann, M., and Dickhuth, H.-H.: Hypertonie, Herz und körperliche Aktivität (Sport). Z. Kardiol., *78*(Suppl. 7):199, 1989.

31. Kinoshita, A., et al.: What types of hypertensives respond better to mild exercise therapy? J. Hypertension, *6*(Suppl. 4):S631, 1988.

32. Klaus, D.: Management of hypertension in actively exercising patients. Implications for drug selection. Drugs, *37*:212, 1989.

33. Lee, W.R., Fox, L.M., and Slotkoff, L.M.: Effects of antihypertensive therapy on cardiovascular response to exercise. Am. J. Cardiol., *44*:325, 1979.

34. Lehmann, M., Dürr, H., Merkelbach, H., and Schmid, A.: Hypertension and sports activities: institutional experience. Clin. Cardiol., *13*:197, 1990.

35. Lund-Johansen, P.: Hemodynamics in early essential hypertension. Acta Med. Scand., *183*(Suppl. 482):1, 1968.

36. Lund-Johansen, P.: Hemodynamics in hypertension at rest and during exercise. J. Cardiovasc. Pharmacol., *10*(Suppl. 11):S1, 1987.

37. Lund-Johansen, P.: Age hemodynamics and exercise in essential hypertension: difference between β-blockers and dihydropyridine calcium antagonists. J. Cardiovasc. Pharmacol., *14*(Suppl. 10):S7, 1989.

38. Martin, N.B., et al.: Comparison of the effects of pindolol and propranolol on exercise performance in young men with systemic hypertension. Am. J. Cardiol., *64*:343, 1989.

39. Messerli, F.H., Kaesser, U.R., and Losem, C.J.: Effects of antihypertensive therapy on hypertensive heart disease. Circulation, *80*(Suppl. IV):-IV-145, 1989.

40. Motz, W., and Strauer, B.E.: Therapy of hypertensive hypertrophy. Scand. J. Clin. Lab. Invest., *49*(Suppl. 196):62, 1989.

41. Nudel, D.B., et al.: Exercise performance of hypertensive adolescents. Pediatrics, *65*:1073, 1980.

42. Nyberg, G., Vedin, A., and Wilhelmsson, C.: Heart rate and blood pressure response to isometric exercise after sublingual nitroglycerine in hypertensive male subjects: a controlled study of propranolol and labetalol for two weeks. Curr. Ther. Res, *25*:400, 1979.

43. Omvik, P., and Lund-Johansen, P.: Comparison of the hemodynamic effects of five calcium channel blockers at rest and during exercise in essential hypertension. Ann. Clin. Res., *20*(Suppl. 48):23, 1988.

44. Omvik, P., and Lund-Johansen, P.: Comparison of long-term hemodynamic effects at rest and during exercise of lisinopril plus sodium restriction versus hydrochlorothiazide in essential hypertension. Am. J. Cardiol., *65*:331, 1990.

45. Pearson, S.B., Banks, D.C., and Patrick, J.M.: The effect of β-adrenoceptor blockade on factors affecting exercise tolerance in normal man. Br. J. Clin. Pharmacol., *8*:143, 1979.

46. Pickering, G.: High Blood Pressure. London, J. & A. Churchill Ltd., 1968.

47. Priebe, U.: Physisches Training bei Hypertonie. Z. Ärztl. Fortbild., *83*:177, 1989.

48. Report of a WHO Expert Committee: Arterial hypertension. WHO Technical Report Series. No. 628. Geneva, Switzerland, 1978.

49. Rogers, G.G., Rosendorff, C., Goodman, C., and Radford, H.M.: Effects of angiotensin converting enzyme inhibition and β-blockade on exercise responses in hypertensive patients. J. Hypertens., *6*(Suppl. 4):S662, 1988.

50. Sannerstedt, R.: Hemodynamic response to exercise in patients with arterial hypertension. Acta Med. Scand, *180*(Suppl. 458):1, 1966.

51. Sannerstedt, R., Wasir, H., Henning, R., and Werkö, L.: Systemic haemodynamics in mild arterial hypertension before and after physical training. Clin. Sci. Mol. Med., *45*:145s, 1973.

52. Sannerstedt, R.: Rehabilitation in arterial hypertension. Adv. Cardiol., *24*:164, 1978.

53. Sannerstedt, R., and Julius, S.: Systemic haemodynamics in borderline arterial hypertension: responses to static exercise before and under the influence of propranolol. Cardiovasc. Res., *6*:398, 1972.

54. Schmieder, R.E., et al.: Efficacy of four antihypertensive drugs (clonidine, enalapril, nitrendipine, oxprenolol) on stress blood pressure. Am. J. Cardiol., *63*:1338, 1989.

55. Stenberg, J., et al.: Hemodynamic response to work with different muscle groups, sitting and supine. J. Appl. Physiol., *22*:61, 1967.

56. Turjanmaa, V.M.H., Kalli, S.T., and Uusitalo, A.J.: Blood pressure level changes caused by posture change and physical exercise: can they be determined accurately using a standard cuff method? J. Hypertens., *6*(Suppl. 4):S79, 1988.

57. WHO/ISH Subcommittee: 1989 Guidelines for the management of mild hypertension: memorandum from a WHO/ISH meeting. Bull. WHO, *67*:493, 1989.

58. Wiechmann, H.W.: Beeinflussung der Ruhe- und Belastungshämodynamik bei essentieller arterieller Hypertonie durch Antihypertensiva. Dtsch. Med. Wochenschr., *112*:1566, 1987.

59. Wijnen, J.A.G., et al.: Variations in exercise systolic blood pressure in physically active middle-aged men with normal and elevated blood pressure. Int. J. Sports Med., *9*:412, 1988.

60. Wollam, G.L, Gifford, R.W. Jr., and Tarazi, R.C.: Antihypertensive drugs: clinical pharmacology and therapeutic use. Drugs, *14*:420, 1977.

61. Wong, H.O., Kasser, I.S., and Bruce, R.A.: Impaired maximal exercise performance with hypertensive cardiovascular disease. Circulation, *39*:633, 1969.

62. Wu, S.C., et al.: Beta-blocker versus diuretic for control of the blood pressure response to stress in hypertensive patients. Eur. Heart J., *7*:885, 1986.

63. Yamauchi, K., et al.: Effects of enalapril on the cardiovascular response to treadmill exercise in patients with mild to moderate systemic hypertension. Clin. Ther., *11*:755, 1989.

17
CHAPTER

Children With Heart Disease

by
Gordon R. Cumming

CARDIAC ANOMALIES IN CHILDREN

Incidence

Congenital heart disease is present in about 5 per 1000 school age children; only 1 or 2 per 1000 have disease of any significance as far as sports participation is concerned by the time they reach school age.[42] Rheumatic heart disease is present in only 1 per 1000 school children in most North American communities, and in most instances valvular damage is mild. Cardiomyopathy, myocarditis, such hereditary syndromes as the Marfan syndrome, and other heart problems occur in less than 1 per 1000 school age children. A bicuspid aortic valve is found in 1% of children and is not an important lesion as far as exercise is concerned, as is the case for 99% of cases of mitral valve prolapse found in 1 to 10% of adolescents. Wolff-Parkinson-White (WPW) syndrome occurs in about 2 per 1000 children; 20 to 30% of these youths may have a history of rhythm disorder. Excluding post-cardiac surgery patients, significant rhythm disorder is present in less than 1 per 1000 children. Significant congenital coronary anomalies occur in only about 2 per 100,000 children. There is no place for the *routine* exercise testing of children, either as a means to detect heart disease or to assess the safety for exercise activities.

Heart Murmurs

Eighty percent of children aged 4 to 10 years have a heart murmur. In most of these children, the murmur is soft and clearly normal (innocent or functional). Some normal murmurs are sufficiently loud or there are possible additional auscultatory changes to lead the examiners to doubt whether the heart is normal. Significant organic heart disease in these patients can usually be excluded by an experienced examiner with auscultation and, when necessary, with supplemental information from chest roentgenography, electrocardiography, and echocardiography.

The child with a normal murmur is normal, and vigorous sports training is obviously permissible. The child with a "borderline" murmur either has a very mild heart defect or no defect at all; vigorous sports training should also be allowed. There are still occasional cases of sports programs in which children with normal murmurs are unnecessarily restricted because of hesitancy on the part of physicians to give complete clearance or because of anxieties and uncertainties created in parents.

Bergmann and Stamm reviewed a series of school children listed as having suspect congenital heart disease, and found significant abnormalities in only 18%.[6] Many of the children without disease were being unnecessarily restricted in physical education and sport. This restriction is simply bad medical care. Most children with definite mild heart defects can take part safely in intense sport training, so why impose any restrictions on the child who may or may not have a minor defect? Measurement of exercise capacity is of no value in deciding whether a heart murmur is normal, because children with mild or moderately severe heart defects may have above-average exercise capacities.

ECHOCARDIOGRAPHY

A major change has occurred in the evaluation of heart murmurs in the past 15 years. No longer is the advice of an experienced cardiologist considered good enough, and most patients end up being referred for ultrasound studies. Ultrasonography is a major advance in clinical cardiology in children, but there is a tendency to overdiagnosis, and often normal or trivial examination findings may seem important when the ultrasonographic report is taken verbatim. A proven example is the overdiagnosis of valve regurgitation by Doppler ultrasonography.

Up to 20% of normal children may show minimal degrees of regurgitation at one or all three of the pulmonary, mitral, and tricuspid valves. Less than 5% will have mild leakage at the aortic valve. When a child with an innocent murmur is referred for ultrasonography and the report returns "mitral regurgitation," it is important to remember that the heart can still be normal and that the regurgitation is physiologic; the murmur is not caused by the trivial normal valve leak.

Valve lesions that are important with regard to exercise participation usually produce heart chamber enlargement, loud and typical murmurs, and radiologic changes in cardiac contour.

CONGENITAL HEART DISEASE

Congenital heart lesions can be classified as those with left-to-right shunts (atrial septal defect (ASD), ventricular septal defect (VSD), patent ductus arteriosus); those with obstruction (aortic and pulmonary stenosis (AS and PS) and coarctation of aorta); and complex lesions (including tetralogy of Fallot and transposition of the great arteries). These eight defects constitute 85% of the pathologic findings in congenital heart disease. A discussion of these defects in relation to exercise pathophysiology follows.

Atrial Septal Defects

In most children with ASD, pulmonary artery pressures are normal, right ventricular pressures are normal or slightly elevated, and heart failure or other symptoms are rare. The defect may remain undetected during childhood. Some of these children are underweight, some have frequent respiratory tract infections, and most are asymptomatic and take part normally in sports and physical education activities. Most children with ASD are not receiving any medication.

Maximal treadmill exercise tests in these children reveal exercise capacities well within the normal range; some are above average, but only occasionally are treadmill endurance times in the top 10% of normal values. These children do not need to be restricted from competitive sport. There are no special precautions with maximal exercise testing, and they are not at risk for bacterial endocarditis.

Some children with ASD develop mitral valve prolapse and may have exercise-induced arrhythmias; this occurrence is less common in children than in adults. The primum type ASD is often associated with a cleft in the mitral valve, usually with relatively mild mitral regurgitation. Occasionally, the regurgitation is of moderate severity and these patients have symptoms of exercise limitation.

Surgery is currently recommended for patients with ASD when there is any cardiac enlargement or when the shunt flow exceeds 40% of pulmonary blood flow. Surgery is most commonly performed when the patient is between 5 and 10 years of age; most patients are asymptomatic at the time of surgery. Resumption of physical education is possible 6 weeks after surgery and intense sports participation may commence 3 months after surgery. With encouragement from the physician and the parents, children get back into full activities without the need for rehabilitation programs. Some teenage youths with ASD have been involved in serious athletic competition prior to discovery of the defect and can gradually resume their training activities within 4 to 6 weeks of surgery.

Intracardiac pressures are usually normal in patients with ASD, pulmonary blood flow is usually twice normal, and 50% of this flow is due to the shunt from the left to the right atrium across the defect. During exercise, this left-to-right shunt generally falls to 30% of pulmonary blood flow, and any right-to-left shunt remains very small so that arterial oxygen saturation remains normal.[3] In some older patients, and in patients living at altitudes above 1500 m, pulmonary artery pressures are increased at rest and with exercise. In one third of patient groups, left ventricular (LV) output during maximal exercise is subnormal and may remain so even 5 years after surgery.[21] Hemodynamics are more likely to be normal if the ASD is repaired before rather than after age 10 years.

Isolated Ventricular Septal Defects

The seriousness of an isolated VSD is dependent on its size. Small defects (3 mm or less in diameter) usually cause no serious problems. Defects get smaller, not larger, as the child ages. Small defects never require surgical repair, and at least 30% of them close spontaneously. Children with small defects can take part normally in competitive sport. They have normal exercise capacities and can have capacities well above average levels. There are no problems encountered with maximal exercise testing.

In patients with a small VSD, resting cardiac pressures are normal and blood crosses the septum from left to right. The shunt flow may vary from less than 1% to 30 or 40% of pulmonary blood flow, depending on the size of the hole. During light and moderate exercise, the shunt flow may remain at about the same amount as it was at rest, so that it becomes a smaller proportion of the total lung blood flow. With severe exercise, shunt flow may increase.[4,34] Pulmonary artery pressures remain normal or are only slightly increased during maximal exercise.

To prevent bacterial endocarditis, patients with a small VSD are advised to take antibiotics prior to those surgical procedures likely to cause bacteremia, and are advised to treat all bacterial infections with extra caution and respect.

A large VSD is one that is greater than one half of the diameter of the aorta. There is free transmission of LV pressure across the large hole to the right ventricle and pulmonary artery, so that systolic pressures (SBP) become equal in the ventricles and in the aorta and pulmonary artery. Surgical closure of these defects may be required in infancy because of persisting heart failure and failure to thrive. If a large defect is left untreated, pulmonary vascular resistance gradually increases because of medial (and subsequent intimal) thickening of the pulmonary arterioles and the volume of the left-to-right shunt decreases. A point is eventually reached between 2 to 12 years of age when the pulmonary arterioles are severely and irreversibly damaged and pulmonary vascular resistance exceeds systemic vascular resistance. The shunt changes, to right to left, carrying low oxygen, right ventricular (RV) blood across the defect into the LV and out through the aorta.

Patients with VSD and high pulmonary artery pressures should have their defects repaired when between the ages of 2 and 24 months. Occasional patients have multiple defects that are difficult to repair in infancy and corrective surgery may be delayed. For these patients, pulmonary artery banding is the palliative measure. The parents of the occasional child may not seek medical care until pulmonary vascular resistance is 85% of systemic resistance, when surgery is ill advised because of lung damage.

Patients who have had pulmonary hypertension because of VSD (or patent ductus arteriosus) and have had surgical closure of their ventricular defects may be left with residual damage to the lung arterioles. Pulmonary vascular resistance usually does not change with closure of the defect. Lung blood flow normally increases to three or four times the resting value during exercise, with an increase in pulmonary artery pressure of only 5 or 10 mm Hg. After surgical repair of the VSD, patients who have some residual pulmonary vascular disease may show pressure increases of 10 to 60 mm Hg above normal levels with exercise.[52,55] Arterial oxygen pressure (pO_2) may fall with exercise because of ventilation-perfusion inequalities, and exercise capacity may be below normal levels. Except in severe cases of residual pulmonary hypertension, normal recreational sports and physical education activities are permissible. These children usually know their limitations and do not wish to take up serious training in sports with a high aerobic component.

Exercise in patients with unoperated large VSD and approximately equal pulmonary and systemic vascular resistance causes an increase in the right-to-left shunt and in cyanosis.[55] Pulmonary artery and aortic SBP remain equal because of the large hole connecting the right and left sides of the heart, but the damaged lung arterioles cannot handle the exercise-induced increased venous return to the right ventricle. As a result, the right-to-left shunt increases, causing cyanosis. Exercise capacity becomes considerably limited when cyanosis occurs.

Some children have intermediate VSD between the very small and very large. Their pulmonary artery SBP is 40 to 60 mm Hg, the left-to-right shunts are 40 to 65% of pulmonary blood flow, pulmonary blood flow is 1.8 to 3.0 times greater than the systemic blood flow, and the shunt is entirely left to right. During exercise, the shunt flow usually does not change, whereas systemic and pulmonary blood flows increase in proportion to the exercise load. Pulmonary artery pressures increase slightly with exercise. Exercise capacity is either in the lower range of normal or just below normal. Surgery is indicated for these children, ideally by age 3 to 4 years, when it becomes obvious that spontaneous reduction in the size of the defect is not going to occur. Asymptomatic 5-year-old children with VSD, a pulmonary artery SBP value under 35 mm Hg, and left-to-right shunts less than 40% of pulmonary blood flow can be followed conservatively to see if the defect becomes smaller with time. These children have normal exercise capacities and can be allowed to take part in competitive sports. In most of these children, the defects gradually decrease in size and surgery is not necessary. After surgery for VSD, children may have arrhythmias, subtle ventricular dysfunction that may impair exercise function, and elevations in pulmonary artery SBP with exercise.[52]

Pulmonary Stenosis

Obstruction to RV outflow may occur in the outflow tract, at the pulmonary valve, or beyond the valve. Valvular pulmonary stenosis (PS) is the most common isolated lesion. At rest, there may be a peak pressure gradient of 5 to 10 mm Hg across the normal pulmonary valve; a larger gradient indicates PS. With severe obstruction, RV pressure may exceed 225 mg Hg, and pulmonary artery pressures are low at 15/7 mm Hg. Resting cardiac output ($\dot{Q}$) is usually normal in children with mild or moderate PS, whereas exercise $\dot{Q}$ is in the lower range of normal. Patients with mild stenosis (RV-SBP of 30 to 60 mm Hg) increase the RV-SBP by 20 to 40 mm Hg with exercise. Patients with moderate stenosis (RV-SBP of 60 to 90 mm Hg) often increase their RV pressures by as much as 100 mm Hg with exercise, with maximal recorded pressures of 225 to 250 mm Hg. Patients with long-standing severe stenosis have impaired RV function and decreased maximal $\dot{Q}$.[56,66]

Right ventricular end-diastolic pressure is increased when RV muscle mass is increased; there is a parallel, corresponding increase in the right atrial "a" wave. If the foramen ovale is patent, right atrial pressure may exceed that in the left atrium during atrial systole, and desaturated blood will go from the right to the left atrium, causing a varying degree of arterial oxygen desaturation. Arterial oxygen content will fall further during exercise as the right to left shunt increases, sometimes to a major degree. In most patients, the degree of desaturation is mild (with oxygen saturation remaining around 90%), but the right-to-left shunt is quite large in some patients and saturation can fall below 70% with exercise.

Intervention is recommended for patients with PS if RV pressure exceeds 80 mm Hg, whereas patients with lesser degrees of stenosis usually do not require surgical repair and may take part in all exercise activities. Although some individuals may not have the potential to achieve above-average aerobic fitness levels, all levels of sports participation should be allowed. Exercise testing is considered quite safe, even in patients with severe PS. Occasionally, exercise $\dot{Q}$ falls well below required levels and exercise hypotension, syncope, or both may occur.

Formerly, all patients requiring intervention had surgery. Today, nearly all can be adequately treated at the time of heart catheterization by expanding a balloon in the valve orifice, which splits the valve (balloon angioplasty).

Two or three years may be required before RV muscle mass decreases after ballooning or surgical correction of severe PS. There may be a secondary obstruction to RV outflow due to hypertrophied muscle that takes a few years to subside. Young PS patients are ordinarily back at school 2 to 4 weeks after surgery and within 2 days after ballooning. They can gradually resume physical education activities 6 weeks after surgery and full sports activities within 3 months. With ballooning, regular physical education is permissible within 1 week and, depending on the result, full sports participation is permissible in 1 month. If the surgery involved ventriculotomy, these times are delayed on an individual basis. Ideally, most children with significant PS have had surgery before they reach school age. There may still be some postoperative impairment in RV function that limits exercise performance.[13] Even so, these children can engage in intense sport training to reach their full potential.

Aortic Stenosis

Congenital aortic stenosis (AS) is of four types: valvar, subvalvar, supravalvar, and idiopathic hypertrophic subaortic stenosis (IHSS). The hemodynamics of the first three types are similar. There is a fixed obstruction to LV outflow, causing a high pressure in the ventricular cavity proximal to the obstruction and a slightly reduced pressure in the aorta.

The pressure drop across the obstruction is inversely proportional to the area of the narrow zone and is directly proportional to the square of the rate of blood flow during systole $(ml \cdot sec^{-1})$. In mild AS, peak LV pressure is 10 to 40 mm Hg above aortic SBP. This peak pressure gradient is 41 to 60 mm Hg in moderate stenosis and over 60 mm Hg in severe stenosis. The increased LV work causes hypertrophy without dilatation, so that the LV cavity becomes smaller. Valvular aortic stenosis tends to worsen with time, with fibrous thickening of the leaflets and subsequent calcification. Valves are replaced only as a last resort in children or young adults. Obstruction can be partially relieved surgically, but a thickened bicuspid valve cannot be transformed into a normal one. Although a subvalvular ridge can be removed, there frequently is some residual obstruction after surgery for subvalvar stenosis as well. Ideally, children with AS should have surgery before symptoms develop. The decision to operate is based on the pressure gradient across the valve, i.e., patients with peak gradients of 60 mm Hg or more are recommended for surgery, patients with peak gradients of 40 mm Hg or less are not, and patients with gradients of 40 to 60 mm Hg are considered possible surgical candidates on the basis of the anatomy of the obstruction, ECG and ultrasonographic changes, and possibly the exercise response.

During exercise, the LV peak SBP in children with AS increases by 20 to 120 mm Hg, whereas aortic SBP may not rise or may increase to a lesser extent than in normal children. Left ventricular end-diastolic pressure may be elevated at rest and may show a further increase with exercise. Resting and exercise Q̇ are usually in the lower range of normal.

Clinical exercise testing has been suggested as a means of assessing the severity of AS.[1,14] Failure of brachial artery pressure to increase by more than 15 mm Hg with exercise suggests a gradient of over 50 mm Hg, but false-positive results are common.

The electrocardiogram performed during exercise frequently shows ST depression in patients with AS.[12,33,60] A depression of over 0.2 mV with a downsloping segment is highly suggestive of a gradient of over 50 mm Hg, but there are false-positive and false-negative responses. Thus, clinical decisions should not be made entirely on the presence or absence of ST change. Kveselis et al. calculated the LV oxygen supply ratio and suggested that ST depression in AS patients is due to reduced myocardial oxygen supply.[45]

Most children with AS are asymptomatic, with symptoms first appearing with strenuous exercise. Angina occurs because coronary perfusion pressure is less than intramyocardial pressure, while myocardial demands are increased because of increased work and myocardial mass. Lightheadedness or syncope on exertion occurs because of low cerebral blood flow from a restricted exercise output or because of cardiac slowing. Sudden unexpected death may occur on exertion either because of cardiac standstill or ventricular fibrillation. It is this latter possibility, even though uncommon, that makes AS a dangerous lesion and makes one overly cautious in allowing these children to participate in competitive sport.

Patients with clinically mild AS and a negative exercise ECG can be allowed unrestricted sports activities. If the stenosis is moderate, regular physical education is permitted with unrestricted sports activity up until age 11 years; after that age, intramural and recreational sports are allowed. Regardless of the exercise ECG pattern, serious sports training seems unwise in the teen years. If the peak gradient is over 40 mm Hg, intense running or

other aerobic activities are best avoided, especially if ST changes are present in the exercise ECG. If the peak gradient is over 60 mm Hg, surgery is usually recommended and exercise activity should be curtailed.

Surgery often leads to some degree of aortic insufficiency. If the preoperative resting gradient was 80 mm Hg, a postoperative gradient of 25 mm Hg and a regurgitant fraction of 15% is commonly encountered. Postoperatively, the exercise peak gradient may still be over 60 mm Hg, and the exercise ECG often shows 0.2 to 0.4 mV ST depression. These patients are advised to take part in recreational sports activities but to avoid competitive activities with high cardiac demands. It must be emphasized that surgery in these patients is only palliative; close medical supervision is required and valve replacement may be necessary between 1 and 15 years after the initial surgery.

Some patients cannot be helped surgically because of the severity of their valve lesion and a small aortic root; most exercise activities need to be curtailed for these patients.

Idiopathic hypertrophic subaortic stenosis (IHSS) is part of a diffuse myocardial disease with asymmetric hypertrophy of the ventricular septum causing obstruction to aortic outflow. The condition may be very mild or very severe in childhood. Sudden death occurs more often in the severe cases, but occasionally occurs when the disease seems relatively mild. Exercise testing can be performed safely in these patients, but has no value in diagnosis or prognosis. Exercise capacities can be average or even above average when the disease is mild, but intense sports participation is considered unwise. Because there is a strong hereditary factor, all members of a family should be screened by ECG and echocardiography to detect occult cases.

IHSS is one of the common conditions found at autopsy in a series of unexpected sudden death occurring during sports activities. Therefore, it is generally recommended that these patients should engage only in recreational activities.

Coarctation of the Aorta

The main clinical features of coarctation of the aorta are elevated arm blood pressure with brisk brachial and radial pulses, and low leg pressure with diminished or absent femoral and pedal pulses. At age 6 years, arm blood pressure may be borderline at 115/75 or as high as 225/110 mm Hg. Blood pressures that are borderline at age 6 years tend to increase with age, and most patients have a resting SBP of 180 mm Hg by age 20 years.

It has been known for some time that exercise leads to a marked elevation of arm SBP in patients with coarctation. A child with a SBP at rest of 140 mm Hg may have a SBP during exercise as high as 250 or 270 mm Hg; in adults, SBP may be pushed over 300 mm Hg by exercise but most laboratories stop exercise tests when pressure exceeds 250 mm Hg. The main cause of the elevated blood pressure at rest is the mechanical factor of the aortic narrowing, but additional humoral and neurogenic factors seem to be operative in some patients.

Resting leg blood flow is normal in patients with coarctation, but is below normal during exercise. To compensate for this deficiency, leg muscles extract more oxygen from the blood and the pO_2 of femoral vein blood is reduced to less than 10 torr during exercise. Some patients experience easy leg fatigue during exercise, but many (the majority are boys) have an athletic build with a large chest, broad shoulders, narrow hips, and a subtle decrease in leg development.

The marked elevation of upper body blood pressure in the young coarctation patient is potentially dangerous. Some patients develop small aneurysms of the arteries in the circle of Willis, such that marked exercise-induced hypertension may rupture one of these aneurysms and produce a fatal cerebral hemorrhage, even before the age of 10 years.

Exercise testing is of clinical value for the evaluation of coarctation patients before and after surgery. For example, the blood pressure response to exercise may help to decide the timing of surgery. After surgery, the exercise blood pressure response may provide information as to the need for postoperative angiography or possible reoperation, and regarding sport participation.

In coarctation patients, resting blood pressure should be measured in both arms; the side with the higher value should be used to follow pressure during exercise. Blood pressure in the leg can be measured at rest and immediately after exercise with either a large thigh cuff and auscultation over the popliteal fossa or a cuff on the calf and Doppler recording of the posterior tibial blood flow. If blood pressure readings are to be compared in the arm and leg, it is best to have the patient supine immediately post-exercise and have two observers measure arm and leg pressures simultaneously.

The left subclavian artery may be involved in the coarctation and, occasionally, this artery will be involved in the repair of the coarctation. As a result, left arm pressure values may not accurately reflect upper body blood pressure. Occasionally, the right subclavian artery arises below the aortic narrowing, so that neither arm accurately reflects upper body blood pressure; diagnosis may then be difficult. The normal differences between the brachial artery and central aortic pressure curves are accentuated in coarctation, especially during exercise. Brachial artery SBP may be 25 mm Hg above aortic SBP at rest, with a difference of 50 mm Hg during exercise.

The exact significance of the exercise arm-to-leg pressure difference after coarctation surgery is uncertain. Hansen monitored intra-arterial pressures during submaximal and maximal exercise in 19 male subjects several years after coarctation surgery, and reported the following SBP values (mm Hg): arm 159, leg 133 at rest; arm 207, leg 131 at 100 W exercise and arm 219, leg 141 at maximal exercise of 150 to 250 W, a difference of 78 mm Hg.[18] Corresponding mean pressures, however, were: arm 99, leg 96 at rest; arm 109, leg 99 at 100 W; and arm 123, leg 101 mm Hg at maximal work. The difference in mean pressures was only 22 mm Hg, with most of the difference noted only in systole; this finding may be due more to reduced aortic compliance at the anastomosis and a distortion of the peripheral pressure waves rather than to any residual narrowing that should be repaired. Hansen found no correlation between SBP or gradients and the aortic diameter at the anastomosis.[31] In contrast, Markel et al. found that an arm to leg pressure difference greater than 35 mm Hg was helpful in recognizing patients with significant residual aortic narrowing only if the resting gradient was at least 15 mm Hg.[51] When the resting gradient was less than 15 mm Hg, a high exercise systolic pressure and a high arm:leg gradient did not signify aortic narrowing. Leg exercise was superior to arm exercise in unmasking residual coarctation. Zellers and Driscoll surveyed the current thinking of the value of exercise blood pressure measurements in deciding whether to intervene in patients with prior repair of coarctation.[74] They presented the case of a 10-year-old-boy with a resting gradient of 15 mm Hg, and an exercise systolic pressure of 200 mm Hg. If the exercise gradient was 60 mm Hg, 60% of the experts favored intervention. If the exercise systolic pressure reached 280 mm Hg, 94% favored intervention. Intervention in these patients can consist of balloon angioplasty, repeat direct operation on the aortic anastomosis, or a bypass graft from the left subclavian artery to the aorta distal to the coarctation. Exercise tests may help to decide the type of operation that is best for coarctation: end-to-end anastomosis, patch grafting, or subclavian arterioplasty. In one series, arm-to-leg SBP difference was 32 mm Hg for those with end-to-end anastomoses and only 10 mm Hg for those with patch grafts.[65]

Should there be a cut-off point determined for blood pressure values at which exercise is terminated in patients with coarctation of the aorta? Because directors of exercise laboratories obviously do not want to cause a subarachnoid hemorrhage, it seems prudent to halt exercise tests when SBP is about 240 mm Hg. We have allowed a few asymptomatic patients to exercise with a SBP over 250 mm Hg.

Should there be an exercise pressure level that dictates abstinence from sports in children? There is no scientific information on which to draw to answer this question. Before surgery, we do not restrict children with resting pressures below 140/90 mm Hg and exercise pressures below 180/100 mm Hg. After surgery, which usually takes place before the age of 10 years, normal physical education and recreational sports activities can be allowed in patients with pressures less than 140/90 mm Hg at rest and exercise pressures under 220/100 mm Hg. The tendency today is for earlier surgery, that is, by 4 years in asymptomatic patients and in infancy in symptomatic patients. Youths with exercise pressures over 220/100 mm Hg should be discouraged from strenuous athletic training. Patients with persistent elevation of resting and exercise SBP after surgery to correct coarctation can be treated with one or more drugs, such as beta blockers and diuretics or angiotensin-converting enzyme inhibitors, with good reduction in exercise blood pressure.

For example, Cotton et al. gave beta blockers to 10 patients (mean age 18 years) who had resting arm to leg gradients of less than 15 mm Hg, but exercise arm pressures over 220 mm Hg.[13] Mean exercise systolic blood pressure fell from 229 to 196 mm Hg, and the gradient dropped from 84 to 51 mm Hg without altering peak exercise time. It is important to have at least yearly postoperative blood pressure follow-up for all coarctation patients, and to have yearly exercise pressures for patients taking part in vigorous physical activity.

EXERCISE ECG IN COARCTATION. Ischemic-type downsloping ST depression often occurs in the exercise ECG of coarctation patients, both before and after surgery. This change has no bearing on how the exercise test is conducted, even when the ST depression exceeds 0.3 or 0.4 mV. The significance of this change is uncertain, as it may be the nonspecific response of a hypertrophied myocardium. In young adults, this finding may be a manifestation of early coronary disease.

Cyanotic Congenital Heart Disease

The "blue baby" is one of the more dramatic presentations of heart disease. Fortunately, many of these patients can have corrective surgery so that they are normal or nearly normal by the time they reach school age, and thus will have no special requirements for physical education. Some children do not have a favorable lesion and corrective surgery is not possible. Such surgery can involve the use of prosthetic conduits or valves and is best postponed until growth is nearly complete. These children do have cyanosis and moderate to marked limitation of exercise capacity.

Some patients with arterial oxygen saturation of 75 to 90% are not cyanotic at rest, but intense cyanosis may develop with exercise if these patients are willing to push themselves to the point of severe symptoms. They may stop exercising on the treadmill because of severe dyspnea or air hunger, but they often stop because of general or local fatigue. Severe headache commonly occurs at the point of severe fatigue or shortly after exercise ceases, and an unpleasant weak or sick feeling may occur. Cyanotic patients uncommonly develop anginal pain during maximal exercise.

Left on their own, young children with cyanotic heart disease perform many physical activities during the day that bring on cyanosis and dyspnea, after which they rest a few minutes and begin again. The appearance of severe cyanosis (especially when the cyanosis occurs with marked air hunger, pinched facial expression, or a greyish pallor) can be rather alarming to the inexperienced observer. In the last 20 years, we have routinely had children with cyanotic heart disease exercise to the point of severe fatigue, and there have been no adverse reactions. Recovery from the dyspnea occurs within 5 minutes, but headache and weakness may last for 30 minutes or more if the subject makes a near-maximal effort.

Arterial oxygen saturation can be monitored during exercise with an ear oximeter, pulse oximeter, with a transcutaneous pO_2 electrode, or with blood from the warmed fingertip, earlobe, or indwelling arterial catheter. Although the exercise end point varies from patient to patient, the lower the oxygen saturation at rest, the lower generally is the saturation when the patient stops exercise. In addition, the dominant factors are patient motivation and the tenacity and experience of the exercise technologist. Patients with blood oxygen saturation of over 80% at rest usually stop exercise at saturations of about 60%. Those individuals with resting saturations of 60 to 70% stop exercise at saturations of 45 to 50%, whereas those with resting saturations of 50% stop exercise at saturations of 25 to 35%. On the other hand, Motram and colleagues found no correlation between resting oxygen saturation and saturation during exercise.[57] Some patients will drive themselves until arterial oxygen saturations fall as low as 20 to 25% (arterial pO_2 = 20 mm Hg).

In cyanotic patients, the exercise pO_2 of femoral vein blood rapidly falls to 10 mm Hg early in exercise and is less than 6 mm Hg when symptoms of fatigue begin. At these levels, it can be presumed that tissue oxygen pressure is below the critical value established in animal experiments for normal muscle function. The fatigue these patients experience seems to be due to lack of oxygen in the exercising muscles, even though there may be a considerable amount of oxygen remaining in the arterial blood coming into the muscles.

Because of muscle hypoxia, one would think that lactate would be formed in great quantity by the exercising muscles in these patients. Surprisingly, lactate values determined 2 minutes after cessation of exercise may be only 4 to 6 mmol·L^{-1}, whereas values of 8 to 12 mmol·L^{-1} are reached by children with non-cyanotic heart disease. There is the possibility that lactate is not as readily released by the exercising muscles of these patients, because high muscle lactate levels have been reported.[7]

MECHANISM OF THE EXERCISE INCREASE IN CYANOSIS. In patients with tetralogy of Fallot (large VSD plus infundibular PS), the magnitude of the right-to-left shunt is dependent on the resistance to blood flow through the narrow RV outflow tract compared to that out the aorta and through the systemic resistance vessels. Total peripheral resistance declines during exercise because of vasodilation of muscle blood vessels. Tachycardia and catecholamine release increase the unfunctional narrowing of the RV outflow tract, making it more difficult for blood to go to the lungs. Both the decrease in systemic resistance and the increase in RV outflow obstruction act together to increase the amount of RV blood that goes through the VSD and out the aorta. Given that the blood returning to the right atrium and RV from the exercising muscles is almost totally depleted of oxygen and that the volume of this blood is increased, it is obvious that the arterial blood oxygen content will fall quite dramatically during exercise in these patients.

SQUATTING. Young patients with tetralogy of Fallot instinctively learn to squat, getting into a flat-footed baseball catcher's stance when they are fatigued. This posture increases the tension in the leg muscles, reduces blood flow to the leg muscles, raises peripheral resistance and blood pressure, and decreases the right-to-left shunt. Post-exercise heart rate falls more rapidly with squatting, and the time required for arterial blood oxygen saturation to return to pre-exercise values is shortened when the squatting position is assumed.

EXERCISE TESTING FOR THE CYANOTIC PATIENT. The objectives of an exercise test are the same as for other patients, i.e., to assess exercise capacity, to observe whether any arrhythmias develop, to follow the patient's progress objectively with regard to exercise capability, and to show some patients and parents that a certain amount of activity is possible. The exercise test usually reveals that the patient is more limited than expected on the basis of the exercise history provided by the parents or by the older child. The apparent reason for this greater degree of limitation is that exercise activities of children are usually intermittent and the frequent rest pauses allow sufficient recovery. The exercise test, however, involves continuous activity and many children with cyanotic heart disease have $\dot{V}_{O_2max}$ values below 15 ml·kg^{-1}·min^{-1}. Thus, the initial exercise load should be as low as 2 METs.

The exercise ECG in the cyanotic patient may show alarming degrees of ST depression. We do not consider this change to be an indication to stop exercise. Some patients with cyanotic heart disease have no ST-segment change with exercise, and the significance of any change is uncertain. Many patients with cyanotic heart disease have peaked P waves measuring 0.3 to 0.6 mV, due to right atrial overload. These P waves increase in amplitude during exercise (reaching a level as high as 1.2 mV). These tall P waves may be mistaken by the inexperienced observer as bizarre QRS complexes or may be identified as an R wave by the on-line minicomputers connected to many exercise ECG systems.

After surgery, patients with cyanotic heart disease seldom have completely normal hearts when detailed physiologic studies are done at rest and especially with exercise. Despite major changes in ventricular function, the majority of patients are asymptomatic, can perform exercise tests quite well, and can take part in recreational sports without any problem. For example, patients with transposition of the great arteries after the Mustard or Rastelli operations frequently show definite abnormalities of both RV and LV function when evaluated with radionuclide angiography.[59] Patients after the Fontan operation for tricuspid atresia or single ventricle fail to increase their LV ejection fraction during exercise.[68] Maximal cardiac index during exercise is often less than 60% of average normal levels, and submaximal exercise is compensated for by greater oxygen extraction in the working muscles.

EXERCISE TESTING OF CHILDREN WITH DISORDERS OF CARDIAC RHYTHM

Exercise testing can be used to evaluate the heart's response to physical activity in patients with known rhythm disorders and to bring out occult arrhythmias in patients in whom there is a high frequency of rhythm disturbance. Exercise testing is also used to assist in the diagnosis of arrhythmia in patients with intermittent symptoms of palpitation, syncope, and light-headedness, and to assess the safety of sport for patients with known or potential rhythm disorders.

Exercise testing and ambulatory ECG monitoring (Holter) complement one another. The exercise test gives an instant answer and provides information on near-maximal or maximal exercise. The Holter provides a higher yield of rhythm changes because the duration of monitoring is 24 hours, during which sleep and activities of daily living are monitored, even though a period of intense physical activity is often not included.

Congenital Heart Block

Congenital blockage of atrial impulse transmission to the ventricles most often occurs in children whose hearts are otherwise normal. Although in most patients the ventricles are paced from the low atrio-ventricular (A-V) node or HIS bundle, the pacing site can be lower in one of the main HIS branches or down in the ventricles. In infancy, ventricular rate is about 80 beats·min^{-1} at rest, gradually slowing to 30 to 40 beats·min^{-1} by age 16 to 20 years. Resting $\dot{Q}$ is normal; stroke volume (SV) is about twice that of normal and compensates for the slow rate. With maximal exercise, most of these patients can increase their heart rate (HR) to 80 to 120 beats·min^{-1} and maximal $\dot{Q}$ is in the low normal range of 8 to 10 L·min^{-1}·m^{-2}, as is $\dot{V}_{O_2max}$ and treadmill endurance time.[35] Although asymptomatic, about 10% of these children have symptoms from the slow rate and eventually need demand pacemakers. The exercise response does not necessarily predict which patients will need pacing, as the symptoms often appear at rest and not with exercise.[41] Results of more recent radionuclide studies suggest that LV ejection fraction may not increase normally with exercise in patients with congenital heart block.[30]

Some children develop bigeminal rhythm with exercise or other patterns of ventricular ectopy.[71] They have a subnormal exercise $\dot{Q}$ and cannot keep up with their peers. This development may predate the need for pacing and is one of the uses of exercise testing.

When children receive a pacemaker set at 80 to 90 beats·min^{-1} and are able to achieve this HR on their own with exercise, their exercise capacity is not improved. If HR is limited to 50 to 60 beats·min^{-1} and pacing increases it to 90 beats·min^{-1}, exercise performance is then improved. Ideally, these patients should have sequential atrioventricular pacing.

Children with congenital A-V block have large hearts well suited to maintaining $\dot{Q}$ with a large SV. When heart block is acquired (the most common cause is surgical injury to the conduction system), this adaptation has not taken place and pacing is usually necessary. Exercise HR will be the same as the resting pacing rate (generally 70 to 90 beats·min^{-1}) and exercise $\dot{Q}$ is impaired. If these children remain active and try to improve themselves by exercise training to the point of fatigue and dyspnea, they usually have exercise capacities in the low normal range. Experience with the newer dual chamber pacing units in children is most encouraging, for when the atrial impulse can be delivered to the ventricles and both atrial and ventricular rates increase with exercise, exercise performance is enhanced.

Exercise Response in Children with Other Arrhythmias at Rest

Patients with 2:1 or partial A-V block often increase the level of block with exercise (e.g., to 4:1) and have reduced exercise tolerance. Children with atrial flutter and a 4:1 block (ventricular rate about 75) increase their rates suddenly to 2:1 (rate

150), and occasionally 1:1 conduction occurs with rates of 260 to 300. In patients with structurally normal hearts, this occurrence is surprisingly well tolerated for 5 to 10 minutes while exercise continues.

Children with atrial fibrillation respond to exercise in the same manner as do adults (i.e., HR increases in a chaotic way at low exercise loads), but the exercise tolerance is mostly dependent on the underlying pathologic process. Digoxin does not adequately control the exercise HR, but low doses of beta blocker or Verapamil may be effective.

Ventricular Extrasystoles

Ryujin et al. performed exercise tests on 196 children with ventricular ectopy on their resting ECG.[64] The degree of ectopy increased in 29 patients, and the test was considered useful in recognizing those with potentially serious rhythm disturbances. If PVCs are suppressed by exercise and the heart is clinically normal, no further assessment is required. Although it is possible to assess this in the medical office with running on the spot or other similar exercise, the suppression of PVCs by this submaximal exercise may be misleading. A few children may have suppression of PVCs by light exercise, only to develop ventricular tachycardia with more severe exercise. In a 7-year follow-up study, Jacobsen et al. found that in 17 patients with rest PVCs and with suppression on exercise, 8 patients continued to have rest PVCs; this arrhythmia was suppressed again by repeat exercise testing.[36]

More than 90% of patients with frequent ventricular ectopic beats at rest have their arrhythmia cease during exercise. In most patients, this cessation will occur during the initial states of the test; in others, near maximal exercise is required. There is usually no contraindication to exercise testing or sports in these patients.

Supraventricular Tachycardia (PAT)

This is sometimes brought out by exercise testing, allowing a firm diagnosis. In one center, PAT occurred in about 1 per 100 exercise tests.[8]

Exercise in patients with a WPW ECG pattern may lead to supraventricular tachycardia, the delta wave may disappear during exercise,[9] or there may be partial normalization of QRS but some retention of the delta wave.

Patients with disappearance of pre-excitation during exercise can be expected to have a long effective refractory period in the accessory pathway and be at low risk for serious arrhythmias.

Ventricular Tachycardia (VT)

Fulton et al. performed exercise tests on 26 children with VT.[25] Seven had VT at rest, and sinus rhythm was restored with exercise. Rocchini and co-workers performed exercise tests on 21 children with VT.[63] Patients with symptoms showed increased severity of the arrhythmia on exercise. In those who were asymptomatic, exercise decreased the severity of the arrhythmia.

Ventricular tachycardia secondary to arrhythmogenic right-ventricular dysplasia will frequently develop arrhythmia during exercise testing.[32]

There is a condition termed "benign" VT, associated with a HR of 150 to 180 beats·min^{-1}. If this rhythm is present at rest, reversion to sinus rhythm occurs as soon as the exercise HR exceeds the ectopic rate, and exercise performance will be normal.

In most children with resting atrial or ventricular ectopic arrhythmias, exercise restores sinus rhythm, but the arrhythmia reappears (often to an accentuated degree) within 1 or 2 minutes of stopping exercise.

Rhythm Disorders Precipitated by Exercise When No Arrhythmia is Present at Rest

A common rhythm disorder in children is paroxysmal supraventricular tachycardia (PAT), which is often due to accessory atrioventricular conduction pathways, with or without W-P-W patterns in the resting prearrhythmia ECG. Exercise may bring out the W-P-W pattern when it is not present at rest, and be of diagnostic value. Exercise often causes partial or total normalization of QRS, and Bricker et al. have suggested that these children do not require further electrophysiologic study.[6] Exercise may also precipitate PAT and be of diagnostic value.

Exercise-induced ventricular extrasystoles (VES) or VT occur infrequently in children without evidence of structural heart disease. Exercise-induced VES has been known to occur after ventricular incisions have been made, e.g., after surgery to correct VSD or tetralogy. The significance and need for treatment of exercise-induced VES is uncertain. Sudden death occurs in patients who have undergone operative repair of tetralogy, even 5, 10, or 20 years after surgery. Most of these deaths have occurred in individuals with obvious RV dysfunction, or in those with resting ventricular arrhythmias. Exercise testing may be of value in determining subjects that are at risk for life-threatening arrhythmia, and in evaluating the efficacy of anti-arrhythmic therapy.

Exercise testing may lead to the recognition of children who have problems in sinus node function or the conduction systems, but it is not nearly as sensitive as electrophysiologic testing in recognizing abnormal sinus node function.[10]

SUDDEN DEATH

During Exercise in Patients Under Age 20 Years

Lambert et al. enlisted the cooperation of personnel from 20 major cardiac centers in North America, Europe, and Israel, and collected 254 cases of patients 1 to 21 years of age who died suddenly and unexpectedly while out of the hospital.[47] In the 186 patients who had never had cardiac surgery, various types of myocardial disease accounted for 29% of the sudden deaths. Other causes included AS (18%), Eisenmenger's syndrome (15%), cyanotic heart disease with PS (10%), Ebstein's disease (6%), congenital heart block (4%), and primary pulmonary hypertension (2%). Only one patient had rheumatic heart disease. Fifty-eight per-

cent of the deaths occurred during sleep or with the patient at rest, 32% occurred during leisure play activity, and only 10% occurred during sport. One half of the group of patients who died during or shortly after sports activity had severe AS or obstructive cardiomyopathy.

Patients with severe AS, obstructive cardiomyopathy, or other forms of myocardial disease may enjoy fairly good health and may not have any symptoms that they consider significant. As a consequence, they may place their lives in jeopardy with vigorous exercise activities. Patients with cyanotic heart disease or pulmonary hypertension have obvious symptoms with exercise and seldom enter into structured competitive sport situations. Results of this study by Lambert et al. indicate that exercise activities (including competitive sports) constitute little or no risk for young patients with mild and moderate congenital heart disease or for patients with rheumatic heart disease.

After Surgery for Congenital Heart Disease

Unfortunately, sudden death occurs even 5 and 10 years after apparently successful surgery for congenital heart disease. Patients who had large VSDs, tetralogy of Fallot, transposition of the great arteries, or such complex anomalies as double-outflow RV or single ventricle are at particular risk. Most patients have resting evidence of cardiac strain including enlargement, failure, gallop rhythm, resting conduction disturbances or ventricular ectopic beats, pulmonary hypertension, and history of A-V block in the postoperative period. By showing runs of ventricular tachycardia or ectopies, it has been suggested that exercise tests may be useful for detecting those individuals at high risk.[27,28,38,40,70,72] Whether exercise really adds anything to what can be determined from resting or ambulatory ECG studies is unproven, however. A real dilemma exists in knowing 1) whether to initiate anti-arrhythmic drug therapy and if so, what agents and for how long; and 2) whether the treatment is achieving anything.

EXERCISE TESTING

Test Protocols

I have found the Bruce treadmill test so satisfactory for children 4 to 16 years of age that I would not advocate any other protocol for routine clinical testing. For maximal tests, treadmill speed should reach levels that require the child to run. In children, Balke-type walking protocols give lower maximal values of HR and $\dot{V}_{O_2}$. For children with severe disease, 1.7 mph at 0% grade and 1.7 mph at 5% grade become the initial stages of the Bruce protocol, allowing observation of even the severely impaired child for 7 to 8 minutes of exercise.

Bicycle exercise is not entirely suitable for maximal performance tests in children under age 9 years, but it is ideal for special studies of blood pressure, $\dot{Q}$ with the use of a rebreathing technique, and special hemodynamic measurements during which the reproducible calibrated power outputs and lack of motion can be used to advantage. The bicycle power outputs should likely be based on body weight (not height or surface area) and small increments in work loads are required in young children. Loads should be about 3 minutes in duration to avoid fatigue and be incremented by 0.5 to 1.0 $W \cdot kg^{-1}$.

The maximal HR of normal children ranges from 185 to 238 beats$\cdot$min^{-1}. As a result, submaximal tests based on HR are difficult to interpret. Tests to establish PWC_{170} (i.e., the power output at a HR of 170 beats$\cdot$min^{-1}) cannot be used to compare different subjects, but can be used to follow the progress of the same individual. Most exercise tests should be continued until the point of severe fatigue or until symptoms or untoward signs develop.

ECG Criteria to Indicate When to Stop an Exercise Test

Fortunately, there are no reported instances of ventricular fibrillation, myocardial infarction, or death occurring in a pe-

diatric exercise facility. Although we have never stopped a pediatric patient because of ST-segment depression and do not think it is necessary, other investigators think otherwise. If the child looks and feels well, other ECG changes occurring with exercise are only relative indications to stop. Ventricular tachycardia develops in a few children with light to moderate exercise, but if the rate is under 180 beats$\cdot$min^{-1}, we have recommended the well child continue exercise, and the rhythm often reverts to a sinus pattern at high power outputs; the same principle is true for multifocal, frequent ventricular extrasystoles. Although these rhythm disturbances would be an indication to stop exercise in a patient with cardiomyopathy or AS, it is not necessarily the case in the child with a structurally normal heart or with mild congenital disease. Many of these seemingly ominous ventricular arrhythmias occur after the child has already stopped exercise, during the first few minutes of recovery.

Exercise ECG Patterns

Just as in adults, there is controversy over which ECG leads to use to monitor and record information in children with heart disease. For routine exercise testing, I have used only lead CM-5, and have thought it useful to have a 13-lead or Frank vector exercise ECG in only a few special situations. Other researchers will argue the need to monitor right precordial leads in patients with RV overload. Because we pay no attention to ST changes in these patients, however, these precordial leads are usually superfluous for diagnosis or monitoring. For the detection of arrhythmias, it is advantageous to have at least two simultaneous leads. In adult patients undergoing coronary arteriography for atypical chest pain, Chaitman et al. found that lead CM-5 performed better than any or all of 14 other leads in terms of specificity, sensitivity, and accuracy for predicting the presence or absence of significant coronary disease; CM-5 was found to be sufficient to assess ischemia from congenital coronary anomalies.[11]

ST changes in lead CM-5 are not common in normal children. About 3% of teenage girls have 0.2 mV or more horizontal depression of ST persisting 0.08 sec after the peak of the R wave. Such changes occur in less than 1% of boys. Although these changes are said to be more prevalent in children with hyperlipidemias, there is no proof that these changes are of any predictive or prognostic value. In 103 normal children, James found that 7% of normal boys and 14% of normal girls had 0.1 to 0.2 mV ST depression in their exercise ECG.[39] Most of the changes were present in lead V5 or V6 and would likely have been detected by lead CM-5.

The criteria for a positive or abnormal ST-segment response to exercise in adults have been the subject of considerable debate. There is no debate about this response in children because the significance of any change is uncertain. The criteria of 0.1 mV or greater ST depression 60 msec after the J-point without regard for ST slope, as suggested by James, would seem to be too sensitive a criterion, i.e., any change that occurs in 11% of absolutely normal children is obviously not satisfactory.[37] Coronary artery anomalies (congenital or acquired) that are present in less than 1 in 10,000 children and ST criteria need to be fairly stringent to avoid a tremendous number of false-positive assessments. In geographic areas that demonstrate a prevalence for Kowasaki's disease, which causes potentially permanent changes in the coronary arteries, exercise testing may be of additional value.

In three patients with pulmonary artery origin of the left coronary artery who were tested in our laboratory, ST depression was over 0.5 mV and the segment was downsloping. Children with simple or mild congenital anomalies do not usually show ST depression. Patients with LV myocardial disease, AS or coarctation of the aorta do develop ST depression, which is information of some value when assessing disease severity. Patients with severe RV overload may show ST depression reaching 0.5 to 0.8 mV in lead CM-5, but there is no consistent pattern and none that is of known prognostic importance.

Maximal Heart Rate

Children with mild and moderately severe heart lesions without cyanosis have maximal HR in the range of 180 to 220 beats·min^{-1}, with a mean of 200 beats·min^{-1}.[16] Reports of a mean maximal HR less than 200 in patients with mild or moderate heart disease are suspect. In many of these studies, the observers failed to obtain near-maximal efforts from their patients. Occasionally, these patients have nodal pacemakers, producing a lower maximal HR. Many children with severe non-cyanotic heart disease have maximal HR close to 200 beats·min^{-1}, but some stop exercising because of severe fatigue when their HR is only 160 to 170 beats·min^{-1}. Average maximal HR is still about 190 beats·min^{-1} in this group.

Children with cyanotic congenital heart disease have a maximal HR of 140 to 220 beats·min^{-1}.[16] Some patients have arterial oxygen saturation as low as 25%, are severely fatigued and distressed with dyspnea, and yet have a HR of only 150 beats·min^{-1}. If really pushed, these patients might get their HR up another 30 or 40 beats·min^{-1}, but most laboratory personnel will not push the child to this extent, if for no other reason than compassion, and also because of safety concerns. The mean maximal HR for children with cyanotic heart disease in our laboratory is 178 ± 12 beats·min^{-1}.

When a low HR is reported, the post-exercise lactate level should be above 6 mmol·L^{-1} in children under age 10 years and over 8 mmol·L^{-1} in children over age 10 years to confirm that the exercise test was indeed near maximum. Laboratory staff conducting exercise capacity studies should utilize serum lactate measurements to confirm that near-maximal tests have been obtained.

EXERCISE CAPACITY
Normal Children

The mean exercise capacities for children tested in a hospital laboratory who proved to not have heart disease are listed in Table 17–1. The oxygen requirement for stages 1, 2, 3, 4, and 5 of the Bruce protocol in 10-year-old subjects are 18, 27, 36, 48, and 57 ml·kg^{-1}·min^{-1}—about 7% higher than those values reported for adults.[15] It is important that normal values be established within each laboratory, because the results are dependent on the skill of the technicians, as well as on the population and the philosophy of the laboratory staff.

Children with Heart Defects

Most school children with heart defects are not sickly. Those children who would be in this category have had surgery and have hearts that function almost normally by the time they enter school. The distribution of maximal treadmill or bicycle performances of children with heart defects differ little from that of the general population, except for the 5 to 10% of school age patients with significant unresolved problems leading to cyanosis, pulmonary hypertension, or borderline heart failure.

Demonstration of the normal exercise capacity of most children with heart disease requires the choice of a valid maximal exercise test; the selection of a suitable comparative normal population; the testing of cardiac patients and normal children under similar circumstances; having skilled test supervisors who are not at all reticent about encouraging cardiac patients to push close to exhaustion; and having children coming from a community in which it is the norm for children with cardiac anomalies to play and exercise with their friends, rather than being restricted or made to worry by overanxious physicians, parents, and school authorities.

In Table 17–2, low fitness has been defined as having a treadmill endurance time on the Bruce test below the 10th percentile line for the normal population based on age and gender.[16] The 10th percentile is used because of the relatively small number of subjects (327 normal subjects and 830 patients) and the arbitrary decision that subjects below the 10th per-

centile values should be considered unfit. Only 21% of the group of cardiac patients fell below the 10th percentile; these individuals had septal defects, severe valve lesions, or cyanosis. Of the entire patient group, 47% had treadmill endurance times above the 50th percentile line; endurance times above the 90th percentile line (expected in 10% of the population) were found in 4% of the cardiac patients. This survey of fitness levels in a cardiac clinic population showed that the majority of cardiac patients can keep up with their peers, and that above-average endurance times are possible, even with the presence of significant disease.

EXERCISE TRAINING

Miller et al. presented the results of a 5-week training experiment with 12 children after repair of various heart defects.[54] Control subjects had a $\dot{V}_{O_2max}$ of 41.2 ml·kg^{-1}·min^{-1} before training, and showed a 12% improvement. Cardiac patients had a $\dot{V}_{O_2max}$ of 35.3 ml·kg^{-1}·min^{-1} before training and failed to improve. Maximal HR was 199 and 193 beats·min^{-1} in the control subjects and 183 and 174 beats·min^{-1} in the cardiac patients before and after training, respectively. It could be argued that the cardiac patients probably did not exercise maximally with these low maximal HRs (especially after training), and that the entire experiment was dependent on achieving maximal efforts from the children.

In children who have had surgery for Fallot's tetralogy, James found that those patients who had the operation at a young age and then took part normally in sports activities ended up with normal average exercise capacities.[40]

A 6-week home exercise program involving the use of a Monark ergometer in 16 postoperative patients with tetralogy of Fallot and 10 postoperative patients with VSD improved ergometer exercise capacity 25%; $\dot{V}_{O_2max}$ did not improve.[29]

Galioto et al. reported that 24 training sessions over a period of 12 weeks given to eight children after complex heart surgery improved resting and peak exercise $\dot{Q}$ by

TABLE 17-1. **Exercise Values for Normal Children Tested in a Hospital Clinic**

| Age (years) | Bruce Treadmill Time (Min) | | | | Bicycle Ergometer: Maximal Power Output (kpm·kg⁻¹) | | Work 0.85 (kpm·kg⁻¹)* | |
| | Mean | | 10th Percentile | | | | | |
	Males	Females	Males	Females	Males	Females	Males	Females
4–5	11.5 ± 1.5	11.0 ± 1.4	9.5	9.5	15.6 ± 5.0	14.8 ± 4.6	9.8 ± 2.5	9.7 ± 2.9
6–7	12.5 ± 1.2	12.3 ± 1.2	10.8	11.0	19.8 ± 5.1	18.8 ± 5.3	12.8 ± 3.8	10.4 ± 2.9
8–9	13.2 ± 1.4	12.2 ± 1.1	12.0	10.5	21.2 ± 4.3	19.0 ± 5.0	13.2 ± 3.2	10.5 ± 2.2
10–12	13.5 ± 1.7	12.1 ± 1.3	11.0	10.5	23.4 ± 4.1	18.8 ± 4.8	13.2 ± 3.0	10.2 ± 2.1
13–15	13.8 ± 1.4	11.1 ± 1.7	12.0	9.0	21.3 ± 4.7	17.5 ± 4.2	12.4 ± 3.1	9.5 ± 2.2
16–20	14.3 ± 2.3	11.6 ± 1.7	10.5	9.2	21.4 ± 5.4	16.7 ± 2.9	12.7 ± 2.9	9.5 ± 1.8

*Work 0.85 = power output at 85% of actual maximal HR (equal to W170 if maximal HR is 200).

TABLE 17-2. Distribution of Treadmill Endurance Times of Children with Heart Disease

Defect and Severity	Subjects with Endurance Times Categorized by Bruce Test Percentile Ranges*			
	<10%	11–50%	51–90%	>90%
VSD				
Small	6	43	48	4
Medium	18	23	56	3
Large	29	53	14	5
Postoperative	9	44	45	2
ASD				
Small	11	34	49	7
Medium	3	35	55	8
Large	33	55	11	0
Postoperative	9	49	38	5
PDA				
Postoperative	0	50	50	0
AS				
Mild	0	47	39	14
Moderate	0	45	55	0
Severe	14	50	35	0
Postoperative	22	60	19	0
PS				
Mild	2	42	34	0
Moderate	0	31	38	13
Severe	0	80	20	0
Postoperative	1	60	20	0
Coarctation				
Preoperative	13	37	46	4
Postoperative	22	60	17	0
Tetralogy				
Unoperated	67	33	0	0
Palliation only	90	10	0	0
Post open-heart repair	19	60	22	0
Other cyanotic conditions	92	8	0	0
Rheumatic heart disease				
Normal heart	8	40	48	4
Mild and moderate	12	34	42	14
Severe valve disease	47	53	0	0
TOTAL	21%	40%	43%	4%

* Established for 327 children with innocent heart murmurs. VSD = ventricular septal defect; ASD = atrial septal defect; PDA = patent ductus arteriosus; AS = aortic stenosis; PS = pulmonary stenosis.

25% and improved treadmill time.[26] Koch and co-workers reported increased flexibility in children receiving special instructions after heart surgery.[44]

I personally doubt there is much of a need for structured in-hospital cardiac rehabilitation programs for children after surgery. With proper instructions to children and parents, the children can resume free exercise activities within a few weeks of surgery, and nearly all can take part in all free-time activities with their friends within months of surgery.

Exercise in Children After Heart Surgery

Most children with significant heart defects will have had heart surgery before they start school. The physical educator or physician confronted with a child with a potential heart problem in relation to exercise most often finds a well-looking child with a median sternotomy or other thoracic scar. If the surgery was performed in infancy, the current attending physician, and even the parents, often do not know the nature of the underlying condition or the type of surgery. It is necessary to refer back to the original treatment center for this information and to obtain results of the last heart catheterization data if postoperative studies were done, the last echocardiogram, and (if possible) a recent treadmill test.

In general, patients who had successful surgery for patent ductus, ASD (secundum), uncomplicated VSD, or pulmonary stenosis can be considered close to normal and allowed unrestricted sport activity even though there may be subtle changes in function.[67] Patients after surgery for coarctation need evaluation of exercise blood pressure, as outlined above. Surgery in childhood for AS is palliative and unrestricted; intense sport training is generally not advisable except for the few with ideal results. After surgery for tetralogy of Fallot, many can have normal functional capacities, but others have limitations.[69] Patients with more-complex lesions need individual consideration. Most will not be able to achieve high levels of cardiovascular fitness; they can often be normal average, but not supernormal.[2,19]

Increasing numbers of children in the school system have had excellent surgical results for problems that were uniformly fatal 30 years ago. Patients with transposition who have had the Mustard (or Senning) operation and patients with a variety of lesions who have had the Fontan operation are of special interest. These children have hearts that are clearly abnormal, they have definite limitations in their chronotropic and hemodynamic responses to exercise, yet they often function at near-normal levels in the school system and with regular physical education.

Exercise Function After the Mustard Operation for Transposition of the Great Arteries

The Mustard operation suddenly provided normal lives for many infants with transposition of the great arteries who previously never reached their first birthday. This operation redirects the venous return to the heart so that oxygenated blood enters the right ventricle and then the aorta, while venous blood enters the left ventricle and then the pulmonary artery. There are two areas of interest in relation to exercise: sinus node dysfunction and rhythm problems, and the fact that the right ventricle is not the ideal systemic pump. Benson et al.[5] and Parrish et al.[59] studied exercise right ventricular function using nuclear angiography. Normal resting right ventricular ejection fraction is about 45%, and was 44% in these patients. Normally on exercise, right ventricular ejection fraction increases by at least 5%. Eight of 19 of the patients studied by Benson et al. showed a normal increase, 5 had a below-normal increase, and 6 had a major decrease in right ventricular ejection fraction on exercise.

By age 10, up to 50% of patients with the Mustard operation have cardiac rhythm problems. Maximal HR during exercise is reduced below 170 beats·min^{-1} in up to 75% of patients. Despite this treadmill performance, endurance time is average or better in at least one-third of patients, and below 2 standard deviations of normal in only a few. Mathews reported on 71 exercise tests with 46 patients after the Mustard procedure.[53] Maximal $\dot{V}_{O_2}$, exercise time, and HR were about 80% of normal, with values tending to decrease with age. With sinus rhythm at rest, 10% had arrhythmias on exercise, including junctional rhythms, aortoventricular block, supraventricular tachycardia, atrial and ventricular premature beats, and multifocal ventricular premature beats. Despite these problems, most of these patients remained free of symptoms.[20] Unfortunately, there are occasional late deaths even 10 years after the Mustard operation, but these are seldom related to exercise activities. Most of the patients who died had known rhythm problems, residual defects, or significant problems with myocardial function. Despite the problems with right ventricular function and rhythm, most of these patients are asymptomatic. They seldom admit to any problems with physical education in school. They do not participate in competitive aerobic sports but seldom need to drop out of regular physical education activities. Although some of these patients do run into significant problems with right ventricular function and/or arrhythmia, and their activities need to be curtailed, the majority have no restrictions, other than avoidance of serious athletic training.

Exercise After the Fontan Operation

Various complex congenital heart problems are now palliated very effectively by the Fontan procedure, in which right atrial blood is delivered to the pulmonary artery by connecting the right atrial appendage to the pulmonary artery, or to the outflow area of the right ventricle. Patients may or may not have had a previous connection between the superior vena cava and the right pulmonary artery. Such major defects as tricuspid atresia and single ventricle can be palliated to a degree where there is no cyanosis and a reasonable (if not completely normal) exercise performance.

In one recent report, Rhodes et al. found that peak workload, peak $\dot{V}_{O_2}$, and peak $\dot{Q}$ were about 65% of control or less, whereas patients after surgery for tetralogy of Fallot studied in the same laboratory had peak workloads 83% of control and peak $\dot{Q}$ 98% of control.[62] The exercise capacity of the Fontan patients was unrelated to technical differences in the procedure, to underlying lesion, or to prior surgeries. The Fontan patients had inappropriately high ventilation volumes in relation to workload and $\dot{V}_{O_2}$.[19] A good clinical result depends on preservation of ventricular function, as measured with nuclear angiography.[68']

Cumming reported on catheterization studies after the Fontan procedure.[17] The mean gradient from right atrium to pulmonary artery was only 3 mm Hg, and maximal cardiac index was 6.2 L·min^{-1}·m^2 (a little below 60% of normal); the low output was partially compensated by an increased oxygen extraction by the working muscles and a greater reliance on anaerobic function. The correlation coefficient between maximal $\dot{Q}$ for supine ergometer work at catheterization and treadmill endurance time was only 0.40. The limited exercise capacity of the patients was likely related to reduced blood flow to the exercising muscles.

Although patients after the Fontan operation have exercise capacities that are 60% of normal, they often keep up with their peers in most physical education classes, and it is appropriate to allow them free activities with the provision that they rest or slow down when they are dyspneic. Exercise does not seem to precipitate serious arrhythmias or other problems in this group of patients.

Exercise studies have been carried out on children with other cardiac lesions such as pulmonary atresia,[2] Ebstein malformation of the tricuspid valve, and such chest wall deformities as pectus excavatum[73] and severe scoliosis.

After surgery for congenital heart disease, there are many reasons for some potential impairment of cardiopulmonary function, despite the achievement of a good anatomic correction. Ventricular function and SV can be limited by ventriculotomy scars, myocardial fibrosis, architectural changes in the myocardium or residual hypertrophy, inadequate volume development, or mild A-V valve regurgitation. There may be residual obstruction to ventricular outflow, with gradients across the right or left ventricular outflow tracts or at the site of coarctation. Circulation in the lung may have permanent impairments because of small arteries, kinking and obstruction of arteries after surgery, thrombotic or embolic obstructions, or pulmonary hypertensive vascular disease. Electric conduction delays may occur within the atria or ventricles and maximal HR may be reduced in some patients. The studies of Epstein et al. in adults showed that even after surgery for such a simple lesion as ASD, exercise $\dot{Q}$ may be abnormally low for a given $\dot{V}_{O_2}$.[21]

Cardiac output is measured by rebreathing techniques in some pediatric cardiology research laboratories on a regular basis, generally using a CO_2 method, but also using acetylene.

In general, $\dot{Q}$ tends to be 10 to 15% below normal in patients with repaired noncyanotic lesions and 15 to 25% below normal in patients with repaired cyanotic lesions.[24] Even in patients with such simple lesions as ASD, VSD, or pulmonary stenosis, exercise $\dot{Q}$ tends to range from low normal to below normal.[22]

Despite the findings of impaired output, most of these children can, when pushed, do as much as normal children in terms of treadmill work. Reasons for this may include partial compensation by greater arteriovenous oxygen difference, greater use of anaerobic sources, more efficient exercise, and altered muscular function. Measuring $\dot{Q}$ adds to the complexity of exercise testing and may reduce treadmill or bicycle endurance times, especially in patients given only one test.

To achieve functional normalcy, it is probably important that surgery be performed at as young an age as possible for correction of most lesions to ensure proper cardiac growth and development. Surgery before school age allows the child to take part in all activities with his or her peers without the interruption of major surgery. The operative repair must be meticulous and myocardial preservation should be complete. Whenever possible, palliative procedures that cause circulatory changes in the lungs should give way to early corrective procedures.

Depending on the procedure performed, we have conducted near-maximal exercise tests 4 to 10 weeks after surgical correction of congenital heart defects to show the child and parent that a return to normal activities is permissible. Most children with repair of ASD, anomalous pulmonary venous return, PS, AS, or coarctation are encouraged to walk 3 days after surgery; go back to school 14 to 20 days after surgery; walk, bicycle, or swim within 3 to 4 weeks of surgery; and return to regular physical education training within 2 to 4 months of surgery. Children with repair of large VSD or tetralogy of Fallot usually require some delay from the previous recommendations. After complex surgery involving conduits and prosthetic valves, individual advice concerning progression into exercise activities is required.

Children who had cyanosis and limited functional capacities were able to exceed their preoperative levels of activity within 2 weeks of surgery. Parents are advised to give the child freedom to choose his or her own activities for the first few weeks after leaving hospital in the firm belief that if it hurts or causes harm, the child will find out and avoid the activity without external advice.

The attitude toward activity should be a positive one, i.e., the child should be encouraged to do what his or her friends are doing in as short a time as seems reasonable. With this approach, most children achieve normal exercise capacities and many can experience whatever sports participation they choose. Although there is usually no need for detailed exercise prescription or for supervised rehabilitation programs for most children after heart surgery, workers at the Hospital for Sick Children in Toronto have shown that formal instructions given to children and parents led to improved fitness test results.[48,49] When problems exist, the cardiac status should be reviewed and a maximal treadmill test should be obtained; when appropriate, remedial exercises can be prescribed by the physician and supervised by the parents. A few children may require exercise prescriptions based on HR for safety and avoidance of arrhythmia. When children who have had heart surgery wish to take on intense sports training in physically demanding sports, they should have regular maximal exercise tests to assess cardiac rhythm and physiologic responses.

PREVENTION OF ADULT CORONARY DISEASE

Coronary heart disease very likely starts in childhood or adolescence. Exercise, with its accompanying lifestyle, has been shown to be helpful in weight control, blood pressure control, raising HDL, reducing LDL cholesterol, and avoidance of smoking in pediatric populations. Unfortunately, a 60-year study involving 20,000 children to assess whether vigorous aerobic exercise started in childhood would prevent or delay the onset of coronary disease will likely never take place because of the cost and other logistical hurdles.

By the criteria of an American task force, hypertension is defined as a blood pressure above the 95th percentile for age and gender.[61] Results of exercise studies in children with mild hypertension showed that SBP did not increase as much in these patients as in the control group, that SBP at maximal exercise rarely exceeded 220 mm Hg, and that no symptoms or rhythm disturbances occurred.[23,43] Children who are normotensive at rest but who have a higher than normal increase in exercise blood pressure may be prone to develop hypertension in later years, but current reports are preliminary and such studies require 10 to 30 years of follow-up data.

Sixty percent of children with hypertension are overweight, which may partially account for their decreased aerobic fitness; these children often are just as active as their peers. Asymptomatic children with mild or moderate hypertension generally have normal SBP and HR responses to dynamic exercise. Some hypertensive adolescents may have higher exercise HR and higher serum epinephrine and lactate values.[43]

Many writers have cautioned against the performance of isometric exercises and weight lifting in patients with heart disease or hypertension. There have been no facts to prove adverse effects, however, and SBP can be higher with dynamic exercise when compared to SBP associated with isometric exercise. In one study in hypertensive adolescents, 2 months of weight training did not alter the resting blood pressure determination or echocardiographic heart dimensions.[46]

ATTITUDE TOWARD SPORT, PHYSICAL EDUCATION, AND EXERCISE

Physicians, school authorities, physical educators, coaches, and some parents want a safe approach to everything. They will play safe to cover their own tracks, even if it unnecessarily restricts the child who does not need restrictions, and even if these restrictions may interfere with the normal social, physical, and mental development of the child.

Most children with heart disease or who have had surgery for heart disease require no restrictions whatsoever from recreational sports activities, physical education, and even joining in competitive sports. This does not mean children with significant structural heart disease should be encouraged to aim for a career in professional sports or for the next Olympic Games. It does mean, however, that very few children under the age of 10 or 11 years need to be restricted. The child should be the judge of what to join and when to stop exercising. Even children with such severe heart malformations as inoperable pulmonary atresia can carry on in this way. Children limited by their heart defects usually decide on their own that they are not destined for sports activities requiring tremendous endurance or strength. They can continue to participate in whatever activity they choose at recreational levels, however, and they need never be placed in a situation in which they are singled out as being different or inferior. These children need never be given a list of DO's and DON'Ts. I have given this advice to parents and children for over 25 years in a busy practice of pediatric cardiology without a single instance of regret.

Children with a cardiomyopathy or chronic myocarditis are steered away from all competitive sports situations and many exercise activities (as are those patients with moderate AS) because of a proven relationship between intense exercise activity and sudden death. In patients with the Marfan's syndrome, we do not know whether the restrictions we suggest are followed in the child's free time, nor whether restrictions delay the dilatation of the aorta, with the eventual development of severe aortic regurgitation, dissection, or rupture. Common sense indicates that weight training or strenuous exercise has a strong likelihood of being harmful, but even in these children, total abstinence from physical activities is not required.

REFERENCES

1. Alpert, B.S., et al.: Exercise blood pressure response—a predictor of severity of aortic stenosis in children. J. Pediatr., 98:763, 1981.
2. Barber, G., Danielson, G., Page, C., et al.: Pulmonary atresia with ventricular septal defect. Preoperative and postoperative responses to exercise. J. Am. Coll. Cardiol., 7:630, 1986.
3. Bay, G., Abrahamsen, A.M., and Muller, C.: Left to right shunt in atrial septal defect at rest and during exercise. Acta Med. Scand., 190:205, 1971.
4. Bendien, C., et al.: Hemodynamic effects of dynamic exercise in children and adolescents with moderate to small ventricular defects. Circulation, 70:929, 1984.
5. Bensen, L.N., Bonet, J., McLaughlin, P., et al.: Assessment of right ventricular function during supine bicycle exercise after Mustard's operation. Circulation, 65:1052, 1982.
6. Bergman, A.B., and Stamm, S.J.: The morbidity of cardiac nondisease in school children. N. Engl. J. Med., 276:1008, 1967.
7. Bjarke, B., Eriksson, B.O., and Saltin, B.: ATP, CP, and lactate concentrations in muscle tissue during exercise in male patients with tetralogy of Fallot. Scand. J. Clin. Lab. Invest., 33:255, 1974.
8. Bricker, J.T., and Vargo, T.A.: Advances in exercise testing. In Pediatric Cardiology: Its Current Practice. J.T. Bricker and D.G. McNamara. London, Edward Arnold, 1988, pp. 99–111.
9. Bricker, J.T., Garson, A., Paridon, S.M., and Vargo, T.A.: Exercise correlates of electrophysiologic assessment of sinus node function in young individuals. Pediatr. Exerc. Sci., 2:163, 1990.
10. Bricker, J.T., et al.: Exercise testing in children with Wolff-Parkinson-White syndrome. Am. J. Cardiol., 55:1001, 1985.
11. Chaitman, B.R., et al.: The importance of clinical subsets in interpreting maximal treadmill exercise test results: the role of multiple-lead ECG systems. Circulation, 59:560, 1979.
12. Chandramouli, B., Ehmke, D.A., and Lauer, R.M.: Exercise-induced electrocardiographic changes in children with congenital aortic stenosis. J. Pediatr., 87:725, 1975.
13. Cotton, J.L., Kavey, R.W., and Blackman, M.S.: B-Blocker therapy for exercise induced hypertension after coarctation repair. Circulation, 78 (Suppl. II):200, 1988 (Abstract).
14. Cueto, L., and Moller, J.H.: Hemodynamics of exercise in children with isolated aortic valvular disease. Br. Heart J., 35:93, 1973.
15. Cumming, G.R., Everatt, D., and Hastman, L.: Bruce treadmill test in children. Normal values in a clinic population. Am. J. Cardiol., 41:69, 1978.
16. Cumming, G.R.: Maximal exercise capacity of children with heart defects. Am. J. Cardiol., 42:613, 1979.
17. Cumming, G.R.: Maximal exercise hemodynamics after the Fontan procedure. In Pediatric Cardiology. Edited by E.E. Doyle, M.A. Engle, W.M. Gersony, W.J. Rashkind, and N.S. Talner. New York, Springer-Verlag, 1986, pp. 257–266.
18. Driscoll, D.J.: Exercise rehabilitation programs for children with congenital heart disease. A note of caution. Pediatr. Exerc. Sci., 2:191, 1990.
19. Driscoll, D.J., Mottram, C., and Danielson, G.: Spectrum of exercise intolerance in 45 patients with Ebstein's anomaly and observations on exercise tolerance in 11 patients after surgical repair. J. Am. Coll. Cardiol., 11:831, 1988.
20. Ensing, G., Heise, C., and Driscoll, D.: Cardiovascular response to exercise after the Mustard operation for simple and complex transposition of the great vessels. Am. J. Cardiol., 62:613, 1988.
21. Epstein, S.E., et al.: Hemodynamic abnormalities in response to mild and intense exercise following operative correction of an atrial septal defect or tetralogy of Fallot. Circulation, 45:1065, 1973.
22. Finnegan, P., et al.: Hemodynamic studies at rest and during exercise in pulmonary stenosis after surgery. Br. Heart J., 36:913, 1974.
23. Foxler, D.E., et al.: Response of hypertensive adolescents to dynamic and isometric exercise stress. Pediatrics, 64:579, 1979.
24. Franklin, W.H., Heise, C.T., and Barber, G.: What is the cardiac output response to exercise after repair of congenital heart disease? Pediatr. Exerc. Sci., 1:171, 1988.
25. Fulton, D.R., Chung, K.J., Tabakin, B.S., and Keane, J.F.: Ventricular tachycardia in children without heart disease. Am. J. Cardiol., 55:1328–1331, 1985.
26. Galioto, F.M., Tomassoni, M.A., Vaccaro, P., and Vaccaro, J.: Effect on cardiac output of a cardiac rehabilitation program in children after surgical repair of congenital heart disease. J. Am. Coll. Cardiol., 11:250A, 1988 (Abstract).
27. Garson, A., Gillette, P.C., and McNamara, D.G.: Control of late postoperative ventricular arrhythmias with phenytoin in young patients. Am. J. Cardiol., 46:290, 1980.
28. Garson, A., et al.: Stress-induced ventricular arrhythmias after repair of tetralogy of Fallot. Am. J. Cardiol., 46:1006, 1980.
29. Goldberg, B., et al.: Effect of physical training on exercise performance of children following surgical repair of congenital heart disease. Pediatrics, 68:691, 1981.
30. Hannon, J., Danielson, G., Page, F., et al.: Cardiorespiratory response to exercise after repair of tetralogy of Fallot. Texas Heart Inst. J., 12:393, 1985.

31. Hansen, E.: Coarctation of the aorta. A long term followup after surgery. Scand. J. Thorac. Cardiovasc. Surg., *14* (Suppl. 24):1, 1980.
32. Hesslein, P.S.: Noninvasive arrhythmia diagnosis. *In* The Science and Practice of Pediatric Cardiology. Edited by A. Garson, Jr., J.T. Bricker, and D.G. McNamara. Philadelphia, Lea & Febiger, 1990, pp. 1737.
33. Hossack, R.F., and Neilson, G.H.: Exercise testing in congenital aortic stenosis. Aust. N. Z. J. Med., *9*:169, 1979.
34. Hugenholtz, P.G., and Nada, A.S.: Exercise studies in patients with congenital heart disease. Pediatrics, *32*:760, 1963.
35. Ikkos, D., and Hanson, J.S.: Response to exercise in congenital complete atrioventricular block. Circulation, *22*:583, 1960.
36. Jacobsen, J.R., Garson, A., Jr., Gillette, P.C., and McNamara, D.G.: Premature ventricular contractions in normal children. J. Pediatr., *92*:36–38, 1978.
37. James, F.: Exercise ECG in Children. Edited by E.K. Chung. Baltimore, Williams & Wilkins, 1979.
38. James, F.W., and Kaplan, S.: Unexpected cardiac arrest in patients after surgical correction of tetralogy of Fallot. Circulation, *52*:691, 1975.
39. James, F.W., et al.: Maximal exercise stress testing in normal and hyperlipidemic children. Atherosclerosis, *25*:85, 1976.
40. James, F.W., et al.: Response to exercise in patients after total surgical correction of tetralogy of Fallot. Circulation, *54*:671, 1976.
41. Karpawich, P.P., Gillette, P.C., Garson, A., Jr., et al.: Congenital complete atrioventricular block: clinical and electrophysiologic predictors of need for pacemaker insertion. Am. J. Cardiol., *48*:1098, 1981.
42. Keith, J.D., Rowe, R.D., and Vlad, P.: Heart Disease in Infancy and Childhood. New York, MacMillan, 1978.
43. Klein, A.A., et al.: Sympathetic nervous system and exercise tolerance response in normotensive and hypertensive adolescents. J. Am. Coll. Cardiol., *3*:381, 1984.
44. Koch, B.M., Galioto, F.M., Vaccaro, P., et al.: Flexibility and strength measures in children undergoing a cardiac rehabilitation program. Phys. Sports Med., *16*:139, 1988.
45. Kveselis, D.A., et al.: Hemodynamic determinants of exercise-induced ST-segment depression in children with valvular aortic stenosis. Am. J. Cardiol., *55*:1133, 1985.
46. Laird, W.P., Foxler, D.E., and Swanborn, C.D.: Cardiovascular effects of weight training in hypertensive adolescents. Med. Sci. Sports, *11*:78, 1979 (Abstract).
47. Lambert, E.C., et al.: Sudden unexpected death from cardiovascular disease in children. A cooperative international study. Am. J. Cardiol., *34*:89, 1974.
48. Longmuir, P., et al.: The benefits of a postoperative exercise program for children with congenital heart disease. Clin. Invest. Med., *5* (Suppl. 1): 45, 1983 (Abstract).
49. Longmuir, P., Turner, J., Rowe, R., and Olley, P.: Postoperative exercise rehabilitation benefits children with congenital heart disease. Clin. Invest. Med., *8*:232, 1985.
50. Manno, B.V., et al.: Left ventricular function at rest and during exercise in congenital complete heart block. A radionuclide angiographic evaluation. Am. J. Cardiol., *52*:92, 1983.
51. Markel, H., Rocchini, A.P., Beekman, R.H., et al.: Exercise-induced hypertension after repair of coarctation of the aorta: arm versus leg exercise. J. Am. Coll. Cardiol., *8*:165, 1986.
52. Maron, B.J., et al.: Postoperative assessment of patients with ventricular septal defect and pulmonary hypertension. Response to intense upright exercise. Circulation, *48*:864, 1973.
53. Matthews, R.A., Fricher, F.J., Beerman, C.B., et al.: Exercise performance after the Mustard operation for a complete transposition. *In* Perspectives in Pediatric Cardiology. Edited by R.H. Anderson. New York, Futura, 1988, pp. 261.
54. Miller, W.W., et al.: Physical training in children with congenital heart disease. *In* Frontiers of Activity and Child Health. Limites de la Capacité Physique chez l'Enfant. Edited by H. Lavallée and R.J. Shephard. Quebec, Pelican, 1977.
55. Mocellin, R., et al.: Funktionelle Untersuchungen in Ruhe und während Belastung bei Kindern und Jugendlichen mit Ventrikelseptumdefekt und pulmonarer Hypertonie. Z. Kardiol., *64*:1036, 1975.
56. Moller, J.H., Rao, S., and Lucas, R.V.: Exercise hemodynamics of pulmonary valvular stenosis. Circulation, *46*:1018, 1972.
57. Motram, C.D., Staats, B.A., and Driscoll, D.J.: Patterns of oxygen desaturation during exercise in patients with congenital heart disease. Pediatr. Exerc. Sci., *2*:178, 1990 (Abstract).
58. Paridon, S.M., Ross, R.D., Kuhns, L.R., and Pinsky, W.W.: Myocardial performance and perfusion during exercise in patients with coronary artery disease caused by Kawasaki disease. J. Pediatr., *116*:52–56, 1990.
59. Parrish, M.D., et al.: Radionuclide angiographic evaluation of right and left ventricular function during exercise after repair of transposition of the great arteries. Circulation, *67*:178, 1983.
60. Pernot, C., et al.: L'épreuve d'effort dans les sténoses aortiques congénitales. Arch. Mal. Coeur, *71*:517, 1979.
61. Report of the Task Force on Blood Pressure Control in Children. Pediatrics, *59* (Suppl. 5):797, 1977.
62. Rhodes, J., Garofano, R.P., Bowman, F.O., Jr., et al.: Effect of right ventricular anatomy on the cardiopulmonary response to exercise. Circulation, *81*:1811, 1990.
63. Rocchini, A.P., Chun, P.O., and Dick, M.: Ventricular tachycardia in children. Am. J. Cardiol., *47*:1091, 1981.
64. Ryujin, Y., Arakaki, Y., Takahashi, O., and Kamiya, T.: Ventricular arrhythmias in children: the validity of exercise stress tests for their diagnosis and management. Jpn. Circ. J., *48*:1393, 1984.
65. Smith, R.T., et al.: Stress testing for comparison of synthetic patch aortoplasty with resection and end-to-end anastomosis for repair of coarctation in childhood. J. Am. Coll. Cardiol., *4*:765, 1984.
66. Stone, F.M., et al.: Pre and postoperative rest and exercise hemodynamics in children with pulmonary stenosis. Circulation, *49*:1102, 1974.
67. Tomassone, T., Galioto, F.M., Vaccaro, P., and Vaccaro, J.: Effects of exercise training on exer-

cise tolerance and cardiac output in children after repair of congenital heart disease. Sports Train. Med. Rehab., *1*:327, 1990.

68. Torso, S.D., et al.: Radionuclide assessment of ventricular contraction at rest and during exercise following the Fontan procedure for either tricuspid atresia or single ventricle. Am. J. Cardiol., *55*:1127, 1985.

69. Wessel, H., Cunningham, W., Paul, M., et al.: Exercise performance in tetralogy of Fallot after intracardiac repair. J. Thorac. Cardiovasc. Surg., *80*:582, 1980.

70. Wessel, H.U., et al.: Prognostic significance of arrhythmia in tetralogy of Fallot after intracardiac repair. Am. J. Cardiol., *46*:843, 1980.

71. Winkler, R.B., Freed, M.D., and Nada, A.S.: Exercise-induced ventricular ectopy in children and young adults with complete heart block. Am. Heart J., *99*:87, 1980.

72. Wolfe, G.S., Rowland, T.W., and Ellison, R.C.: Surgically induced right bundle branch block with left anterior hemiblock. Circulation, *46*:587, 1972.

73. Wynn, S.R., Driscoll, D.J., Ostrom, N.K., et al.: Exercise cardiorespiratory function in adolescents with pectus excavatum. Observations before and after operation. J. Thorac. Cardiovasc. Surg., *99*:41, 1990.

74. Zellers, T.M., and Driscoll, D.J.: Utility of exercise testing to assess aortic recoarctation. Pediatr. Exerc. Sci., *1*:163, 1989.

18
CHAPTER

Valvular and Congenital Heart Disease in Adults

by
Gordon R. Cumming

VALVULAR HEART DISEASE IN ADULTS

Disease of the heart valves in adults is due to three main causes: previous acute rheumatic fever; degenerative changes in previously normal valves or valves with congenital abnormalities; and infection. Valve abnormalities may be detected by clinical examination in 2% of the population by 40 years of age and in 5% by 70 years of age. Mitral valve prolapse (present in 5 to 10% of female patients) and bicuspid aortic valve (present in 1% of subjects) are excluded from these estimates. Doppler ultrasonography will identify trivial or very mild tricuspid, pulmonary, or mitral regurgitation in up to 20% of the normal population and the aortic valve in 0 to 5%. In the absence of long-term studies, these subjects should be regarded as normal. Valvular stenosis causes obstruction to blood flow and the chamber behind the narrow valve must produce extra work to sustain cardiac output ($\dot{Q}$). Stenosis develops or progresses gradually, and because the normal valve orifice is larger than is necessary, stenosis is usually severe before exercise symptoms occur. Valvular leakage (also called incompetence, regurgitation, or insufficiency) may develop slowly, the heart gradually dilates in response to the increased volume of work, and severe degrees of incompetence are possible in the absence of major symptoms. Valvular

incompetence may also develop acutely; the heart cannot adapt rapidly to the increased volume work and acute heart failure results. Chronically deformed valves may be both stenotic and incompetent, so that the functional change is mixed.

Minimal degrees of valvular incompetence or stenosis produce characteristic heart murmurs, allowing the clinical detection of very mild valvular malfunction. Patients with mild valvular lesions have no symptoms, they can usually exercise vigorously without symptoms, and they can take part in intense sports activities without adverse effects. Patients with severe valve lesions are candidates for valve replacement or reconstruction. Valve replacement, formerly reserved for the patient with severe disease, is now undertaken at an earlier point in the disease process to prevent potentially irreversible myocardial damage.

A major advance is assessing valvular disease has been the use of Doppler echocardiography. This is displayed as a graph of velocity against time. Velocity increases when blood traverses a narrowed valve; the pressure drop across the valve is related to this velocity using the formula, $P = 4 V^2$. The more recent two-dimensional ultrasonographic machines superimpose the velocity information on the two-dimensional echo image with a color-coded display of Doppler flow patterns. This display can be used to assess the severity of aortic regurgitation by measuring the length and/or area of the color flow regurgitant jet. Similarly in mitral regurgitation, the superimposed color flow image can be used to quantify the degree of mitral regurgitation, but technical factors make this estimate more difficult.

Mitral Stenosis

Mitral stenosis (MS) is usually a sequela of rheumatic fever. In the most severe form of MS, the mitral orifice is filled with a funnel-shaped mass of fibrous tissue bearing little resemblance to the delicate normal mitral apparatus. The normal mitral valve orifice measures 4 cm^2. Symptoms of dyspnea with intense exertion occur when the valve orifice is reduced to 2 to 2.5 cm^2; dyspnea occurs with ordinary walking when the orifice area is less than 1 cm^2.

In MS, a pressure gradient develops across the mitral orifice that is proportional to orifice size and the square of the rate of blood flow across the valve. With an orifice size of 1 cm^2, a normal $\dot{Q}$ and resting heart rate (HR) of 70 beats/min, the mean left atrial pressure is about 25 mm Hg (normal is 10 mm Hg). Blood flow across the mitral valve occurs only in diastole, and the time for diastole is reduced when HR is increased. With physical exercise, $\dot{Q}$ and HR increase, and marked increases in left atrial pressure may occur with valve orifices of less than 1.5 cm^2. An elevated left atrial pressure is transmitted retrograde to the lung capillaries, and pulmonary edema occurs when this capillary pressure exceeds the oncotic pressure of the blood (25 mm Hg). Patients with significant MS frequently have increased left atrial pressure, to a level greater than 40 mm Hg during exercise; with sustained exercise, severe and potentially fatal pulmonary edema can occur. These patients limit their physical activities to levels low enough to avoid dyspnea, and should be given stress tests or exercise programs with caution.

The right ventricle pumps the systemic venous return through the pulmonary circulation to the left atrium. Normally, there is a pressure drop across the pulmonary vascular bed of about 7 mm Hg (i.e., if mean left atrial pressure is 10 mm Hg, mean pulmonary artery pressure would be about 17 mm Hg). Thus, in MS the expected mean pulmonary artery pressure would be 32 mm Hg, with an elevation of left atrial pressure to 25 mm Hg. In some patients with longstanding MS, functional and anatomic changes in the small pulmonary blood vessels increase the resistance to flow across the pulmonary vascular bed, and pulmonary artery pressure may be considerably higher than left atrial pressure, e.g., with a left atrial pressure of 25 mm Hg, the mean pulmonary artery pressure may be 60 mm Hg, with the pulsatile pressure at 95/30. Pulmonary vascular resistance increases even further during exercise, with left atrial mean pressure reaching 40 mm Hg and mean pulmonary artery pressure possibly exceeding 100 mm Hg (135/60). The right ventricle cannot function effectively against this high an afterload. Thus, stroke volume (SV) falls. The patient may not complain of dyspnea, only fatigue on exertion due to a low $\dot{Q}$. The right ventricle becomes the limiting factor; if it cannot pump the venous return through the lungs, there is less chance of pulmonary edema and less dyspnea. Thus, this failure of the right ventricle actually protects the patient from pulmonary edema. Muscular fatigue from a low $\dot{Q}$, not dyspnea from lung congestion, limits exercise performance.

When the mitral valve area is less than 1.25 cm^2, SV falls during exercise due to inadequate left ventricular filling. The increase in HR reduces the diastolic filling period; the increase in left atrial pressure cannot fully compensate for this reduction, and diastolic filling of the left ventricle is reduced. The $\dot{Q}$ response to exercise is reduced because of the low SV, even though HR is abnormally rapid at low work loads. The lungs are stiff, the work of breathing is increased, and ventilation is disproportionately increased at light exercise loads. Because of the reduced $\dot{Q}$, muscle perfusion is reduced and lactate is produced at low work loads. Maximal oxygen uptake ($\dot{V}_{O_2max}$) is considerably below normal levels, with usual values of 12 to 20 ml·kg^{-1}·min^{-1}. Maximal HR may be reduced because dyspnea is the cause of premature termination of exercise. Exercise systolic blood pressure (SBP) may reach only 130 mm Hg because of the low output. Chapman et al. reported $\dot{V}_{O_2max}$ values of 22 ml·kg^{-1}·min^{-1} before and 27 ml·kg^{-1}·min^{-1} after mitral valvotomy, normal values being about 39 ml·kg^{-1}·min^{-1} for the subjects studied.[10] Blackmon et al. found mean $\dot{V}_{O_2max}$ values of 18 and 26 ml·kg^{-1}·min^{-1} before and after mitral commisurotomy, respectively.[6] Median treadmill times were 4 minutes before and 6.5 minutes after surgery, as opposed to 9 minutes for age-matched normal persons following the standard Bruce treadmill protocol. A "plateau" occurred in the $\dot{V}_{O_2}$ during incremental exercise tests in about two-thirds of MS patients.

Arterial oxygen pressure and oxygen saturation levels are normal at rest and with light exercise, but they may fall during exercise at loads sufficient to cause dyspnea and lung edema. Because of the low $\dot{Q}$, mixed venous blood oxygen content is low at rest and during exercise, and visceral blood flow is reduced. Exercise capacity in patients with MS and sinus rhythm can be improved by slowing HR and prolonging diastolic filling period with the use of beta blocking agents. Some caution is necessary, however.[24]

Mitral valve surgery is recommended if the patient's symptoms are sufficiently severe that they want surgery; if there is arrhythmia; if there is developing pulmonary hypertension; or if there is a thromboembolic problem. The mitral valve is far from normal after palliative mitral valve operations and exercise gradients are present after valve replacement. Myocardial function may remain impaired and there may be abnormalities of other valves or residual pathologic lung changes. The degree of improvement in exercise capacity depends on the degree of residual dysfunction, presence or absence of arrhyth-

mia, the age of the subject, and the effort made to improve exercise capacity.

Aortic Stenosis

In adults, aortic stenosis (AS) is caused by gradual fibrosis and calcification of a normal valve, of a congenital bicuspid or stenotic valve, or of a valve damaged by rheumatic fever. The patient is asymptomatic until the valve deformity and narrowing are severe. Many patients reach 60 to 80 years of age before AS becomes symptomatic.

The obstruction of outflow from the left ventricle causes its peak SBP to increase in proportion to the degree of narrowing and the rate of systolic ejection. The obstruction may cause a lowering of the pressure in the aorta downstream from the valve. The severity of AS is generally assessed by the magnitude of the peak SBP difference (gradient) between the left ventricle and the aorta. In mild stenosis, the gradient is 30 mm Hg or less; in moderate stenosis the gradient is 40 to 60 mm Hg, and in severe stenosis a value over 60 mm Hg is noted when $\dot{Q}$ is normal. The follow-up of patients with AS has been simplified with the advent of accurate, noninvasive assessment of hemodynamics using Doppler ultrasonography to measure aortic jet velocity. Those with a velocity of over 4 m·sec^{-1} require valve replacement, whereas those with a velocity of less than 3 m·sec^{-1} do not (maximal gradient under 36 mm Hg). The maximal jet velocity can be used to calculate peak and mean gradients and aortic valve area but there is little additional clinical value in doing so, except in the borderline cases with velocities between 3 and 4 m·sec^{-1}.

Adults with AS are asymptomatic until their disease is far advanced. Once symptoms develop, the prognosis without surgery is grim, e.g., 2 to 5 years with angina, 2 years with exercise-induced syncope, and 1 year or less once cardiac failure occurs. Aortic valve surgery is strongly recommended once symptoms develop. To prevent sudden death or myocardial problems, surgery is often recommended in AS patients prior to the development of

319

symptoms on the basis of deterioration shown by electrocardiography, cardiac enlargement, changes in wall thickness and ventricular function from ultrasonographic studies, reduced exercise capacity, detection of arrhythmias, a peak gradient measurement of over 50 mm Hg across the valve, or evidence of deteriorating left ventricular function in response to exercise.

Symptomatic AS patients are not candidates for exercise programs because of the danger of sudden death. Asymptomatic patients should be carefully screened before increasing their physical activity, and for most, exercise intensity should be mild.

Patients with mild or moderate degrees of AS may have a normal exercise capacity and an increase in $\dot{Q}$ during exercise that is in the lower range of normal. The peak gradient across the valve may increase by 20 to 50 mm Hg during exercise, with peak left ventricular pressures reaching 200 to 300 mm Hg. In moderate, fully compensated AS with normal high resting ejection fractions, exercise may lead to a fall in ejection fraction and changes in isovolumic contraction and relaxation, presumably because of subendocardial ischemia.[27]

In AS patients with impaired left ventricular function, left ventricular end-diastolic pressures are increased and $\dot{Q}$ fails to increase normally with exercise. Aortic blood pressure may not increase or may even fall with exercise, possibly leading to exercise-induced syncope. The rising end-diastolic pressure produces pulmonary congestion and dyspnea; the inadequate $\dot{Q}$ causes fatigue.

Coronary perfusion pressure is the pressure in the aorta; it may be 50 to 150 mm Hg below the intramyocardial tension during exercise in AS patients. This decrease in coronary perfusion pressure relative to the intramyocardial pressure, plus the hypertrophied myocardium with increased oxygen requirements, leads to subendocardial ischemia, despite widely patent coronary arteries. Angina occurring with exercise is a common symptom when the lesion is severe.

The mechanism of exercise-induced sudden death is uncertain. Marked cardiac slowing may occur with the severe increase in intramyocardial tension, leading to standstill or ventricular tachycardia and fibrillation.

Mitral Regurgitation

Scarring of the mitral valve after rheumatic fever once was the major cause of mitral regurgitation. Now other factors are more frequently involved, including congenital anomalies, myxomatous degeneration, mitral prolapse syndrome, papillary muscle dysfunction, chordal rupture, bacterial destruction, and annular disease. Mild mitral regurgitation produces no symptoms and no pressure changes in the heart. Life span may be unaffected and exercise capacity is normal.

Moderately severe mitral regurgitation leads to increased left atrial and left ventricular volumes. The V wave in the left atrial pressure curve is increased, but mean left atrial pressure is only slightly increased; pulmonary venous and arterial pressures are nearly normal. Exercise $\dot{Q}$ may be slightly below normal levels. Severe mitral regurgitation causes marked left atrial enlargement. The distensibility of the left atrial cavity may allow considerable valve leaks to occur without major increases in left atrial or pulmonary artery pressures. On the other hand, some patients have V waves in the left atrium of 40 to 60 mm Hg, as well as an elevation of mean left atrial pressures to 25 to 40 mm Hg. A volume overload on the left ventricle may be well tolerated for a number of years and left ventricular end-diastolic pressure may remain normal. This volume overload may overburden the left ventricle, with eventual elevation in left ventricular end-diastolic pressures and mean left atrial pressures. In turn, high left atrial pressures cause pulmonary venous congestion, elevation in pulmonary artery pressures, and dyspnea.

Mitral regurgitation increases when aortic blood pressure is increased, as during an isometric muscular contraction. Mitral regurgitation increases during isotonic exercise in part because of the increase in HR, i.e., the more time the heart spends in systole, the greater is the total volume of regurgitation. This increase may be offset to some degree by the reduction in peripheral resistance during light and moderate rhythmic exercise. Exercise performance is improved by such vasodilating drugs as hydralazine or captopril, which reduce the resistance to the left ventricular ejection via the aorta.

Patients with mitral regurgitation complain of dyspnea on exertion because of an increased left atrial pressure and of exercise-induced fatigue because of a reduced $\dot{Q}$. Atrial fibrillation frequently develops in patients with distended left atria secondary to longstanding mitral regurgitation, but these patients tolerate the fibrillation better than do patients with MS.

Surgery (usually valve replacement) is performed when symptoms become significant to the patient; if there is demonstrable deterioration in the patient's status (such as increasing heart size shown radiographically, decreasing exercise capacity, or cardiac arrhythmias); or if deteriorating ventricular function at rest or during exercise is demonstrated by nuclear scanning.

Serial exercise testing has some role in patient evaluation by objectively demonstrating a decrease in exercise performance. Exercise testing with the measurement of left ventricular ejection fraction by nuclear angiography has been found to be a sensitive, noninvasive method to assess left ventricular function.[7]

Mitral Valve Prolapse

The mitral valve prolapse syndrome is the most common of the valvular abnormalities, affecting as much as 10% of the population. In most instances, the condition is mild and is of little or no importance, but some patients with this syndrome are prone to exercise-induced arrhythmias. The common underlying cause of mitral prolapse is disruption of the collagen fibrils and myxomatous change in the chordae tendineae as they insert into the mitral valve leaflet. In the mildest cases, the valve bulges back into the left atrium in the last third of systole, producing a characteristic clicking noise in late systole, but no valve leak. A very mild, late systolic mitral leak develops as the next stage; the regurgitant volume is not sufficient to cause any hemodynamic change. Severe mitral regurgitation may occur in about 2% of cases of mitral prolapse.

Population surveys involving echocardiography yielded results that suggest a 6% incidence of mitral prolapse in healthy young men and 17% in young women, with 99% of these subjects being asymptomatic. Patients may report to the physician's office with palpitations, chest pain not resembling angina, angina-like pain, and anxiety. Whether the symptoms are related to the disease is often debatable. There has been a suggestion that these symptoms may be due to autonomic nervous system dysfunctions, which have been demonstrated in many of these patients.

Patients with mitral prolapse may have resting ventricular premature contractions or ventricular tachycardia. There is a high frequency of left atrial bypass conduction pathways or classical WPW syndrome. Paroxysmal tachycardia that is difficult to control may also occur.

In 24 consecutive cases of children with mitral valve prolapse seen in a cardiac clinic, Kavey et al. reported exercise-induced ventricular premature contractions in 27% of patients, with bigeminy in one subject, multifocal ventricular tachycardia in one subject, R-on-T wave in three subjects, and unifocal ventricular premature contractions in three other subjects.[21] In adults, potentially life-threatening arrhythmias occur in as many as 75% of patients, but these are a select series of patients with symptoms severe enough to precipitate referral to a major cardiac center. Holter monitoring is likely to show more arrhythmias than is exercise testing.[34]

Patients occasionally develop malignant rhythm disorders, and sudden death is a possible complication. There is a problem in giving exercise advice to these patients for whom the rhythm is not controlled by propranolol. It should be emphasized that most patients with mitral prolapse have mild forms of the lesion, and they can take part in all sports activities, including intense competitive sport.

Aortic Regurgitation

When cardiac systole ends, the aortic valve should completely prevent the flow of aortic blood back into the left ventricle. A leakage during diastole is referred to as aortic regurgitation or aortic insufficiency. The main causes of aortic regurgitation are congenital anomalies, rheumatic fever, and valve destruction from bacterial infection. Less common causes include syphilis, trauma, Marfan's syndrome, and rheumatoid spondylitis. Long-standing hypertension or aging can cause dilatation of the aortic root and mild aortic regurgitation. When aortic regurgitation develops gradually, the left ventricle compensates by both dilatation and enough hypertrophy to keep a normal ratio of wall thickness to cavity size. This compensation keeps the patients with significant aortic regurgitation almost asymptomatic for a number of years. Eventually, however, the left ventricle fails to stand up under the chronic overload, and symptoms of exertional and nocturnal dyspnea appear. Exertional angina in the absence of coronary artery narrowing may occur and is explained by the low coronary perfusion pressure in diastole, the increased muscle mass, and increased myocardial oxygen requirements.

Systolic blood pressure may be elevated to 140 to 170 mm Hg because of the large SV, and diastolic pressure is reduced to 30 or 40 mm Hg because the aortic valve does not sustain the diastolic aortic pressure. When measuring blood pressure by sphygmomanometry, brisk arterial sounds may be present down to zero cuff inflation, and an accurate diastolic pressure is not possible unless a clear muffling of the sounds is evident. This finding is particularly true with post-exercise pressure measurements.

Mild to moderate aortic regurgitation is well tolerated for years and patients can enjoy normal recreational pursuits. In moderate or severe degrees of aortic regurgitation, there is a gradual deterioration in left ventricular performance, and surgical intervention (aortic valve replacement) is indicated before the development of significant left ventricular impairment.

Aortic regurgitation occurs during diastole. Thus, there may be considerable reduction in the volume of the aortic valve leak when HR rises with exercise and total time in diastole is reduced. This situation accounts for the observation that patients with aortic regurgitation can have a nearly normal exercise capacity, despite having extremely hyperdynamic left ventricles, bounding peripheral pulses, and considerable cardiac enlargement. Patients with mild to moderate aortic regurgitation have a decrease in left ventricular end-diastolic volume during exercise, in keeping with the reduced regurgitant fraction that occurs with exercise.[19]

Asymptomatic patients with aortic regurgitation may show a reduced shortening fraction due to increased left ventricular systolic diameter during isometric exercise, as well as an increased SBP when compared to that of normal subjects.[16] Most patients with severe aortic regurgitation have reduced ejection fractions during exercise, but this sign is not the important prognostic factor as initially suspected, because surgical results can be excellent in these patients.[14] The significance of a reduction in left ventricular ejection fraction during exercise in patients with aortic regurgitation is related to several factors other than myocardial contractility alone, such as age, blood pressure change, and HR. By itself, a decrease rather than the expected increase in ejection fraction is not an indication for surgery.

At some stage, the left ventricle may be unable to compensate for the continuous volume overload of aortic regurgitation; left ventricular end-diastolic pressure then increases, further dilation occurs, and the ejection fraction starts to fall. At this stage, patients experience dyspnea, early fatigue, and excess sweating with exercise.

Isometric exercise increases peripheral resistance and the volume of aortic regurgitation, but this occurrence is not a particular worry in most patients. In patients with aortic regurgitation that is due to weakening of the aortic wall (as in the Marfan's or Ehlers-Danlos syndromes or syphilitic aortitis), all strenuous exercise should be avoided.

Tricuspid Valve Disease

Anatomic or functional tricuspid regurgitation occurs in patients with severe mitral valve disease. Such patients are usually not candidates for exercise testing or rehabilitation until after valve surgery. Tricuspid stenosis is uncommon.

Combined Valvular Lesions

Aortic and mitral valve lesions frequently occur together, causing an added hemodynamic burden. Patients with mitral regurgitation tolerate AS poorly because the increased left ventricular pressure caused by the AS increases the volume of mitral regurgitation. Patients with combined mitral and aortic regurgitation do poorly because aortic blood leaks back into the left atrium. Mitral stenosis limits left ventricular filling and $\dot{Q}$, and may diminish the signs of aortic valve disease.

Hemodynamic Change Common To All Valvular Disease

When valvular disease becomes severe, the heart is unable to maintain $\dot{Q}$ at the level usually required to perform a given activity; SV either fails to increase or falls as HR increases, and blood pressure tends to fall. The body compensates for the low $\dot{Q}$ by vasoconstriction in those organs not vital for the immediate performance, e.g., gut and viscera, kidney, skin, and nonexercising muscles. At light exercise loads, a greater proportion of the limited $\dot{Q}$ goes to the working muscles. Oxygen is almost completely removed from blood traversing the working muscles in patients with restricted $\dot{Q}$; pO_2 falls to under 8 mm Hg

and the oxygen saturation is reduced to less than 5% in the venous effluent, even at low work loads. This nearly complete oxygen extraction from the working muscles, plus the reduced blood flow to the nonworking parts, leads to very low oxygen levels in mixed venous (pulmonary artery) blood, and pulmonary artery oxygen saturation falls to 15 to 20% at low work loads. This more complete oxygen extraction allows the exercise to proceed despite the low $\dot{Q}$, but it is a compensatory mechanism that has considerable limitation and does not permit high work levels.

Exercise and Heart Failure

Heart failure is the end-stage of many forms of heart disease, including hypertensive heart disease, coronary artery disease, primary cardiomyopathy, and overload from valvular and congenital heart problems. Heart failure is defined as the inability of the heart to meet the requirements of the person, or as the inability to do so at normal cardiac filling pressures. Congestive heart failure (CHF) patients have congestion of neck veins, lungs, and liver, as well as fluid retention due to impaired heart function.

In the past, CHF patients have been advised to rest and avoid all exercise except that required for subsistence living; CHF also was a relative contraindication for exercise testing. In the past 5 years, there have been hundreds of exercise studies in patients with compensated heart failure. The word compensated implies that they are stable (usually on medication), they have no current lung congestion, they are not short of breath at rest, and they have no peripheral edema (often because they avoid salt and take diuretics).

At rest, these patients have a low $\dot{Q}$, a wide arteriovenous oxygen difference, a low SV, a reduced rate of ventricular ejection, and a high left ventricular end-diastolic pressure. Blood pressure may be normal, and peripheral vascular resistance is raised. Resting HR is in the range of 85 to 100 beats $\cdot$ min^{-1} and atrial fibrillation may be present. With exercise, working capacity is reduced, often to below 5 METs, exercise $\dot{Q}$ is low but usually increases above resting, and ejection fraction can either decrease, remain unchanged, or increase. Maximal exercise HR often is considerably diminished. Stroke volume most commonly decreases with exercise. End-diastolic pressure and pulmonary artery capillary wedge pressure and mean pulmonary artery pressures increase.

The patient often stops exercise because of dyspnea, which is related to the increasing pulmonary capillary wedge pressure, increasing lung fluid, and stimulation of lung "J" receptors. Respiration is rapid. Generally, there has not been a close correlation between hemodynamic measures and limitation of exercise, leading to other hypotheses to explain the exercise limitation.

Muscle blood flow is reduced at rest and during exercise in patients with heart failure, and muscle vessels do not dilate normally in response to exercise. Patients who vasodilate better than others with exercise may have higher exercise capacities. Muscles in the CHF patient rely to a greater extent on the glycolytic pathways during exercise, and muscle fibers may show signs of atrophy. These factors may lead to early fatigue, which is the other symptom that limits exercise performance.

Patients with cardiac impairment have slower $\dot{V}_{O_2}$ kinetics, perhaps because of the low $\dot{Q}$, which fails to deliver oxygen to the tissues. Tissue extraction of the oxygen that does reach the muscles is increased by the slow transit time and a shift of the oxyhemoglobin dissociation curve to the right because of acid metabolites.

To sustain work activity, patients must work below their anaerobic threshold, as measured using breath-to-breath gas exchange measurements or by direct determination of arterial lactate. Work protocols to measure anaerobic threshold in impaired subjects using the gas exchange method must increase work intensity at a rate sufficient to increase the rate of lactate production, but not at a rate that will fatigue the subject so rapidly that a break in the ventilation slope cannot be recognized.

Maximal oxygen uptake is a defined physiologic end point. It is the $\dot{V}_{O_2max}$ the patient can attain and is reached only when it can be shown that a further increase in exercise workload fails to increase $\dot{V}_{O_2}$ above a minimal defined amount. In cardiac patients, it is often unwise to encourage exercise to the point of truly achieving $\dot{V}_{O_2max}$, and such terms as peak $\dot{V}_{O_2}$ or symptom-limited $\dot{V}_{O_2max}$ should be used instead of $\dot{V}_{O_2max}$.

Early in exercise, subjects with impaired cardiac function have a slow increase in oxygen utilization, but a rapid increase in CO_2 output and an increase in the respiratory exchange ratio.

The reduction in systemic blood flow in chronic heart failure leads to vasoconstriction (mediated by adrenergic nerves, circulating norepinephrine, angiotensin II, and vasopressin) and to reduced blood flow to the kidney, gut, skin, and limbs.

Patients with heart failure are currently treated with such angiotensin converting enzyme (ACE) inhibitors as captopril or enalapril to reduce peripheral resistance, decrease lung congestion, improve other hemodynamic parameters, and allow more exercise with fewer symptoms in the majority of patients. Life may be prolonged in many patients, and the fear of difficult breathing is controlled. There is immediate improvement in central hemodynamics. ACE inhibitors can dramatically improve the CHF in patients with mitral and/or aortic insufficiency.

Although $\dot{V}_{O_2max}$ is often not immediately improved by ACE inhibitors, lessening of symptoms allows the patients to walk and exercise more. This eventually leads to an improvement in muscle function and a subsequent improvement in exercise performance, including $\dot{V}_{O_2max}$ and anaerobic threshold. There have been various reports of training programs in patients with CHF, with modest gains in peak $\dot{V}_{O_2}$ of 3 to 4 ml$\cdot$kg$^{-1}\cdot$min^{-1}.

Exercise testing now has a place in monitoring the safety and effectiveness of low-intensity exercise activities in patients with heart failure due to various causes. It was felt previously that exercise testing had no or limited value in the assessment and management of these patients. Anaerobic threshold and time-related changes in $\dot{V}_{O_2}$ are not frequently measured outside the research laboratory at present. In training programs for patients with significant cardiac impairment, it is useful to allow them to monitor a safe work intensity with instructions to carry on with exercise as long as breathing allows them to continue a conversation or using a modified Borg scale with such descriptive terms as "somewhat hard." In these patients with marked myocardial damage and very limited cardiac reserve, it may not be useful to have a target HR (it can be as low as 10 beats·min^{-1} above the resting value) or to know a safe workload based on the ECG because the ECG may show severe changes at rest or there may be a left bundle-branch block. In any exercise test situation, the exercise loading must be low (e.g., treadmill stages requiring only 2, 3, 4, or 5 METs, or cycle ergometer stages requiring 20, 30, or 40 watts).

There is often a poor correlation between treadmill work time and severity of heart disease as measured by ejection fraction, end-diastolic pressure, pulmonary artery pressure, or heart size (by radiologic or ultrasonographic methods). Whether a person can perform useful physical work depends on the delivery of oxygen to the mitochondria in the working muscles and on whether the circulation can maintain the internal environment of these mitochondria. These latter functions are related as much to circulation in the tissues as they are to the output of the heart. The only way to measure what the patient can do is to have objective measures of exercise function whether the problem is CHD, primary myocardial disease, or valvular heart disease.

Association of Valvular Heart Disease with Coronary Heart Disease

Angina can occur in patients with AS or aortic regurgitation in the absence of obstructive lesions of the coronary arteries. When this situation occurs, the valvular disease is usually severe. Because ischemic-type ST changes can be observed in the exercise ECG of these patients in the absence of CHD, routine exercise testing does not assist in the detection of CHD in these patients. Thallium scanning may be of value, and most patients selected for valvular surgery have coronary angiography to determine whether coronary bypass and valve replacement should be performed at the same time.

Anginal pain may occur in patients with MS but these individuals usually have severe MS and pulmonary hypertension. If the MS is mild or moderate, coincident coronary artery lesions are likely present if angina is noted.

CHD may be the cause of mitral regurgitation on the basis of papillary muscle dysfunction or chordae rupture, i.e., previous infarction may have occurred. Exercise testing may reveal ischemic ECG changes or produce anginal pain that is not expected on the basis of the degree of mitral regurgitation present, leading to strong suspicion of CHD. Patients with the mitral prolapse syndrome may have various types of chest pain (including pain that mimics angina) and may exhibit exercise ECG changes typical for ischemia in the absence of anatomic narrowing of the coronary arteries.

The patient whose heart is overworked because of a mechanical problem with the valves has need of a larger than normal coronary blood flow. The presence of CHD does not contraindicate valve replacement surgery; rather, the presence of CHD may be an added indication that surgery should be performed. Aggressive management would include the completion of coronary bypass during and in addition to valvular surgery.

EXERCISE TESTING

Functional Capacity of Patients with Valvular Disease

For many years, cardiologists have used the New York Heart Association (NYHA) grading system to classify patients as to functional capacity. This classification system is based on the appreciation of symptoms by the patient (Table 18–1) and the care with which the history is obtained.

Patterson et al. suggest that Class 4 patients have $\dot{V}_{O_2max}$ values below 12 $ml \cdot kg^{-1} \cdot min^{-1}$ (3.5 METs); Class 3 patients have values in the range of 10 to 16 $ml \cdot kg^{-1} \cdot min^{-1}$ (3 to 5 METs); Class 2 patients have $\dot{V}_{O_2max}$ values between 16 and 23 $ml \cdot kg^{-1} \cdot min^{-1}$ (4.5 to 7 METs); and Class 1 patients have values above 23 $ml \cdot kg^{-1} \cdot min^{-1}$ (or greater than 7 METs).[30] The NYHA classification system does not differentiate between patients who are asymptomatic with a sedentary lifestyle and a $\dot{V}_{O_2max}$ of 24 $ml \cdot kg^{-1} \cdot min^{-1}$ and those who are super fit, with a $\dot{V}_{O_2max}$ of over 60 $ml \cdot kg^{-1} \cdot min^{-1}$. The system is designed mainly to assess disease severity in patients whose functional capacity varies from being able to walk at moderate speed without symptoms to being bedridden.[29]

Some patients deny all symptoms, yet they have severe disease and very low exercise capacities. These individuals subconsciously or consciously reduce their activities so that symptoms do not occur.

Value of Exercise Tests

Although exercise testing is not of diagnostic value in patients with valvular heart disease, considerable information can be provided by a graded exercise test continued until symptoms occur. The purposes and values of such a test in these patients follow.

1. Provide an objective evaluation of exercise capacity.
2. Use exercise capacity to counsel patients concerning occupational and recreational physical activities and rehabilitation.
3. Observe the patient when symptoms are present and evaluate exercise symptoms of dyspnea, fatigue, cough, weakness, dizziness, and palpitation.
4. Observe cardiac rhythm during and after exercise; modify anti-arrhythmic treatment based on the response, if necessary.
5. Monitor any deterioration or improvement with serial testing. Use the results to advise the patient concerning the need for surgical intervention or a change in medical management.
6. Objectively evaluate surgical treatment or changes in medical treatment.
7. Assess the need for cardiac catheterization, surgery, or a regimen of rhythm-controlling drugs.
8. Evaluate chest pain in patients with valvular disease and the possibility of associated CHD.
9. Evaluate the possibility of associated peripheral vascular disease and claudication as factors limiting exercise.
10. Use exercise in the physician's examining room to augment cardiac murmurs.

TABLE 18–1. **Functional Classification—New York Heart Association***

Class	Description
0	No heart disease.
I	Patients with heart disease but without limitation of physical activity. "Ordinary" physical activity does not cause undue fatigue, palpitation, dyspnea, or anginal pain.
II	Patients with heart disease resulting in slight limitation of physical activity. "Ordinary" physical activity results in fatigue, palpitation, dyspnea, or anginal pain.
III	Patients with heart disease resulting in marked limitation of physical activity. Less than ordinary activity brings on symptoms.
IV	Patients with cardiac disease unable to carry out any physical activity without discomfort. Symptoms may be present at rest.

* Adapted from Pardee.[29]

11. Assess ventricular function during exercise with nuclear angiography.
12. Assess myocardial perfusion during exercise with thallium scanning.

In some medical circles, there is a curious attitude toward the objective assessment of a patient's functional capacity. In one report, as recent as 1976, concerning a simple noninvasive, symptom-limited ergometer test before and after valve replacement, there is the comment, "All the patients agreed to perform the exercise test after it had been explained to them that it did not form part of the normal investigation or management of their disease."[15] An objective measurement of functional capacity should be a routine part of care, for how else can the patient be completely evaluated and how else can the results of medical or surgical treatment be objectively assessed? Measurements of working capacity should be used by physicians giving advice on employability or on degrees of impairment.

Termination of Exercise Tests

Exercise is usually stopped in patients with valvular disease for the same reason as it is in healthy adults. Patients continue exercise until they wish to stop because of dyspnea or fatigue. It is usually safe to have the patient continue until the respiratory distress is obvious and the patient communicates the desire to stop. It should be emphasized that pulmonary edema can be produced by exercising beyond a certain point in these patients, particularly those persons with MS. Pulmonary congestion induced by exercise may cause coughing rather than dyspnea, and exercise should cease if the coughing becomes significant.

Fatigue, weakness, and pallor are signs of an inadequate $\dot{Q}$ for the demands of the exercise. These signs and symptoms are partly subjective, although the patient in distress is easily recognized. It is a judgment decision as to how far to allow these patients to continue exercise.

Chest pain in patients with rheumatic heart disease can be worrisome, because it may indicate myocardial ischemia or pulmonary hypertension, or it may be an unimportant symptom arising from the chest wall. Signs of inadequate cerebral blood flow (severe facial pallor, confusion, dizziness, and unsteady gait) may occur in patients with valvular disease and are indications to terminate a test. ST depression occurs frequently in patients with valvular disease. These patients frequently receive digitalis preparations, which accentuate or cause ST depressions. I do not recommend termination of an exercise test on the basis of even 0.4 to 0.5 mV ST depression in patients with aortic or mitral regurgitation, when symptoms are absent, the patient appears well, and the test observer has considerable experience in exercising patients with serious valvular disease. In the patient with AS that clinically may be of major degree, a major ST change could be a sign to stop the test. Some laboratory personnel may wish to stop all exercise tests when ST depression is greater than 0.1 to 0.2 mV.

The appearance of certain arrhythmias is another indication to stop an exercise test in patients with rheumatic valvular disease, but the exact criteria used for termination may differ from one laboratory to another and from one patient to another. There should be greater concern for the AS patient than for patients with other valve abnormalities. The rhythm criteria that indicate that an exercise test should be halted may be the same as those recommended in patients with suspect CHD.

Although increasing numbers of premature ventricular contractions (PVC) may be used as a signal to stop an exercise test, the choice of a number (i.e., more than 15 per minute or more than one every four sinus beats) is arbitrary. I have continued exercise in many patients after bigeminal rhythm has appeared, because this arrhythmia seems to be benign and often disappears after HR increases.

Multifocal PVCs are another relative indication to discontinue a test. Many patients, however, may have a few PVCs of differing morphology at light exercise loads and can continue exercising without worsening of the arrhythmia. When such a rhythm appears at a low work load that is easily tolerated by the patient, it seems reasonable to continue the test. This recommendation is especially valid if the patient is active and it is likely that equal or greater physical tasks are performed as part of the daily routine.

The same situation is true for occasional short runs of ventricular tachycardia. In a patient with significant AS, any couplet of ventricular ectopics is cause for worry, and three or more sequential PVCs should be a firm indication to stop the test. On the other hand, in a younger patient with mild mitral regurgitation and especially in patients with the mitral valve prolapse syndrome, frequent short runs (3 to 10 beats) of ventricular tachycardia are experienced without any serious problems. If the purpose of the test is to measure the patient's maximal exercise capacity, the hemodynamic impairment due to a valvular lesion, and the possible dangers of near-maximal work, premature termination because of arbitrary arrhythmia criteria negates that purpose. This discussion is not meant to underplay the potential seriousness of PVCs; the safety of the patient must be the major concern in any exercise laboratory.

Patients with valvular disease may develop atrial fibrillation during an exercise test. Ventricular rate generally is rapid and the test should be terminated. The same maxim holds true for the appearance of supraventricular tachycardia or atrial flutter. These arrhythmias may be transient or prolonged and require cardioversion.

Patients with aortic valve disease may develop left bundle-branch block (LBBB) on exercise. Listed by some authors as an indication to terminate a test, this is a relative indication. If LBBB appears with light exercise and the patient is in no distress, the test can be continued. If the patient is active and frequently exercises at a higher intensity than the load producing the LBBB, then early termination seems unnecessary and negates the value of the test. The same patient may experience in-termittent LBBB at rest, in that the intraventricular conduction problem may be rate dependent.

The appearance of second degree atrio-ventricular block during exercise when atrioventricular conduction was normal at rest is another relative indication to terminate a test. If ventricular rate is adequate and the patient exhibits no distress, the test may be continued with caution.

Many patients with valvular heart disease have resting arrhythmias. Frequent PVCs are not a contraindication to beginning a test, because useful information can be obtained by observing the exercise response. As in normal subjects, the PVCs most commonly decrease or disappear as HR increases with exercise. Another common arrhythmia in patients with valvular disease, particularly mitral disease, at rest is atrial fibrillation. The resting ventricular rate may be well controlled and fairly regular, the resting rate may be as high as 150 or 170 beats·min^{-1}, or there may be extreme variability in the R-R intervals. In patients with a resting HR that exceeds 130 beats·min^{-1}, the exercise test is best postponed until the ventricular rate is better controlled. When the resting ventricular rate is controlled (with or without medication), exercise in the patient with atrial fibrillation may cause abrupt increases in rate that are quite striking, e.g., the rate may jump from 70 beats·min^{-1} at rest to 180 or 190 beats·min^{-1} with the first stage of a multistage test. Nevertheless, the patient may be able to continue exercising for another two stages, reaching maximal rates of 200 to 260 beats·min^{-1}. The patient with atrial fibrillation that has an inappropriately rapid HR response to light exercise may benefit from cautious increases in digoxin dose or from the addition of low doses of a beta blocking agent or verapamil.[22] Exercise testing is of value when monitoring these patients. Conversion to a sinus rhythm in these patients with DC cardioversion or quinidine leads to considerable reduction in exercise HR, and exercise capacity can be significantly improved.[31]

The patient with atrial flutter at rest should exercise with caution. At first examination, atrial flutter may seem to be a sinus or a junctional rhythm, particularly if only one ECG lead is used (i.e., lead CM5). The ventricular rate may be well controlled at 60, 75, or 100 beats·min^{-1} because of 5:1, 4:1, or 3:1 atrioventricular conduction blocks. The ventricular rate may suddenly increase during exercise, with the lessening or even the complete disappearance of the block. These very rapid ventricular rates are poorly tolerated by the patient with severe MS or AS, and are especially dangerous in patients with associated CHD.

Maximal Heart Rate

Patients with mild rheumatic valvular disease who have normal or near normal exercise capacities usually have a maximal HR in the same range as normal (220 minus age in years, with a standard deviation of 12). Patients with symptomatic valvular disease usually have a maximal HR that is about 20 or 30 beats·min^{-1} below the expected value. The possibility of a reduced maximal HR invalidates the prediction of $\dot{V}_{O_2max}$ by using submaximal power outputs and HR, and makes uncertain the use of HR to establish whether patients exercise close to their maximum.

ST Changes in the Exercise Electrocardiogram

ST depression is observed in the exercise ECG of as many as 50% of patients with valvular heart disease in the absence of associated CHD. In patients with coronary arteries that appear normal angiographically, Aronow and Harris found "ischemic" ST changes in 37% of AS patients and in 20% of MS patients during submaximal treadmill exercise.[2] The presence of ST depression in the exercise ECG is of no value in making a positive diagnosis of associated CHD in patients with valvular heart disease. On the other hand, a normal ST segment in the exercise ECG of a patient with valvular disease should give reasonable assurance of the integrity of the coronary circulation, especially if

exercise capacity is nearly normal. ST segment depression may be an indication of strained myocardial function. ST depression in the exercise ECG of patients with aortic regurgitation indicates a greater likelihood of reduced rest and exercise ejection fraction as well as increased end-systolic wall stress and diameter.[25]

Many patients with valvular heart disease receive digitalis preparations, and ST segment changes may be caused by this drug, rather than by any hemodynamic or myocardial factor. The cause of exercise-induced ST depression in patients who are not receiving digitalis is unknown. It is commonly assumed with exercise that relative ischemia may occur in the hypertrophied myocardium or in the myocardium having a greater wall tension. Although ST changes occur more commonly in patients with severe disease who soon require valve surgery, this point is not always valid.

P-wave changes also occur during exercise in patients with valvular disease, with increased voltage or increased degree of bifid P waves. Q-wave and R-wave voltage changes occur in different directions than normal, but do not have enough consistency to be of clinical value.

Exercise Capacity and Severity of Valve Lesions

Exercise capacity measurements provide only a gross assessment of the severity of the hemodynamic derangement associated with valvular heart disease. Not surprisingly, the exercise tolerance of patients with AS or MS and valve areas less than 1 cm^2 is significantly less than that of patients with valve areas over 1 cm^2. The correlations, however, between pulmonary artery pressure, wedge pressure, valve gradient, resting cardiac index, left ventricular end-diastolic pressure, or ejection fraction and the objective measurements of exercise tolerance are surprisingly low. Good performance on a treadmill test does not necessarily indicate that the patient has mild valvular disease or that surgery is not advisable. Similarly, poor performance on a treadmill test does not necessarily indicate that the valvular disease is severe and that surgery is indicated. There are many reasons for these correlations.

Body build is an important determinant of exercise capacity, expressed as treadmill endurance time, $\dot{V}_{O_2max}$ per kilogram body weight, or maximal ergometer power output per kilogram of body weight. The lean subject with severe valve disease may score higher in fitness than the fat subject with a mild valvular lesion.

Some patients with valvular disease avoid physical activity as much as possible; they never exercise to the point of dyspnea and stop in the middle of an exercise test with the first symptoms of fatigue, breathlessness, or muscular discomfort. These symptoms appear at light loads in subjects unaccustomed to any physical activity, regardless of the severity of the valvular disease. Other more stoic patients force themselves to remain on the job, they ignore mild or even severe symptoms of fatigue and dyspnea, and are willing to continue an exercise test despite moderately severe symptoms that are everyday experiences to them. Therefore, tolerance to symptoms and current exercise habits are important determinants of performance in a progressive exercise test.

The status of the myocardium is another important variable in exercise impairment relative to valvular heart disease. Severe aortic regurgitation is well tolerated for many years until myocardial weakness occurs. In all forms of heart disease, the healthy myocardium can compensate for the hemodynamic burden imposed by mechanical faults, and can maintain the systemic blood flow at near normal levels. In patients with myocardial disease or associated CHD, this compensation is not possible, and patients have lower exercise capacities, regardless of the severity of the valvular problem.

Other variables that influence exercise capacity include changes in pulmonary circulation and lung diffusion; blood hemoglobin concentration; cardiac rhythm; total blood volume and its changes with diuretic drugs; regional blood flow in the exercising muscles; and metabolic factors in the muscles. With all of these variables, we should not be disappointed that such gross measurements as $\dot{V}_{O_2max}$ or treadmill endurance time fail to provide even a rough assessment of the function of a heart valve. With the exercise test, only the capacity of the patient to perform that specific exercise at the time of testing can be assessed.

Improvement in Symptoms After Surgery and in Functional Capacity

History alone does not reliably indicate whether a given therapeutic intervention has produced an improvement in functional capacity, even when the intervention is as dramatic as a heart operation, because patients tend to overestimate their improvement. The lack of correlation between subjective improvement in exercise symptoms and objective improvement in exercise capacity was reported by Bergy and Bruce in 1955 for closed mitral commissurotomy.[4] They reported that only 16 of 31 subjects improved in fitness measurements, whereas 29 of the 31 individuals reported subjective improvement.[4]

Work Classification and Rheumatic Heart Disease

The exercise stage that the subject can reach *without* significant symptoms of fatigue and blood pressure or ECG changes allows some guide to occupational capabilities. Table 18–2 is a list of the four general work classifications, the approximate $\dot{V}_{O_2}$ required for each work classification, and the equivalent exercise intensity in the laboratory. As an example, to do light work, the subject should be able to do Stage I of the Bruce protocol without symptoms, and an 80-kg man should be able to work at 400 kpm·min^{-1} on the ergometer.

VALVE SURGERY

Valve Replacements

Mechanical valves in current use include the Starr-Edwards cloth-covered

TABLE 18-2. **Work Classification.**

Class	Examples	Oxygen Requirement $(\text{ml} \cdot \text{kg}^{-1} \cdot \text{min}^{-1})$	Bruce Treadmill Stage	Bicycle Ergometer $(\text{kpm} \cdot \text{min}^{-1})$	
				55 kg	80 kg
I (Sedentary)	Desk work Clerical	7	0 grade	80	120
	Housework Hospital			280	400
II (Light)	Retail sales	14	Stage I		
	Light industry		Stage II	440	640
III (Medium)	Agriculture Light construction	20	(1-2 min)		
	Mining Heavy industry			630	920
IV (Heavy)	Forestry Dock work	27	Stage III (1-2 min)		

valve, available since 1974; the Starr-Edwards model 6120 with a silastic-ball prosthesis available since 1966; the Bjork-Shiley valves available since 1969 and subsequently, the St. Jude valves and others. Problems with these valves include the need for life-long anticoagulant therapy (with warfarin) to prevent thrombosis on the valve, embolism, or both, as well as a variable degree of obstruction because of the ball or disc sitting in the valve orifice. Mechanical failures have been virtually eliminated, except for one unfortunate model of the Bjork-Shiley valve.

Bioprostheses include porcine or pericardial valves (Hancock and Carpentier-Edwards) and cadaver aortic homografts. The bioprostheses have definite immediate advantages over the mechanical prostheses in that anticoagulation is not necessary for patients with aortic bioprostheses or for patients with mitral prostheses and sinus rhythm. In addition, the valve orifices are larger. Unfortunately, bioprostheses may fail and they do so at an accelerated rate in young patients. It is estimated that if inserted at age 10 years, 50% of bioprosthetic valves will have failed by age 20 years, whereas if inserted at age 65 years, only 15% will have failed at age 75 years. Controversy still exists as to the best valve to use in any given patient.[23]

The valve orifice for mechanical prostheses may be narrow enough to cause significant pressure gradients at the rate of blood flow encountered with vigorous exercise.[13] With a $\dot{Q}$ of 15 $\text{L} \cdot \text{min}^{-1}$, the Angell-Shiley valve in the mitral position will have a pressure gradient of 22 mm Hg. The Bjork-Shiley valve in the aortic position will cause a peak gradient of about 50 mm Hg at a $\dot{Q}$ of 10 $\text{L} \cdot \text{min}^{-1}$. Some of the older valves and some of the smaller valve sizes may lead to valve gradients of up to 35 mm Hg in the mitral position and 75 mm Hg in the aortic position during vigorous exercise.[5,33]

Bioprostheses are much superior in this regard. In the mitral position, the Hancock valve leads to a gradient of only 12 mm Hg at a $\dot{Q}$ of 15 $\text{L} \cdot \text{min}^{-1}$. With the 21 to 23-mm size Carpentier-Edwards bioprostheses in the aortic position, Chaitman et al. found peak gradients of only 10 mm Hg at a $\dot{Q}$ of 12 $\text{L} \cdot \text{min}^{-1}$.[9] The same make of valve in the mitral position allowed a 4-mm gradient at a $\dot{Q}$ of 6.8 $\text{L} \cdot \text{min}^{-1}$, but smaller bioprostheses in the mitral position were associated with mitral gradients as high as 30 mm Hg. These figures indicate that certain types and sizes of valves cause significant obstruction at blood flow rates encountered during strenuous exercise.

Doppler Study of Prosthetic Valves

Nearly all prosthetic valves have a trivial to mild degree of insufficiency on color-flow Doppler examination. Moderate to severe insufficiency indicates valve malfunction. The aortic valve is more easily assessed than is the mitral valve. It may be necessary in some cases to use the transesophageal route to assess the mitral valve. All prosthetic valves cause some degree of narrowing, and the peak instantaneous pressure gradient can be measured by using continuous-wave Doppler technology. Normally functioning prosthetic valves have a wide range of gradients (10 to 40 mm Hg) for the same size and valve mode. Postexercise gradients may reach 75 mm Hg with normally functioning prostheses.

Ballooning of Valvular Stenosis

Mitral stenosis can currently be managed by percutaneous ballooning, sometimes delaying indefinitely the need for various surgical interventions. When the mitral valve is pliable, noncalcified, and without a major subvalvular component, excellent long-term results follow ballooning. In valves that are calcified with considerable rigidity extending into the subvalve area, ballooning is more controversial, but major improvement can still be expected in 70% of patients. Ballooning for AS is less successful because by the time intervention is necessary, the valves are heavily calcified and do not readily split or stretch. This treatment for AS is reserved for the elderly and frail who may not tolerate valve surgery. After uncomplicated valve ballooning, a return to normal activities is possible within 5 to 7 days.

Exercise After Valve Replacement

Severe AS causes marked left ventricular hypertrophy, which may persist for some years after aortic valve replacement; a gradual reduction in left ventricular mass occurs over 2 or 3 years. The exercise-induced symptoms of angina and light-headedness or syncope disappear immediately after valve replacement. Easy fatiguability with exercise is related to muscular weakness and should lessen with increased physical activity. Dyspnea on exertion is relative, and if left ventricular function improves after valve replacement, this symptom should improve, with greater exercise capacity and less dyspnea for a given amount of exercise.

Valve replacement or effective palliative valve surgery for severe MS immediately eliminates the congestive changes in the lungs as left atrial pressure falls toward normal levels. There should be an immediate improvement in exercise capacity, a reduced ventilatory effort for a given power output, and less dyspnea. Pathologic changes in the lungs and in the right ventricle may take several years to resolve.

Functional Capacity After Valve Surgery

The improvement in functional capacity after valve surgery is related to many interdependent factors. For example, how severe were the symptoms before surgery? Many patients avoided symptoms by staying away from precipitating events, including physical activity. Was the surgery done before or after severe myocardial changes occurred? How reversible was the myocardial deterioration, if present? Is cardiac arrhythmia present after surgery? Does the arrhythmia cause a problem during exercise, such as an unusually rapid ventricular rate with atrial fibrillation or ventricular tachycardia? Is there disease of the other valves and how does this respond to the valve replacement?

Mild to moderate mitral regurgitation may be benefited by aortic valve surgery, because the left ventricular load is reduced. Moderate aortic valve disease may become of greater importance after mitral valve replacement for severe MS, because left ventricular SV is increased. Was there associated CHD and was this treated? How much functional overlay is there? Does the patient wish to retire, regardless of how good the heart is after surgery? Are exercise capacity tests performed poorly to allow favorable disability income rulings?

Rehabilitation Programs

After valve replacement, many patients get into the normal swing of life (including occupations that require moderate physical work) and into leisure time sports activities or personal fitness programs without any formal effort at rehabilitation programs. Gradual walking programs can be carried out by these patients at home 10 to 30 days after surgery as well as it can be done in a rehabilitation center.

Many subjects gain confidence and improve more rapidly with structured exercise programs, and may enroll in programs designed primarily for patients after a myocardial infarction or coronary bypass surgery. In some centers, all postoperative heart patients are routinely encouraged to enroll in rehabilitation programs, regardless of the type of heart disease; this practice is especially important for those patients unwilling to carry on with home programs.

Important aspects of all rehabilitation programs are the patients' mental attitudes and compliance rates. Hellerstein et al. compared a number of variables in two subgroups of patients with CHD and rheumatic heart disease who attended a work classification clinic.[18] Both groups showed similar attitudes toward death, life, physicians, work attitude, activity, and fellow workers, and there were no important differences. On the whole, both patient groups viewed themselves as self-sufficient and were optimistic that they could lead normal lives. Both groups had similar results in Minnesota multiphasic personality index (MMPI) tests. There was an excess of depression in both groups, but a larger number of the CHD subjects seemed preoccupied with symptoms and sudden death.

EXERCISE PROGRAMS

Results in Patients Without an Operation

The mechanical function of a valve will not improve with exercise. Exercise programs should be able to improve the working capacity of the skeletal muscles, if these were a limiting factor, and might improve patient confidence concerning physical activity. The results of exercise programs in unoperated patients have not been too impressive. For example, Rulli et al. evaluated 37 rheumatic valvular disease patients, aged 19 to 38 years, with a progressive exercise test. Work load was increased by 10 W·min^{-1} until fatigue.[32] According to the NYHA functional classification, 9 subjects were Class I, 26 were Class II, and only 2 were Class III. There was no significant improvement in mean maximal power output after 5 to 6 weeks of a training regimen of 4 to 5 days per week, working for 5 minutes at 50% of the maximal load and at 70% of the maximal load until the maximal HR was reached. Submaximal and maximal HR decreased and oxygen pulse increased.

Anderson and Zohman had five MS patients perform 5 minutes of supine bicycle exercise every other day for 5 weeks.[1] Mean oxygen pulse (ml·beat^{-1}) increased from 5.2 to 5.7 in the first week, but increased only insignificantly, to 5.9, over the next 4 weeks. In a study by Auchincloss and Gilbert, seven women with rheumatic heart disease exercised daily for 30 to 60 minutes for 8 days.[3] There was no resultant increase in $\dot{V}_{O_2max}$, but endurance time for treadmill walking at 2 mph (with the grade increasing at a rate of 6%·min^{-1}) increased from 2.3 to 2.7 minutes. The authors attributed the change to familiarity with the test and motivational factors.

Results of these short-term training investigations do not rule out the possibility that significant improvement in submaximal working capacity can be brought about by long-range, systematic increases in physical activity in previously sedentary subjects with rheumatic valvular disease.

Possible Adverse Effects

The acute problems of exercise (cardiac arrhythmia, anginal pain, acute heart failure and pulmonary edema, and exercise-induced hypotension or syncope) are not specific for patients with valvular disease. The effects of chronic exercise are not really known. Will a person with mild or moderate valvular disease increase the rate of valvular fibrosis and calcification by chronic, intense sport training? Does the myocardium that is already under a chronic overload because of the mechanical handicap of the valve lesion have a greater chance of developing fibrosis or excess dilatation if the patient exercises frequently to the point of severe dyspnea and manifestation of other symptoms? Will enlargement of the heart proceed at a more rapid rate in someone with a significant valve problem who exercises vigorously? What is the optimal amount of daily exercise for these patients? Would they be better off doing nothing more vigorous than walking? Will atrial stretching and hence atrial fibrillation occur sooner in patients who push themselves to do physical work or in those who purposely avoid any physical activity that might cause fatigue or dyspnea? Answers to these questions are not available.

Patients with the hemodynamic burden of a malfunctioning valve who increase their physical activity need to be watched for signs of incipient heart failure, which can be caused by exercise loads in a heart with a borderline level of function. Slight puffiness of the ankles at the end of the day, nocturia, mild nocturnal dyspnea, unexpected weight gain, or more than the usual amount of fatigue can be minor symptoms that are passed over unless specifically sought. Obviously, there comes a point when the myocardium is almost fully taxed by the hemodynamic overload from the valve malfunction, and the additional strain from participation in an exercise program is unwise.

CONGENITAL HEART DISEASE IN ADULTS

Ninety percent of children born with a congenital heart defect will survive to adult years, either because the lesion did not cause a significant problem or because medical and surgical treatment allowed survival. About 7 adults of every 1000 will have, or have had, a congenital heart defect. Some adults are still found to have a cardiac defect that was present since birth but has remained unrecognized until even age 60 years or later. Lesions for which this possibility exists are listed in Table 18–3. Atrial septal defect is by far the most common lesion in this category, and accounts for 50% of congenital heart defects reported in adults.

Unfortunately, some congenital cardiac defects cannot be corrected or can be only partially corrected surgically. Many of these patients, with or without surgical palliation, can survive into their adult years. Most of these patients have very limited exercise capacities and are not usually candidates for exercise programs.

Many of the patients with significant congenital heart disease who have had surgery performed during infancy or childhood have residual hemodynamic problems; the lesions and these problems are listed in Table 18–4. The exercise pathophysiology is the same in these adults as it is in children, except that myocardial reserve may be less; exercise blood pressure is often greater; exercise capacity may be low because of years of physical inactivity; and rhythm disturbances occur more frequently. The older patient who has had surgery for congenital heart disease is more subject to malignant cardiac arrhythmias that may occur at rest or be induced by exercise. Years of hemody-

TABLE 18–3. **Frequently Undetected Lesions in Asymptomatic Patients**

Mild and moderate aortic stenosis (valvular or subvalvular)

Mild and moderate aortic regurgitation

Mild or moderate pulmonary stenosis

Coarctation of the aorta

Atrial septal defect

Ventricular septal defect (small)

Patent ductus arteriosus (small)

Congenital coronary artery anomalies

Mild Ebstein's malformation of the tricuspid valve

Bicuspid aortic valve (may occur in 1% of population)

TABLE 18-4. **Residual Problems Related to Surgical Repair of Lesions**

Lesion	Remaining Defect
Aortic stenosis	Residual stenosis or regurgitation, with gradual deterioration
Coarctation of the aorta	Hypertension with or without residual aortic narrowing; bicuspid aortic valve and complications; cerebral aneurysm
Primum atrial septal defect	Residual mitral valve regurgitation
Ventricular septal defect (VSD)	Residual defect due to incomplete repair; residual pulmonary hypertension induced by exercise
Tetralogy of Fallot	Residual VSD or residual pulmonary stenosis; pulmonary regurgitation; pulmonary artery and pulmonary perfusion problems; ventricular arrhythmia
Transposition of great arteries	Residual VSD or pulmonary stenosis; baffle narrowing; impaired right ventricular function; atrial arrhythmias; heart block
Pulmonary atresia with VSD, Rastelli operation for transposition	Conduit narrowing

namic overload may cause a gradual deterioration in myocardial function. Pulmonary vascular disease may be gradually progressive and the incidence of bacterial endocarditis is greater in older patients. These complications are listed in Table 18-5.

Exercise testing is of considerable help when assessing functional status and in observing cardiac rhythm of these older patients during physical stress. The earliest sign of cardiac deterioration may be the development of exercise rhythm changes or the reduction in exercise capacity.

Frick et al. reviewed the exercise capacities of adults with congenital heart disease in relation to a normal population, using PWC_{150} (power output on the bicycle ergometer at a HR of 150) as the measure of fitness.[12] This method was valid only if the maximal HR of these patients were normal, which is likely in the cases studied. Using PWC_{150} per kilogram of body weight as the criterion, the fitness of the patients was compared to that of normal subjects (see Table 18-6). Patients with low exercise capacities tended to be older, to have such arrhythmias as atrial fibrilla-

TABLE 18-5. **Possible Complications of Congenital Heart Disease in Adults**

Cardiac arrhythmias (all types), atrioventricular blocks, and ventricular tachycardia occur at rest or induced by exercise, ventricular fibrillation

Impaired myocardial function

Bacterial endocarditis, with myocardial weakening or valve dysfunction

Pulmonary vascular disease (frequency and severity increases with age)

Progressive valvular calcification and fibrosis changing mild valve dysfunction into a major hemodynamic problem

Development of systemic hypertension (may accelerate problems because of pre-existing left ventricular dysfunction)

Development of CHD (symptoms appear earlier in process because of chronic hemodynamic overload)

Degenerative changes in prosthetic valves and conduits.

TABLE 18-6. **Physical Work Capacity of Adults with Congenital Heart Disease***

Lesion	Number of Subjects	Work Capacity Level		
		% 2 SD Below Normal	% Above Mean	% Below Mean
Coarctation of aorta	15	0	33	67
Patent ductus arteriosus and ventricular septal defect	35	31	13	56
Atrial septal defect		18	20	63
Preoperative	56			
Postoperative	38	5	26	68
Total		21	19	60

*From Frick et al.[12]

tion, or to have extra large hearts. After surgery, only 5% of the patients with atrial septal defect demonstrated capacities below the normal range. Some of the patients showed major improvements in exercise capacity, but in the majority of individuals, the improvement was slight. Before surgery, 20% of the subjects had values above the normal mean; after surgery, only 26% had above normal values.

Adults who had surgery for coarctation of the aorta during childhood were thoroughly studied by Hanson.[17] $\dot{V}_{O_2max}$ for these patients was well within the normal range for the population but tended toward the low side (42 versus 47 $ml \cdot kg^{-1} \cdot min^{-1}$). The muscle lactate concentration of coarctation patients during and after exercise was higher than that of the normal subjects, which is suggestive of impaired muscle perfusion. Adult subjects with atrial septal defect studied by Epstein ét al. had a mean $\dot{V}_{O_2max}$ of 23.2 $ml \cdot kg^{-1} \cdot min^{-1}$ before and 28.5 $ml \cdot kg^{-1} \cdot min^{-1}$ after surgery.[11] Adult subjects with tetralogy of Fallot had a mean $\dot{V}_{O_2max}$ before and after surgery of 21.8 and 29.3 $ml \cdot kg^{-1} \cdot min^{-1}$, respectively. These postoperative values are much lower than those obtained from patients who underwent surgery in early childhood. When surgery is carried out before the age of 6 years, near normal $\dot{V}_{O_2max}$ values can be expected 2 to 5 years later. Aerobic training of four patients after surgery for tetralogy of Fallot with a mean age of 8 years

increased their $\dot{V}_{O_2max}$ from 42.7 to 54.7 $ml \cdot kg^{-1} \cdot min^{-1}$.[8] No similar information is yet available from adults, aged 30 to 50 years, who had surgical repairs of their cardiac defect in infancy or early childhood. Maron et al. found that the older is the patient at repair of ventricular septal defect (VSD), the greater is the likelihood of an abnormal response to intense upright exercise, including a low maximal $\dot{Q}$ and an increase in pulmonary artery and pulmonary artery wedge pressures.[28] These authors emphasized that results of hemodynamic studies with these patients at rest were normal and did not reveal the often significant abnormalities that were detailed in patients during exercise. Jablonsky et al. measured ventricular function with radionuclide angiography in three groups of adults with VSD: unoperated and small; postoperative; and Eisenmenger's syndrome.[20] Individuals in all three groups had a fall in left ventricular ejection fraction during supine exercise; in the latter two groups, abnormally low ejection fractions were noted with the patients at rest. The mean maximal power output, even in the patients with small VSD, was well below that level noted for the sedentary control subjects. There was no adequate explanation for this difference; children with similar hemodynamics from VSD have normal exercise capacities, and repair of these defects is currently not recommended. Adults with significant pulmonary stenosis show more deterioration in exercise performance than do children.[26] Although these patient groups differ statistically from normal by demonstrating functional abnormalities on detailed testing, most are able to lead normal lives and to take part in recreational sports activities. These functional changes may be of no practical importance in terms of daily living, participation in fitness classes, or longevity.

Reports dealing with long-term results of patients after heart surgery often describe functional capacity in terms of the NYHA classification system. Most postoperative patients who had congenital heart lesions are determined as in Class I; they are not impaired in their daily lives and have no symptoms. This description usually means they are not very active, because even patients with a maximal $\dot{Q}$ that is 40% of the normal value will fit into Class I. Ideally, such objective data as $\dot{V}_{O_2max}$, $\dot{Q}$ max, and ejection fraction should be available for research studies concerning long-term results for any type of heart disease. When such detailed studies are conducted, some degree of functional impairment is usually found.

REFERENCES

1. Anderson, A.D., and Zohman, L.R.: Exercise training in the supine position in patients with mitral stenosis. Am. J. Med. Sci., 245:464, 1967.
2. Aronow, W.S., and Harris, C.N.: Treadmill exercise test in aortic stenosis and mitral stenosis. Chest, 68:507, 1975.
3. Auchincloss, J.H., and Gilbert, R.: Short term physical training in patients with rheumatic heart disease. Chest, 64:163, 1973.
4. Bergy, G.G., and Bruce, R.A.: Discrepancy between subjective and objective responses to mitral commissurotomy. N. Engl. J. Med., 253:887, 1955.
5. Bjork, V.O., et al.: Clinical and hemodynamic results of aortic valve replacement with the Bjork-Shiley tilting disc valve prosthesis. Scand. J. Thorac. Cardiovasc. Surg., 5:177, 1971.
6. Blackmon, J.R., et al.: Physiologic significance of maximal oxygen uptake in pure mitral stenosis. Circulation, 36:497, 1967.
7. Borer, J.S., et al.: Exercise induced left ventricular dysfunction in symptomatic and asymptomatic patients with aortic regurgitation. Assessment with radionuclide cineangiography. Am. J. Cardiol., 42:351, 1978.
8. Bradley, L.M., et al.: Effect of intense aerobic training on exercise performance in children after surgical repair of tetralogy of Fallot or complete transposition of the great arteries. Am. J. Cardiol., 56:816, 1985.
9. Chaitman, B.R., et al.: Hemodynamic evaluation of the Carpentier-Edwards procine xenograft. Circulation, 60:1170, 1979.
10. Chapman, C.B., et al.: Maximal oxygen intake test in patients with predominant mitral stenosis. Circulation, 22:4, 1960.
11. Epstein, S.E., et al.: Hemodynamic abnormalities in response to mild and intense upright exercise following operative correction of an atrial septal defect or tetralogy of Fallot. Circulation, 47:1065, 1973.
12. Frick, M.H., Punsar, S., and Somer, T.: The spectrum of cardiac capacity in patients with nonobstructive congenital heart disease. Am. J. Cardiol., 17:20, 1966.
13. Gabbay, S., et al.: In vitro hydrodynamic comparison of mitral valve prostheses. Circulation, 60 (Suppl. 1):62, 1979.
14. Gee, D.S., et al.: Prognostic significance of exercise-induced left ventricular dysfunction in chronic aortic regurgitation. Am. J. Cardiol., 56:605, 1985.
15. Gilmour, D.G., et al.: Exercise tests before and after heart valve replacement. Br. J. Dis. Chest, 70:185, 1976.
16. Gumbiner, C.H., and Gutgesell, H.P.: Response to isometric exercise in children and young adults with aortic regurgitation. Am. Heart J., 106:540, 1983.
17. Hanson, E.: Coarctation of the aorta—a long term follow-up study after surgery. Scand. J. Thorac. Cardiovac. Surg. [Suppl. 24], 14:1, 1980.
18. Hellerstein, H.K., et al.: A comparison of the personality of adult subjects with rheumatic heart disease and with arteriosclerotic heart disease. In Rehabilitation of Non-Coronary Disease. Edited by H. Denolin, et al. Brussels, Belgium, International Society of Cardiology, 1970.
19. Iskandrian, A.S., et al.: Left ventricular function in chronic aortic regurgitation. J. Am. Coll. Cardiol., 6:1374, 1983.
20. Jablonsky, G., et al.: Rest and exercise function in adults with congenital ventricular septal defects. Am. J. Cardiol., 51:293, 1983.
21. Kavey, R.W., Sondheimer, H.M., and Blackman, M.S.: Detection of dysrhythmia in pediatric patients with mitral valve prolapse. Circulation, 62:582, 1980.
22. Khalsa, A., and Olsson, S.B.: Verapamil-induced ventricular regularity in atrial fibrillation. Acta Med. Scand., 205:509, 1979.
23. Kirklin, J.W.: Replacement of cardiac valves. N. Engl. J. Med., 304:291, 1981.
24. Klein, H.O., et al.: Effects of atenolol on exercise capacity in patients with mitral stenosis with sinus rhythm. Am. J. Cardiol., 56:598, 1985.
25. Kligfield, P., et al.: The exercise electrocardiogram in aortic regurgitation. Circulation, 72:II: III, 1985 (Abstracts).
26. Krabill, K.A., et al.: Rest and exercise hemodynamics in pulmonary stenosis: comparison of children and adults. Am. J. Cardiol., 56:360, 1985.
27. Krayenbuchl, H.P., et al.: Physiologic or pathologic hypertrophy. Eur. Heart J., 4(Suppl. A):29, 1983.

28. Maron, B.J., et al.: Postoperative assessment of patients with ventricular septal defect and pulmonary hypertension. Circulation, *48*:864, 1973.
29. Pardee, H.E. (chairman): Nomenclature and criteria for diagnosis of diseases of the heart and blood vessels. New York Heart Association, New York, 1955.
30. Patterson, J.A., et al.: Treadmill exercise in assessment of the functional capacity of patients with cardiac disease. Am. J. Cardiol., *30*:757, 1972.
31. Resnekov, L.: Circulatory effects of cardiac dysrhythmias. Cardiovasc. Clin., *2*:23, 1970.
32. Rulli, V., et al.: Experience in the rehabilitation of patients with valvular heart disease. *In* Rehabilitation of Non-Coronary Disease. Edited by H. Denolin, et al. Brussels, Belgium, International Society of Cardiology, 1970.
33. Thormann, J., et al.: Hemodynamic alterations induced by isoproterenol and pacing after aortic valve replacement with the Bjork-Shiley or St. Jude medical prothesis. Circulation, *63*:895, 1981.
34. Wrinkle, R.A., et al.: Arrhythmias in patients with mitral valve prolapse. Circulation, *52*:73, 1975.

19
CHAPTER

Low Functional Capacity

by

Henry S. Miller, Jr. and Deborah L. Morley

Patients with poor functional capacity have specific problems that must be addressed and considered before exercise testing and training. The focus of this discussion is on those individuals with a functional capacity of 5 METs or less (New York Heart Association Classification of Class III–IV) due to cardiovascular disease.[4]

CARDIOVASCULAR AND ANATOMIC PROBLEMS

Myocardial impairment leading to markedly decreased functional capacity is related to coronary atherosclerotic heart disease (CHD) in 80 to 85% of cases. Leading this list are problems associated with coronary artery occlusion that result in myocardial infarction. The resultant scar, which is noncontractile or akinetic, severely impairs muscle contraction. Other scarring may result in an aneurysm of the ventricular wall, which not ony contracts inappropriately, but dilates during contraction of the ventricle, further reducing cardiac output ($\dot{Q}$). Angina pectoris, another frequent consequence of coronary atherosclerosis, is a sensation of heavy pressure, usually felt in the chest, neck, or upper extremities, and is associated with increased work of the heart, e.g., during exercise, meals, or excitement. Angina is related to an inadequate supply of blood to the heart muscle. On one hand, coronary blood supply may be sufficient to preserve muscle viability, but it is inadequate to supply the myocardium with sufficient oxygen or to remove lactate during an increased work load. These conditions may result in ischemic pain.

Fortunately, both medical and surgical interventions may improve this condition. There are, however, patients who are inoperable, who have poor results with surgical and medical therapy, who refuse surgery or adequate medical therapy, or who are markedly impaired by their ischemic pain. Those patients with low functional capacities can benefit from an appropriately prescribed exercise program.

Other problems associated with the heart and vascular system represent only 15 to 20% of the reasons for poor functional capacity. Cardiomyopathies and valvular heart disease produce most of the noncoronary patients. Patients with cardiomyopathy (whether ischemic, idiopathic, hypertrophic, or congestive) are living longer and have greater functional capacities as a result of advances in medical therapy. Although very limited, these patients can benefit from exercise.

The hypertrophic cardiomyopathies are congenital and frequently result in aortic outflow tract obstruction. The congestive forms of cardiomyopathy are caused by inflammation of the heart muscle (commonly the Coxsackie virus) or by toxic agents (primarily alcohol) and result in a poorly contracting, dilated heart. The valvular disease problems may be congenital or acquired through rheumatic fever; they are discussed in Chapters 17 and 18.

Atherosclerotic disease may cause obstruction of blood flow in the lower extremities and produces painful intermittent claudication. Aorto-ileo-femoral arterial obstruction is frequently associated with CHD and cerebrovascular atherosclerotic disease, whether or not it is symptomatic. Claudication due to peripheral vascular disease or transient ischemic attacks in patients with cerebrovascular disease may limit functional capacity, particularly when there is concomitant coronary artery disease.

COMMON SIGNS AND SYMPTOMS

Patients with low functional capacity often have chronic heart failure. Congestive heart failure may result from many disease states, but in the majority of cases the cause is underlying obstructive coronary artery disease. Primary myocardial disease accounts for the remaining cases. Heart failure is a pathophysiologic state in which abnormal cardiac function results in an inability of the heart to pump enough blood to meet the body's metabolic demand, and there may be pulmonary, hepatic, and systemic congestion. Patients with chronic heart failure have poor exercise tolerance because of the inability of the heart to provide oxygenated blood to the working muscles. Exercise intolerance is used to grade the severity of heart failure according to the New York State Heart Association Guidelines or classifications based on oxygen consumption measures.[15]

The primary symptom is shortness of breath with mild exertion, which may be due to an impaired left ventricle that is unable to contract completely, resulting in an elevated left ventricular end-diastolic pressure and an accumulation of blood and increased pressure in the pulmonary circulation. The inability of the lung to empty itself of blood results in congestion and shortness of breath. This inadequate emptying may decrease the blood supply to such vital organs of the body as the brain and heart itself. As even mild exercise continues under these circumstances, the demand for blood flow to the skeletal muscles increases, while the blood pressure

begins to decrease, rather than increase, due to a limited $\dot{Q}$. Symptoms of dizziness, confusion, and sudden weakness due to inadequate blood flow to the brain may result. Changes in heart size during exercise when the myocardium is functionally impaired may result in cardiac arrhythmias. When heart chambers dilate and failure ensues, supraventricular tachyarrhythmias frequently occur. These bouts are most commonly paroxysmal episodes of atrial tachycardia, atrial fibrillation, or atrial flutter. Dilatation of the left ventricle with exercise similarly produces frequent premature ventricular and atrial beats. Patients with ventricular aneurysms may be more prone to the development of arrhythmias.

Myocardial ischemia due to an inadequate blood supply more frequently results in ventricular arrhythmias. These arrhythmias are usually single unifocal or multifocal premature ventricular beats, but they may be more complex, producing episodes of ventricular tachycardia (occurring in groups of three to six beats). Ventricular tachycardia of a sustained nature frequently results in ventricular fibrillation and cardiac arrest. Bundle branch block is another common electrocardiographic (ECG) change associated with obstructive coronary disease. This block may be intermittent and occur with an increase in heart rate (HR), or it may be sustained. The right or left conduction bundle may be blocked and may be associated with an increase in atrioventricular node conduction, resulting in prolongation of the P-R interval. Atrioventricular dissociation may occur when the ventricular rate fails to increase appropriately with the sinoatrial node impulse, because of inadequate blood supply to the conduction system of the heart.

As frequently mentioned, symptoms associated with decreased central nervous system blood flow are quite common in individuals with poor ventricular function. Dizziness and even syncope can occur during exercise sessions. Therefore, standing after exercise should be avoided. This problem is usually detected during the testing, when blood pressure fails to increase with activity.

These patients frequently have associated carotid and vertebral artery obstructive disease. If this disease is present, a small decrease in blood pressure may cause a significant decrease in blood flow, resulting in a transient ischemic attack or a more sustained cerebrovascular accident. The platelet thrombi associated with plaques in the carotid arteries may occur more frequently with a decrease in blood pressure and flow, leading to cerebral emboli. Additionally, sudden fatigue and lethargy may occur with exercise or in the post-exercise state due to decreased cerebral blood flow. This low-flow state may be due to carotid artery obstruction or decreased $\dot{Q}$, and may not be associated with localizing cerebral sensory or motor symptoms.

Although there are many other anatomic problems that can cause poor functional capacity and related symptoms, the major categories have been mentioned. The impairment of day-to-day living is evident. Having angina or shortness of breath with such routine daily activities as taking a shower, climbing a flight of stairs, or eating a bit excessively detracts significantly from the quality of life. Difficulties in performing such pleasurable acts as golf, mixed doubles tennis, walking, or even sightseeing can also be uncomfortable at the 2 to 3-MET capacity level. Sexual intercourse without angina or shortness of breath is almost impossible. Therefore, for an individual to live comfortably and to be gainfully employed, the exercise capacity must be improved as much as possible.

DIAGNOSTIC AND THERAPEUTIC MEASURES

Comprehensive rehabilitative therapy can be prescribed properly only following accurate assessment of the patient. Certain problems that occur during hospitalization give the physician a clue to further complications that may develop: arrhythmias that occur 2 to 3 days after the heart attack; development of chest pain 3 or 4 days after the event; myocardial functional impairment, as manifested by increasing shortness of breath; or an inability to do mild activity. Persons who exhibit significant ST-segment depression and who experience angina during low level exercise testing (9 to 10 days after infarction) are more likely to experience reinfarction or sudden death within the first year after the infarction.[13]

Ischemia, arrhythmias, and left ventricular function can be assessed fairly simply. The resting and exercise ECGs performed before or shortly after discharge can detect the presence of ischemia, both adjacent to and away from the primary infarcted area. A patient with an exercise capacity of less than 7 METs, because of ischemia and angina should be further evaluated with radionuclide or angiographic studies. With the same exercise test, it is possible to determine the ability of the patient to increase HR and blood pressure appropriately with exercise. Although beta blockers and other drugs may affect HR, a plateau or drop in blood pressure with increased exercise is a good indication of problems with left ventricular function; if present, further evaluation should be conducted and more appropriate therapy should be instituted. Arrhythmias can be assessed both at rest and during activity with the use of an exercise ECG or ambulatory monitoring. More complex arrhythmias are associated with an increased occurrence of sudden death and recurrent infarction.[14]

The foregoing information is included to make the reader more aware of the need for early testing to evaluate problems that herald catastrophic events. Even though all details are not included, we stress that early testing is important, particularly in patients with low functional capacity. Frequently, the exercise test performed 2 to 3 weeks after the event will suffice to establish an initial safe exercise level for the patient in the rehabilitation program.

Radionuclide (resting and exercise) and echocardiographic studies allow further assessment of myocardial blood flow and contractility, as well as heart valve function. Coronary arteriography is a valuable anatomic test to assess the degree of obstructive coronary disease and left ventricular contractility.

Once the patient has been evaluated and details of the degree of infarction, coronary occlusive problems, and left ventricular function are established, the graded exercise test is an excellent means to evaluate the progress made by the patient through his rehabilitative course. By the time a patient enters the program, therapeutic decisions should have been made. Those individuals with severe obstructive disease will probably have had coronary bypass surgery or balloon angioplasty of the coronary lesion. Those persons who have developed ventricular aneurysm with large akinetic and dyskinetic areas may require surgery (with or without coronary artery bypass grafting) for their removal. Stenotic and significantly regurgitant valves, as well as peripheral vascular obstructive disease, will have been repaired when possible. It is the group of patients that fails to respond to surgery or in which surgery cannot be accomplished that comprises a large portion of those patients in the rehabilitative program with low functional capacity. The specifics concerning medical therapy in this group should be assessed very carefully. The physician and exercise professional should know about the medications the patient is taking upon entering the program and any utilized previously. This knowledge should include an understanding of the reasons for any discontinuation of or changes in prescribed medications. Familiarity with the action of the drugs on HR and blood pressure at rest, as well as during exercise, is extremely important. The appropriateness of the prescribed drugs in relation to the patient's history, diagnosis, and present symptomatology should be considered. If a patient has supraventricular arrhythmias, one should look not only at anti-arrhythmic drugs but also at drugs that improve cardiac function. Digitalis preparations, as well as some diuretics, may be more effective in controlling these

arrhythmias than such drugs as quinidine or other anti-arrhythmic agents. The problem may be associated with dilatation of the heart (i.e., changes due to congestive failure), rather than with irritable foci.

The use of angiotensin-converting enzyme (ACE) inhibitors in the management of patients with heart failure and low functional capacities has become commonplace. Patients who have chronic failure generally have an increased systemic vascular resistance, due in part to vasoconstriction resulting from activation of the renin-angiotensin system. ACE inhibitors are prescribed to patients with heart failure to reduce the systemic vascular resistance and are effective in controlling hypertension whether alone or concomitant with other disease. The major consideration for exercise in patients taking ACE inhibitors is the possibility of hypotension and accompanying arrhythmias. These problems can be addressed by maintaining proper hydration and by altering dosages and the use of concomitant medications.

A new class of drugs, called phosphodiesterase (PDE) inhibitors, is now being studied for use in patients with low functional capacity. PDE inhibitors are inotropic and appear to have microvascular vasodilator properties as well. The adverse effects of these agents are an increase in the incidence of ventricular arrhythmias and hypotension. Several clinical studies are currently in progress to evaluate their effectiveness. Thus, the patient taking either of these drugs should be monitored carefully during exercise testing and training.

Therapeutic Considerations

The therapeutic approach to patients who have markedly limited function should begin by determining the nature of cardiac dysfunction. Does the patient have severe angina pectoris that stops activity almost immediately? Does shortness of breath occur soon after exercise is begun? Does the patient develop multiple arrhythmias with activity or does HR slow precipitously with activity? Does pain develop in the lower extremities or hip area with activity? Obviously, the therapeutic approach to each of these problems is different, even though the decreased level of activity may be identical in all.

In patients who are limited by angina pectoris, an initial history should determine the time of day, the circumstances surrounding the onset (e.g., after medications, with stress, or on exertion), and the relationship of medication dosage and timing to anginal attacks. Perhaps by limiting food intake before an exercise event; by delaying such early morning activities as shaving, showering, or breakfast; or by altering the time that anti-anginal drugs are taken, the patient's ability to exercise comfortably without angina may be improved. In general, our patients are asked to take only liquids in the morning before exercise to prevent dehydration and a drop in blood pressure. Their medications are taken upon arising, which is usually 30 minutes before they arrive at the exercise program. Most patients delay the morning bath until after exercise and thereby eliminate their early morning increase in activity level before medications are effective.

Patients with congestive failure manifested by exertional shortness of breath are also asked to medicate themselves some 30 minutes before exercise, minimize the amount of food eaten before exercise, and hydrate themselves appropriately. Bronchospasm associated with exercise in some patients can be alleviated by the use of bronchodilator inhalant or oral drugs now available. Weight loss is an important factor in these individuals, as is elimination of all inhalants that may impair ventilation, such as cigarettes.

The observation of cardiac rhythm during exercise may reveal that patients tend to have more frequent arrhythmias at rest and low levels of exercise than they do at a higher level of exercise. The reverse may also be true if the coronary circulation is more compromised during activity. Treatment of arrhythmias is usually an around-the-clock necessity. Therefore, taking anti-arrhythmic drugs and other controlling medications at a regular time (e.g.,

30 min to 1 hour before exercise) is important. Patients with pacemakers should be observed very closely as they exercise to assess carefully the point at which the fixed HR is unable to provide an adequate $\dot{Q}$.

Many patients with fixed pacemakers are able to increase their HR with exercise, allowing $\dot{Q}$ to rise to meet the demand of activity. This HR response should be evaluated by a graded exercise test. Currently, pacemakers are available that pace both the atria and the ventricles (dual-chamber pacemakers). With an increased atrial rate with exercise, the pacemaker will pace the ventricle at the same rate. Additionally, pacemakers that increase their pacing rate as a response to exercise (e.g., Activitrax) are now commonly used. They increase HR according to the rise in respiratory rate, chemical changes in the blood, or by detecting other changes associated with exercise. They may pace both the atria and the ventricles or the ventricles alone, producing the higher $\dot{Q}$ needed for exercise.

The improvement in pacemakers has allowed this patient population to be significantly more physically active at work and during recreation. Exercise conditioning programs are tolerated very well and are limited only by the underlying heart disease and left ventricular function.

General rules concerning salt intake and the aforementioned caloric restrictions, as well as the fact that overall good nutrition is more effective than fad diets in achieving weight loss or gain, should be stressed to these patients. A diet that ensures proper hemoglobin and vitamin levels are maintained is important in supporting the oxygen-carrying capacity of the blood and the function of the heart and other muscles.

The effect of smoking on the oxygen-carrying capacity of the blood (i.e., the increase in hemoglobin and hematocrit), the effect of nicotine on arterial constriction in some individuals, and the effect of carbon monoxide in smoke on the oxygen-carrying capacity of blood may be important factors further impairing patients with very limited functional capacity.

The use of drugs, particularly alcohol, should be discussed with these patients. Although alcohol gives one a sense of feeling better, it is not associated with any benefit in coronary blood flow. Recent evidence shows that in concentrations equal to two to four glasses of beer, alcohol causes direct coronary artery constriction.[11] This vasoconstriction may explain the relationship between ethanol and sudden coronary ischemia that is seen clinically. The evidence of an increase in HDL cholesterol with small amounts of alcohol has provided an excuse for many patients to continue to overindulge. Patients with poor functional capacity frequently have decreased myocardial function. Moreover, the depressive effect of excessive alcohol on the function of myocardial cells decreases myocardial contractility and can be quite disabling. Chronic abuse of ethanol is also related to a higher incidence of hypertension, which may in turn increase the stress placed on the heart. Hence, it is particularly important that the patient with poor functional capacity understand the consequences of alcohol intake.

These points are but a few to consider in the medication routines and overall therapeutic attempts made with these patients. We hope to emphasize, however, that maximal medical and surgical therapies are necessary, and that the need for continual reassessment in patients with low functional capacity is to be maximized. In many of these poorly functioning patients, adequate rehabilitative therapy is the additional help they need. The improvement of functional capacity from a 2 to 4-MET activity level can have a very significant effect on the ability of these persons to carry on daily activities.

EFFECTS ON THE ABILITY TO EXERCISE

The fact that patients with extensive myocardial damage, severely depressed left ventricular function, and poor coronary circulation have limited exercise capabilities and are at increased risk for morbid events has been discussed. In addition, there has been doubt cast by many authors as to the ability of patients with functional capacities of less than 5 METs to achieve any training effect, given their low exercise levels. In more recent studies, this contention has been refuted. It has been shown that there can be an improvement in functional capacity, even in those persons with poor ventricular function.[2,5,8,10] It is true, however, that exercise regimens for these patients require special considerations in planning.

EXERCISE TESTING AND PRESCRIPTION

Results of studies are available that support the efficacy and safety of exercise testing in patients with low functional capacities.[1] In these patients, an exercise prescription should be formulated only when clinical information is available from an adequate exercise test. It is important, however, to be aware of the possible adverse reactions that may result from exercise testing. As has been outlined, those abnormalities that cause a decrease in exercise tolerance are often functionally evidenced by chronotropic incompetence (as noted with heart block), exertional hypotension, and significant arrhythmias. The exercise testing staff must be on the alert for these reactions, and should be prepared to handle such situations properly.

Modifications in the usual methods of graded exercise testing may provide more useful information when studying the severely impaired patient. Subjects who are extremely limited usually begin to experience symptoms (e.g., dyspnea and chest pain) at 14 $ml \cdot kg^{-1} \cdot min^{-1}$ (4 METs) or less. Symptoms in those persons with incapacitating angina, however, have been found to appear at 2 or 3-MET levels.[3] Therefore, it is essential to begin the graded exercise test at a very low level. For the particular type of patient in question, the test should begin at 1.0 or 1.5 METs.

Because changes in MET capacity, HR, and blood pressure may occur quickly due to medications or the general lack of impairment, the progression of exercise stages must be carefully considered. Due to the importance of documenting the exact onset of symptoms in this patient population, an increase of 0.5 MET per 2-minute exercise stage is recommended. A gradual increase in exercise level will improve the sensitivity of the stress test for detecting symptoms or hemodynamic changes, and should reduce excessive muscle fatigue. The test may then be terminated due to cardiorespiratory reasons, rather than by local muscle fatigue.

Intermittent testing protocols may also be of value for studying patients with low functional capacity. Exercise interspersed with rest may delay muscle fatigue and allow the patient to tolerate symptoms more effectively, both physically and psychologically. As a result, the patient may reach an exercise level that more truly represents the actual individual functional capacity. In particular, intermittent testing designs are recommended for patients who suffer from claudication.[3]

During exercise testing, many patients are limited by such symptoms as angina pectoris, severe shortness of breath, or electrocardiographic changes of ischemia or arrhythmias, rather than by reaching an exercise level limited by general fatigue. Accordingly, these end points must be considered when the exercise prescription is calculated. These patients should not be made to exercise to a predetermined level according to a specific HR or MET level. As noted, the exercise level may be quite low and seemingly not capable of producing a training effect, but with care and patience it will.

The question of whether individuals with ischemic heart disease should exercise at a level that produces ST-segment depression has been somewhat controversial. We believe that this practice is acceptable if the exercise test proves that the degree of ST-segment depression is safe from the standpoint of arrhythmias and blood pressure stability. In our particular program, patients are allowed to exercise with an ST-segment depression of as much

as 0.2 mV, and even to a greater degree under special circumstances. These patients must be carefully supervised, with frequent monitoring of the HR response, as well as with frequent blood pressure evaluations. We have not found it necessary, however, to monitor the patient with functional limitations continuously after they have been appropriately assessed and the exercise prescription has been carefully calculated.

The standard guidelines of 60 to 85% of symptom-limited HR range may be applicable. Often, the prescribed exercise intensity should be set at 30 to 50% of the symptom-limited functional capacity to allow the patient to become acclimated to exercise. This prescription generally can be upgraded to 60 to 80% after 3 months of exercise training. It is often wise to set the prescription at approximately 1 MET less than that calculated, so that the patient can adapt to exercise and the exercise specialists can become familiar with the patient's response to activity. Frequently, disability associated with deconditioning results in a restriction of the exercise level for the first 1 to 2 months of participation in the program.

Exercise programs for patients with a low functional capacity should emphasize lower intensities of greater duration, greater frequency, or both. When the functional capacity is less than 3 METs, several 5 to 10-minute daily sessions are recommended; one to two daily sessions of 15-minute duration may be desirable for those persons with a 3 to 5-MET capacity. Patients who are severely limited by symptoms or who experience claudication will benefit from intermittent aerobic activity. The duration of exercise should be increased before intensity, the patient being encouraged to work gradually toward continuous aerobic activity. The individual with a functional capacity of 3 to 5 METs should engage in a defined activity program (e.g., walking a specific distance in a certain time eliciting a specified HR or pedalling a bike at a given work load eliciting a specified HR). This procedure provides the subject with a constant work load and better documents changes in symptomatology. It is important that these patients be acutely aware of symptoms and that they report them immediately to the exercise personnel.

The energy requirements of daily exercise or other activity should not exceed an intensity of 80% of the individual's symptom-limited maximal level. Through training, patients should be encouraged to develop functional capabilities that will allow them to perform self-care activities and, when possible, recreational activities that do not exceed their maximal capacity. The achievement of this goal will not only contribute to a successful physical rehabilitation, but also will enhance the control of psychologic symptoms of the severely impaired individual.

Effect of Medication on Exercise Testing and Training

As noted, the problems associated with ischemia (i.e., angina pectoris and poor left ventricular function) and manifested by shortness of breath, extreme fatigue, arrhythmias, or intermittent claudication are all treated with medications that may lead to undesirable effects associated with exercise. These patients are usually medicated with multiple drugs for their symptoms. The exercise test should be performed while the patient is receiving medications, and the exercise prescription should be carefully formulated according to the HR, blood pressure, and arrhythmic responses shown during the graded exercise test. It is extremely important that a dialogue concerning medication be established involving the patients, the medical director, and the exercise leader. There should be an absolute requirement that any changes in medication made by the patient's personal physician should be relayed to the rehabilitation personnel. Changes in HR response when patients are placed on or taken off beta blocker therapy and the development of arrhythmias with alterations in digitalis or anti-arrhythmic therapy are but two important reasons to discuss all medication changes.

More detailed information on potential problems associated with drugs can be found in the American College of Sports Medicine book entitled, Guidelines for Graded Exercise Testing and Exercise Prescription, 4th Edition.[3] Such established time-honored drugs as digitalis have very specific effects. In one patient, it may induce myocardial irritability stimulated by exercise, whereas in another person, profound bradycardia may occur, due to an atrioventricular conduction defect. The effects of digitalis on ST segment changes in the exercise ECG are well known. Probably a more important group of drugs are those that affect blood pressure, particularly in the post-exercise state. Almost all anti-hypertensive drugs (including diuretics that may have a dual action of peripheral dilatation and volume depletion) can at times have a profound effect on post-exercise blood pressure. The decreased myocardial contractility (negative inotropic effect) commonly associated with beta blocker and anti-arrhythmic drug therapy needs to be considered. Calcium antagonists (e.g., nifedipine, verapamil, and diltiazem) are associated with changes during and after exercise.[7] Heart rate at rest and with exercise is increased with nifedipine, whereas myocardial function may be minimally depressed with verapamil and diltiazem. These popular drugs, like all other agents, have direct effects, side-effects, and interactions with other cardiac drugs. These effects and interactions should be studied, because they may alter exercise test results and the ensuing exercise prescription.

TRAINING EFFECTS

There are few data regarding chronic exercise training in patients with low functional capacity and/or heart failure. Previously, these patients were treated with bed rest. Only recently have physicians felt that the potential benefits of exercise training might outweigh the probability of deleterious effects. Carefully prescribed regular exercise may reduce the effects of deconditioning, especially on the peripheral vasculature/musculature, while improving the quality of life.

Recently, Sullivan and colleagues studied the effects of exercise training on 16 patients with chronic heart failure and a mean ejection fraction of 24%.[11,12] Patients exercised for 1 hour 3 to 5 times per week for 16 to 24 weeks at a HR equivalent to that seen at 75% of each patient's symptom-limited maximal oxygen consumption (V_{O_2max}). The mode of activity varied and included walking, jogging, cycle ergometry, and stair climbing. Only one patient discontinued the program because of exacerbation of heart failure. Peak values for V_{O_2}, work load, and exercise time increased, whereas HR dropped both at rest and during an absolute amount of submaximal exercise. Stroke volume at maximal exercise increased but there was no significant change in $\dot{Q}$. Resting arteriovenous oxygen difference was greater. Ventilatory anaerobic threshold occurred at a higher work load, and lactate levels were reduced. During submaximal exercise, the respiratory quotient, carbon dioxide production, ventilation, and ventilatory drive were lower. There was no improvement in leg blood flow, in spite of reductions in lactate. Results of this study indicate that beneficial training effects do occur in patients with chronic heart failure and low functional capacities.

This study and others examining training in patients with severe left ventricular dysfunction support the tenet that although these patients do benefit from regular exercise, adaptations occur primarily in the peripheral vasculature and musculature. A number of studies provide evidence of functional improvements in those persons with significantly compromised functional capacities as a result of training. Most of the research has dealt with subjects who had severely depressed left ventricular function. Conn et al. showed a mean improvement of 1.5 METs after training in patients with initial functional capacities in the range of 4.5 to 9.0 METs.[5] They concluded that improvements were due to an increased oxygen pulse, as the left ventricular ejection frac-

tion did not show a significant change. Six of seven patients who were initially classified as Class III functional capacity (NYHA) improved to Class II after 6 weeks of walking/jogging at 70 to 85% of their symptom-limited maximal HR.[2] Conditioning caused a decrease in functional aerobic impairment, resting HR, and HR at submaximal workloads, but did not affect left ventricular end-diastolic pressure or volume, ejection fraction, or cardiac index. Therefore, it was concluded that the increase in work capacity was a result of improved peripheral adaptations, because there was no change in the resting hemodynamic parameters. Similar conclusions were reached by investigators who trained patients with ejection fractions of less than 45% for 2 months with a variety of aerobic activities.[8] After training, the hemodynamic and angiographic parameters were essentially unchanged, but the rate-pressure product (HR $\times$ systolic blood pressure) was improved. The increase in this value suggests an improvement in circulation, again indicating that although the ventricular myocardium may not improve, peripheral adaptations may allow an increase in work tolerance. Redwood et al. reported the improvement of the average threshold of limiting angina from 9.6 to 15.1 ml·kg^{-1}·min^{-1} after 6 weeks of bicycle ergometer training.[10]

The period of exercise training in these studies was relatively short for individuals of such limited capacity, yet some improvement was noted. Even for studies in which adult fitness participants were used as subjects, 6 and 8 weeks of exercise provided little, if any, training effect, even though the subjects did improve. The question of whether ventricular functional improvement, increased collateral circulation in the myocardium, or further central hemodynamic changes may occur with longer duration of activity is not yet answered. Hopefully, studies involving training of longer duration and with appropriate follow-up and hemodynamic measurements will be accomplished. In our program, patients who were functionally limited (Class III or less than 4.5

METs) improved by approximately 1.5 METs over 1 year, with most of the effect noted in the first 3 months. Again, there was a higher total MET capacity and a decreased HR at submaximal workloads. The percent improvement in functional capacity was significant, and patients reached levels that allowed them to be comfortable in terms of their symptoms with daily and low level leisure activities. It should be noted that left ventricular evaluative studies were not accomplished.

It appears that the severely impaired patient can benefit from training in that daily life activities are better tolerated. Although the absolute changes are not impressive, the relative improvements in these poorly functional patients are high. The advantages of carefully prescribed and supervised exercise for patients with low functional capacity are both physical and psychologic. It must be recognized that the upper limits of improvement will be dictated by the nature of the particular functional impairment, despite the quality of treatment. It is most important to have a comprehensive rehabilitation program, which not only considers the benefits of exercise but also the marked functional improvement that may occur with weight loss and the need for counteracting depression in every possible way.

Low functional capacity may be a result of numerous anatomic and functional abnormalities of the cardiovascular system. These conditions can often be improved significantly by medical and surgical therapy. In many patients, however, specific rehabilitative problems exist. Although exercise testing has been shown to be safe when properly accomplished, the possible adverse reactions that may occur in this group of patients should not be forgotten. Low level tests with 0.5 to 1-MET increments and intermittent protocols until the end points are reached should be considered to allow the greatest possible yield of information from exercise testing. Exercise prescriptions must begin with a low intensity to accommodate the marked deconditioning that is usually present in a patient of low functional capacity. Greater

duration or frequency with less intensity of exercise is beneficial. Activities should be of an aerobic nature and should not overtire the patient; all attempts should be made to not discourage exercise training before conditioning can occur. Improved functional capacity as a result of training in this impaired group of patients seems to be due mainly to changes in peripheral mechanisms. Despite the relative lack of hemodynamic improvement, exercise training, if properly handled, has definite benefits for these "special" patients. Being able to carry on daily activities without symptoms and to resume such recreational games as golf, doubles tennis, or nature trail walks is beneficial, both psychologically and physiologically.

REFERENCES

1. Almendral, J.M., et al.: Treadmill stress testing in the evaluation of patients with valvular heart disease. Cardiology. 69:42, 1982.
2. Alpert, P.L., et al.: Long-term effects of physical training on coronary patients with impaired ventricular function. Circulation, 60:1519, 1979.
3. American College of Sports Medicine: Guidelines for Graded Exercise Testing and Exercise Prescription. 4th Ed. Philadelphia, Lea & Febiger, 1990.
4. Committee on Exercise of the American Heart Association: Exercise Testing and Training of Apparently Healthy Individuals. A Handbook for Physicians. New York, American Heart Association, 1972.
5. Conn, E.H., Williams, R.S., and Wallace, A.G.: Exercise responses before and after physical conditioning in patients with severely depressed left ventricular function. Am. J. Cardiol., 49:296, 1982.
6. Criqui, M.H., Langer, R.D., and Reed, D.M.: Dietary alcohol consumption and potassium. Independent and combined effects on blood pressure. Circulation, 80:609, 1989.
7. Hanrath, P., Kremer, P., and Bleifeld, W.: Influence of nifedipine on left ventricular dysfunction at rest during exercise. Eur. Heart J., 3:325, 1982.
8. Letac, B., Criber, A., and Desplanches, J.F.: A study of left ventricular function in coronary patients before and after physical training. Circulation, 56:375, 1977.
9. Morley, D., and Bove, A.A.: Moderate concentrations of ethanol constrict human coronary arteries. Clin. Res., 88:431A, 1990.
10. Redwood, H.R., Rosing, D.R., and Epstein, S.E.: Circulatory and symptomatic effects of physical training in patients with coronary artery disease and angina pectoris. N. Engl. J. Med., 286:959, 1972.
11. Sullivan, M.J., Higginbotham, M.B., and Cobb, F.R.: Exercise training in patients with severe

left ventricular dysfunction: hemodynamic and metabolic effects. Circulation, *78*:500, 1988.

12. Sullivan, M.J., Higginbotham, M.B., and Cobb, F.R.: Exercise training in patients with chronic heart failure delays ventilatory anaerobic threshold and improves submaximal exercise performance. Circulation, *79*:324, 1989.

13. Theroux, P., et al.: Prognostic value of exercise testing soon after myocardial infarction. N. Engl. J. Med., *301*:341, 1979.

14. Vismara, L.A., Anderson, E.A., and Mason, D.T.: Relation of ventricular arrhythmias in the late hospital phase of acute myocardial infarction to sudden death after hospital discharge. Am. J. Med., *59*:6, 1975.

15. Weber, K.T., and Janicki, J.S.: Pathophysiologic response to exercise in patients with chronic cardiac failure. Heart Failure, *18*:140, 1985.

20
CHAPTER

End-Stage Renal Disease

by

Patricia Painter

Chronic renal failure (CRF) results from structural renal damage and progressively diminished renal function. Once initiated, the disease typically progresses to end-stage renal disease (ESRD), in which there is inadequate or nonexistent kidney function, requiring some form of renal replacement therapy such as dialysis or transplantation. In 1989, there were nearly 120,000 patients treated with dialysis in the United States. Another 9000 received kidney transplants.[16]

The initial damage to the kidney may be the result of long-standing hypertension, vascular changes associated with diabetes mellitus, autoimmune processes, chronic infection, congenital abnormalities, or other unknown causes. Although the rate of progression to end-stage is variable, the biochemical, endocrine, and metabolic disorders associated with decreased renal function are similar, regardless of the initial cause of dysfunction. Progressive renal failure results in the loss of both excretory and regulatory functions of the kidney. The gradual deterioration of function is monitored clinically by serum levels of blood urea nitrogen (BUN) and creatinine. The inability to excrete substances results in a condition known as uremia, which is characterized by fatigue, nausea, malaise, anorexia, and subtle neurologic symptoms. Uremia secondarily impairs the function of other metabolic and organ systems.[30]

Treatment of progressive renal failure consists of medical management (with aggressive dietary protein restriction) until serum creatinine clearance is <5 ml·min^{-1}, at which time some form of renal replacement therapy is required—either dialysis or transplantation.

There are two forms of dialysis available to patients with CRF. Hemodialysis is the most common form,[5] with approximately 79% of all patients treated in a clinical center or at home. This is a process of ultrafiltration (fluid removal) and clearance of excess toxic solutes from the blood. It necessitates the placement of an arteriovenous (a-v) fistula in the arm or leg, from which the blood is removed from the body at a rate of 200 to 300 ml·min^{-1} (the total amount of blood extracorporeal at one time never exceeds 500 ml). The blood is passed through a dialyzing chamber, across a semipermeable membrane that separates the blood from a dialysis fluid. The osmotic gradient and osmolar concentration of this dialysis fluid is controlled in order to draw specific molecular weight substances and excess fluids from the blood. The blood is then returned to the body through the a-v fistula. The hemodialysis treatment requires between 2.5 and 4 hrs to complete and must be done 3 times per week. Side effects of the treatment may include fatigue, hypertension, cramping, and general feelings of malaise.

Hemodialysis therapy requires such additional therapeutic measures as anticoagulants, replacement of vitamins and other required substances that may be removed by dialysis, and administration of human recombinant erythropoietin for increasing red blood cell production.

Another form of dialysis, which is used by approximately 14% of patients with CRF, is peritoneal dialysis.[27] This therapy utilizes the peritoneal membranes for ultrafiltration of fluids and clearance of toxic substances by introduction of a dialysis fluid into the peritoneal cavity through a permanent catheter placed in the abdominal wall. This fluid is introduced over a 12-hr period by a machine that cycles the fluid continuously (continuous cycling peritoneal dialysis) or manually through 2-L bags, which are changed every 4 hrs during the day by the patient (continuous ambulatory peritoneal dialysis).

Although dialysis therapy is life-sustaining, patients still experience significant clinical problems including renal osteodystrophy with significant orthopedic concerns, decreased growth, muscle weakness and cramping, peripheral neuropathy, hypertension, accelerated atherosclerosis, anemia, and a wide variety of electrolyte imbalances and hormonal/metabolic derangements. Cardiovascular dysfunction in dialysis patients is common and is secondary to several factors: such hemodynamic factors as pressure and volume overload; such metabolic factors as acidosis, anemia, electrolyte abnormalities, abnormal lipid metabolism, and uremic toxins; and such pathologic factors as coronary artery disease, infectious endocarditis, left ventricular hypertrophy, pericardial disease, and myocardial calcification. Any or all of these may be present and result in electrocardiographic abnormalities, cardiomegaly, congestive heart failure, and/or dysrhythmias. Additionally, there are significant psychosocial issues that patients and their families must face as a part of dealing with a chronic, life-threatening disease, and dependence on the health care community and a machine for maintenance of life.[5]

Renal transplantation has become the treatment of choice for most patients with ESRD.[26] Approximately 7 to 10% of all patients receive transplants. Kidneys are obtained from either a living relative (family member) or a cadaver. Patients with severe cardiac, cerebrovascular, or pulmonary disease and neoplasia are not considered appropriate candidates for transplant. Extensive immunologic studies are performed on recipients and donors to minimize the immunologic response to the transplanted kidney that results in rejection of the organ. When an appropriate immunologic match is found, it is placed in the extrailiac position, attached to the iliac artery. Following the transplant, patients must take immunosuppressive medications, which typically includes prednisone and cyclosporine, although the combinations and dosages may vary between centers. Most metabolic, endocrine, and biochemical derangements of uremia are corrected following transplantation. Complications following kidney transplantation are primarily related to immunosuppressive therapy, with infection and side-effects of the medications becoming problematic for many patients.

Transplant recipients are at a higher risk for developing cardiovascular disease than the general population. This risk is associated independently with cumulative dosage of prednisone, lipid abnormalities, hypertension, and smoking.[19] Weight gain is a significant problem following transplant and may be a result of one or a combination of factors: the increased appetite secondary to prednisone, removal of restrictions in the diet, and food tasting better. Long-term corticosteroid therapy may result in osteonecrosis, particularly affecting the hip, knee and shoulder joints. Although psychosocial issues may be less evident following transplant, the stress of uncertainty of rejection is consistently present. Additionally, patients experience financial stresses associated with employment and medical insurance payment of medications.

FUNCTIONAL STATUS

The functional status of patients with ESRD is not optimal. Gutman et al. reported that in 2481 dialysis patients interviewed, the percentage of those capable of physical activity beyond caring for themselves was only 50% in the nondiabetic population and 23% in diabetic patients.[12] Significant efforts have been made by the Batelle Human Affairs Institute to evaluate the functional status in ESRD patients.[2,3,8,14] In questionnaires and interviews of over 800 patients in eight centers, Evans et al. found that significant numbers of patients report limitations in various physical tasks.[2,3] They showed that over 80% of dialysis patients are limited in vigorous activities, and a significant percentage (62 to 79%) of patients treated with dialysis are limited in tasks that require only minimal energy expenditure, such as walking several blocks or climbing stairs. Even 40% of transplant recipients report limitations in these simple physical tasks. In addition, the symptoms of tiring easily and fatigue are prevalent in most patients (67 to 82% of dialysis patients and 43% of transplant recipients).

EXERCISE CAPACITY

Cardiorespiratory fitness levels in patients treated with dialysis are reported to be low (Fig. 20–1). Direct measurement of maximal aerobic power ($\dot{V}_{O_2max}$) reports values only half of those expected for normals of the same age. $\dot{V}_{O_2max}$ values reported in "the best" (i.e., no other coexisting medical conditions) hemodialysis patients range from 15.3 to 21.0 ml·kg^{-1}·min^{-1}.[7,11,32,36,37,39,40] One study reported somewhat higher values in 10 patients, averaging 28.6 ml·kg^{-1}·min^{-1}.[23] Patients treated with peritoneal dialysis do not differ significantly from hemodialysis patients,[4,32] with average $\dot{V}_{O_2max}$ levels of 21.1 ml·kg^{-1}·min^{-1}. Exercise capacity may be even lower in patients with other coexisting medical problems, which are more representative of the general dialysis populations.[29,34] Symptom-limited cycle ergometer testing performed on 171 hemodialysis patients was performed as pre-exercise screening. The average estimated peak exercise capacity was 3.5 METS, and 89% of the tests were terminated because of leg and/or general fatigue.[29,34]

One of the major limiting factors to exercise in ESRD may be anemia. The correction of the anemia of CRF with human recombinant erythropoietin (EPO) has resulted in significant increases in exercise capacity (about 17%). Even with correction of the anemia, $\dot{V}_{O_2max}$ levels remain low (17.6 ml·kg^{-1}·min^{-1}).[36]

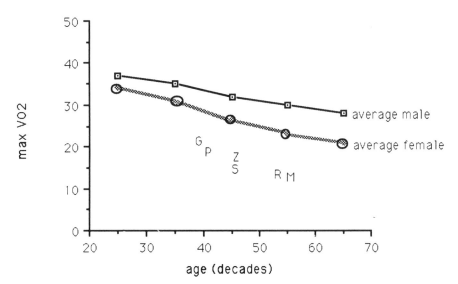

Fig. 20–1. Reported $\dot{V}_{O_2max}$ values (ml·kg^{-1}·min^{-1}) of hemodialysis patients compared to values for normal sedentary males and females. Sedentary normal levels are as reported by the American Heart Association. G = Goldberg et al.[12]; P = Painter et al.[14]; Z = Zabetakis et al.[13]; S = Shalom et al.[15]; R = Robertson et al.[18]; and M = Moore et al.[26]

Other conditions that may limit exercise capacity in dialysis patients include autonomic dysfunction, which may limit the increase in heart rate (HR) during exercise; cardiovascular dysfunction, which may limit the stroke volume increase during exercise; and abnormal peripheral metabolism and/or skeletal muscle function. Thus, both central and peripheral limitations may exist.[30,35]

Diesel et al. reported a more significant relationship between isokinetic muscle strength and V_{O_2max} than between $\dot{V}_{O_2max}$ and such oxygen transport factors as hemoglobin and hematocrit.[7] This suggests that peripheral mechanisms are most important to exercise limitations in this patient group and is consistent with the subjective reports of patients who experience significant muscle weakness with minimal activity.

At least part of the exercise limitation may be physical inactivity, because few patients receive counseling or encouragement to participate in exercise training. We found that only 8% of our in-center hemodialysis patients participated in a regular exercise program at home, which involved activities other than necessary daily tasks (unpublished data).

Exercise capacity increases dramatically following successful kidney transplantation.[9,31] The removal of the uremic state may in some way remove some of the physiologic limitations to exercise mentioned above in dialysis patients, because most metabolic, endocrine, and biochemical derangements are corrected with transplant. The initial increases in exercise capacity may be related only to the physiologic improvements resulting from transplantation, because it has been reported that physical activity levels do not spontaneously increase. Kelly and Gallagher reported initial increases in exercise capacity soon after transplant, but there were no further increases over the next 6 months.[9] Similarly, patient participation in regular physical activity did not increase.

EXERCISE TRAINING EFFECTS

Exercise conditioning programs have been shown to consistently increase exercise capacity in hemodialysis patients (Fig. 20-2). Increases in $\dot{V}_{O_2max}$ between 21 and 42% have been reported following training programs lasting 3 to 12 months.[11,37,39,40] In patients with other coexisting medical problems, the magnitude of improvement in peak exercise capacity may be less. However, when starting at such low levels of exercise capacity, any increase will be significant in terms of how it impacts the individual's ability to function during activities of daily living. Moore et al. reported a significant correlation between increase in $\dot{V}_{O_2}$ peak and a "health index," which was a score that quantifies overall wellness by weighting the number of medications, the number of other diseases, and excess weight (dietary compliance and resulting fluid overload).[25] Those patients with the lowest health index (the healthier patients) showed the greatest improvement in $\dot{V}_{O_2max}$ with 3 months of exercise training.

Improvement in cardiovascular risk factors has also resulted from exercise training in this patient group; this includes improved lipid profiles (decreased triglycerides and VLDL-cholesterol plus increased HDL-cholesterol); improved glucose metabolism (decreased fasting insulin with improved insulin binding and glucose disappearance rates); increased hematocrit and hemoglobin levels;[10,15] and improved psychological profiles (reduced anxiety, hostility, and depression).[6]

Renal transplant recipients respond to exercise training with increases in $\dot{V}_{O_2max}$.[20,24] Exercise training results in increased skeletal muscle strength in these patients,[17,20] which is important, because prednisone therapy results in significant muscle weakness (e.g., renal transplant patients have quadricep strength values that average only 70% of normal sedentary levels.[17] Transplant recipients have been shown to normalize muscle strength through strength training.[17] No studies of the effects of exercise training on cardio-

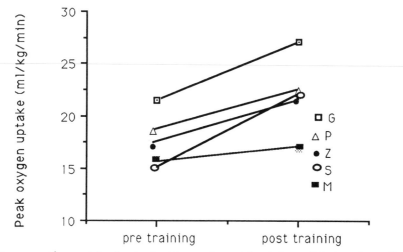

Fig. 20–2. Changes in $\dot{V}_{O_2max}$ ml·kg^{-1}·min^{-1}) with exercise training in hemodialysis patients. G = Goldberg et al.[11]; P = Painter et al.[32]; Z = Zabetakis et al.[40]; S = Shalom et al.[39]; and M = Moore et al.[25]

vascular risk factors in transplant recipients have been reported.

EXERCISE TESTING CONSIDERATIONS

The utility of exercise testing in patients with ESRD prior to starting an exercise program is difficult to assess.[38] Assuming that the reasons for performing an exercise test prior to initiating exercise training are to define the degree of risk associated with increasing exercise intensity and to establish the appropriate exercise intensity for exercise prescription, the dialysis patient presents some specific challenges to some basic principles of exercise testing for the following reasons (summarized in Table 20–1).

TABLE 20–1. **Factors that May Complicate ECG Interpretation in Renal Dialysis Patients**

Long-standing left ventricular hypertrophy
Electrolyte abnormalities
Attenuated heart rate responses to exercise (maximal heart rates < 85% of age-predicted values)
Peripheral limitations to exercise
Very low peak exercise capacity
Medications (e.g., digitalis preparations)

1) The peak exercise capacity in this patient group is very low and, in most cases, similar to the metabolic cost of activities of daily living. Thus, if patients do not present with symptoms during activities of daily living, it is predictable that exercise testing may not provide more information about their cardiac status. The limitation to exercise for most patients is skeletal muscle fatigue, which prevents them from attaining a level of myocardial stress adequate to induce electrocardiographic changes or symptoms, thereby limiting the diagnostic information obtained. In terms of exercise prescription, the results of an exercise test on one day may not apply on another day when the patient is fluid-overloaded because of dietary indiscretion, or when the patient is volume-depleted by aggressive dialysis treatment. The changing physiology of these patients poses problems in applying the test results to all possible days.

2) Most studies of dialysis patients report low peak exercise HRs, which average less than 75% of age-predicted levels. In a group of 337 patients tested on the cycle ergometer, the average was 70% of age-predicted levels.[34] This is well below the 85% of age-predicted levels needed to assure adequate myocardial stress diagnos-

tic reliability of the test. The sensitivity of exercise testing was studied by Orie et al. in a group of 20 uremic patients whose renal failure was the result of juvenile onset diabetes.[28] These patients performed symptom-limited thallium stress tests and underwent cardiac catheterization soon thereafter. Eleven patients had significant CAD, as determined by angiography, but only 2 of these 11 had positive exercise electrocardiograms (ECGs). Eighteen patients had nondiagnostic exercise ECGs, most likely because of the low peak HRs achieved. Thus, the specificity of the exercise ECG was 100%, and the sensitivity was only 18%. The thallium scans increased the exercise test sensitivity to 73%. The likelihood of disease in these patients was high, considering that their diabetic microangiopathy had progressed to renal failure. However, the autonomic neuropathy and/or peripheral limitations make the exercise ECG unreliable as a diagnostic criterion for CAD. Because nondiabetic uremic patients have similar blunted HR responses and peripheral limitations to exercise, it might be expected that similar limitations in the exercise ECG would be seen.

3) Most patients on hemodialysis exhibit abnormal resting ECGs, which may affect the interpretation of ischemia during exercise. Conditions (e.g., long-standing left-ventricular hypertrophy, electrolyte abnormalities, and digitalis preparations) may be present and result in exercise ECGs that are uninterpretable for ischemia. Dysrhythmias noted at rest or during exercise may actually be related to the electrolyte and/or acid-base status of the patient at that given time; this could change following a dialysis treatment and may not be the result of a underlying cardiac pathology. Some authors have expressed concern about serum potassium in exercising dialysis patients.[13] Recent studies have shown that increases in potassium with maximal exercise in these patients are minimal and are well tolerated, without increased frequency of dysrhythmias.[18,22]

4) Blood pressure responses to exercise may also be affected by the changing physiologic status, in that a) the fluid status of the patient may fluctuate dramatically, depending on compliance to dietary and fluid recommendations, as well as on the fluid removal during dialysis, and b) antihypertensive therapy may include a prescription of medication to be taken at or above a given systolic pressure or a prescription to skip a dose before dialysis in order to avoid dialysis-related hypotension and/or removal of the medication by dialysis. In our experience, only 36% of 337 patients had resting systolic pressures < 140 mm Hg.[34] Half of these patients had a hypertensive systolic pressure response to exercise (> 10 mm Hg increase per MET, as recommended by the American Heart Association[1]). The average increase in systolic pressure was 22 mm Hg/MET. This excessive blood pressure response to very low level exercise is typical and illustrates the difficulty in regulating blood pressure in these patients.

Patients tolerate symptom-limited exercise testing well. In 337 patient tests performed immediately prior to dialysis, only 9% were stopped because of blood pressure responses, angina, dysrhythmia, shortness of breath, or claudication.[34] All other tests were terminated because of leg fatigue or orthopedic limitations.

Obviously, the requirement for exercise testing prior to initiating exercise training is the decision of the medical director of the dialysis or transplant unit and/or of the exercise therapy program. If an exercise test is performed on dialysis patients, it may be more useful in terms of instruction, experience of exercise, and developing the exercise training program than for diagnostic purposes. Whenever testing is performed, the following should be considered.

1. *Timing of the test.* Most patients feel best and are more "normal" physiologically on a nondialysis day. Testing immediately prior to dialysis may result in more frequent dysrhythmias, more symptoms of shortness of breath, and

lower exercise tolerance due to excess fluid and electrolyte elevations. Testing immediately following dialysis has been done without problems by some,[37] but our experience with 12 tests has been a high incidence of symptomatic postexercise hypotension. This was probably due to volume depletion from dialysis with maximal vasoconstrictive compensation for maintenance of blood pressure. When exercise was applied and the vasodilation occurred, the patient was unable to further compensate to maintain pressure.

2. *The test protocol.* The test should start at a very low exercise intensity (probably 1.5 METs) and increase very gradually with 0.5 METs per stage. This protocol will allow a greater number of stages and more physiologic measurements. It also provides psychological encouragement for the patient that he/she can actually exercise and allows progress at a reasonable pace. Patient experiences with the Bruce protocol typically are negative and discouraging, because they are unable to stay with the protocol for any length of time because of the inappropriate starting levels and large increments in intensity per stage.

3. *Type of testing.* Because leg fatigue is the primary end point, treadmill exercise may be most appropriate because of the localized leg fatigue associated with cycle ergometry. However, in patients who have bone or joint discomfort with weight-bearing activities, cycle ergometry may be more appropriate.

4. *Physiologic measurements.* Standard physiologic measurements should be made during exercise testing. In light of the changing physiologic conditions of these patients, the use of a rating of perceived exertion (RPE) scale is also highly recommended and should be fully explained to the patient, with the goal of understanding how this measure can be an important guide for regulating exercise training intensity.

Standard practice for exercise testing should be applied to renal transplant recipients. The only modifications in exercise protocol would be in the case of patients with orthopedic limitations, for whom the mode of exercise testing should be non–weight-bearing (e.g., cycle ergometry).

EXERCISE PRESCRIPTION

Exercise training in patients treated with dialysis will be very low-level, and should progress gradually according to individual tolerances. The exercise training should begin as soon as the patient is stabilized on dialysis. Following transplant, the exercise training should begin as soon as clinically appropriate (within 1 week) after surgery to assure that regular exercise is considered by the patient and family as an integral part of the transplant therapy. The following are specific considerations.

TYPE OF PROGRAM. Hemodialysis patients have a high prevalence of cardiac risk factors, and the prevalence of cardiac disease is also high. Thus, according to available guidelines, they should probably exercise in a supervised setting with personnel trained to respond to a medical emergency. However, there may be problems in recommending such an approach in this population. First, there are very few such programs available and because Medicare (which covers 80% of their medical costs) does not cover supervised exercise training, the cost of participation in a cardiac rehabilitation program will be prohibitive for the majority of patients. Second, considering the amount of time devoted to their disease and treatment (at least 3 hrs per treatment, 3 days per week), it may be unreasonable to require patients to exercise in a supervised setting on 3 other days of the week. Third, considering the low peak exercise capacity, the level of prescribed exercise intensity will be very low and the initial duration will be very limited, making the risk of the exercise program no more than that associated with the patient's daily activities. Thus, requiring the patient to participate in a supervised setting may be unreasonable.

357

An acceptable and highly recommended approach to exercise training for hemodialysis patients and one that alleviates many of these concerns is to have the patient use an exercise bicycle during the dialysis treatment.[29,33] This will not involve any extra time, because patients are essentially a "captive audience" and guaranteed to be there 3 times per week. It does not affect the dialysis treatment in any way, especially if performed within the first hour of treatment. The dialysis staff is prepared to respond to any emergency related to dialysis, which can include cardiac arrest, myocardial infarction, or other cardiovascular emergencies. Such a program is cost-effective in that the dialysis staff can be trained to set up the bicycle and help to motivate patients to participate and progress with their programs. Such a program does not necessarily incur additional costs, depending on the personnel involved. Exercise training during dialysis has been shown to be effective in increasing exercise capacity and modifying some cardiovascular risk factors.[33] It has produced surprisingly high participation rates[29,33] and was well accepted by patients and staff in a large multicenter clinical program.[29]

If the dialysis clinic is unable to provide the opportunity to exercise during the treatment, home exercise (or at such community programs as the YMCA) must be encouraged. In this case, the following considerations are appropriate and are summarized in Table 20–2.

TIMING OF EXERCISE. Patients on hemodialysis may feel more like exercising on their nondialysis day. However, considering their low exercise capacity, patients should exercise daily, as tolerated. Patients treated with peritoneal dialysis may consider exercising during a dialysis "exchange" when the abdomen is empty of fluid. This may be more comfortable and may facilitate exercise at a higher intensity. Exercising "empty" may also reduce any risk of increased intra-abdominal pressures causing leaks around the catheter.

TYPE OF EXERCISE. As discussed, exercise training during the dialysis treatment can be performed only using a stationary cycle. Exercise off dialysis may incorporate any other mode of exercise. The only consideration would be for those with orthopedic problems to use a non–weight-bearing activity. Also, patients who are severely deconditioned may require muscle strengthening exercises prior to being able to perform other activities for adequate conditioning.

Patients treated with peritoneal dialysis may participate in most activities, but swimming will require special hygienic care of the catheter site. The dialysis staff should be consulted concerning this catheter care prior to starting a swimming program.

Transplant recipients should be very aware that activities that place significant stress on the joints (e.g., jogging) may cause problems secondary to prednisone. Because only a few patients experience joint deterioration after transplant, jogging and such activities are not contraindicated, but the need for increased awareness of the body's response to exercise suggests that education on appropriate footwear and choice of exercise surfaces is essential. Strength training and/or stair exercise may also be important for patients following transplant, because the large muscle groups of the legs are most affected by the muscle-wasting properties of prednisone.

FREQUENCY OF EXERCISE. Exercise should be performed 4 to 6 days per week, although exercise on dialysis days may be at a lower intensity. Most patients state that some type of physical activity every day helps prevent joint stiffness and bone pain. Initially after transplant, two sessions of exercise per day may be most appropriate to increase caloric expenditure. Leg muscle weakness may limit most patients in exercising continuously for an adequate duration to counteract the increased caloric intake experienced after transplant.

DURATION OF EXERCISE. Patients on dialysis typically have such a limited exercise capacity that interval exercise may have to be incorporated (work intervals of 2 min, followed by rest intervals of 1 min

TABLE 20-2. **Special Considerations for Exercise Prescription for Each of the Treatment Modes of End-Stage Renal Disease**

Consideration	Hemodialysis	Peritoneal Dialysis	Transplant
Timing of Exercise	Off-dialysis days During dialysis	During dialysis exchange	Start early post transplant
Type of Exercise			
Walking	No problems	No problems	No problems
Walk/jog	Bone/joint concerns Low exercise capacity	Bone/joint concerns Low exercise capacity	Bone/joint concerns
Stationary cycle	No problems	No problems	No problems
Swim	Low exercise capacity	Special catheter care Low exercise capacity	No concerns
Stair exercise	Low exercise capacity	Low exercise capacity	Recommended
Aerobics	Bone/joint concerns Low exercise capacity	Bone/joint concerns Low exercise capacity	Bone/joint concerns
Frequency	4–5 times/week	4–5 times/week	4–6 times/week
Duration			
Warm-up	3–5 min	3–5 min	3–5 min
Conditioning			
Initial	2–3 min/intervals	4–5 min/intervals	5–10 min/continuous
Goal	30 min/continuous	30 min/continuous	30+ min/continuous
Cool-down	5 min (longer during dialysis)	5 min	5 min
Intensity			
Warm-up	RPE 8–9	RPE 8–9	RPE 8–9
Conditioning	RPE 12–13	RPE 12–13	RPE 13–14 (65–85% max HR)
Cool-down	RPE 8–9	RPE 8–9	RPE 8–9
Other considerations	Slow progression Realistic goals	Home program Weight control Slow progression Realistic goals	Strength training Weight control "Normal activities"

and repeated as tolerated). The patient should then gradually increase the duration of the work intervals, gradually working toward 30 min of continuous exercise.

Given that transplant patients typically are limited initially by leg muscle fatigue, exercise sessions starting with 5 min and progressing by 2 to 3 min each day (two sessions/day) are tolerated very well by most and assure appropriate skeletal muscle adaptation to the increasing levels of exercise.

EXERCISE INTENSITY. Prescribing exercise intensity to dialysis patients should be done using the perceived exertion scale because of their abnormal HR responses to exercise. The relationship between the percentage of maximal HR and percentage of $\dot{V}_{O_2max}$ is 20% lower than in normal subjects[21] The changing fluid status of these patients may also change the HR response to exercise. If exercise is performed during the dialysis treatment, the very rapid changes in fluid may alter the HR responses. In eight patients in our center,[30] a standard exercise workload was performed for 15 min immediately before dialysis and for 15 min during each of the 3 hrs of the treatment. The exercise HR was 115 and RPE was 13 prior to dialysis. During the third hour, HR was 139 and RPE was 16. This is most likely due to the removal of fluid during that time, which resulted in a compensatory increase in HR and vasoconstriction to maintain blood pressure. Exercise obviously challenges this compensatory mechanism, and it may be necessary to decrease the intensity of exercise if exercise is performed in the latter 2 hours of treatment. This intensity reduction may be even more important for patients who use the new dialysis machines called "high-flux" or high-efficiency dialysis, which decreases the time required for treatment to 2 to 2.5 hrs.

Autonomic dysfunction of uremia typically normalizes within 6 months of transplantation, making intensity prescription by HR appropriate at that time. Initially after transplant, however, medications are being adjusted, the patient is adjusting to a new physiology with the transplanted kidney, and it may be best to use RPE. This will accommodate the "ups and downs" experienced following transplant and will assure that patients are "tuned in" to their bodies during the exercise session. Patients seem to understand the use of RPE and use it appropriately in most cases.

GENERAL CONSIDERATIONS

End-stage renal disease is a chronic condition that will result in death if some form of renal replacement therapy is not successfully and consistently implemented. Patients treated with dialysis are constantly confronted with their disease, which often results in significant psychological adjustments. Thus, it is prudent to assess the psychological status of the patient prior to initiating exercise training. For some, this intervention may definitely help in the adjustment, providing a way to make them feel "more normal." In others, however, the psychological adjustment to chronic disease may be overwhelming, making participation in exercise training inappropriate and unreasonable until a later time.

Patients treated with dialysis are often fatigued and experience frequent hospitalizations, sometimes making it difficult for them to continue to make progress with their exercise. They will often find themselves "starting over." Encouragement and support from the health care staff is essential in this ongoing process. Patients may also change modalities of therapy. Some patients may choose or have to change dialysis therapies secondary to infection or complications associated with the current treatment. Many dialysis patients (often the most healthy) will be called for transplant. Some of these may experience rejection of the transplanted kidney, necessitating the return to dialysis to maintain life. Thus, appropriate modifications of the exercise prescription must be made as the treatment changes.

After transplant, patients may experience mild rejection episodes, which are often treated with medications that have side effects of varying severity. Patients often leave the hospital with the new kidney and progress extremely well with exercise, only to return for treatment of rejection. The medications cause the patient to have severe flu-like symptoms, which cause significantly reduced energy levels lasting up to 6 to 8 weeks after the treatment. Patients must be encouraged to participate as tolerated and to progress gradually until the effects of the medications subside.

With any of these patients, it is essential to be realistic in what benefits will be gained with exercise. Not all patients will increase their hematocrits or be able to control their blood pressures with regular exercise. However, there are data showing that these positive benefits are possible and are therefore worth seeking. The most certain result of regular exercise is the increase in functional capacity, making activities of daily living easier. Most patients experience feelings of increased energy (especially transplant recipients) with regular exercise and general feelings of well-being. Exercise is an excellent way to focus attention and energy on health and away from disease. Exercise provides something patients *can* do and should be presented as a positive part of their medical therapy. For patients who depend on the medical community and a machine for their lives and who live with many restrictions, taking responsibility for their physical functioning may be the part of the treatment that has been missing.

REFERENCES

1. American Heart Association Committee on Exercise: Exercise Testing and Prescription for Patients with Heart Disease or at High Risk for Its Development: A Handbook for Physicians. Dallas, American Heart Association, 1975.
2. Battelle Human Affairs Research Centers. Edited by Evans, R.W., Manninen, D.L., Garrison, L.P., and Hart, L.G.: Treatment of ESRD in the United States: Selected Findings from the National Kidney Dialysis and Transplant Study. Seattle, 1985.
3. Battelle Human Affairs Research Centers. Edited by Evans, R.W., Manninen, D.L., Thompson, C.: A Cost and Outcome Analysis of Kidney Transplantation: The Implications of Initial Immunosuppressive Protocol and Diabetes. Seattle, 1989.
4. Beasley, R.W., Smith, A., and Neale, J.: Exercise capacity in chronic renal failure patients managed by continuous ambulatory peritoneal dialysis. Aus. N. Z. J. Med., 16:5, 1986.
5. Brenner, B.M., and Stein, J.H. (eds.): Contemporary Issues in Nephrology: Chronic Renal Failure. New York, Churchill Livingston, 1981.
6. Carney, R.M., McKevitt, P.M., Goldberg, A.P. et al.: Psychological effects of exercise training in hemodialysis patients. Nephron, 33:179, 1983.
7. Diesel, W., Noakes, T.D., Swanepoel, C., and Lambert, M.: Isokinetic muscle strength predicts maximum exercise tolerance in renal patients on chronic hemodialysis. Am. J. Kidney Dis., 16:109, 1990.
8. Evans, R.W., Manninen, D.L., Garrison, L.P., et al.: The quality of life of patients with end-stage renal disease. N. Engl. J. Med., 312:553–559, 1985.
9. Gallagher, S.: Longitudinal evaluation of functional capacity and activity levels in kidney transplant patients. Anna J., 18:378–382, 1991.
10. Goldberg, A.P., Geltman, E.M., Gavien, J.R., et al.: Exercise training reduces coronary risk and effectively rehabilitates hemodialysis patients. Nephron, 42:311–316, 1986.
11. Goldberg, A.P., Geltman, E.M., Hagerg, J.M., et al.: Therapeutic benefits of exercise training for hemodialysis patients. Kidney Int., 516:S303–S309, 1983.
12. Gutman, R.A., Stead, W.W., and Robinson, R.R.: Physical activity and employment status of patients on maintenance dialysis. N. Engl. J. Med., 304:309–313, 1981.
13. Hagberg, J.: Exercise testing and prescription for the end-stage renal disease patient. In Exercise in Modern Medicine: Testing and Prescription in Health and Disease. Edited by B. Franklin, S. Gordon, and G. Timmis. Baltimore, Williams & Wilkins, 1989.
14. Hart, L.G. and Evans, R.W.: The functional status of ESRD patients as measured by the sickness impact profile. J. Chron. Dis., 40(Suppl. 1):117–130, 1987.
15. Harter, H.R., and Goldberg, A.P.: Endurance exercise training: an effective therapeutic modality for hemodialysis patients. Med. Clin. North Am., 69:159–174, 1985.
16. Health Care Financing Administration (Bureau of Data Management and Strategy): ESRD Facility Survey Tables. Washington, August 31, 1991.
17. Horber, F.F., Scheidegger, J.R., Gunig, B.E., and Frey, F.J.: Evidence that prednisone-induced myopathy is reversed by physical training. J. Clin. Endocrinol. Metab., 61:83–88, 1985.
18. Huber, W., and Marquard, E.: Plasma potassium and blood pH following physical exercise in dialysis patients. Nephron, 40:383–384, 1985.
19. Kassiske, B.L.: Risk factors for accelerated atherosclerosis in renal transplant recipients. Am. J. Med., 84:985–992, 1988.
20. Kempeneers, G.L.G., Myburgh, K.H., Wigins, T., et al.: The effects of an exercise training programme in renal transplant recipients. Am. J. Kidney Dis., 16:57–65, 1990.
21. Kettner, A., Goldberg, A.P., Hagberg, J.M., et al.: Cardiovascular and metabolic responses to submaximal exercise in hemodialysis patients. Kidney Int., 26:66–71, 1984.
22. Lundin, A.P., Stein, R.A., Brown, C.D., et al.: Fatigue, acid-base and electrolyte changes with exhaustive treadmill exercise in hemodialysis patients. Nephron, 46:57–62, 1987.
23. Lundin, A.P., Stein, R.A., Frank, F., et al.: Cardiovascular status in long-term hemodialysis patients: an exercise and echocardiographic study. Nephron, 28:234–238, 1981.
24. Miller, T.D., Squires, R.W., Gau, G.T., et al.: Graded exercise testing and training after renal transplantation: a preliminary study. Mayo Clin. Proc., 62:773–777, 1987.
25. Moore, G.E., Painter, P.L., Brinker, K.R., and Mitchell, J.H.: Exercise training for hemodialysis patients: selection of appropriate participants. (Submitted for publication.)
26. Morris, P.J.: Outcomes and complications of renal transplantation. In Diseases of the Kidney. 4th Ed. Edited by R.W. Schrier and C.W. Gottschalk. Boston, Little Brown, 1988.
27. Nissenson, A.R., and Fine, R.N. (eds.): Dialysis Therapy. St. Louis, C.V. Mosby, 1986.
28. Orie, J.E., Jabi, H., Glass, N., et al.: Thallium 201 myocardial perfusion imaging and coronary arteriography in asymptomatic patients with end-stage renal disease secondary to juvenile onset diabetes mellitus. Transplant. Proc., 27:1709–1710, 1986.
29. Painter, P.L.: Exercise during hemodialysis: participation rates. Dialysis Transplant., 17:21–26, 1986.
30. Painter, P.L.: Exercise in end stage renal disease. Exerc. Sports Sci. Rev., 16:305–339, 1988.
31. Painter, P.L., Hanson, P., Messer-Rehak, D.L., et al.: Exercise tolerance changes following renal transplantation. Am. J. Kidney Dis., 10:452–456, 1987.
32. Painter, P.L., Messer-Rehak, D.L., Hanson, P., et al.: Exercise capacity in hemodialysis, CAPD and renal transplant patients. Nephron, 42:47–51, 1986.
33. Painter, P.L., Nelson-Worel, J.N., Gill, M.M., et al.: Effects of exercise training during hemodialysis. Nephron, 43:87–92, 1986.
34. Painter, P.L., Sepsis, P.G., Coplon, N., and Gottheiner, T.: Use of exercise testing for screening

for exercise training in hemodialysis patients. (Submitted for publication.)

35. Painter, P.L., and Zimmerman, S.W.: Exercise in end-stage renal disease. Am. J. Kidney Dis., 7:386–394, 1986.

36. Robertson, H.T., Haley, N.R., Guthrie, M., et al.: Recombinant erythropoietin improves exercise capacity in anemic hemodialysis patients. Am. J. Kidney Dis., 15:325–332, 1990.

37. Ross, D.L., Grabeau, G.M., Smith, S., et al.: Efficacy of exercise for end-stage renal disease patients immediately following high-efficiency hemodialysis: a pilot study. Am. J. Nephrol., 9:376–383, 1989.

38. Rostrand, S.G.: Management of ischemic heart disease, heart failure, and pericarditis in patients on hemodialysis. In Dialysis Therapy. Edited by A.R. Nissenson and R.N. Fine. St. Louis, C.V. Mosby, 1986.

39. Shalom, R.J.A., Williams, R.S., McMurray, R.G., and Dennis, V.W.: Feasibility and benefits of exercise training in patients on maintenance dialysis. Kidney Int., 25:958–963, 1984.

40. Zabetakis, P.M., Gleim, G.W., Pasternak, F.L., et al.: Long-duration submaximal exercise conditioning in hemodialysis patients. Clin. Nephrol., 18:17–22, 1982.

21
CHAPTER

Pregnancy

by
Larry A. Wolfe

Pregnant women constitute a unique exercising population for several important reasons. First, pregnancy is a normal but exceedingly complex biologic process that has profound effects on maternal regulatory functions. Pregnancy, recovery following childbirth, and lactation involve dynamic structural and functional adaptations that occur according to a predictable time sequence. These occur over approximately 12 months to accommodate the changing needs of the developing child. Physical conditioning is also a complex process that may augment, diminish, or have no effect on the magnitude of gestational physiologic changes, depending on the specific variable concerned.[121]

Unlike disease conditions or other developmental and aging processes, the well-being of the fetus and of the exercising woman must be considered. The possibility that the increased physiologic demands of maternal exercise may result in competition between the mother and fetus for such things as blood flow, fuel substrate availability, and heat dissipation has been the basis of traditional medical advice that pregnant women should rest.[64,67] However, existing research supports the view that healthy women experiencing normal pregnancies can benefit from regular exercise.[121] In theory, maternal metabolic and cardiopulmonary reserve can be maintained by regular, appropriately prescribed exercise, whereas chronic inactivity may result in loss of adaptive reserve.

The safety and efficacy of exercise during pregnancy depend on the relationship between exercise quantity and quality and the extent of maternal-fetal physiologic reserve. If exercise exceeds this level of reserve, then fetal development may be affected adversely. Conversely, if the level of exercise stress is insufficient, then beneficial adaptive changes may not occur (Fig. 21-1). The reader can therefore appreciate the importance of pre-participation health screening, individualized exercise prescription, and ongoing medical monitoring to ensure that exercise is both safe and beneficial. This chapter summarizes current views on optimal methods for the conduct of prenatal exercise programs.

ANATOMIC AND PHYSIOLOGIC CHANGES

Biologic effects of pregnancy on maternal systems occur in response to an array of endocrine changes, including alterations in maternal anatomy and in the regulation of maternal metabolic and cardiopulmonary functions. An overview of the most important of these relationships is provided below.[75,96,98]

Endocrine System

Because of the influence of placental gonadotrophins (principally human chorionic gonadotrophin, or hCG), the ovarian corpus luteum enlarges and secretes estrogen, progesterone, and relaxin. Endocrine functions of the corpus luteum are essential to support the first 6 weeks of

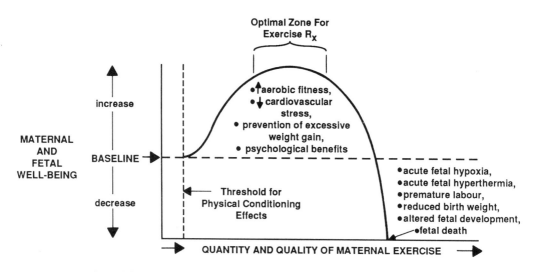

Fig. 21-1. Hypothetical dose-response relationship for exercise during pregnancy.[64,67,121] Exercise performed within the normal range of maternal-fetal physiological reserve will increase maternal metabolic and cardiopulmonary reserve. Conversely, excessive physical activity may jeopardize fetal well-being. (From Wolfe et al.[122])

gestation. The output of the corpus luteum declines after approximately 8 weeks as estrogen and progesterone synthesis by the placenta increases. Placental estrogen and progesterone secretion then continues to rise until just before delivery, whereas hCG production regresses after the initial increase in early gestation. The effects of hCG include luteinizing, luteo-trophic, and thyroid-stimulating actions. Secretion of another placental hormone (human chorionic somatomammotrophin, or hCS) gradually increases during gestation. It has effects similar to those of growth hormone, including nitrogen, potassium, and calcium retention, and reduced glucose metabolism.

During the first two pregnancy trimesters, increasing blood levels of estrogen and progesterone promote pancreatic beta-cell hyperplasia and greater insulin sensitivity to a glucose load, resulting in augmented insulin secretion.

The thyroid gland enlarges slightly in association with an augmented level of plasma thyroxin-binding proteins and an increase in the concentration of circulating thyroxine. However, blood levels of unbound thyroxine and tri-iodothyronine are not greatly augmented, suggesting that pregnancy does not involve a hyper-thyroid state. Increases in circulating thyroid hormone levels and binding proteins appear in approximately the second month and may be caused by augmented circulating estrogen levels.

Adrenal adjustments to pregnancy are complicated and are not completely understood. There are increases in circulating levels of cortisol-binding globulin (transcortin), total cortisol, and free cortisol. The rate of cortisol secretion is not increased, but its clearance rate appears to be reduced. Levels of adrenocorticotrophic hormone are reduced in early pregnancy, but increase gradually along with circulating free cortisol levels during the course of gestation. These effects are probably partially mediated by estrogen and may be an adaptation to reduced tissue sensitivity to cortisol. Aldosterone secretion is also markedly increased during the first trimester and may help to compensate for the natriuretic effects of progesterone.

Prolactin (PL) levels increase, possibly as a consequence of higher estrogen levels. Controversy exists concerning the effects of pregnancy on circulating parathyroid hormone levels. In this regard, plasma levels of ionized calcium are reportedly unchanged or only slightly augmented.

However, plasma levels of 1,25 dihydroxyvitamin D levels are elevated and promote increased intestinal absorption of calcium; this increase may be promoted by hPL and estrogen. Higher levels of plasma calcitonin appear to protect the maternal skeleton from bone reabsorption related to increased plasma levels of 1,25 dihydroxyvitamin D or possible rises in parathyroid hormone secretion.

Body Weight and Composition

Weight gain during pregnancy averages about 12 kg.[17,86] Of this, the fetus accounts for approximately 3.5 kg, increased size of the uterus 1.0 kg, larger breasts 1.5 kg, placenta 0.7 kg, amniotic fluid 0.8 kg, additional maternal fluid gain 2.0 kg, and higher maternal fat 2.5 kg.

Weight gain accelerates during the course of gestation. During the first trimester, an increase of 1 to 3 kg is usually observed. During the second trimester, the normal increase is 6 to 8 kg. Weight gain in the third trimester averages 3.5 to 4 kg and tends to plateau near term.[17,86] Weight gain of less than 1 kg/month during the last two trimesters is usually a cause for clinical concern.[3]

Maternal body fatness rises gradually as a result of hyperinsulinemia and other endocrine and metabolic changes. In late gestation, maternal adiposity tends to decrease in association with greater fetal energy needs and maternal insulin resistance.[33,58] In general, women with greater body fatness deliver heavier infants than women with lower body fatness.

Musculoskeletal Systems

The physical changes of pregnancy and body weight gain dictate significant changes in balance, posture, and locomotion. The pregnant uterus weighs approximately 6 kg at term, and its development results in abdominal protrusion, upward displacement of the diaphragm, and compensatory changes in spinal mechanics and pelvic rotation.

As compensation for the upward displacement (about 4 cm) of the diaphragmatic mid-position, the anteroposterior and transverse diameters of the thoracic cage increase approximately 2 cm. The substernal angle increases from 70 to 105°, and thoracic cage circumference increases by 5 to 7 cm.[97]

Although more study is needed, it is widely assumed that pregnancy displaces the woman's line of gravity forward and dictates the need for exaggerated lumbar lordosis, forward flexion of the cervical spine, anterior pelvic tilt, and slumping abduction of the shoulders. Presumably as a result of increased lumbar lordosis, lowback pain is experienced by approximately 50% of pregnant women.[6,70]

As a result of increased production of estrogens and relaxin, there is increased laxity of connective tissue, which may predispose pregnant women to joint and ligament damage, as well as to overuse orthopedic injury. Round and broad ligament strain, as well as pubic joint pain, are commonly encountered during pregnancy. Diastasis recti is also frequently observed and involves splitting of the rectus abdominis muscles and protrusion of the anterior uterine wall through the opening.[96]

Metabolic Rate

Resting oxygen intake ($\dot{V}_{O_2}$) rises gradually during gestation to a level 20 to 30% above that of the nonpregnant state.[8,13,14,59,90,104] The magnitude of change is approximately proportional to the increase in fat-free body mass resulting from fetal growth plus the maternal anatomic changes described above.[104] Such factors as increased cardiac work and oxygen cost of breathing also contribute.[11]

As described above, more insulin is secreted in early gestation, resulting in augmented carbohydrate utilization, increased lipogenesis, reduced lipolysis, and greater maternal adiposity. In late gestation, insulin resistance develops because of the influence of hCS and other "anti-insulin" hormones, resulting in reduced carbohydrate utilization, greater lipolysis, and a reduction in maternal fat stores.[33,58] Because glucose is the primary fetal metabolic fuel and crosses the placenta by facilitated diffusion, the apparent purpose of such insulin resistance is to ensure adequate glucose availability to the fetus. If insulin resistance is excessive, a state of gestational diabetes may develop. Fetal morbidity related to maternal diabetes can include macrosomia and neonatal hypoglycemia, hypocalcemia, hyperbilirubinemia, and respiratory distress.[61]

Cardiovascular System

Endocrine influences lead to important changes in cardiovascular function. Secondary to increased aldosterone secretion and associated sodium and water retention, there is a gradual increase in blood volume to a level 40 to 50% above that seen in the nonpregnant state.[63] Because red cell volume increases to a lesser extent, hematocrit and hemoglobin concentrations decrease, and a relative state of anemia ensues.[68,103] The greater blood volume is accompanied by venous relaxation, enlargement of the pelvic veins, and greater venous capacitance.[43,44] These effects appear to be mediated by estrogen and progesterone.[32]

The heart itself dilates as a result of the direct influence of estrogen and/or chronic hemodynamic loading related to an increased blood volume and augmented venous return.[48,54] Left ventricular end-diastolic volume increases in association with little or no change in wall thicknesses, resulting in a lower thickness-to-radius ratio and only a moderate rise in left ventricular mass.[54,72,99] Because left ventricular performance is slightly augmented,[99] stroke volume (SV) is increased as a result of a larger left ventricular end-diastolic volume and moderately improved contractile performance.[46,116]

Resting heart rate (HR) increases by 5 to 10 beats/min during the first month of gestation, possibly because of the influence of hCG.[24] As pregnancy progresses, peripheral vascular resistance decreases because of the development of the vascular shunt caused by the growing uteroplacental unit, as well as by the vessel-dilating effects of reproductive hormones.[115] Because hCG levels decline after early gestation, further progressive increases in resting HR are thought to be the result of hemodynamic reflexes aimed at maintaining adequate blood pressure.[24] Because increases in resting cardiac output ($\dot{Q}$) tend to balance the reduction in peripheral vascular resistance during the first two trimesters, systolic and diastolic blood pressures are maintained or only slightly reduced compared to nonpregnant values.[99,111]

In the third trimester, venous return is often reduced as a result of mechanical compression of the inferior vena cava by the gravid uterus.[56] This effect is greatest in the supine posture and least evident in the left lateral decubitus position. Postural hypotension is commonly observed in late gestation and is only partly compensated by further increases in resting HR.[116]

Pulmonary Ventilation

Remodeling of the chest cage and upward displacement of the diaphragm changes lung volumes and capacities. These effects include reduction in residual volume, expiratory reserve volume, and functional residual capacity. However, inspiratory capacity is increased, and vital capacity is not significantly changed. Thus, total lung capacity is only moderately reduced, and resting pulmonary function is generally well-preserved.[2,59,97]

Apart from the anatomic changes just cited, the most important effect of pregnancy on the pulmonary system is an increase in ventilatory sensitivity, apparently mediated by higher circulating progesterone levels. The response threshold is reduced, and sensitivity to carbon dioxide is increased,[69] resulting in a larger tidal volume and minute ventilation.[2,8,16.59,91] As a result of increased pulmonary ventilation, arterial PO_2 levels rise to about 100 mm Hg, and arterial PCO_2 levels drop to 30 to 32 mm Hg. The resulting respiratory alkalosis is only partly compensated by excretion of bicarbonate by the kidney; blood pH remains at approximately 7.46.[8,50,91,94]

Augmented work of breathing related to more diaphragmatic work and greater use of accessory muscles of respiration is partly offset by decreased bronchial smooth muscle tone and reduced pulmonary resistance.[38]

MATERNAL ADAPTATIONS TO ACUTE AND CHRONIC EXERCISE

Submaximal Exercise

The magnitude of changes in energy requirement for submaximal exercise depends on whether the exercise is weight-supported (e.g., stationary cycling, swimming) or weight-dependent (e.g., walking, running). Available research supports the concept that the net oxygen cost of weight-supported exercise is not significantly changed, whereas the net energy requirement of weight-dependent activities rises in proportion to gains in body weight.[4,8,46,59,91,104] Thus, conventional equations to predict the energy cost of such standard exercise tasks as cycling and treadmill walking or running are probably valid during pregnancy, provided that revised estimates of resting $\dot{V}_{O_2}$ are incorporated where applicable. The energy cost of activities that require agility or stabilization of the body would be expected to be higher than that predicted from changes in body weight alone.

Fuel metabolism during submaximal exercise is a subject of much controversy. Some evidence suggests that maternal carbohydrate utilization at any given percentage of maximal $\dot{V}_{O_2}$ ($\dot{V}_{O_2max}$) is increased in late gestation and may result in postexercise hypoglycemia.[25] On the other hand, insulin resistance that develops in late gestation would tend to promote greater dependence on fat than on carbohydrate metabolism.[33,58] Further study is needed to resolve controversy in this area.

Changes in cardiopulmonary responses to standard steady-state exercise in the upright posture are in the same direction as those seen in the resting state. These include higher values for HR,[5,39] SV,[46,117] $\dot{Q}$,[46,117] tidal volume, minute ventilation ($\dot{V}E$), and ventilatory equivalent for oxygen.[59,85,91]

Arterial PCO_2 values are significantly reduced and arterial PO_2 values are moderately increased compared to those seen in the nonpregnant state.[8,46,59,91] Systolic and diastolic blood pressures are usually unchanged or slightly reduced at any absolute submaximal $\dot{V}_{O_2}$.[10,123] Despite changes in the regulation of cardiopulmonary functions, perception of exertion at any given submaximal power output is similar to that found in the nonpregnant state.[84]

In late gestation, SV and $\dot{Q}$ during standard weight-supported exercise may be reduced compared to values measured in early and mid-pregnancy. As in the resting state, this effect is attributed to compression of the inferior vena cava by the gravid uterus, impeding venous return. This effect is most evident during exercise in the supine posture. Dyspnea is commonly experienced by pregnant women both at rest and during exercise,[40,41,94] and may be inversely correlated with alveolar PCO_2 levels.[40,41]

$\dot{V}_{O_2max}$

Knowledge concerning the effects of pregnancy on maximal aerobic power is limited for several reasons. First, few investigators have used progressive maximal exercise testing protocols to measure $\dot{V}_{O_2max}$ in this population because of ethical concerns for fetal well-being. Second, existing studies have accepted $\dot{V}_{O_2}$ at volitional fatigue as representing true $\dot{V}_{O_2max}$, rather than using a plateau in $\dot{V}_{O_2}$ during graded exercise testing as the criterion measure.[8,100,101,107] Peak exercise HRs in such studies have been lower than age-predicted maximal HRs for nonpregnant subjects. Because sympathetic responses to exercise are reportedly blunted in late gestation, these data may, in fact, represent true maximal responses.[12,120] On the other hand, it may be more difficult to achieve a true maximal effort if the ability to employ anaerobic glycolysis for supplemental energy during heavy exercise is reduced as a result of insulin resistance in late pregnancy.[8] Thus, existing data on $\dot{V}_{O_2max}$ in pregnancy must be viewed with caution. Finally, because of the higher submaximal HR and the possibly lower maximal HR in late pregnancy,[120] predicting

$\dot{V}_{O_2max}$ from submaximal exercise data is probably not a valid practice.

Based on available data,[121] it appears that absolute $\dot{V}_{O_2max}$ ($L \cdot min^{-1}$) is not greatly affected by pregnancy and may vary in accordance with changes in physical activity habits during the course of gestation. Values expressed as $ml \cdot kg^{-1} \cdot min^{-1}$ usually decline significantly as a result of maternal weight gain.

Maternal Physical Conditioning Effects

In view of the profound changes in the regulation of metabolic and cardiorespiratory functions that occur in pregnancy, it is logical to expect that maternal responses to physical conditioning may be different. Unfortunately, controlled longitudinal physical conditioning studies of pregnant women are few in number. Nevertheless, existing published reports[28,31,51,53,60,78] and preliminary communications from my laboratory[26,39,84,85,123] suggest the following:

1. Absolute $\dot{V}_{O_2}$ ($L \cdot min^{-1}$) at any given exercise HR can be increased substantially by physical conditioning in the second and third trimesters.

2. At rest and during mild steady-state exercise, the hemodynamic effects of pregnancy appear to dominate those of physical conditioning. HR is not significantly reduced and SV is not markedly increased at any given exercise power output.

3. During moderate and heavy steady-state exercise, HR reduction at any given external power output in response to physical conditioning becomes more evident than at rest or during mild exercise.

4. The rate-pressure product (HR $\times$ systolic blood pressure $\times 10^{-2}$), an index of myocardial oxygen demand, is reduced during moderate to heavy steady-state exercise at any given absolute power output.

5. Perception of effort at any given exercise power output is reduced by physical conditioning. This effect becomes more evident as exercise intensity increases.

6. Reduction in body fatness is usually observed following endurance conditioning in nonpregnant women. Body fatness, as reflected by skinfold thicknesses, may not decrease in response to moderate aerobic conditioning during pregnancy.

7. Ventilatory demand and carbohydrate utilization are reduced at any given submaximal exercise power output.

In summary, it appears that aerobic performance and cardiopulmonary reserve during exercise are enhanced as a result of endurance-type physical conditioning in pregnancy. It follows that physically fit pregnant women may better satisfy fetal physiologic demands during exposure to metabolic, environmental, or physiologic stresses. Important areas for future study include endurance conditioning effects on maternal responses to nonsteady state and maximal exercise, thermoregulation, carbohydrate tolerance, maximal anaerobic power, and maternal psychologic status.[122] Specific effects of muscular conditioning regimens, including strenuous weight training, also remain for future study. Finally, physical conditioning effects on such medical conditions as gestational diabetes and low-back pain should be investigated.

FETAL RESPONSES TO ACUTE MATERNAL EXERCISE

The most important concerns for fetal well-being during acute maternal exercise are related to uteroplacental blood flow and oxygen delivery, heat dissipation, prevention of fetal hyperthermia, and availability of glucose for fetal metabolism[121] (Fig. 21–2).

Data from exercising laboratory animals and a limited amount of human data suggest that the absolute level of uteroplacental blood flow is reduced during maternal exercise and that the magnitude of this reduction is related directly to the intensity and duration of maternal exercise.[65,76] Mechanisms that may compensate for this reduction and that may minimize fetal hypoxia include hemoconcentration of

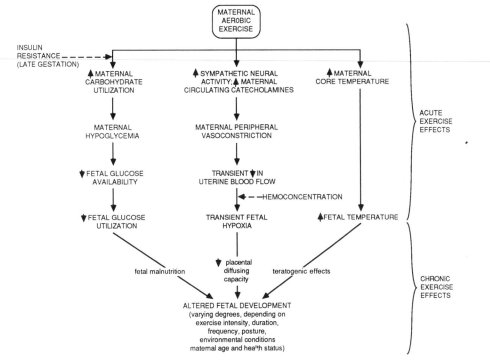

Fig. 21–2. Postulated ill effects of strenuous maternal exercise on fetal glucose availability, oxygen delivery, and heat dissipation. Chronic exercise that exceeds maternal-fetal physiologic reserve may alter fetal development. (From Wolfe et al.[121])

maternal blood during exercise, redistribution of uteroplacental blood flow to favor the cotyledons at the expense of myometrial flow,[27,45,49] and increased uteroplacental arteriovenous oxygen difference.[64] Fetal bradycardia is an early response to moderate hypoxia and appears to be a reflex response mediated by fetal arterial chemoreceptors to minimize fetal oxygen demand. Development of transient fetal bradycardia during or following acute maternal exercise has been reported from several laboratories in women with normal, healthy pregnancies.[7,21,118] Thus, it appears that both maternal and fetal mechanisms exist during normal pregnancy to compensate for exercise-induced reductions in uteroplacental blood flow, but the extent of this adaptive reserve is not clearly documented.

Although specific data on exercise are not available, concern has been expressed that fetal hyperthermia associated with increased maternal body temperature could result in fetal developmental defects. In particular, teratogenic effects have been reported in relation to maternal fever[93,110] and chronic temperature stress in animals[30] during closure of the neural tube in early pregnancy, resulting in central nervous system defects. Maternal core temperature is the most important determinant of fetal temperature. At rest, fetal temperature is about 0.5 °C higher than maternal core temperature.[1] During exercise, fetal temperature rises more slowly than maternal core temperature, reversing the maternal-fetal temperature gradient.[66] The magnitude of the rise in fetal temperature is directly related to the intensity and duration of maternal exercise, and values may not return to pre-exercise baseline for as much as 1 hour after cessation of maternal exercise.[66]

Glucose is the primary fuel for fetal metabolism, and its availability is critical for fetal well-being and growth.[33,58] Utilization of carbohydrate by skeletal muscle increases as a function of exercise intensity. Therefore, combined maternal-fetal demands during strenuous exercise in late gestation may lead to postexercise hypoglycemia[25] and reduced fetal glucose uptake.[114]

Evaluation of fetal oxygen supply, temperature, and carbohydrate metabolism is problematic in exercising human subjects. However, fetal HR (FHR) has been used as an index of fetal well-being because FHR is the primary determinant of fetal $\dot{Q}$ and because gross changes in FHR patterns are often associated with fetal distress.[88] In particular, fetal bradycardia (FHR at baseline < 120 beats·min for > 2 min) and other deceleratory patterns are common reactions to hypoxic stress. Tachycardia (FHR at baseline > 160 beats·min^{-1}) is also observed during mild hypoxia or during recovery from hypoxia.[88]

Available information suggests that the normal fetal response to maternal aerobic-type exercise is a gradual increase in FHR baseline, with a subsequent return to pre-exercise baseline within about 20 min after exercise.[7,21,87,119,121] The magnitude of FHR acceleration appears to be related to the intensity and duration of exercise, but such factors as increased fetal temperature or state of wakefulness may also contribute. Fetal bradycardia is a sign of fetal hypoxic distress, but is occasionally observed during or following exercise in healthy women with normal pregnancies.[7,21,119] The likelihood of such reactions appears to increase as a function of exercise intensity.[21]

PHYSICAL CONDITIONING AND PREGNANCY OUTCOME

A central issue for exercise during pregnancy is whether chronic maternal exercise improves or worsens fetal development. On one hand, it is well documented that heavy exercise coupled with inadequate nutrition can result in reduced maternal weight gain and unacceptably low infant birth weights.[80,112] Similarly, several studies of forced exercise in laboratory animals have reported such findings as reduced placental weight, lower placental

diffusing capacity, and lighter fetal body and organ weights. Evidence also exists that such effects are dose-dependent and tend to increase with the level of chronic exercise stress.[42,81,110] However, the applicability of conclusions generated from animal studies to predict findings in exercising women may be limited because of known anatomic and physiologic differences between humans and various animal species. Use of forced exercise in animal studies, failure of some researchers to familiarize animals with the exercise regimen before pregnancy, and difficulties comparing the quantity and quality of exercise in animal studies to that employed in prenatal exercise programs may also have affected experimental findings.[121]

Completed studies of fitness-type conditioning generally support the hypothesis that carefully prescribed exercise is not associated with increased pregnancy complications, shortened gestation, or other undesirable effects.[47,60,118,121] A recent meta-analysis of published studies suggested that the only effects of exercise are significant trends toward less weight gain and a slightly lower birth weight.[62] However, the mean weight gains and infant birth weights reported were well within normal limits for a healthy pregnancy. These results could also be related to selection factors because women who choose to exercise may have lower pre-pregnancy weight and body fatness and might be expected to gain less weight and to deliver lighter infants. Further study is definitely needed to clarify the relationship between physical conditioning and pregnancy outcome.

PRE-PARTICIPATION MEDICAL SCREENING

Existing research supports the concept that a healthy woman experiencing a normal pregnancy can participate in a moderate physical conditioning program without jeopardizing her own health or that of her developing fetus.[62,67,121] As a result of the many anatomic and physiologic changes of pregnancy, sufficient adaptive reserve apparently exists to accommodate basic maternal and fetal needs, as well as the additional demands of exercise.[62] However, fetal development may be altered if a normal level of physiologic reserve does not exist or if exercise exceeds the limits of existing adaptive reserve. Factors that may reduce physiologic reserve include maternal metabolic and cardiopulmonary diseases,[111] infectious disease processes, significant obstetric complications, inadequate nutrition, alcohol use, smoking, or multiple pregnancy (e.g., triplets). In the presence of such conditions, it is prudent for pregnant women to forgo strenuous exertion (Table 21–1).

Other factors that may alter the risk/benefit ratio for exercise appear in Table 21–2 and include a poor obstetric history, metabolic or cardiopulmonary conditions of mild to moderate severity, medications, low physical fitness, or the presence of twins in late gestation. In such instances, a decision to increase exercise quantity and quality or to continue a vigorous exercise program should be made with the advice and consent of a qualified physician. A sample form for pre-participation medical screening appears in Figure 21–3. Part A includes basic information on the woman's past and present obstetric history, general health status (adapted from the PAR-Q form, British Columbia Ministry of Health) and current health habits.[89,122] In Part B, the physician is asked to confirm the accuracy of information provided in Part A and to identify specific obstetric or general health conditions that may contraindicate the individual's participation. If none exists, written clearance is provided for the woman to begin participation in a prenatal exercise class. This form should be retained and handled in a confidential manner by the exercise class instructor.

Given that the participant's health status may change during pregnancy, the physician is encouraged to withdraw his/

TABLE 21–1. **Absolute Contraindications for Exercise in Pregnancy**[3,18,19,34,35,37,64,79,105]

1. Severe structural heart disease, ventricular dysfunction or cardiac arrhythmias
2. Peripheral vascular disease, uncontrolled hypertension or thyroid disease, other serious systemic disorder (e.g., hepatitis, mononucleosis)
3. Diagnosis of incompetent cervix
4. Two or more consecutive spontaneous abortions in previous pregnancies
5. Bleeding or diagnosis of placenta previa
6. Ruptured membranes or premature labor in current pregnancy
7. Development of pre-eclampsia/eclampsia in current pregnancy
8. Smoking or excessive alcohol intake (> 2 drinks/day)
9. Very low body fatness, poor nutrition, history of eating disorders
10. Multiple pregnancy (triplets, etc.)

Adapted from Wolfe et al.[122]

TABLE 21–2. **Relative Contraindications for Exercise in Pregnancy**[3,18,19,34,35,37,64,97,105]*

1. Mild structural heart disease, ventricular dysfunction or cardiac arrhythmia
2. Significant pulmonary disease (e.g., asthma)
3. Anemia or iron deficiency (Hb $<$ 10.5 g·dl^{-1})
4. Medications that can alter cardiac output or blood flow distribution
5. Type I or Type II diabetes mellitus
6. History of premature labor or intrauterine growth retardation in previous pregnancies
7. Bleeding during current pregnancy; breech presentation in third trimester
8. Presence of twins (after 24 weeks gestation)
9. Very low physical fitness, poor nutrition

* Risks may exceed benefits of aerobic conditioning and decision as to whether or not to exercise should be made in accordance with advice of a qualified physician.
Adapted from Wolfe et al.[122]

371

Patient's name: .... Address ....
Last First Initial
....

Date..................... Age (yr): .... Phone: ....

Part A: (to be completed by participant)

1. Date of last physical examination: .... 2. First day of last menstrual period: ....
3. Estimated date of delivery: .... 4. Is this your first pregnancy? (circle answer) **Yes** No
5. In earlier pregnancies, did you have any medical difficulties or complications? **Yes** No
If **Yes**, please describe these briefly below and ask your physician to describe them specifically in Part B.
....
6. In your present pregnancy, have you experienced any of the following? (please circle)

Vaginal bleeding	Pain or swelling in the calf of a leg	Any gush of fluid from the vagina	Severe nausea or vomiting	Infection (colds, viral or bacterial infections)
Unexplained abdominal pain	Unusual fatigue or lack of energy	Sudden swelling of face, hands or feet	Severe headaches	

7. Do you or have you in the past experienced any of the following? (please circle)

Problems with your heart	Problems with your breathing	Pains or palpitations in your heart or chest	High blood pressure	Pains or problems with bones or joints	Diabetes

Other medical problems which might affect your ability to exercise:
....
8. Please list any drugs or medications that you are currently taking: ....
9. At the present time, do you smoke cigarettes? (circle answer) **Yes** No
If **Yes**, please estimate the number of packs/day: ....
10. At the present time, do you consume any alcohol? (circle answer) **Yes** No
11. At the present time, do you participate in any form of physical exercise? (circle answer)
Regularly Occasionally Seldom Never Type of exercise: ....

Part B: (to be completed by participant's personal physician or obstetrician)

1. To the best of your knowledge, is the information provided in PART A by your patient complete and medically accurate? (circle answer) **Yes** No
2. Has your patient experienced any of the following specific medical symptoms or conditions in this pregnancy or in previous pregnancies which might suggest that participation in an exercise programme is unusually risky or dangerous? (circle applicable items)

Premature labour	History of spontaneous abortion	Anaemia	Incompetent cervix	Intrauterine growth retardation	Pre-eclampsia Toxaemia	Infection or other systemic disorder

3. Does your patient have any additional medical symptoms or conditions (e.g. multiple pregnancy, diabetes, hypertension, heart disease, pulmonary disease, arthritis) which would make it inadvisable for her to participate in an exercise programme during pregnancy? (circle answer) **Yes** No
If **Yes**, please explain: ....

Part C: *Please check one of the following:

.... The above-named person is in good general health and information currently available suggests that she can safely participate in fitness and pregnancy classes conducted by a qualified instructor.

.... The above-named person should not participate in fitness and pregnancy classes since medical risks may outweigh the expected benefits.

Additional comments: ....
Signed: .... M.D. address: ....
Phone: ....

***Note:** If your patient's medical status changes during the course of her pregnancy, you are free to withdraw medical approval of her participation. The instructor will inform you of any unusual symptoms observed in relation to exercise classes.

Fig. 21-3. Sample pre-participation medical screening form for prenatal exercise programs. (From Wolfe et al.[122])

her approval for participation by informing both the exercising woman and exercise instructor if the risk of exercise increases. In addition, the instructor and participants should know signs and symptoms of such conditions as toxemia, preeclampsia, phlebitis, severe anemia, intrauterine growth retardation, and premature labor, which necessitate immediate medical consultation[122] (Table 21-3). Note that the screening and safety procedures outlined above are provided only as a sug-

1. Any signs of bloody discharge from the vagina
2. Any "gush" of fluid from the vagina (premature rupture of membranes)
3. Sudden swelling of the ankles, hands, and face
4. Persistent, severe headaches and/or visual disturbance; unexplained spells of faintness or dizziness
5. Swelling, pain, and redness in the calf of one leg (phlebitis)
6. Elevation of pulse rate or blood pressure that persists after exercise
7. Excessive fatigue, palpitations, chest pain
8. Persistent contractions (> 6 to 8/hour) that may suggest onset of premature labor
9. Unexplained abdominal pain
10. Insufficient weight gain (< 1.0 kg/month during last two trimesters)

* Participants and the exercise instructor should know these signs and symptoms, and the participant should consult the physician monitoring her pregnancy if any are encountered. Women who develop pre-eclampsia, eclampsia, severe anemia, phlebitis, significant infection, signs of fetal intrauterine, growth retardation, or other significant medical problems should discontinue participation in the exercise program.
Adapted from Wolfe et al.[122]

gested model and may require modification to comply with local standards of medicolegal practice.

EXERCISE TESTING PROCEDURES

Possible applications of exercise testing in pregnancy include the following:

Cardiac diagnosis
Evaluation of aerobic fitness
Detection of uteroplacental insufficiency
Research

The risk/benefit ratio of maximal exercise testing is debatable in view of the fact that such testing may result in fetal hypoxia, as suggested by frequent occurrences of fetal bradycardia, when healthy pregnant women are evaluated.[21] However, maximal exercise testing may be useful from a medical diagnostic viewpoint to evaluate chest pain and other cardiovascular symptoms, pulmonary function, and medication effects. Unfortunately, the possibility of fetal injury is higher in many women with suspected cardiopulmonary disease, and the decision to perform an exhaustive exercise test should be made in accordance with the risk/benefit ratio for individual patients. It should be kept in mind that the incidence of coronary artery disease in women of child-bearing age is low, and the value of an exercise electrocardiogram to detect coronary artery disease is questionable because of the high incidence of false-positive test results in young women.

Risks to the fetus of submaximal exercise testing appear to be significantly lower than those with maximal testing.[21] However, the ability to accurately estimate functional capacity ($\dot{V}_{O_2max}$) from submaximal HR versus power output relationships is questionable because the basic assumptions of conventional tests are altered. In this regard, HR at rest and during standard submaximal exercise increases progressively during pregnancy. On the other hand, maximal HR may be reduced in late gestation,[120] possibly because of blunted sympathetic nervous system responses to strenuous exertion.[12] Thus, maximal HR reserve ($HR_{max} - HR_{rest}$) is reduced, and the magnitude of HR change in response to exercise is decreased.[92] Finally, $\dot{V}_{O_2}$ during standard exercise is moderately increased at any given exercise power output as a result of such factors as increased cardiorespiratory work. The oxygen cost of exercise may also be further augmented as a result of inefficient movement mechanics in late pregnancy. Because the error involved in predicting $\dot{V}_{O_2max}$ by procedures such as the Åstrand nomogram is 10 to 15% in healthy, nonpregnant adults,[9] violation of basic assumptions probably introduces an unacceptable level of error in pregnant women.

An alternative procedure to estimate aerobic fitness is to calculate the physical work capacity in watts at a HR of 150 or 170 (PWC_{150} and PWC_{170}, respectively) from the regression of power output as a function of HR during steady-state submaximal exercise.[106] Although this procedure may overestimate maximal aerobic power during late gestation, peak values are reasonably stable during the course of normal pregnancy and improve significantly in response to a progressive exercise regimen initiated at the start of the second trimester.[84,85] Because aerobic-type exercise can reduce uterine blood flow and because changes in FHR patterns are commonly observed during fetal hypoxic stress, exercise testing with postexertional FHR monitoring has been suggested for early detection of uteroplacental insufficiency.[95] Unfortunately, the normal range of FHR responses to standard maternal exercise has not been fully described, and the sensitivity, specificity, and safety of such testing in women with suspected uteroplacental incompetence has not yet been confirmed.

The acceptability of maximal exercise testing for research purposes has been a subject of considerable debate during the past decade.[121] Although FHR deceleratory responses are not unusual following exercise tests to volitional maternal fatigue,[21] several laboratories have reported the use of "maximal" testing protocols without apparent fetal or maternal ill effects.[21,100,101,107] Thus, maximal testing may be justifiable for the study of healthy women under carefully controlled conditions. However, critical examination by a qualified human investigation committee of safety precautions and the risk/benefit ratio of procedures to be employed is definitely indicated.

Exercise Testing Modalities and Protocols

The most useful exercise testing modalities during pregnancy include treadmill walking and upright leg cycling because the chance of injury is low, physiologic monitoring is not complicated by excessive vertical movement, and the effects of the conceptus on maternal biomechanics are minimized. Both treadmill running and bench stepping are less convenient in these respects. Arm cranking ergometry is also feasible for the study of physiologic functions[53] and may minimize postexercise uterine contractions,[29] but is less useful for the measurement or estimation of $\dot{V}_{O_2max}$ because a relatively small muscle mass is employed.

Because most sedentary pregnant women have low capacities for non–weight-supported exercise, treadmill protocols (e.g., the modified Bruce, Naughton, or Balke protocols) are most appropriate[36] (Table 21–4).

Cycling tests may involve one or more steady-state submaximal power outputs[85,86,123] or progressive increases in power output of 15 to 30 watts every 1 to 2 min. Pedalling frequency should be 60 to 80 rpm to avoid local fatigue of the anterior thigh muscles. The total length of a progressive exercise test on the treadmill or cycle ergometer should not exceed 10 to 12 min in order to minimize the reduction of uterine blood flow.

All exercise test protocols should incorporate a warm-up at a very low exercise level for 3 to 5 min, as well as a gradual cool-down to avoid venous pooling of maternal blood, arterial hypotension, and reduced uterine blood flow. To minimize thermal stress, the testing environment should be at a moderate temperature (18 to 20 °C) and low humidity for all types of dynamic exercise testing.

Strength and Flexibility Assessment

Given that the main purpose of prenatal exercise regimens is to promote maternal-fetal health, rather than to maximize increases in physical performance, the value of specific strength or flexibility tests is questionable. With respect to the former, gestational hormones cause increases in the laxity of maternal connective tissue and could predispose pregnant women to musculoskeletal injury in the process of determining their maximal range of joint movement. Also, because joint flexibility is temporarily altered and because the gravid uterus may interfere mechanically with some common tests (e.g., sit-and-

TABLE 21–4. **Recommended Treadmill Walking Protocols for Exercise Testing During Pregnancy**[36]

Protocol	Stage	Speed (mph)	Grade (%)	Time (min)
Naughton	1	2	0	2
	2	2	3.5	2
	3	2	7.0	2
	4	2	10.5	2
	5	2	14.0	2
	6	2	17.5	2
Balke	1	3	0	2
	2	3	2.5	2
	3	3	5.0	2
	4	3	7.5	2
	5	3	10.0	2
	6	3	12.5	2
	7	3	15.0	2
	8	3	17.5	2
	9	3	20.0	2
	10	3	22.5	2
Modified Bruce	0	1.7	0	3
	½	1.7	5	3
	1	1.7	10	3
	2	2.5	12	3
	3	3.4	14	3
	4	4.2	16	3

reach test), the validity and usefulness of the data obtained seem doubtful.

The efficacy of common tests of muscular strength and endurance (e.g., pushups or situps) is often reduced by maternal anatomic and biomechanical factors. Testing of maximal isometric or isotonic strength also involves the pressor response, with its associated changes in blood pressure and peripheral blood flow, which may be undesirable, especially in late gestation. These effects may be exacerbated if the Valsalva maneuver is employed.[124]

Body Composition and Nutritional Assessment

Because maintenance of sufficient maternal energy stores is critical to ensure normal fetal growth, monitoring of maternal body fatness, weight gain, and nutritional status is very important. Excessive gains in maternal body fatness are also undesirable and may result in maternal obesity following childbirth[106]. Specific norms

are available for optimal maternal weight gain. Maternal body weight should be measured frequently and charted as part of ongoing health monitoring procedures (Fig. 21–4).

The most promising method for evaluation of body fatness is the skinfold technique, whereas changes in body fluid volumes will invalidate conventional equations used in underwater weighing and electrical impedance methods. Skinfolds can be measured at representative torso and limb sites, with the sum of individual skinfolds being used as an index of maternal adiposity. Unfortunately, optimal measurement sites have not yet been identified and norms have not been developed to use when monitoring prenatal fitness programs. These should be formulated by researchers working in this area of study.

Dietary analysis should be conducted by qualified professionals, and advice should be given in accordance with published

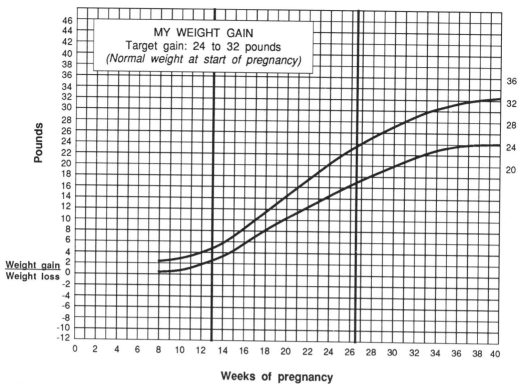

Fig. 21–4. Target weight gain chart for pregnancy. (From Brown, J.E.[17])

guidelines.[17,57,86] In general, nutritional requirements are similar qualitatively to those for nonpregnant women. Meals should include appropriate choices from the four major food groups and should contain approximately 70% carbohydrate, less than 25% fat, and approximately 10% protein. The additional energy requirements of pregnancy are approximately 10, 85, and 215 kcal/day during the first, second, and third trimesters, respectively. Energy intake should also be adjusted in accordance with increases or decreases in occupational or recreational physical activity.

Pregnant women may require specific vitamins and minerals. In particular, iron and folacin supplements can help prevent and treat gestational anemia (hemoglobin less than 10.5 g·dl^{-1}). Calcium supplementation is often recommended, particularly if the individual is lactose intolerant, has milk-protein allergy, or has low dietary calcium intake. Pregnant women with low

intake of pasteurized milk may also be prescribed a daily vitamin D supplement. If intake of animal protein is low, vitamin B$_{12}$ supplementation is often recommended. Finally, vitamin B$_6$ supplementation may be recommended unless the diet is very high in protein or low in cereal, fruit, or vegetables.

PRESCRIPTION OF EXERCISE

Exercise prescription and monitoring during pregnancy requires knowledge and expertise from the fields of obstetrics and exercise physiology, as well as specialized knowledge on the interactive effects of pregnancy and exercise on maternal-fetal biologic and psychosocial functions. Thus, a team approach is recommended in which the woman's obstetrician performs ongoing monitoring of her health status and suggests general limits that should be placed on the exercise regimen as gestation progresses. Ideally, an exercise specialist with a thorough knowledge of maternal-fetal exercise physiology would then formulate a specific exercise prescription based on this medical advice and in accordance with recent exercise test results. The woman's lifestyle and exercise preferences should be considered, and she should be actively involved in the day-to-day monitoring of her exercise program. Three-way communication of this nature is essential for safe and effective prenatal exercise programs.

Prenatal exercise classes usually involve muscular and aerobic conditioning components, as well as appropriate warm-up and cool-down/relaxation periods.[3,34,35] The muscular conditioning phase incorporates specific strengthening exercises to help prevent such conditions as diastasis recti, low-back pain, and urinary incontinence, and also to strengthen muscles involved in the labor process.[34,35] Aerobic conditioning is designed to increase cardiopulmonary adaptive reserve and to aid in the prevention of maternal obesity.[106] It may also contribute to the prevention of gestational diabetes.[53,122] Both muscular and aerobic conditioning exercises appear to have significant psychosocial benefits.[47,122]

Muscular Conditioning

Given that comprehensive treatments of this topic have been published,[34,35] a brief overview of major exercise categories is provided in Table 21–5.

In general, strengthening exercises during pregnancy should involve moderate resistance and the performance of several repetitions to achieve muscular fatigue. To avoid gross changes in venous return and $\dot{Q}$, the Valsalva maneuver should be avoided and the participant should avoid exercising or positioning herself in the supine position. This is particularly important in late gestation when the gravid uterus may impede venous return, resulting in arterial hypotension.

Aerobic Conditioning

Because strenuous aerobic exercise can reduce uterine blood flow, increase maternal core and fetal temperatures, and augment carbohydrate utilization by maternal skeletal muscle, recommendations for aerobic exercise prescription from medical and scientific authorities tend to be conservative and reflect major disagreement on several important issues.[122]

One area of controversy is whether a previously sedentary woman should begin a new aerobic exercise during pregnancy. As discussed in a recent review,[122] evidence suggests that it is safe for healthy women experiencing normal pregnancies to begin a new exercise program after 15 weeks. Exercise intensity and duration are then increased during the course of the second trimester when the discomforts of pregnancy and potential for conflicting demands of pregnancy and exercise are lowest. Because chronic exposure to high temperature may disrupt closure of the neural tube in early pregnancy, it is prudent to avoid any increase in exercise quantity and quality prior to the fifteenth week. Similarly, exercise should not be in-

TABLE 21–5. Muscular Strengthening Exercises for Pregnant Women[34,35]

Category	Purpose	Example
Upper back	Promotion of good posture	Shoulder shrugs, shoulder blade pinch
Lower back	Promotion of good posture	Pelvic tilts, pelvic rocks
Abdomen	Promotion of good posture, prevent low-back pain, prevent diastasis recti, strengthen muscles of labor	Abdominal tightening, abdominal curl-ups
Pelvic floor ("Kegels")	Promotion of good bladder control, prevention of urinary incontinence	"Faucet," "wave," "elevator"
Upper body	Improve muscular support for breasts	Shoulder rotations, arm circles
Buttocks, lower limbs	Facilitation of weight-bearing, prevention of varicose veins	Pelvic tucks, pelvic lifts, pliés, standing leg lifts

creased after the twenty-eighth week when the potential for conflicting maternal and fetal demands during exercise are greatest.[22] On any given day, exercise intensity and duration should be reduced or exercise should be cancelled in late gestation if the individual feels fatigued prior to a scheduled exercise session.

EXERCISE MODALITY. Common sense dictates that pregnant women should not participate in aerobic games or activities that involve significant risk of traumatic injury, as well as those activities which involve hyperbaric (e.g., scuba diving) or hyperthermic environmental stress.[3,82]

Because gestational hormones increase the laxity of connective tissue throughout the body, activities that emphasize weight-bearing or repeated bouncing movements (e.g., running, aerobic dance) may predispose the individual to overuse musculoskeletal injury. Conversely, the most desirable activities are those in which the body is partly supported or that minimize vertical displacement of the center of gravity. These include walking, upright leg cycling, arm cranking exercise, low-impact aerobics, and "aquafit" exercises.

Exercise in the water may be particularly appropriate because the body weight is supported by the buoyant effect of water. Plasma volume expansion during immersion may help maintain uterine blood flow[55,74] and heat dissipation may be facilitated if the water temperature is less than skin temperature.

FREQUENCY OF EXERCISE. Good agreement exists among medical authorities that aerobic conditioning should be conducted on a regular basis, while allowing sufficient time for recovery between sessions.[3,34,122] Initially, a previously inactive woman might exercise a minimum of 3 days per week, with alternating days of exercise and rest. As exercise tolerance improves, this can be increased to 4 to 5 days per week, with no more than 2 consecutive days of strenuous aerobic exercise.

EXERCISE INTENSITY AND DURATION. The interaction of intensity and duration of exercise is important because

both factors reportedly contribute to reducing uterine blood flow and increasing maternal core and fetal temperatures.[65,66]

Prescription and monitoring of exercise intensity is complicated by alterations in the control of both cardiovascular and pulmonary functions during pregnancy. As discussed previously, resting HR rises throughout pregnancy, and maximal HR is reported to be reduced in late gestation. Thus, pregnant women function within a reduced range of HR reserve,[92] and the use of conventional age-predicted HR target zones is less reliable than when used in the nonpregnant state. Revised HR target zones for exercise are provided in Table 21–6. Although these are suitable for the fitness conditioning of most healthy pregnant women, they may underestimate exercise intensity in late gestation.

Perception of exertion is closely correlated with the percentage of maximal mechanical power output under a variety of conditions[20] and appears to be a viable alternative or adjunct to the use of a revised HR target zone for exercise.[84] In my experience, a range of 12 to 14 ("somewhat hard") on Borg's 6 to 20 RPE scale is a suitable target intensity range for most exercising pregnant women.

An additional procedure to avoid overexertion is to employ the "talk test."[34] This test indicates that intensity is too high if the pregnant woman cannot carry on a verbal conversation while exercising. Because the ventilatory equivalent for oxygen ($\dot{V}_E / \dot{V}_{O_2}$) is increased significantly during exercise in pregnancy,[59] this procedure tends to be conservative and

TABLE 21–6. Suggested Heart Rate Target Zones for Aerobic Exercise in Pregnancy*

Maternal Age (Years)	Heart Rate Target Zone
Less than 20	140–155
20–29	135–150
30–39	130–145
Greater than 40	125–140

* Values apply to most healthy pregnant women. Exercise at the lower part of the recommended HR range when initiating a new exercise program and in late gestation.

may ensure safety at the expense of the effectiveness of exercise as a conditioning stimulus. Safe prescription of exercise duration depends on the intensity selected. If exercise intensity is high, then duration should be reduced to prevent significant restriction of uterine blood flow and to avoid any risk of fetal hypothermia. Assuming that exercise intensity is determined in accordance with the procedures outlined above, a minimal duration of 15 min per session is recommended to ensure an adequate conditioning stimulus. Previously sedentary women can then gradually increase the duration of aerobic exercise by 1 to 2 min per week during the second trimester to a maximum of 25 to 30 min per session[84,85,123] (Table 21–7).

It is particularly important for participants to avoid exercising in warm or humid environments during the aerobic exercise component. In this regard, metabolic heat production and increases in maternal core temperature depend directly on the intensity and duration of exercise. Because the effects of pregnancy on maternal thermoregulatory capacities are not well documented,[25,52,73] it is prudent to reduce exercise intensity and duration or forgo exercise altogether if ambient temperature or relative humidity exceed 22 °C or 75%, respectively. Another useful recommendation has been to limit aerobic exercise to intervals of 10 to 15 min with intervening rest periods of 2 to 3 min under all environmental conditions.[87] Pregnant women should drink water before and after aerobic exercise to ensure adequate hydration and normal thermoregulatory adaptive capacity. Finally, during such stationary activities as cycle ergometry, the use of fans to increase convective and evaporative heat loss may help to prevent fetal hyperthermia.

In summary, the procedures outlined above are recommended guidelines for aerobic exercise prescription that are suitable for most healthy pregnant women. However, an individualized approach for exercise prescription is strongly advised because optimal procedures may vary, depending on maternal age, occupation, socioeconomic factors, physical fitness, nutrition, and personal exercise goals. Attention to the safety of aerobic exercise is essential in all circumstances, and recommended safety precautions should be well known and implemented by the class leader and participants (Table 21–8).

WARM-UP AND COOL-DOWN. Initial warm-up before muscular and aerobic conditioning activities should include moderate range-of-motion exercises for all major joints. Mild static stretching exercises should also be included for all major muscle groups.

Cool-down following aerobic exercise should be gradual, especially in late gestation when Q̇, arterial blood pressure, and splanchnic blood flow may fall precipitously with abrupt cessation of muscular contraction, owing to the impedance of venous return by the gravid uterus. After exercise cessation, mild static stretching

TABLE 21–7. **Example of Gradual Increase in Aerobic Exercise Quantity During the Second Trimester for a Previously Sedentary Woman**

Week of Gestation	Duration (Minutes/ Session)	Frequency (Sessions/ Week)
Do not begin a new exercise program or increase habitual quantity and quality prior to the 15th week.		
16	15	3
17	16	3
18	18	3
19	20	3
20	20	4
21	22	3
22	22	4
23	23	3
24	23	4
25	24	3
26	24	4
27	25	3
28	25	4
Do not increase exercise duration or frequency after the 28th week of gestation. If necessary, reduce exercise quantity and quality to avoid chronic fatigue in late gestation.		

Obtain medical clearance before participation

Non–weight-bearing exercise modalities (e.g., cycling, swimming) are preferable to weight-bearing exercise modalities (e.g., jogging)

Exertion levels should be prescribed on an individual basis

Avoid strenuous exertion during the first trimester. Do not increase exercise quantity or quality prior to the 15th week or after the 25th week

Increases in exercise quantity and quality during the second trimester should be *very* gradual for previously inactive women

Avoid exercise or positioning the individual in the supine posture—particularly in late gestation

Avoid exercise in warm/humid or hyperbaric environments

Drink liquids before and after exercise to ensure adequate hydration

Do not exercise when fatigued—particularly in late gestation

Periodic rest intervals may help minimize hypoxic or thermal stress to the fetus

Know reasons to discontinue exercise and consult a qualified physician immediately if they occur

Adapted from Wolfe et al.[122]

and relaxation exercises that stress diaphragmatic breathing are recommended to conclude the exercise session.[34]

POSTNATAL PHYSICAL CONDITIONING

Postulated benefits of exercise during pregnancy include facilitation of labor and faster recovery from labor.[122] Although more study is needed, one recent study supports the validity of these claims.[47] Unfortunately, little or no information currently exists concerning the safety and efficacy of exercise participation in the postpartum or immediate postnatal period.

Physiologic changes associated with parturition are profound and include regression at varying rates of anatomic and physiologic changes induced and maintained during pregnancy by gestational hormones. Immediate weight loss is 5 to 7 kg, due to expulsion of the fetus, the placenta, and body fluids. However, body fatness requires 3 to 12 months to return toward prepregnancy levels. Blood volume returns rapidly to preconception levels, whereas anatomic changes of the heart and vasculature regress more slowly. Ventilatory sensitivity also returns rapidly to nonpregnant levels because of withdrawal of the effects of elevated progesterone production. Finally, endocrine and metabolic functions are altered by the process of lactation.

Advantages of early postnatal exercise include gradual strengthening of muscle groups stressed during pregnancy and strained during labor, as well as prevention of deconditioning and physiologic deterioration related to bed rest. Such exercises can begin soon after delivery and include walking and such bed exercises as abdominal tightening, pelvic floor (Kegel) exercises, recumbent pelvic tilts, and deep breathing, as well as other mild static contractions and range-of-motion exercises.[35] Between the third postpartum day and 6 postpartum weeks, the degree of ambulation and intensity of muscular conditioning can be increased gradually. Women with diastasis recti should avoid strenuous abdominal exercises until abdominal muscle separation is closed in accordance with her physician's advice.[35]

Women who have had Caesarean sections recover more slowly than those who have had vaginal deliveries. Because the individual rate of recovery varies greatly, specific exercises and the speed of progression should be determined in accordance with medical advice.[35] Other complications that may delay resumption of physical activity include anemia, vaginal bleeding following delivery, and fatigue in women who are nursing.[35]

Controversy exists concerning the optimal time for resumption of normal exercise patterns following pregnancy. This probably occurs because the time varies with maternal age, health status, predelivery physical fitness, whether or not a woman breast feeds, psychologic and lifestyle factors, and the woman's desire to return to her customary level of activity. Thus, return to pre-pregnancy activity levels can range between 6 weeks and 6 months.

SUMMARY

Pregnancy is an exceedingly complex biologic process that results in hormonally mediated changes in maternal anatomy, as well as in altered regulation of metabolic and cardiopulmonary functions. Adaptations to standard submaximal exercise include increases in HR, $\dot{Q}$, and pulmonary ventilation. The maximal capacity for weight-supported exercise ($\dot{V}_{O_2max}$, $L \cdot min^{-1}$) is not greatly affected by pregnancy, but the capacity for weight-dependent exercise ($\dot{V}_{O_2max}$, $ml \cdot kg^{-1} \cdot min^{-1}$) gradually decreases as a function of gestational weight gain.

Maternal responses to aerobic conditioning differ from those of nonpregnant women. Such women do not appear to develop bradycardia, and body fat stores may be protected as a result of hyperinsulinemia. Expected increases in submaximal exercise SV may be masked by gestational effects on blood volume and venous return. However, HR responses to heavy submaximal exercise are significantly reduced by aerobic conditioning owing to a widened arteriovenous oxygen difference. Further study will be needed to characterize physical conditioning effects on cardiopulmonary responses to maximal exercise.

Concerns for fetal well-being during acute maternal exercise center on the transient reduction in uterine blood flow, interruption of fetal glucose availability, and risk of fetal hyperthermia in early gestation. However, sufficient maternal-fetal physiologic reserve appears to exist in healthy, well-nourished women to accommodate maternal and fetal needs during moderate exercise. In the absence of maternal metabolic and cardiopulmonary disease, environmental or nutritional stress, or uteroplacental insufficiency, physical conditioning appears to improve maternal physiologic reserve without jeopardizing fetal well-being or pregnancy outcome.

The specific value of exercise testing may be reduced because maximal testing may be stressful to the fetus. In addition, submaximal tests to predict $\dot{V}_{O_2max}$ from submaximal HR versus power output relationships are probably invalid in this population because the basic assumptions of such tests are altered by pregnancy.

Physical conditioning programs for pregnant women usually include both muscular and aerobic conditioning components. The purposes of the former include the promotion of good posture; prevention of diastasis recti, low-back pain, and urinary incontinence; and strengthening of specific muscle groups involved in the active stage of labor.

It is generally not recommended that previously sedentary women begin a new aerobic conditioning regimen prior to the fifteenth or later than the twenty-eighth week of gestation. However, exercise quantity and quality can be gradually increased over the course of the second trimester, when the discomforts of pregnancy and risks to fetal well-being are lowest. Exercise intensity can be prescribed and monitored by the combined use of revised HR target zones and conventional perception of exertion scales. The "talk test" is also a useful procedure to prevent overexertion. Minimal and maximal recommended durations for aerobic exercise are 15 and 30 min, respectively. Pregnant women should exercise a minimum of 3 and maximum of 5 days per week.

Safety considerations for exercise in pregnancy include thorough medical screening and ongoing medical surveillance, avoidance of hyperbaric and hyperthermic environments, attention to adequate nutrition and hydration, individualized exercise prescription, and good communication between the exercising woman, her obstetrician, and the exercise instructor.

Postnatal exercise can be resumed immediately after delivery, beginning with mild static exercises and ambulation during the first 3 days and progressing gradually toward more-strenuous muscular and aerobic conditioning activities. The time required for a complete return to fitness conditioning or athletic training varies from 6 weeks to 6 months, depending on individual characteristics, exercise goals, and circumstances.

ACKNOWLEDGEMENTS. The Exercise/ Pregnancy research program at Queen's University has been supported by the Advisory Research Committee (Queen's University), Fitness Canada, the Canadian Fitness and Lifestyle Research Institute, the Ministry of Health (Ontario), the Ministry of Tourism and Recreation (Ontario), the Ontario Respiratory Disease Foundation, and Health and Welfare (Canada).

REFERENCES

1. Abrams, R., Caton, D., Clapp, J., and Bacon, D.H.: Thermal and metabolic features of life in utero. Clin. Obstet. Gynecol., 13:459, 1970.
2. Alaily, A.B., and Carroll, K.B.: Pulmonary ventilation in pregnancy. Br. J. Obstet. Gynecol., 85:518, 1978.
3. American College of Obstetricians and Gynecologists. Pregnancy and the postnatal period. ACOG Home Exercise Programs, 1985.
4. Artal, R., et al.: Exercise prescription in pregnancy: weight-bearing versus non-weight-bearing exercise. Am. J. Obstet. Gynecol., 161:1464, 1989.
5. Artal, R., et al.: Exercise in pregnancy. Maternal cardiovascular and metabolic responses in normal pregnancy. Am. J. Obstet. Gynecol., 140:123, 1981.
6. Artal, R., Friedman, M.J. and McNitt-Gregg, J.L.: Orthopedic problems in pregnancy. Physician Sportsmed., 18:93, 1990.
7. Artal, R., et al.: Fetal heart rate responses to maternal exercise. Am. J. Obstet. Gynecol., 155:729, 1986.
8. Artal, R., Wiswell, R., Romem, Y., and Dorey, F.: Pulmonary responses to exercise in pregnancy. Am. J. Obstet. Gynecol., 154:378, 1986.
9. Åstrand, P.O., and Rodahl, K.: Textbook of Work Physiology. Physiological Bases of Exercise. 3rd Ed. Toronto, McGraw-Hill, 1986.
10. Bader, R.A., Bader, M.E., Rose, D.J., and Braunwald, E.: Hemodynamics at rest and during exercise in normal pregnancy as studied by cardiac catheterization. J. Clin. Invest., 34:1524, 1956.
11. Bader, R.A., Bader, M.E., and Rose, D.J.: The oxygen cost of breathing in dyspneic subjects as studied in normal pregnant women. Clin. Sci., 18:223, 1959.
12. Barron, W.M., et al.: Plasma catecholamine responses to physiologic stimuli in normal human pregnancy. Am. J. Obstet. Gynecol., 150:80, 1986.
13. Blackburn, M.W., and Calloway, D.H.: Basal metabolic rate and work energy expenditure of mature pregnant women. J. Am. Diet. Assoc., 69:24, 1976.
14. Blackburn, M.W., and Calloway, D.H.: Energy expenditure and consumption of mature, pregnant and lactating women. J. Am. Diet. Assoc., 69:29, 1976.
15. Bonica, J.J: Maternal respiratory changes during pregnancy and parturition. Clin. Anest., 10:1, 1974.
16. Briend, A.: Maternal physical activity, birthweight and perinatal mortality. Med. Hypotheses, 6:1157, 1980.
17. Brown, J.E.: Nutrition for your pregnancy. Minneapolis, University of Minnesota Press, 1983.
18. Bullard, J.A.: Exercise and pregnancy. Can. Fam. Physician, 27:977, 1981.
19. Caldwell, F., and Jopke, T.: Questions and answers: ACSM 1985. Physician Sportsmed., 13:146, 1985.
20. Carton, R.L., and Rhodes, E.C.: A critical review of the literature on scales for perceived exertion. Sports Med., 2:198, 1985.
21. Carpenter, M.W., et al.: Fetal heart rate response to maternal exertion. JAMA, 259:3006, 1988.
22. Clapp, J.F., and Dickstein, S.: Endurance exercise and pregnancy outcome. Med. Sci. Sports Exerc., 16:556, 1984.
23. Clapp, J.F. III: The effects of maternal exercise on early pregnancy outcome. Am. J. Obstet. Gynecol., 161:1453, 1989.
24. Clapp, J.F. III: Maternal heart rate in pregnancy. Am. J. Obstet. Gynecol., 152:659, 1985.
25. Clapp, J.F. III, Wesley, M., and Sleamaker, R.H.: Thermoregulatory and metabolic responses prior to and during pregnancy. Med. Sci. Sports Exerc., 19:124, 1987.
26. Collings, C.A., Curet, L.B., and Mullin, J.P.: Maternal and fetal responses to a maternal aerobic exercise program. Am. J. Obstet. Gynecol., 145:702, 1983.
27. Curet, L.B., Orr, J.A., Rankin, J.H.G., and Ungerer, T.: Effect of exercise on cardiac output and distribution of uterine blood flow in pregnant ewes. J. Appl. Physiol., 55:834, 1976.
28. Dibblee, L., and Graham, T.E.: A longitudinal study of changes in aerobic fitness, body composition, and energy intake. Am. J. Obstet. Gynecol., 147:908, 1983.
29. Durak, E.P., Jovanovic-Peterson, L., and Peterson, C.M.: Comparative evaluation of uterine response to exercise on five aerobic machines. Am. J. Obstet. Gynecol., 162:754, 1990.
30. Edwards, M.J.: Congenital defects in guinea pigs following induced hyperthermia during gestation. Arch. Pathol., 84:42, 1967.
31. Erkkola, R.: The influence of physical training during pregnancy on physical work capacity and circulatory parameters. Scand. J. Clin. Lab. Invest., 36:747, 1976.
32. Fawer, R., et al.: Effect of the menstrual cycle, oral contraception, and pregnancy on forearm

blood flow, venous distensibility and clotting factors. Eur. Clin. Pharmacol., *13*:251, 1978.

33. Felig, P.: Fuel metabolism and diabetes mellitus in pregnancy. Med. Clin. North Am., *61*:43, 1977.

34. Fitness Canada. Fitness and Pregnancy. A manual available from Fitness Canada (promotions and communications), 365 Laurier Ave. W., Ottawa, Canada, K1A 0X6.

35. Fitness Ontario. Pre/Post Natal Fitness. Ontario Ministry of Tourism and Recreation Sports and Fitness Branch, Toronto, 1983.

36. Fox, K., and Ilsey, C.D.: The Essentials of Exercise Electrocardiography. London, Current Medical Literature, 1984.

37. Gauthier, M.M.: Guidelines for exercise during pregnancy: too little or too much? Physician Sportsmed., *14*:162, 1986.

38. Gee, J.G.L., Packer, B.S., Millen, J.E., and Robin, E.D.: Pulmonary mechanics during pregnancy. J. Clin. Invest., *46*:945, 1967.

39. George, K.P., et al.: Aerobic training effects on resting hemodynamics during pregnancy. Med. Sci. Sports Exerc., *22*:527, 1990 (Abstract).

40. Gilbert, R., Epifano, L., and Auchincloss, H.J.: Dyspnea of pregnancy. A syndrome of altered respiratory control. JAMA *182*:97, 1962.

41. Gilbert, R., and Auchincloss, H.J.: Dyspnea of pregnancy. Clinical and physiological observations. Am. J. Med. Sci., *252*:270, 1966.

42. Gilbert, R.D., Cummings, L.A., Juchau, M.I., and Longo, L.D.: Placental diffusing capacity and fetal development in exercising or hypoxic guinea pigs. J. Appl. Physiol., *46*:828, 1979.

43. Goodrich, S.M., and Wood, J.E.: Peripheral venous distensibility and velocity of venous blood flow during pregnancy or during oral contraceptive therapy. Am. J. Obstet. Gynecol., *90*:740, 1964.

44. Goodrich, S.M., and Wood, J.E.: The effect of estradiol-17 beta on peripheral venous distensibility and velocity of venous blood flow. Am. J. Obstet. Gynecol., *96*:407, 1966.

45. Greiss, F.C., Jr.: Differential reactivity of the myoendometrial and placental vasculatures: adrenergic responses. Am. J. Obstet. Gynecol., *112*:20, 1972.

46. Guzman, C.A., and Caplan, R.: Cardiorespiratory response to exercise during pregnancy. Am. J. Obstet. Gynecol., *108*:600, 1970.

47. Hall, D.C., and Kaufman, D.A.: Effects of aerobic and strength conditioning on pregnancy outcomes. Am. J. Obstet. Gynecol., *157*:1199, 1987.

48. Hart, M.V., Håsenpud, J.D., Hohimer, A.R., and Morton, M.J.: Hemodynamics during pregnancy and sex steroid administration in guinea pigs. Am. J. Physiol., *249*:R179, 1985.

49. Hohimer, A.R., McKean, T.A., Bissonette, J.M., and Metcalfe, J.: Maternal exercise reduces myometrial blood flow in the pregnant goat. Fed. Proc., *41*:4190, 1982.

50. Hytten, F.E.: Physiological changes in early pregnancy. J. Obstet. Gynecol. Br. Commonw., *75*:1193, 1968.

51. Ihrman, K.: A clinical and physiological study of pregnancy in a material from northern Sweden. VIII. The effect of physical training during pregnancy on the circulatory adjustment. Acta Soc. Uppsala, *65*:335, 1960.

52. Jones, R.L., Bati, J.J., Anderson, W.M., and Bennett, N.L.: Thermoregulation during aerobic exercise in pregnancy. Obstet. Gynecol., *65*:340, 1985.

53. Jovanovic-Peterson, L., Durak, E.P., and Peterson, C.M.: Randomized trial of diet versus diet plus cardiovascular conditioning on glucose levels in gestational diabetes. Am. J. Obstet. Gynecol., *161*:415, 1989.

54. Katz, R., Karliner, J.S., and Resnik, R.: Effects of a natural volume overload state (pregnancy) in left ventricular performance in normal human subjects. Circulation, *48*:434, 1978.

55. Katz, V.L., McMurray, R., Berry, M.J., and Cefalo, R.C.: Fetal and uterine responses to immersion and exercise. Obstet. Gynecol., *72*:1493, 1988.

56. Kerr, M.G.: Cardiovascular dynamics in pregnancy and labour. Br. Med. Bull., *24*:19, 1968.

57. King, J.C., and Butterfield, G.: Nutritional needs for physically active pregnant women. In Exercise in Pregnancy. Edited by R. Artal and R.A. Wiswell. Baltimore, Williams & Wilkins, 1986.

58. Knopp, R.H.: Fuel metabolism in pregnancy. Contemp. OB/GYN, *12*:83, 1978.

59. Knuttgen, H.G., and Emerson, K., Jr.: Physiological response to pregnancy at rest and during exercise. J. Appl. Physiol., *36*:549, 1974.

60. Kulpa, P.J., White, B.M., and Visscher, R.: Aerobic exercise in pregnancy. Am. J. Obstet. Gynecol., *156*:1395, 1987.

61. Landon, M.B., and Gabbe, S.G.: Diabetes and pregnancy. Med. Clin. North Am., *72*:1493, 1988.

62. Lokey, E.A.: The effects of exercise training on pregnancy outcomes.

63. Longo, L.D.: Maternal blood volume and cardiac output during pregnancy: a hypothesis of endocrinologic control. Am. J. Physiol., *245*:R720, 1983.

64. Lotgering, F.K., and Longo, L.D.: Exercise and pregnancy—how much is too much? Contemp. OB/GYN *23*:63, 1984.

65. Lotgering, F.K., Gilbert, R.D., and Longo, L.D.: Exercise responses in pregnant sheep: oxygen consumption, uterine blood flow and blood volume. J. Appl. Physiol., *55*:834, 1983.

66. Lotgering, F.K., Gilbert, R.D., and Longo, L.D.: Exercise responses in pregnant sheep: blood gases, temperatures, and fetal cardiovascular system. J. Appl. Physiol., *55*:842, 1983.

67. Lotgering, F.K., Gilbert, R.D., and Longo, L.D.: Maternal and fetal responses to exercise during pregnancy. Physiol. Rev., *65*:1, 1985.

68. Lund, C.J., and Donovan, J.C.: Blood volume during pregnancy. Significance of plasma and red cell volumes. Am. J. Obstet. Gynecol., *98*:393, 1967.

69. Lyons, H.A., and Antonio, R.: The sensitivity of the respiratory center in pregnancy and after administration of progesterone. Trans. Assoc. Am. Physicians, *72*:173, 1959.

70. Mantle, M.J., Greenwood, R.M., and Curry, H.L.F.: Backache in pregnancy. Rheumatol. Rehabil., *16*:95, 1977.

71. Martin, A.D., Notelovitz, M., Fields, C., and O'Kroy, J.: Predicting maximal oxygen uptake from treadmill testing in trained and untrained women. Am. J. Obstet. Gynecol., *161*:1127, 1989.

72. Mashini, I.S., et al.: Serial noninvasive evaluation of cardiovascular hemodynamics during pregnancy. Am. J. Obstet. Gynecol., *156*:1208, 1987.
73. McMurray, R.G., and Katz, V.L.: Thermoregulation in pregnancy. Implications for exercise. Sports Med., *10*:146, 1990.
74. McMurray, R.G., Katz, V.L., Berry, M.J., and Cefalo, R.C.: The effect of pregnancy on metabolic responses during rest, immersion and aerobic exercise in the water. Am. J. Obstet. Gynecol., *158*:481, 1988.
75. Metcalfe, J., Stock, M.K., and Barron, D.H.: Maternal physiology during gestation. *In* The Physiology of Reproduction. Edited by E. Knobil, Neill, et al. New York, Raven Press, 1988, pp. 2145–2176.
76. Morris, N., Osborn, S.B., Wright, M.P., and Hart, A.: Effective uterine blood-flow during normal and pre-eclamptic pregnancies. Lancet, *2*:481, 1956.
77. Morton, M., et al.: Left ventricular size, output, and structure during guinea pig pregnancy. Am. J. Physiol., *246*:R40, 1984.
78. Morton, M.J., et al.: Exercise dynamics in late gestation: effects of physical training. Am. J. Obstet. Gynecol., *152*:91, 1985.
79. Morton, M.J., Paul, M.S., and Metcalfe, J.: Exercise during pregnancy. Med. Clin. North Am., *69*:97, 1985.
80. Naeye, R.L., and Peters, E.C.: Working during pregnancy: effects on the fetus. Pediatrics, *69*:724, 1982.
81. Nelson, P.S., Gilbert, R.D., and Longo, L.D.: Fetal growth and placental diffusing capacity in guinea pigs following long-term maternal exercise. J. Dev. Physiol., *5*:1, 1983.
82. Newhall, J.F., Jr.: Scuba diving during pregnancy: a brief review. Am. J. Obstet. Gynecol., *140*:893, 1981.
83. Nygaard, I., Dehancey, J.O.L., Arnsdarf, L., and Murphy, E.: Exercise and incontinence. Obstet. Gynecol., *75*:848, 1990.
84. Ohtake, P.J., Wolfe, L.A., Hall, P., and McGrath, M.J.: Physical conditioning effects on exercise heart rate and perception of exertion in pregnancy. Can. J. Sport Sci., *13*:71P, 1988 (Abstract).
85. Ohtake, P.J., Wolfe, L.A., and McGrath, M.J.: Ventilatory responses to physical conditioning during pregnancy. Physiologist, *31*:A158, 1988 (Abstract).
86. Palin, D., and Rankine, D.: Nutrition in pregnancy—national guidelines: a summary. J. Can. Diet. Assoc., *47*:209, 1987.
87. Paolone, A.M., and Worthington, S.: Cautions and advice on exercise during pregnancy. Contemp. OB/GYN, *25*:150, 1985.
88. Parer, J.T.: Fetal heart rate. *In* Maternal-Fetal Medicine: Principles and Practice. Edited by R.K. Creasy and R.I. Resnick. Philadelphia, W.B. Saunders, 1984.
89. PAR-Q Validation Report, British Columbia Ministry of Health, 1978.
90. Pernoll, M.L., et al.: Oxygen consumption at rest and during exercise in pregnancy. Resp. Physiol., *25*:285, 1975.
91. Pernoll, M.L., et al.: Ventilation during rest and exercise in pregnancy and postpartum. Resp. Physiol., *25*:295, 1975.
92. Pivarnik, J.M. et al.: Cardiac output responses of primigravid women during exercise determined by the direct Fick technique. Obstet. Gynecol., *75*:954, 1990.
93. Pleet, H., Graham, J.M., and Smith, D.W.: Central nervous system and facial defects associated with maternal hyperthermia at 4–15 weeks gestation. Pediatrics, *67*:785, 1981.
94. Prowse, C.M., and Gaensler, E.A.: Respiratory and acid-base changes during pregnancy. Anesthesiology, *26*:381, 1965.
95. Pomerance, J.J., Gluck, L., and Lynch, V.A.: Maternal exercise as a screening test for uteroplacental insufficiency. Obstet. Gynecol., *44*:383, 1974.
96. Pritchard, J.A., MacDonald, P.C., and Grant, N.F.: William's Obstetrics. 17th Ed. Norwalk, CT, Appleton-Century-Crofts, 1985.
97. Ratigan, T.R.: Anatomic and physiologic changes of pregnancy: anesthetic considerations. J. Am. Assoc. Nurse, *51*:38, 1983.
98. Romen, Y., and Artal, R.: Physiological and endocrine adjustments to pregnancy. *In* Exercise in Pregnancy. Edited by R. Artal and R.A. Wiswell. Baltimore, Williams & Wilkins, 1986.
99. Rubler, S., Damani, P.M., and Pinto, E.R.: Cardiac size and performance during pregnancy estimated with echocardiography. Am. J. Cardiol., *40*:534, 1977.
100. Sady, S.P., Carpenter, M.W., Thompson, P.D., and Sady, M.A.: Cardiovascular response to cycle exercise during and after pregnancy. J. Appl. Physiol., *66*:336, 1989.
101. Sady, M.A., et al.: Cardiovascular response to maximal cycle exercise during pregnancy and at two and seven months post partum. Am. J. Obstet. Gynecol., *162*:1181, 1990.
102. Sady, S.P., et al.: Prediction of $\dot{V}_{O2max}$ during cycle exercise in pregnant women. J. Appl. Physiol., *65*:657, 1988.
103. Scott, D.E.: Anemia in pregnancy. Obstet. Gynecol. Annu., *1*:219, 1972.
104. Seitchik, J.: Body composition and energy expenditure during rest and work in pregnancy. Am. J. Obstet. Gynecol., *97*:701, 1967.
105. Shangold, M.M., Metcalfe, J., Longo, L.D., and Clapp, J.F. III.: Symposium: exercise during pregnancy-state of the art. Med. Sci. Sports Exerc., *17*:218, 1985 (Abstract).
106. Sheldon, J.H.: Maternal obesity. Lancet, *2*:896, 1949.
107. Sjöstrand, T.: Changes in respiratory organs of workmen at an ore smelting works. Acta Med. Scand. Suppl., *196*:687, 1977.
108. South-Paul, J.E., Rajagopal, K.R., and Tenholder: The effect of participation in a regular exercise program upon aerobic capacity during pregnancy. Obstet. Gynecol., *71*:175, 1988.
109. Smith, D.W., Clarren, S.K., and Harvey, M.A.S.: Hyperthermia as a possible teratogenic agent. Pediatrics, *92*:878, 1978.
110. Smith, A.D., Gilbert, R.D., Lammers, R.J., and Longo, L.D.: Placental exchange area in guinea pigs following long-term maternal exercise: a stereological analysis. J. Dev. Physiol., *5*:11, 1983.
111. Sullivan, J.M., and Ramanathan, K.B.: Management of medical problems in pregnancy—se-

vere cardiac disease. N. Engl. J. Med., *313*:304, 1985.

112. Tafari, N., Naeye, R.L., and Gobeze, A.: Effects of maternal undernutrition and heavy physical work during pregnancy on birth weight. Br. J. Obstet. Gynecol., *87*:222, 1980.

113. Templeton, A., and Kelman, G.R.: Maternal blood gases. (PA_{02}-Pa_{02}), physiological shunt and VD/VT in normal pregnancy. Br. J. Anaesth., *48*:1001, 1976.

114. Treadway, J.L., and Young, J.C.: Decreased glucose uptake in the fetus after maternal exercise. Med. Sci. Sports. Exerc., *21*:140, 1989.

115. Ueland, K., and Parer, J.T.: Effect of estrogen on the cardiovascular system of the ewe. Am. J. Obstet. Gynecol., *96*:400, 1966.

116. Ueland, K., Novy, M.J., Peterson, E.N., and Metcalfe, J.: Maternal cardiovascular dynamics. IV. The influence of gestational age on the maternal cardiovascular response to posture and exercise. Am. J. Obstet. Gynecol., *104*:856, 1969.

117. Ueland, K., Novy, M.J., Peterson, E.N., and Metcalfe, J.: Cardio-respiratory responses to pregnancy and exercise in normal women and patients with heart disease. Am. J. Obstet. Gynecol., *115*:4, 1973.

118. Webb, K.A., Wolfe, L.A., Tranmer, J.E., and McGrath, M.J.: Pregnancy outcome following physical fitness training. Can. J. Sports Sci., *13*:93P, 1988 (Abstract).

119. Webb, K.A., et al.: Fetal heart rate (FHR) responses to maternal aerobic exercise and physical conditioning. Med. Sci. Sports Exerc., *21*:S32, 1989 (Abstract).

120. Wiswell, R.A., et al.: Hormonal and metabolic response to exercise in pregnancy. Med. Sci. Sports Exerc., *17*:206, 1985 (Abstract).

121. Wolfe, L.A., Ohtake, P.J., Mottola, M.F., and McGrath, M.J.: Physiological interactions between pregnancy and aerobic exercise. Exerc. Sports Sci. Rev., *17*:295, 1989.

122. Wolfe, L.A., et al.: Prescription of aerobic exercise during pregnancy. Sports Med., *8*:273, 1989.

123. Wolfe, L.A., Ohtake, P.J., George, K.P., and McGrath, M.J.: Aerobic training effects on exercise hemodynamics during pregnancy. Med. Sci. Sports Exerc., *22*:S28, 1990 (Abstract).

124. Work, J.A.: Is weight training safe during pregnancy? Physician Sportsmed., *17*:257, 1989.

125. Zaidise, I., Artal, R., and Bessman, S.P.: Fuel metabolism in pregnancy. *In* Exercise in Pregnancy. Edited by R. Artal and R.A. Wiswell. Baltimore, Williams & Wilkins, 1986.

Index

Page numbers in *italics* indicate illustrations; numbers followed by "t" indicate tables.

Environmental factors *(continued)*
  temperature regulation and energy
    balance, 87 – 88
  See also Temperature
Exercise and Children's Health (Rowland), 57
Exercise-induced asthma. *See* Asthma
Exercise-induced bronchoconstriction, 68
Exercise prescription/programs. *See*
    Prescription
Exercise testing. *See* Testing
Exercise Testing in Children (Godfrey), 57
Exertional hypotension, 17 – 19

F

Fatigue, 37
Females
  osteoporosis, 52 – 53
  physiologic response in, 45 – 49, 48t
  physique and body composition, 41 – 45,
    43t, 44t
  training effect in, 50
Fetal response to exercise, 367 – 370
Field testing, 10 – 11
Fitness level, 35
Fitness profile, 30
Fluid balance and heat, 90 – 91
Fontan procedure, 310 – 311
Fractures in osteoporosis, 127, 134 – 135
Frequency of exercise, 32, 82
Friskis & Svettis program, 285 – 287
Frostbite, 93 – 94
Functional capacity, 17
  aging and, 78 – 79
  altitude effects, 97 – 99
  in asthma, 220 – 221
  atmospheric pollution and, 101t, 101 – 102
  in children, 58 – 60, 67
  in chronic obstructive respiratory
    disorders, 231 – 232, *232*
  in congenital heart disease, 305 – 306
  in cystic fibrosis, 245t, 245 – 246
  exercise intensity and, 33, 35 – 36
  low in coronary heart disease, 339 – 347
  in obesity, 198 – 199, *199*
  in pregnancy, 367 – 368
  in renal failure, 352 – 354, *353*
  sex differences, 45 – 49, 48t
  in valvular disease, 325 – 326, 329 – 330
    postsurgical, 332 – 333
Functional restoration in low-back pain,
    147 – 149

G

Gait effects of exercise, 134
Gender. *See* Sex
General principles
  aging
    deconditioning and disease, 77
    general effects, 75 – 77
    prescription, 80 – 85, 81t, 84t
    testing methods, 77 – 80, 79t
  child/adult differences
    methodologic considerations, 65 – 69
    patient selection, 64 – 65
    in physiologic response, 57 – 63
    prescription, 69 – 71
  environmental factors
    altitude, 97 – 100
    cold exposure, 93 – 97
    heat exposure, 88 – 93
    interstressor exposure, 104 – 106
    pollutant exposure, 100 – 104, 101t
    thermoregulation and energy balance,
      87 – 88
  male/female differences
    acute physiologic response, 45 – 49, 48t
    in aging, 52
    chronic adaptation, 49 – 52
    environmental factors, 54
    menstruation, 53 – 54
    osteoporosis, 52 – 53
    physique and body composition, 41 – 45,
      43t, 44t
  of prescription
    aging, 80 – 85, 81t, 84t
    basic components of exercise programs,
      32 – 34
    child/adult differences, 69 – 71
    compliance, 40
    general knowledge, 29 – 30
    individual refinements, 35 – 37
    individual vs. group exercise, 38
    male/female differences, 55
    need, 30 – 31
    overuse problems, 37 – 38
    supervision, 38 – 39
    training principles, 31 – 32
  of testing
    clinical applications, 12 – 22
    instrumentation, 12
    legal implications, 22 – 23
    physiologic, 3 – 5
    protocols, 8 – 12, 12t, 13t
    type of exercise, 5 – 8
Girls. *See* Females; Sex
Glucocorticosteroids in asthma, 218
Group exercise, 38, 121, 201
Growth hormone deficiency, 68 – 69

U.S. Air Force School of Aerospace Medicine, 9

V

Vagal reflex in cold exposure, 95
Valsalva maneuver, 7 – 8
Valvular heart disease
  in adults
    pathophysiology, 317 – 318
      aortic regurgitation, 322 – 323
      combined lesions, 323
      congestive heart failure and exercise, 323 – 324
      hemodynamics, 323
      mitral regurgitation, 320 – 321
      mitral stenosis, 318 – 320
      mitral valve prolapse, 321 – 322
      tricuspid disease, 323
    work classification, 330, 331t
  in children. See Congenital heart disease
  prescription
    adverse effects of exercise, 334
    postsurgical rehabilitation, 333
    results without surgery, 333
  surgical treatment
    balloon valvuloplasty, 332
    exercise following, 332 – 333
    functional capacity after, 332 – 333

valve replacement, 331 – 332
testing
  functional capacity (NYHA classifications), 325 – 326, 326t
  maximal heart rate, 329
  postprocedure, 330
  ST-segment changes, 329
  termination, 327 – 329
  value, 326 – 327
Ventilatory failure, 231
Ventricular dysrhythmias, 302, 328
  exercise-induced, 20
Ventricular septal defects, 293 – 294
Very low-density lipoproteins (VLDL), 161 – 162, 170
VO_{2max}. See Functional capacity

W

Walking regimens in obesity, 201 – 202, 202t
Water exercise, 202 – 203
Wet bulb globe temperature index (WBGT), 92 – 93
Wingate Anaerobic Test, 67 – 68, 68t
Wolfe-Parkinson-White syndrome, 302 – 303
Work classifications in valvular disease, 330, 331t
Work defined, 34
World Health Organization (WHO) hypertension criteria, 275 – 278